THE
Texture
OF Life

Occupations and Related Activities

4TH EDITION

Edited by

Jim Hinojosa, PhD, OT, BCP, FAOTA, and
Marie-Louise Blount, AM, OT, FAOTA

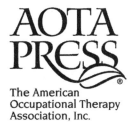

AOTA PRESS

The American
Occupational Therapy
Association, Inc.

AOTA Centennial Vision

We envision that occupational therapy is a powerful, widely recognized, science-driven, and evidence-based profession with a globally connected and diverse workforce meeting society's occupational needs.

Mission Statement

The American Occupational Therapy Association advances the quality, availability, use, and support of occupational therapy through standard-setting, advocacy, education, and research on behalf of its members and the public.

AOTA Staff

Frederick P. Somers, *Executive Director*
Christopher M. Bluhm, *Chief Operating Officer*

Chris Davis, *Director, AOTA Press*
Ashley Hofmann, *Development/Production Editor*

Rebecca Rutberg, *Director, Marketing*
Jennifer Folden, *Marketing Specialist*
Amanda Goldman, *Marketing Specialist*

American Occupational Therapy Association, Inc.
4720 Montgomery Lane
Bethesda, MD 20814
Phone: 301-652-AOTA (2682)
TDD: 800-377-8555
Fax: 301-652-7711
www.aota.org
To order: 1-877-404-AOTA or store.aota.org

Disclaimers

This publication is designed to provide accurate and authoritative information in regard to the subject matter covered. It is sold or distributed with the understanding that the publisher is not engaged in rendering legal, accounting, or other professional service. If legal advice or other expert assistance is required, the services of a competent professional person should be sought.
—From the Declaration of Principles jointly adopted by the American Bar Association and a Committee of Publishers and Associations

It is the objective of the American Occupational Therapy Association to be a forum for free expression and interchange of ideas. The opinions expressed by the contributors to this work are their own and not necessarily those of the American Occupational Therapy Association.

ISBN: 978-1-56900-352-7

Library of Congress Control Number: 2014933154

Cover Design by Debra Naylor, Naylor Design, Inc., Washington, DC
Composition by Maryland Composition, Laurel, MD
Printed by Automated Graphic Systems, Inc., White Plains, MD

CONTENTS

ACKNOWLEDGMENTS

For all of their joint and individual efforts in the preparation of this book, the editors sincerely thank the faculty and staff of the Department of Occupational Therapy, Steinhardt School of Culture, Education, and Human Development at New York University. Special thanks are extended to the authors and contributors to this work. We thank Christina A. Davis who, as Director AOTA Press, encouraged and supported all of our efforts. Finally, we thank Ashley Hofmann, Development/ Production Editor for AOTA Press, who was there at every aspect of the project. We are grateful for her continual support.

Marie-Louise Blount profoundly appreciates the love and support of Elena and Wesley Blount and family members Barry Levinson, Meyer Levinson-Blount, Ari Levinson-Blount, and the family's newest member, Guy Ezra Levinson-Blount, who have made all of her endeavors worthwhile. Jim Hinojosa thanks both his parents, who instilled in him a love for engagement in purposeful, meaningful activity. He sincerely thanks Steven A. Smith for all his support. Additionally, he thanks Dr. Anne C. Mosey, who provided the insight that would refine his thinking about activity and occupational therapy.

To our clients, we are indebted to them because they reaffirmed our beliefs about the value of active engagement and the meaningfulness of occupational therapy. Finally, we are indebted to our students, current and former, who provided the reason for writing this book. We continually learn from them the value of what we do.

ABOUT THE EDITORS

Jim Hinojosa, PhD, OT, BCP, FAOTA, is a professor of occupational therapy in the Department of Occupational Therapy in the Steinhardt School of Culture, Education, and Human Development at New York University. Specializing in pediatrics, he is a strong advocate for family-centered care, believing that everyone benefits when health professionals work closely with families to develop interventions that reflect their needs and values.

Dr. Hinojosa has more than 35 years' experience as an occupational therapist, researcher, and educator. In his role as educator, Dr. Hinojosa has presented and conducted workshops throughout the United States and Canada. He is the co-editor and author of 12 textbooks and has written or published over 200 chapters and articles.

A Fellow of the American Occupational Therapy Association (AOTA), Dr. Hinojosa has served on many of its commissions and boards and was awarded its highest honors, the Award of Merit and the Eleanor Clarke Slagle Lectureship. He also served as director of the American Occupational Therapy Foundation Board and received its Meritorious Service Award.

Marie-Louise Blount, AM, OT, FAOTA, is an occupational therapist with clinical experience and a long career as an educator. She has been an occupational therapist for over 50 years. Retired from the position of professional program director in the Department of Occupational Therapy at the Steinhardt School of Culture, Education, and Human Development at New York University, she held the rank of clinical professor.

Previously, she had held faculty positions at three other universities. In the past, she served on AOTA's Representative Assembly as the representative from Maryland. Currently she works as an editor, primarily as co-editor of the journal *Occupational Therapy in Mental Health.*

ABOUT THE AUTHORS

FRAN BABISS, PHD, OTR/L
Coordinator of Evidence-Based Practice
South Oaks Hospital
Amityville, NY

MARIE-LOUISE BLOUNT, AM, OT, FAOTA
Coeditor, *Occupational Therapy in Mental Health*
Croton-on-Hudson, NY

WESLEY BLOUNT
Editor
Croton-on-Hudson, NY

KAREN A. BUCKLEY, MA, OTR
Clinical Assistant Professor
Department of Occupational Therapy
Steinhardt School of Culture, Education, and
    Human Development
New York University
New York

LISA E. CYZNER, PHD, OTR
Private Pediatric Practitioner
Cyzner Institute
Charlotte, NC

NANCY ROBERT DOOLEY, PHD, OTR
Professor and Occupational Therapy Program
    Director
New England Institute of Technology
East Greenwich, RI

**RITA P. FLEMING-CASTALDY, PHD,
    OTR/L, FAOTA**
Associate Professor
University of Scranton
Scranton, PA

JYOTHI GUPTA, PHD, OTR/L, FAOTA
Professor
St. Catherine University
Departments of Physical Therapy and
    Occupational Science and Occupational
    Therapy
Minneapolis, MN

KRISTINE HAERTL, PHD, OTR/L, FAOTA
Professor
Department of Occupational Therapy and
    Occupational Science
St. Catherine University
St. Paul, MN

**BARBARA J. HEMPHILL, DMIN, MS,
    OTR, FAOTA**
Associate Professor Emeritus
Department of Occupational Therapy
Western Michigan University
Kalamazoo

JIM HINOJOSA, PHD, OT, BCP, FAOTA
Professor
Department of Occupational Therapy
Steinhardt School of Culture, Education, and
    Human Development
New York University
New York

TSU-HSIN HOWE, PHD, OTR, FAOTA
Associate Professor
Department of Occupational Therapy
Steinhardt School of Culture, Education, and
    Human Development
New York University
New York

MARGARET KAPLAN, PHD, OTR
Associate Professor
Occupational Therapy Program
State University of New York
Downstate Medical Center
Brooklyn

PAULA KRAMER, PHD, OTR, FAOTA
Professor and Director of the Doctorate of
    Occupational Therapy Program
Department of Occupational Therapy
Samson College of Health Sciences
University of the Sciences in Philadelphia
Philadelphia

LAURETTE OLSON, PHD, OTR/L, FAOTA
Professor
Graduate Program in Occupational Therapy
Mercy College
Dobbs Ferry, NY

ANITA PERR, PHD, OT, ATP, FAOTA
Clinical Associate Professor
Department of Occupational Therapy
Steinhardt School of Culture, Education, and
    Human Development
New York University
New York

SALLY E. POOLE, OTD, OT/L, CHT
Clinical Assistant Professor
Department of Occupational Therapy
Steinhardt School of Culture, Education, and
    Human Development
New York University
New York
and
Co-owner, Hands-On Rehab
Valhalla, NY

RUTH SEGAL, PHD, OTR
Professor and Chair
Seton Hall University
School of Health and Medical Sciences
Department of Occupational Therapy
South Orange, NJ

JEFF SNODGRASS, PHD, MPH, OTR
Area Chair and Program Director
Associate Professor
Department of Occupational Therapy
Milligan College
Milligan College, TN

JEFF TOMLINSON, MSW, OT, FAOTA
Washington Heights Community Service
    New York and
Adjunct Instructor
Department of Occupational Therapy
Steinhardt School of Culture, Education, and
    Human Development
New York University
New York

SUZANNE WHITE, MA, OTR/L
Clinical Associate Professor
Occupational Therapy Program
State University of New York
Downstate Medical Center
Brooklyn

JUDY URBAN WILSON, MA, OTR
Assistant Director
Department of Occupational Therapy
Bellevue Hospital Center
New York

LIST OF FIGURES, TABLES, EXHIBITS, EXERCISES, CASE EXAMPLES, AND APPENDIXES

Figures

Tables

Exhibits

Exercises

Case Examples

Appendixes

FOREWORD

Barbara A. Boyt Schell, PhD, OT/L, FAOTA

Occupational therapy was founded on a set of core beliefs, chief among them that purposeful activities and engagement in occupation fosters dignity, competence, and health (Peloquin, 2005). From those early days of forging a new set of interventions as well as a new profession, occupational therapy scholars and practitioners continue to engage in ongoing conversations, attempting to elucidate what we mean when we talk about occupation and activity (Crepeau, Schell, Gillen, & Scaffa, 2014). This new edition of *The Texture of Life: Occupation and Related Activities* provides a welcome addition to this conversation.

Although they may not be aware of this history, students and new practitioners quickly come to appreciate that what seems a very straightforward idea (i.e., doing activities is a good way to help people) is in fact a lot more complex in practice. Effective practice requires an appreciation of a mix of personal, contextual, and philosophical perspectives that must be considered in harnessing the use of occupation and purposeful activity for effective therapy outcomes.

The process of writing this foreword has prompted me to recall my first years of practice. I was prepared with knowledge of anatomy, kinesiology, and psychology, as well as human growth and development. I was exposed to an array of medical, psychological, and developmental pathologies. I was equally well versed with knowledge about how to analyze, perform, and grade a wide range of activities. The challenge to me as a new practitioner was how to artfully combine and use all this knowledge to actually help people. This was before the days of the Model of Human Occupation (see Kielhofner, 2008, for lat-

est version) or even *Uniform Terminology* (American Occupational Therapy Association [AOTA], 1979), the precursor to today's *Occupational Therapy Practice Framework: Domain and Process* (AOTA, 2014).

Before the emergence of occupational science, practitioners used the term *purposeful activity* to describe their interventions. Most of the theories of the field were borrowed or adapted from disciplines as diverse as developmental psychology, medicine and industrial management. As a profession, we were deeply focused on trying to understand how various body systems related to performance actions. Although we knew that client interests were very important, we did not have the Canadian Occupational Performance Measure (Law et al., 2005) or indeed many assessments that looked at how people performed their activities of daily life. Thus, we could not systematically measure how our clients were doing in terms of the ultimate goal of engaging in their life activities. It was challenging to define and focus our choice of intervention approaches in concert with our client's goals and to clearly document outcomes.

How I would have loved to have had access to a text like this to guide me in thinking about how to use activity and occupation as therapy. *The Texture of Life* helps practitioners really understand how to "do" occupational therapy by carefully and specifically describing the processes of using activity and occupation as therapy. The editors and their contributing authors have used the skills of activity analysis on the profession itself and, in doing so, have brought to light many concepts, theories, and practical strategies necessary to harness purposeful activities and occupation to promote health and social participation. In my mind, this text serves as a "secret decoder ring," revealing the underlying processes of the profession.

Occupational therapy has been successful in helping clients and society, because those core ideas of occupational therapy on which the profession was founded are continually reimagined in light of the demands of each decade. With each reiteration, we learn more about how to best to "do" occupational therapy. Yes, we must reason carefully, and yes, we must consider many person-based and environmental factors, but ultimately, we must actually do something with our clients, so they can get back to doing their lives. This is not so easily done. Being effective and efficient occupational therapy practitioners requires rigorous analysis combined with creative improvisation. This new edition of *The Texture of Life* brings further clarity and contemporary understandings to that process.

The mindful attention to using terminology that connects to the language of AOTA and the World Health Organization helps to connect the work here to the larger world of ideas about activity. In the Chapter 1, "Occupations, Activities, and Occupational Therapy," Jim Hinojosa and Marie-Louise Blount set out to "define and outline the relationships among the major constructs of the profession: occupation, activity, purposeful activity, and occupational performance" (p. 2). I am particularly appreciative of how they reflect current thinking while challenging the field to consider the implications of choices for the current and future practices of the profession.

Subsequent chapters succeed in addressing the many parameters of using occupation and purposeful activity as therapy. As an effective blend of the tried and true and the newly emerging, the fourth edition of *The Texture of Life* is a gift to the profession.

References

American Occupational Therapy Association. (1979). *Occupational therapy product output reporting system and uniform terminology for reporting occupational therapy services.* Bethesda, MD: Author.

American Occupational Therapy Association. (2014). Occupational therapy practice framework: Domain and process (3rd ed.). *American Journal of Occupational Therapy, 68*(Suppl. 1), S1–S48. http://dx.doi.org/10.5014/ajot.2014.682006

Crepeau, E. B., Schell, B. A. B., Gillen, G., & Scaffa, M. E. (2014). Analyzing occupation and activity. In B. A. B. Schell, G. Gillen, & M. E. Scaffa (Eds.) *Willard and Spackman's occupational therapy* (12th ed., pp. 234–238). Philadelphia: Lippincott, Williams & Wilkins.

Kielhofner, G. (2008). *The Model of Human Occupation: Theory and application* (4th ed.). Philadelphia: Lippincott, Williams & Wilkins.

Law, M., Baptiste, S., Carswell, A., McColl, M., Polatajko, H., & Pollock, N. (2005). *Canadian Occupational Performance Measure.* Ottawa, ON: Canadian Association of Occupational Therapists.

Peloquin, S. M. (2005). Embracing our ethos, reclaiming our heart [Eleanor Clarke Slagle Lecture]. *American Journal of Occupational Therapy, 59,* 611–625. http://dx.doi.org/10.5014/ajot.59.6.611

INTRODUCTION

Jim Hinojosa, PhD, OT, BCP, FAOTA, and
Marie-Louise Blount, AM, OT, FAOTA

A friend asked, "Are there enough changes in occupational therapy to warrant a new edition of *The Texture of Life?*" As of 2014, we can confidently write that the profession of occupational therapy has significantly changed since 2009, and at an extraordinary rate. Research, practice, and education for occupational therapy practitioners have increased in response to constant changes in society, health care, and the educational system. Ongoing research and a commitment to occupation-based intervention has resulted in occupational therapy interventions that are evidence based while also sensitive to the clients' personal needs.

In the fourth edition of The *Texture of Life: Occupations and Related Activities,* the contributors have more clearly defined the importance of occupation, and more clearly described the relationship between occupations and their related activities. In each chapter, contributors have presented up-to-date information, including changes consistent with the American Occupational Therapy Association's (AOTA's; 2014) *Occupational Therapy Practice Framework: Domain and Process* (hereinafter, *Framework*). They have struggled with ideas that are foundational to the profession's core and have written chapters that support clinical reasoning and practice.

The authors' emphasis on occupation reflects a major change in our profession. Occupational therapists and occupational therapy assistants have begun endorsing the term *occupation* and using the terms *activities* and *purposeful activities* less frequently. In this text, authors have addressed many of the implications of expanded use of the term *occupation* by addressing important questions: Do clients and practitioners understand the term *occupation?* How does or doesn't the term influence the occupational therapy profession's practices? Does the term *occupation* affect how consumers and society view occupational therapy? And, most important, how has endorsing the term influenced the profession's philosophical and theoretical development? Even as the authors of this text have addressed these issues, we hope that others will question these ideas and expand them.

In this edition, we challenged the authors to discuss the scope and depth of our profession with a focus on activities. We asked the authors to use the *Framework* (AOTA, 2014) and the *International Classification of Functioning, Disability and Health* (World Health Organization, 2001) as basic references. In addition, we asked them to address occupation as it is being currently used and developed within the profession. We have organized this textbook to reflect the foundational concepts of occupation and related activities. The first three chapters discuss how occupational therapy practitioners define occupation, purposeful activities, and activities. Within the discussion of these concepts is a brief presentation of the perspectives of scholars within the profession.

Next, we present specific knowledge about the characteristics of occupation and activities, and how practitioners conceptualize them for occupational therapy practice. Chapter 4, "Occupation and Activity Analysis," presents activity analysis, which practitioners use to deconstruct occupation and related activities into their component parts.

Chapter 5, "The Occupational Profile," explores the importance of an occupational profile to understand the client, and Chapter 6, "Activity Synthesis as a Means to Structure Occupation," discusses activity synthesis and how practitioners use synthesis to reconstruct an activity for therapy. Chapter 7, "Clinical Reasoning and Reflective Practice," discusses clinical reasoning and reflective practice.

Next, the textbook offers essential information on the therapeutic use of occupations and related activities. Chapters 12 through 16 describe how occupational therapy practitioners apply their understanding of occupation and related activities to enhance and facilitate occupational performance.

The final chapters of this textbook explore important aspects of the domain of concern of occupational therapy. Each chapter covers a specific area, including leisure, work, self-care, and care of others. Chapter 17, "Occupations in the Context of Spirituality," and Chapter 18, "Occupations, Activities, and Empowerment," address the specialized areas of spirituality and empowerment. The text ends with Chapter 19, "Reflections for the Future: Occupation, Purposeful Activities, and Activities," which discusses the importance to occupations and related activities to the profession's future.

We believe that this textbook's contributors have responded to our challenges admirably. We hope that this text will provide a clear understanding of the fundamental concepts of occupational therapy. Furthermore, we hope that it will clarify the language of our profession. Finally, we hope that this text will serve as a foundation for continuing dialogue within our profession, as we continue to refine even our most fundamental ideas.

References

American Occupational Therapy Association. (2014). Occupational therapy practice framework: Domain and process (3rd ed.). *American Journal of Occupational Therapy, 68*(Suppl. 1), S1–S48. http://dx.doi.org/10.5014/ajot.2014.682006

World Health Organization. (2001). *International classification of functioning, disability and health*. Geneva: Author.

CHAPTER 1.

OCCUPATION, ACTIVITIES, AND OCCUPATIONAL THERAPY

Jim Hinojosa, PhD, OT, BCP, FAOTA, and Marie-Louise Blount, AM, OT, FAOTA

Highlights

✧ Foundational concepts
✧ Occupational therapy: The profession's mandate
✧ Tools of the profession
✧ Tools of intervention: Purposeful activities.

Key Terms

✧ Actions of an activity
✧ Activities
✧ Context
✧ Daily occupations
✧ Environment
✧ Goal directed
✧ Human environment
✧ Leisure occupations
✧ Mandate
✧ Meaningfulness
✧ Nonhuman environment
✧ Occupational form

✧ Occupational performance
✧ Occupation-as-means
✧ Occupations
✧ Play
✧ Pluralistic approach
✧ Productive occupations
✧ Purposeful activities
✧ Purposefulness
✧ Self-care activities
✧ Task analysis
✧ Tools
✧ Work

In this chapter, we focus on occupations and purposeful activities as they relate to the practice of occupational therapy today. We define and outline the relationships among the major constructs of the profession: occupation, activity, purposeful activity, and occupational performance. Moreover, we provide the framework for the rest of the book. To appreciate the topics addressed in this book, an understanding of the basic concepts on which it is founded is essential. We explain the terms generally used in occupational therapy that encompass the rationale for the profession's practice. Further, we stress the varying definitions and points of view that have grown around these terms over the years. We also stress our own definitions for these terms and how they are related to each other.

Occupation has come to be the widely accepted term for the foundation of the ideas, theories, and models that govern what occupational therapy practitioners do. Even though other terms, such as *activity*, are widely used in its place, we emphasize *occupation* as a first and overarching principle and subsume other important terms under its umbrella.

Thus, this chapter is organized to provide, first, definitions of the terms as we use them. We also explore some historical bases (Bauerschmidt & Nelson, 2011) for the terms and highlight the variety of approaches to their definitions and applications. The etymology of the term *occupation* provides another avenue to its transition to English, particularly American English.

The chapter emphasizes the crucial importance of purposeful activities, or what some call *occupation-as-means,* to the fundamental practice of occupational therapy. To apply our current approach, we address the foundational topics in the following order: occupation, activity, and occupational performance. At a later point in the chapter, we explore what makes an activity purposeful.

Other aspects of practice that we investigate include the tools of the profession, that is, what occupational therapy practitioners do to use their legitimate tools (Mosey, 1981) and how they have done so in the past. Key to application is an understanding of therapeutic modalities and how they have and will change over time. Thus, we discuss activities of daily living (ADLs), work, and play or leisure as fundamental tools of the therapeutic process, areas agreed upon by most practitioners.

A crucial measure of practice is the meaning and value of occupation, with activity as a secondary element, to the person or client as an individual. Meaningfulness, therefore, is central, and we explore how it is structured and maintained.

Foundational Concepts

Occupational therapy has developed several foundational concepts over the years. Occupation has been a core concept of occupational therapy since its inception in 1917. Founders George E. Barton and William R. Dunton, MD, shared correspondence about the importance of "occupation work." At that time, people commonly used the term *occupation* to describe daily work activities. Thus, Barton proposed a profession devoted to the therapeutic use of occupation, that is, occupational therapy (as cited in Reed & Sanderson, 1999), in which professionals would use both recreation and daily tasks as therapeutic agents. This "work" was not specific to a patient, nor was it related to employment (Harvey-Krefting, 1985).

As occupational therapy has evolved, occupational therapy practitioners and scholars have used different terms, sometimes interchangeably, to describe the profession and its primary therapeutic modalities, that is, *occupation, activity, purposeful activity,* and *occupation-as-means* (Bauerschmidt & Nelson, 2011; Hinojosa & Blount, 2009). It is not surprising that different terms have been used, because the focus and concerns of the profession, as in any profession, have changed in response to the changing needs of society. Because professions exist to meet the needs of society, professions transform as society's knowledge, technology, and values shift. As professions transform, their focus and language change.

Many practitioners strive for unambiguous personal definitions of *occupation, activity, purposeful activity,* and *occupation-as-means.* Although the distinctions among the four terms and their specific uses may be clear to some, to others, the terms describe the same concept: a person's participation in daily life pursuits (American Occupational Therapy Association [AOTA], 2014). In this chapter, we propose distinct definitions that explain the essential characteristics distinguishing each term.

Defining *Occupations* and *Activities*

Occupational therapy practitioners' definitions of *occupation* and *activities* shape their practices. *Occupation* comes from the Latin *occupare*, which "connotes taking hold of (i.e., occupying) time and place" (Kielhofner, 2006a, p. 1175). Kielhofner went on to write that today's discussions of occupation are about how people use their time. *Occupations* are activities that are personally meaningful to the person who voluntarily engages in them out of personal choice or sociocultural necessity. Thus, occupations are unique to each individual, providing personal satisfaction and fulfillment as a result of engaging in them (AOTA, 2014; Pierce, 2001).

Occupations are specific to the people who are engaged in and experiencing them within their sociocultural context and are grounded in place, social group, and cultural meaning (Pierce, 2001). Occupations define a person's identity, instill competence, and provide life satisfaction (Latham, 2008). Kielhofner (2006b) observed that

> the common denominator of occupational therapy practice is involvement of persons in occupations as a means to enhance their well-being. . . . Consequently, occupational therapy focuses on empowering clients to actively influence their own rehabilitation process and outcomes, but selecting their own objectives for the kind of lives clients want to lead. (p. 1175)

As stated previously, occupation is the core concept of occupational therapy. However, Bauerschmidt and Nelson (2011) observed that the use of the term by practitioners has fluctuated over 9 decades of the profession. In their study, Bauerschmidt and Nelson defined *occupations* as things done voluntarily by a person and *activities* as things done voluntarily as part of therapy. Therefore, occupational therapy practitioners provide interventions designed to create conditions in which a person participates in an activity that allows that person to develop skills so that he or she can engage in occupations related to work, play, and activities of daily living (ADLs). In other words, activities are foundational to human occupation.

Defining *Activities* and *Purposeful Activities*

It is important for practitioners to distinguish between the definitions of *activities* and *purposeful activities*. Activities—what we do, the foundation of much of our routine, enterprise, and art—have a unique place in the context of occupational therapy. In fact, mapping the import of activities in occupational therapy shows a varied landscape, one with multiple meanings. *Activities* encompass a wide range of actions that a person takes to accomplish or perform something. They are goal directed (AOTA, 2014; Latham, 2008) and involve doing.

In occupational therapy, when a person participates in a personally important action to realize a goal, he or she is engaged in a *purposeful activity*. Furthermore, when a person engages in activities out of personal choice and values those activities, these clusters of purposeful activities form occupations (Hinojosa, Kramer, Royeen, & Luebben, 2003; Latham, 2008). In occupational therapy, when a practitioner uses an activity therapeutically, the term *purposeful activity* is used to highlight the fact that occupational therapy practitioners use activities that have a function, are therapeutically goal directed, and require the person to participate.

Defining *Purposeful Activities* and *Occupation-as-Means*

Some occupational therapy practitioners define purposeful activities they use therapeutically as *occupation-as-means*. They prefer this term because it reflects occupation-based practice and captures the association between occupation and activity used as a therapeutic medium. It is believed to capture the uniqueness of occupational therapy (Gray, 1998). *Occupation-as-means* denotes that the goal of intervention is the person's ability to engage in the occupation.

In this book, we have chosen to use the term *purposeful activity*, rather than *occupation-as-means*, to describe the therapeutic use of activity. We believe it is more understandable, and by using it, practitioners can clearly understand the relationship between activity and occupation. We support the position that practitioners use the term *occupation* to capture the scope of a fundamental construct of occupational therapy. Included in a person's occupations are the purposeful activities that he or she engages in as part of living. Note that some practitioners choose to use only the concept of occupation (AOTA, 2008, 2014; Nelson, 1997; Nelson & Jepson-Thomas, 2003). In fact, in the 2008 revision of the *Occupational Therapy Practice Frame-*

work: *Domain and Process* (the *Framework*; AOTA, 2008), the authors concluded that although scholars in the field acknowledge differences between the terms *activity* and *occupation,* they have decided to use only *occupation.* In their definition, *occupation* includes activities. Most practitioners, however, continue to use the terms *occupation* and *purposeful activity* interchangeably (Latham, 2008).

In the most recent *Framework* (AOTA, 2014), the authors acknowledged that some practitioners continue to use *activity* and *occupation* interchangeably. The document, however, focuses on the use of *occupation* as the end result and the means of therapy. The term *activities* is used to describe components of occupations that "always hold meaning, relevance, and perceived utility to clients at their level of interest and motivation" (p. S29).

Exercise 1.1. Reflection on Daily Life Activities

Reflect and list the actions in which you have engaged today. Classify them into occupations, activities, and purposeful activities. Identify those that were difficult to categorize. Why were they difficult to categorize? What criteria did you finally decide to use to categorize the unclear activities?

Pluralistic Approach to Understanding Purposeful Activities

Although *purposeful activity* refers to portions of occupations and encompasses a variety of behaviors and performances (AOTA, 1995), the need still exists to discuss, delimit, and understand the behaviors and tasks that are part of the activity and at the same time appreciate the occupations under which the activity is subsumed. In other words, having a definition for a phenomenon does not necessarily simplify one's understanding of it or of the issues it raises.

We suggest, therefore, a *pluralistic approach,* a multidimensional view of purposeful activity, to address these issues recommended by Mosey (1985). Henderson et al. (1991) have also suggested that practitioners embrace a multidimensional view as both an entity and a therapeutic modality. We support Mosey's and Henderson et al.'s acknowledgment that occupational therapy services can and do include approaches and methods other than

---

Exercise 1.2. Range of Activities

Consider other aspects of activities that range from simple to complex, identifying not only the polar ends of a given continuum but also the various stages of complexity that exist along the continuum.

---

purposeful activity. Because purposeful activity is fundamental to occupational therapy practice, practitioners need to understand the many modes in which the term is used.

In occupational therapy, some approaches use the term *purposeful activities* and others use substitute terms such as *occupation-as-means* (Latham, 2008). All approaches, however, include the belief that occupational therapy practitioners use activities in a specific manner. Henderson et al. (1991) also noted that practitioners use a wide range of types and levels of activity in practice. Activities may range from low level (e.g., reaching for an object) to high level (e.g., a simulated work activity). They may also range from simple to complex, for example, on a continuum from gross (e.g., an assembly toy in which a smaller plastic ring is placed on top of a larger plastic ring) to fine (e.g., attaching a small nut to a bolt and screwing it in place), or from very brief (performing a very time-limited activity once) to more lengthy (a demanding work or leisure activity carried out in a concentrated fashion for an hour or more).

As Henderson and colleagues (1991) pointed out, both purposefulness and the varied meanings invested in the term *purposeful activities* are "attributes of persons and not of activities" (p. 370). Henderson and colleagues were rightly concerned that occupational therapy practitioners realize that the *meaningfulness* (i.e., the extent to which an activity is relevant and interesting to the person [Foster, 2008]) and *purposefulness* (i.e., having personal meaning and being goal directed with active engagement [AOTA, 1997]) of an activity are invested in it by the person performing the activity or, sometimes, by the practitioner, often with the client's collaboration. They identified the fact that in acute care settings or any situation in which remediation of disability is the goal of intervention, activities or segments of activities may be a means of attaining that purpose or goal. Their view, which we share, is that all activities have the potential to be meaningful and purposeful.

Many variables—such as the person performing the activity, the context in which it is used, and when in the course of a program or series of activities it is introduced—affect the activity's meaningfulness and purposefulness. In addition, occupational therapy practitioners often use other techniques or tools, with or without activities, as part of their interventions. These techniques or tools often are not meaningful to the client. Nevertheless, the practitioner's concern and goal are to provide an intervention that will eventually facilitate a person's ability to engage by participating in meaningful daily life activities or occupations.

Henderson et al. (1991) identified the relevance to occupational therapy of the profession's historical and traditional applications of activity and its more contemporary expressions of choices or applications of activity. They were concerned not only with the ways in which practitioners view and use activities but also with the ways in which they investigate an activity's therapeutic aspects.

Occupation, activity, and purposeful activities have additional manifestations for occupational therapy practitioners, giving rise to the multiple and varied meanings attributed to these terms. We believe that activities represent the core and the texture of people's daily lives. We propose that no single definition is correct or absolute. In fact, we believe that discussion of the meanings of the terms adds to an understanding and appreciation of the concepts behind them. Ultimately, practitioners' increased understanding of these concepts improves their use of them within the context of therapeutic intervention.

Occupational Therapy: The Profession's Mandate

Before examining the tools that a profession uses, it is important to consider the profession's *mandate*, or its purpose and focus. Professions exist to apply knowledge for the benefit of the members of society (Kielhofner, 1992; Luebben, Hinojosa, & Kramer, 2010; Mosey, 1981, 1996). Although each profession has a unique purpose, professions often overlap in the services they provide and the tools they use as part of their interventions to benefit people

(Kramer, Luebben, & Hinojosa, 2010). Each profession's practice is grounded in the society in which it exists and therefore may vary depending on the region of the country, the city, or the culture in which it is practiced. These differences in a profession's practices sometimes create tension for members of the profession who would like to believe that all members of the profession practice in the same manner with the same goals (Strauss, 2001).

Members of a distinct profession share a specialized training and a unique expertise. They also share a common philosophy and a code of ethics. Occupational therapy practitioners' philosophical beliefs outline how they view the person, society, and people in the context of their environment. The tools practitioners use to intervene with clients are heavily influenced by occupational therapy's philosophical orientation.

In 1979, the AOTA Representative Assembly approved an association policy related to the philosophical base of occupational therapy (AOTA, 1979). In this statement, AOTA articulated the profession's basic beliefs about human nature and adaptation. Moreover, it stated that practitioners believe in the importance of purposeful activity to facilitate the adaptive process. Adoption of this statement highlighted the importance of purposeful activity, which was then considered to be synonymous with occupation. The relationship between purposeful activity and occupation has been the focus of major philosophical discussion within the profession.

In 2012, AOTA adopted a revised philosophical base (AOTA, 2012a) affirming that occupation is the core of occupational therapy and is both the means and end to therapy. At the same time, AOTA (2012b) adopted a policy specifying occupation as the common core of occupational therapy. Although AOTA advocates for the sole use of the term *occupation,* practitioners and scholars continue to write about activities and purposeful activities. The following definitions delineate the terms as they are used in this book.

Occupation

"Occupations are the ordinary and familiar things that people do every day" (AOTA, 1995, p. 1015). The meaningful groupings of activities that people engage in as part of their daily lives are *occupations.*

These occupations give life meaning and have been broadly categorized by practitioners as work, self-care, and play or leisure. The range of activities included in any one occupation is defined by the person who is engaging in the activity, the circumstances around which the activity is performed, and the environment. For example, eating can be a pleasure at a state fair, work at a business lunch, or self-care at home.

The important dimensions of an occupation make it a unique classification for occupational therapy practitioners. First and foremost, occupations have personal, specific meaning to the person. This personal meaning is variable and determined by contextual, temporal, psychological, social, symbolic, cultural, ethnic, and spiritual dimensions. Second, occupations involve mental abilities and skills, and they may or may not have an observable physical dimension. Third, the occupations in which a person engages define him or her. Fourth, as the person interacts with his or her environment, matures, or responds to life conditions, his or her preferred occupations are likely to change (AOTA, 1995).

The principal concern of occupational therapy is to maintain, restore, or facilitate a person's ability to function within his or her daily occupations. We have broadly defined *daily occupations* to include active participation in self-maintenance, work, leisure, and play activities.

Activity

Activities are the actions that people take to accomplish a physical or mental task. The World Health Organization (2001) defines the term more broadly, stating "*activity* is the execution of a task or action by an individual" (p. 10, italics added). Activities suggest an active process and may involve engagement with others, although some are performed alone. Additionally, some activities involve specific objects and space.

People engage in activities because they are expected to do them, because they want to do them, or because they need to do them. Most of the activities that people engage in as a part of daily life are ordinary and mundane. As noted by Cynkin and Robinson (1990), there is nothing dramatic or glamorous about making a bed, fixing a faucet, taking a shower, or washing clothes. For the most part, people are unaware of the many activities

they perform as part of their daily routines; most are performed automatically (Cynkin & Robinson, 1990). People do not even think about the importance of these daily activities until they can no longer perform them.

Purposeful Activity

People engage in purposeful activities as part of their daily routines. "*Purposeful activity* refers to goal-directed behaviors or tasks . . . that the individual considers meaningful" (AOTA, 1993, p. 1081). *Purposeful activities* are tasks or experiences in which the person actively participates. Although engaged in and participating in a purposeful activity, the person directs his or her attention to accomplishing the task (AOTA, 1993). Purposeful activities are one of the foundational elements of an occupation. Unique combinations of purposeful activities link together with the person's personal meanings to form his or her occupations.

Purposeful activities are goal directed in that they involve active participation and require coordination among a person's physical, emotional, and cognitive systems. *Goal directed* means that the person actively engages in actions to meet a personal purpose or need; it does not mean that the end product must be a physical outcome. In occupational therapy, purposeful activities are an important therapeutic tool. They are used alone to address a specific need, or they are used in patterns or groups to help a person develop meaningful occupations (AOTA, 1997).

Occupational Performance

"Occupational performance is the doing, the action, the active behavior, or the active responses exhibited within the context of an occupational form" (Nelson, 1988, p. 634). *Occupational form* refers to the context of action contributing to the meaning and purpose that the occupation brings to the person (Nelson, 1988). The occupational form includes the occupation's essential elements, such as its organizational structures, that influence the person's performance of the occupation. The occupational form has both objective and subjective dimensions. Aspects of the objective dimension may be the physical stimuli involved, the objects and their characteristics, the human context, and the temporal context. The subjective, or perceived, dimension is derived from the sociocultural reality, which is independent of the specific person (Nelson, 1988).

Occupational performance is possible because of the person, environment, and occupation (activity) match. The success of a person in completing an occupation depends on the context in which it is performed (Kielhofner, 2009). Thus, *occupational performance* is a person's action in response to the occupation as the person perceives it and the surrounding environmental factors. Or, as defined by Kielhofner (2009), "occupational performance is doing an occupational form" (p. 170). Occupational therapy practitioners are concerned with occupational performance; in other words, they focus on facilitating a client's ability to participate in occupations, taking into consideration the client's perception of the occupations and the environment

Tools of the Profession

Occupational therapy practitioners use a wide variety of *tools* in their practice. These therapeutic tools are selected to be consistent with well-defined theoretical bases or rationales. Note that practitioners do not conceptualize practice in one universally accepted way. Some view practice on the basis of a model, others suggest paradigms, and others use frames of reference.

In this book, we do not address the issue of how practice is conceptualized. We accept the view that scholars use different organizational structures and view practice differently. What is important is that each of the models, paradigms, or frames of reference provides guidelines for the selection and use of therapeutic tools. Each practitioner selects from a wide assortment of tools with which he or she is both knowledgeable and competent and can use in practice. Specialization of practice has resulted in variations in the tools practitioners use. Whatever tools they choose to use, however, they all share a common goal—the client being able to engage and participate in occupations associated with daily living, work, play, or leisure activities.

The practices and concerns of a profession change over time with the advancement of knowledge and technology. Thus, a profession changes its priorities

and practices in response to changes in society. This continuous change ensures that the profession remains viable and is responsive to the needs of the society that it serves. Occupational therapy's evolution in response to changes in society, knowledge, and technology has indeed made it a viable, dynamic profession that continues to meet its mandate from society.

Yet, change has been difficult for some practitioners. For example, the extensive early use of crafts has been replaced with new modalities such as manual manipulation, computer adaptation, or physical activity (e.g., yoga, lifting weights). Changes in the importance and use of a modality are sometimes seen as not consistent with the profession's philosophical base. Using the previous example, some practitioners continue to believe that "true" occupational therapy must involve active engagement in an activity.

Occupational therapy's mandate has always been to enable people to engage and participate in their own daily life activities. Occupational therapy, a health care profession, has been influenced by the trends and concerns of medicine (Christiansen & Baum, 1997). Although medicine continues to affect the profession's evolution, other, more recent changes in society seem to be having a greater influence. In response to societal change, occupational therapy has moved into education and community-based service delivery models. This change in society's priorities has led to an increase in the number of practitioners working in education-based practices and a change in the site of practice to schools and community settings (Kramer & Hinojosa, 1999). This shift in the site of practice and service delivery models is also evident in other areas of practice. The 1990s saw a shift from clinic settings to more integrated community, classroom, and home settings. These changes have been in response to numerous internal influences (e.g., growth in knowledge, advances in technology) and external influences (e.g., social and government policy, payment practices).

Intervention Tools

The application of any frame of reference (i.e., models, practice guidelines, paradigms) involves the use of a variety of intervention tools. *Tools* are items, actions, means, modalities, methods, or instruments that are used in practice in a theoretically prescribed manner to bring about change. These tools become legitimate in a profession when the profession's members have expertise in their use (Mosey, 1996). Occupational therapy practitioners use a variety of tools, depending on their particular frame of reference (Mosey, 1996). Beyond purposeful activities, other legitimate tools discussed in the literature are the nonhuman environment, the conscious use of self, activity analysis and adaptation, activity groups, teaching–learning processes, stimulus–response interactions, atmospheric elements, physical agent modalities, and technology (Kramer et al., 2010; Mosey, 1986, 1996). In addition to these tools, the profession has others that are very specialized and often specific to one frame of reference (Kramer et al., 2010). A profession's tools change with evolving knowledge, technological advances, and clients' changing needs.

One of the major issues related to tools is that some practitioners consider the tools of the profession to be exceptionally meaningful—some may even consider the tools to be symbolic of the profession as a whole (Kramer et al., 2010). This importance may be the result of the tangible aspects of legitimate tools and because practitioners use them daily as they interact with clients (Mosey, 1986). In addition, many practitioners view the tools of their profession as unique. In reality, however, the legitimate tools are not unique and are shared by other professions. What is unique is the way in which a specific profession applies them. In occupational therapy, this singularity lies in how the tools are used together in the application of the specific frame of reference for intervention.

Exercise 1.3. Personal Hierarchy of Needs

An important concern of educators is what motivates people and how it interrelates with the development of human potential (Maslow, 1971; Maslow, Frager, & Fadiman, 1970). Abraham Maslow, the founder of humanistic psychology, proposed that a person's gratification of needs is the most important single principle underlying development. He proposed seven hierarchical levels of needs: (1) physiological, (2) safety, (3) love and belongingness, (4) esteem, (5) self-actualization, (6) knowing and understanding, and (7) aesthetics. Glover, Bruning, and Filbeck (1983) proposed that a person examines his or her life as a means to understanding that life and the self. Each person fills his or her needs by engaging in occupations.

Reflect on the past 2 days and how you satisfied your personal needs in the following categories of Maslow's hierarchy:

- Physiological needs (food, drink, sleep, survival)
- Safety (avoidance of danger and anxiety, desire for security)
- Love and belongingness (affection, feeling wanted, roots in a family or peer group)
- Esteem (self-respect; feelings of adequacy, competence, mastery)
- Self-actualization (striving for or using talents, capacities, potentialities)
- Knowing and understanding (curiosity, learning about the world)
- Aesthetics (experience and understand beauty for its own sake).

After completing the list, consider the following:

- What needs were being met or not met?
- What activities contributed to the satisfaction of your needs?
- What does the list suggest about your health status?

Activities as Therapeutic Modalities

Practitioners use activities, which are naturally part of people's lives, to facilitate their abilities to engage in occupations. Each day, people engage in numerous activities. They perform some activities to meet their self-care needs, some because they enjoy them, and others in response to expectations or to circumstances that require action. Thus, activities are the things that people do, and they are also the building blocks that people use to construct their lives. Occupational therapy evolved from this context—from the realized importance of how people occupy their time as human beings—thus, the concern with occupations is central to the beliefs of occupational therapy practitioners.

From our perspective, *activities* are those actions that people do to accomplish a goal or function. They consist of groupings of actions or tasks that a person performs as part of accomplishing a goal or fulfilling an expected or required function. Activities are purposeful when they are goal directed and meaningful to the person who is completing the task or action. When practitioners view a pattern of daily activities together that have personal meaning to a client, they categorize them as *occupations.* Thus, *occupations* are fundamentally based on activities (Hinojosa et al., 2003; Kramer & Hinojosa, 1995).

From this perspective, both activities and the resulting occupations are a fundamental and essential aspect of life. People's daily activities and occupations define who and what they are; engagement in purposeful activities gives their lives meaning. Occupational therapy practitioners, in defining their domain of concern, typically view activities as part of occupations (e.g., they divide activities into ADLs, work or productive activities, or play or leisure activities). By viewing activities in this manner, practitioners think about how they relate to the outcome for the person who engages in them. Thus, the same activities may fit into several occupations depending on the goal of the activity, the person's developmental status, and the specific circumstances and context in which the person performs the activity.

The following example illustrates this point: For a school-aged child at camp, writing a letter to his or her parents may be work. For a young person, writing a letter to a girlfriend may be a leisure activity. For an adult, writing a shopping list may be an ADL. The occupations for which writing is a component activity thus include work, leisure, and ADLs. For the professional author, writing is an occupation in both the employment and the occupational therapy senses. In this scenario, the author engages in several writing activities that together are viewed as an occupation.

In the following sections, we outline the unique view of occupational therapy practitioners of purposeful activities and how they relate to ADLs, work or productive occupations, and play or leisure occupations.

Activities of daily living

Each day, all people engage in a variety of occupations of daily living. These occupations are composed of *self-care activities,* which are the means by which people interact with and respond to their personal demands and needs. Not all self-care activities are interesting or enjoyable; in fact, many basic self-care activities are boring, routine, and unexciting. These ordinary daily self-care activities, however, are basic to people's survival as social human beings and crucially important to their self-esteem and self-worth. The ability to feed oneself, dress oneself, or take care of one's own toileting needs provides valued independence. In sum, people's ability to take care of themselves and meet their daily needs is vital to their existence. The multitudes of purposeful activities categorized as self-care are determined by a wide range of factors, including individual attributes and abilities, culture, context, developmental status, and socioeconomic status.

Exercise 1.4. Activities of Daily Living

Look at the activities that you listed in Exercise 1.3, and select the ones that you consider self-care occupations and ADLs. Categorize these activities into groups of those you enjoyed or found interesting and those that were boring, routine, or unexciting. What were the factors for you that characterized whether an activity was enjoyable or unexciting? Reflect on how your answers define who you are as a person.

Work or productive occupations

Work or *productive occupations* are composed of the numerous activities that people engage in to support themselves and their families, to fill time in a socially acceptable fashion, to give expression to their interests, to apply their education and training, to maintain important social status, to alleviate stress, to mitigate loneliness, or to avoid doubts about life's purposes, to name just a few possibilities. Work is an obligation for many people, but in U.S. society, it is not usually a requirement for children, some students, some people with disabilities, and some retirees (Marx, 2012). Still, much of an adult's time is devoted to work and productive activities.

In addition to time spent working, people often devote time to preparing for work and traveling to and from work. Many people have more than one job, and the activities involved in work are extremely varied. Most American workers must adjust to the demands of large, formal organizations and complex technology. Also, and sometimes problematically, often because of the amount of time spent at work, work becomes for many a center of social life. Close friendships, groups with shared interests, loving relationships, and marriages often arise in work settings, leading the workplace to be a locale of many satisfactions and stresses.

Work activities are central to the lives of most adults and become a key focus to what makes many people's lives meaningful. Because work is so central to people's lives, its disruption, in times such as the present, by high levels of unemployment, can be a very disturbing factor in the lives of the unemployed and for those with whom their lives are linked. High unemployment levels are therefore also of consequence to occupational therapy practitioners and those with whom we work.

Exercise 1.5. Work or Productive Occupations

Look at the activities that you listed in Exercise 1.3, and select those that you consider work or productive occupations. Reflect on the amount of time you spent engaged in work or productive occupations. Think about what your answers say about your values and the way you live your life.

Play or leisure occupations

Play or *leisure occupations* include a wide range of activities that a person engages in for their intrinsic pleasure and enjoyment. They can range from solitary and sedentary activities, such as reading, to group activities such as sports. An important characteristic of play or leisure activities is that people engage in them because they want to. As with self-care activities, a wide range of factors—including individual attributes and abilities, culture, context, developmental status, and socioeconomic status—determines a person's play and leisure purposeful activities. Leisure occupations may call for little or a great deal of equipment, for example, ranging from a pair of dice to complex fishing gear. Specific environments and sometimes large amounts of space can be involved in the pursuit of leisure. For certain leisure participants, fishing in a nearby lake might meet the same ends as playing golf on a vast golf course.

Occupational therapy practitioners are concerned with the wide range of activities in which people engage. Activities are fundamental and normal for all humans. Purposeful activities and their associated occupations define what and who people

are, allow people to express feelings, and have personal and social meaning to people. People learn from engaging in purposeful activities and get satisfaction from them. Through purposeful activity, a person can explore interests, satisfy needs, determine and assess capacity and limitations, meet personal and interpersonal needs, and cope with life. Most important, from participating in purposeful activities a person develops and acquires his or her own occupations.

Exercise 1.6. Play or Leisure Occupations

Look at the activities that you listed in Exercise 1.3, and select those that you consider play or leisure occupations. Reflect on the amount of time you spent engaged in play or leisure occupations. Think about what your answers say about your values and the way you live your life. How do you express your feelings through play occupations? Do you currently have a balance of self-care, productive, and play occupations?

Tools of Intervention: Purposeful Activities

Occupational therapy practitioners use purposeful activities as tools of intervention. Therefore, it is crucial that they have more than just an appreciation of them. Not only must practitioners have in-depth knowledge of purposeful activities as the foundation of occupation, but they must also understand the value and benefit of purposeful activities as therapeutic media. Using purposeful activities as therapeutic tools requires an understanding of the component elements of purposeful activities. In addition, because of the larger goal of purposeful activities, practitioners must view them within the context of a person's life, abilities, and life circumstances. In other words, when using purposeful activities, practitioners must always keep in mind the client's broader occupations.

Occupational therapy practitioners have always used activities as part of their interventions with clients, but why do they use purposeful activities? Although specific activities have changed and will continue to change, the following six basic reasons for choosing to use purposeful activities are relatively constant:

1. *Purposeful activities build on a person's abilities and lead to the achievement of personal and functional goals.* For an activity to be purposeful, it must have four qualities. First, the activity must be directed toward a goal that the participant considers important. Second, the participant must be actively engaged in the activity because he or she wants to be. Third, the activity must have personal meaning to the participant (Evans, 1987; Gilfoyle, 1984; Mosey, 1986; Nelson, 1988; Nelson & Jepson-Thomas, 2003). An activity's purposefulness is always dependent on the person who is doing the activity and the situational context in which it is done (Henderson et al., 1991). Fourth, the participant must be capable and have the knowledge, skills, and abilities to engage in the activity. Therefore, practitioners select purposeful activities because they are meaningful to the person and build on his or her capacities to bring about action. The person's ability to complete purposeful activities provides the foundation for his or her occupations. When a person engages in personally chosen purposeful activities, these purposeful activities form occupations.

2. *Purposeful activities offer the person opportunities to act effectively and to achieve a goal.* Therefore, the person must be an active participant. The degree of active participation depends on the person's abilities. When a person cannot physically, cognitively, or mentally complete the activity himself or herself, the person still completes a purposeful activity if he or she actively directs someone else to complete the activity. For example, if a person is physically unable to dress himself but directs a personal assistant as to his choice of clothes and the manner in which he wishes to get dressed, the person's effective action allows him to achieve his goal. The completion of the activity has a result: a physical outcome such as finishing a chore or an intellectual achievement such as acquiring information from reading. An important factor is that the person is fully involved mentally or physically in the activity. Practitioners believe that successful accomplishment will lead to the person's development of abilities and skills and that with improved abilities and skills, the person will then begin or continue to engage in occupations.

3. *Purposeful activities provide opportunities for the person to achieve mastery of the environment and to perform something successfully, thus promoting feelings of personal competence.* By skillfully selecting an appropriate activity, practitioners can match the person's capabilities, potential, and desires with particular tasks. Thus, an appropriate purposeful activity provides an opportunity for a person to master skills, accomplish something, and build self-confidence. Accomplishment of various tasks leads to a successful experience and ultimately to the accomplishment of purposeful activities. These accomplishments, when grouped together, develop into successful achievement of occupations. For example, a person who can master washing his or her face (purposeful activity) and then bathing (purposeful activity) may gradually become capable of independently completing his or her own self-care (occupation). From the person's perspective, the feeling of mastery of the environment is realized as he or she engages in purposeful activities (washing and bathing) as part of the intervention plan.

4. *When engaged in a purposeful activity, the person directs his or her attention to the accomplishment of the activity's end goal.* One major value of this engagement in a purposeful activity is that the person's attention is not on the specific tasks and actions required. For example, a child who is playing with a doll is less likely to attend to the increased upper-extremity range of motion, cognitive challenges, or psychosocial interaction sought by the practitioner; instead, the child's goal is to have fun while engaging in an imaginary activity. When an adult makes a sandwich, he or she may not focus on the pain or limited range of motion associated with arthritis, concentrating instead on the edible product. However, this ability to attend to the activity and not the disability may be interfered with or lost for the client with cognitive impairment. Such a loss of attention may require safety precautions for the elderly client with dementia, for example, who may forget that he is heating water for tea and begin to engage in another activity. A loud whistling teakettle might be an appropriate intervention in such a case.

5. *Engagement in purposeful activities within the context of interpersonal, cultural, physical, and other environmental conditions requires and elicits coordination among the person's sensory, perceptual, motor, and cognitive systems and his or her emotions.* The nature of being involved in an activity (which has a goal and an anticipated outcome and involves several tasks) leads to engagement in a purposeful activity and occurs in complex interactions between the person and his or her environment (Csikszentmihalyi, 1993). Although a practitioner can to some extent control the degree of each factor, the nature of selecting an activity that is meaningful requires multiple levels of processing. The therapeutic value of purposeful activities is enhanced by the complex interaction of factors that stem from involvement in a specific purposeful activity.

6. *Engagement in purposeful activities provides direct and objective feedback about performance to both the practitioner and the client.* Feedback is gathered during the performance of the activity and from the result of the actions. Because the purposeful activities are part of real-life occupations, they provide additional insight into the person's potential to engage in occupations successfully. Feedback from real-life meaningful activities provides valuable information that cannot be obtained from simulated or fabricated tasks.

These six reasons provide the rationale that occupational therapy practitioners have always used to explain their use of purposeful activities. Although the types of activities have continually changed, practitioners are committed to using meaningful, real-life purposeful activities as the best tool for evaluation and intervention.

Practitioners' Examination and Use of Purposeful Activities

To use purposeful activities as part of an intervention, occupational therapy practitioners examine their use from several perspectives. In the following sections, we outline some of the general characteristics of purposeful activities that practitioners consider as they use them as evaluation and therapeutic tools.

Goal of the activity

Each person has goals that drive his or her engagement in an activity. These goals may be immediate or long term. The nature of the goals also varies depending on the person's reason for doing the activity and the time he or she has to complete it. For the occupational therapy practitioner, the person's goal for engaging in the activity is an important factor to consider when judging performance. Practitioners often assume that when the goal for engaging in the activity comes from the person, the person has greater investment in the activity and places more value on it. Likewise, practitioners often assume that if the person is completing the activity for someone else, he or she may not put forth the same effort or have the same investment in the activity.

These assumptions, however, may not be true. When analyzing performance of a task or completion of an activity, one factor that a practitioner must consider carefully is the person's motivation to perform. The practitioner must consider what he or she knows about the person's occupations and, with the person, select purposeful activities that will support these occupations. Another consideration may be the person's ability to perform the activity safely. In addition to the choice of activity, the pace of its performance and the grading of its intensity may be among the considerations for the practitioner.

Meaning and value of the activity

Occupational therapy practitioners use information from the client to select activities for evaluation and intervention that have personal value and meaning for the client. This information includes factors such as his or her personal attributes, culture, lifestyle, and life situation. For example, when working with children, practitioners frequently choose play activities that are meaningful and appropriate to the child. If the child has a physical limitation, comes from a Hispanic background, and lives in a large metropolitan area, practitioners carefully consider each of these factors when selecting a specific activity. In this example, the practitioner, knowing the value of the family eating together, might select imaginary cooking for various dolls with skin color that reflects the child's family.

Knowledge, abilities, and skills required to engage in the activity

Every purposeful activity requires knowledge, abilities, and skills to produce an effective outcome. Occupational therapy practitioners use *task analysis,* which is the examination of the subcomponent parts of an activity and the analysis of the motor, cognitive, or interactive skills required to complete each step and their understanding of the activity to determine what is required to engage in it. On the basis of this analysis, they then select activities that match the person's capacities.

Required objects, articles, or paraphernalia

Most purposeful activities involve the use of objects, articles, or paraphernalia to accomplish the various component tasks. A key point of an *activity analysis* (i.e., identifying the essential information, abilities, skills, and proficiencies necessary to complete each task) is to determine what materials are actually required and to what extent. Practitioners examine the materials that are essential to the task, and at times they modify, adapt, or change the materials required. They try, however, to maintain the integrity of the purposeful activity.

Actions required to engage in the activity

Although many activities are carried out in specific ways, they can often be modified, adapted, or changed if needed. The *actions of an activity* include the structure, rules, organizational features, and timing that each task in the activity requires. Additionally, actions may have to be carried out in a specific way, in a specific order, in a set amount of time, or in a specific time period. Occupational therapy practitioners examine activities in relation to the actions required to engage in and complete them. Such examination requires adept activity analysis skills. Furthermore, people often obtain satisfaction not just from the activity itself but also from the routine and the objects used in the performance.

Required level of engagement with the human environment

Whereas all purposeful activities require that the person who is engaged in the activity partici-pate, many necessitate the participation of other people, that is, the *human environment.* Depending on the activity, others can be a specific person (e.g., mother, spouse, family member, friend), an acquaintance (e.g., peer, colleague, health care provider), or a stranger. Sometimes the activity demands that the people involved have particular knowledge or skills. The specific activity and the context in which it is performed may also influence each person's degree of participation. Practitioners carefully examine the degree and quality of participation required for the whole activity and its component tasks.

Required level of engagement with the nonhuman environment

As discussed previously, most purposeful activities involve the use of objects, articles, or paraphernalia, that is, the *nonhuman environment,* which may also include pets and other animals that may be crucial to the activity. Purposeful activities that involve interaction between the nonhuman elements of the environment and the people included in the activity also vary in terms of degree of involvement. Again, as with the human environment, practitioners carefully examine the degree and quality of participation required for the whole activity and for its component tasks.

Context in which the activity is performed

Performance of a task or an activity can be context dependent. The *context,* sometimes referred to as *environment,* within which an activity is done includes physical, social, cultural, and temporal factors. It can also be used to describe verbal situations or meanings. Both senses of this term are important to practitioners. *Context* may refer to the intervention setting itself, but also to the environment in which the occupation may eventually be performed. It is a complex and multifaceted idea; therefore, it requires careful consideration by the practitioner.

Purposeful Activities in Evaluation and Intervention

When evaluating, therapists use purposeful activities to assess what a person is able and unable to do.

Likewise, intervention uses purposeful activities as the means to motivate and enhance the person's abilities. A person's actual performance in purposeful activities provides insight into his or her ability to engage in occupations and function in the real world. This information, along with other assessment data, is used to develop a comprehensive intervention plan. By definition, selection of purposeful activity is client specific. Thus, activities are selected on the basis of the person's needs, the person's abilities and disabilities, and the activity's inherent characteristics. Once the activity has been selected, the practitioner can grade or adapt it to promote successful performance or elicit a particular response.

Purposeful activities have the potential to facilitate a client's mastery of a new skill, to restore a deficient ability, to provide a means for compensating for a functional disability, to maintain health, and to prevent dysfunction. During intervention, practitioners select activities or modify them in response to crucial changes in the person to provide opportunities for gradual development of skills and other related therapeutic benefits. Aspects of a purposeful activity manipulated as part of the intervention

---

Exercise 1.7. Dunton's Nine Cardinal Principles

According to Peloquin (1991), Dunton (1918) proposed cardinal principles to guide the emerging practice of occupational therapy. Please read them and discuss how they relate to the previous discussion of the use of purposeful activities in occupational therapy. How appropriate are they today?

1. The work should be carried on with cure as the main object.
2. The work must be interesting.
3. The patient should be carefully studied.
4. One form of occupation should not be carried to the point of fatigue.
5. It should have some useful end.
6. It preferably should lead to an increase in the patient's knowledge.
7. It should be carried on with others.
8. All possible encouragement should be given the worker.
9. Work resulting in a poor or useless product is better than idleness. (pp. 733–734)

include sequence; duration; task procedures; the person's position; the position of the tools and materials; the size, shape, weight, or texture of materials; the nature and degree of interpersonal contact; the extent of physical handling by the practitioner during the performance; and the environment in which the activity is attempted. All of these factors are discussed in detail in later chapters.

Summary

Occupational therapy practitioners begin their evaluation of a person with an occupational profile to learn about the person's occupations. As part of intervention, practitioners use purposeful activities to restore function and to compensate for functional deficits (AOTA, 1993). Before using a purposeful activity as part of an intervention plan, practitioners complete an analysis of the activity based on both the client and the context.

When using purposeful activities, practitioners must consider all the information obtained in the occupational profile, including the person's age, occupational roles, cultural background, gender, interests, and preferences. Scrutinizing the context and circumstances surrounding the performance of the activity, practitioners skillfully select purposeful activities within the conditions of the frame of reference that has been selected to guide the intervention. Using activity synthesis, occupational therapists implement purposeful activities that are appropriate and lead to occupational synthesis in which the person naturally engages in occupations.

References

American Occupational Therapy Association. (1979). Philosophical base of occupational therapy, Resolution #531-79. *American Journal of Occupational Therapy, 33,* 785.

American Occupational Therapy Association. (1993). Position paper: Purposeful activity. *American Journal of Occupational Therapy, 47,* 1081–1018. http://dx.doi.org/10.5014/ajot.47.12.1081

American Occupational Therapy Association. (1995). Position paper: Occupation. *American Journal of Occupational Therapy, 49,* 1015–1018. http://dx.doi.org/10.5014/ajot.49.10.1015

American Occupational Therapy Association. (1997). Statement—Fundamental concepts of occupational therapy: Occupation, purposeful activity, and function. *American Journal of Occupational Therapy, 51,* 864–866. http://dx.doi.org/10.5014/ajot.51.10.864

American Occupational Therapy Association. (2008). Occupational therapy framework: Domain and process (2nd ed.). *American Journal of Occupational Therapy, 62,* 625–683. http://dx.doi.org/10.5014/ajot.62.6.625

American Occupational Therapy Association. (2012a). Policy 1.11. The philosophical base of occupational therapy. In *Policy manual.* Bethesda, MD: Author.

American Occupational Therapy Association. (2012b). Policy 1.12. Occupation as the common core of occupational therapy. In *Policy manual.* Bethesda, MD: Author.

American Occupational Therapy Association. (2014). Occupational therapy practice framework: Domain and process (3rd ed.). *American Journal of Occupational Therapy, 68*(Suppl. 1), S1–S48. http://dx.doi.org/10.5014/ajot.682006

Bauerschmidt, B., & Nelson, D. L. (2011). The terms *occupation* and *activity* over the history of official occupational therapy publications. *American Journal of Occupational Therapy, 65,* 338–345. http://dx.doi.org/10.5014/ajot.2011.000869

Christiansen, C., & Baum, C. M. (1997). The occupational therapy context: Philosophy–principles–practice. In C. M. Baum & C. Christiansen (Eds.), *Occupational therapy: Enabling function and well-being* (2nd ed., pp. 26–45). Thorofare, NJ: Slack.

Csikszentmihalyi, M. (1993). Activity and happiness: Towards a science of occupation. *Journal of Occupational Science: Australia, 1,* 38–42. http://dx.doi.org/10.1080/14427591.1993.9686377

Cynkin, S., & Robinson, A. M. (1990). *Occupational therapy and activities health: Toward health through activities.* Boston: Little, Brown.

Dunton, W. R. (1918). *Occupation therapy. A manual for nurses.* Philadelphia: W. B. Saunders.

Evans, K. A. (1987). Definition of occupation as the core concept of occupational therapy. *American Journal of Occupational Therapy, 41,* 627–628. http://dx.doi.org/10.5014/ajot.41.10.627

Foster, A. (2008). Games and motivation to learn science: Personal identity, applicability, relevance and meaningfulness. *Journal of Interactive Learning Research, 19*(4), 597–614.

Gilfoyle, E. M. (1984). Transformation of a profession [Eleanor Clarke Slagle Lecture]. *American Journal of Occupational Therapy, 38,* 575–584. http://dx.doi.org/10.5014/ajot.38.9.575

Glover, J. A., Bruning, R. H., & Filbeck, R. W. (1983). *Educational psychology: Principles and applications.* Boston: Little, Brown.

Gray, J. M. L. (1998). Putting occupation into practice: Occupation as ends, occupation as means. *American Journal of Occupational Therapy, 52,* 354–364. http://dx.doi.org/10.5014/ajot.52.5.354

Harvey-Krefting, L. (1985). The concept of work in occupational therapy: A historical review. *American Journal of Occupational Therapy, 39,* 301–307. http://dx.doi.org/10.5014/ajot.39.5.301

Henderson, A., Cermak, S., Coster, W., Murray, E., Trombly, C., & Tickle-Degnen, L. (1991). Occupational science is multidimensional. *American Journal of Occupational Therapy, 45,* 370–372. http://dx.doi.org/10.5014/ajot.45.4.370

Hinojosa, J., & Blount, M.-L. (Eds.). (2009). *The texture of life: Purposeful activities in the context of occupation* (3rd ed.). Bethesda, MD: AOTA Press.

Hinojosa, J., Kramer, P., Royeen, C. B., & Luebben, A. (2003). The core concept of occupation. In P. Kramer, J. Hinojosa, & C. B. Royeen (Eds.), *Perspectives in human occupation: Participation in life* (pp. 1–17). Philadelphia: Lippincott Williams & Wilkins.

Kielhofner, G. (1992). *Conceptual foundations of occupational therapy.* Philadelphia: F. A. Davis.

Kielhofner, G. (2006a). Occupation. In G. L. Albrecht (Ed.), *Encyclopedia of disability* (Vol. 3, pp. 1174–1175). Thousand Oaks, CA: Sage.

Kielhofner, G. (2006b). Occupational therapy. In G. L. Albrecht (Ed.), *Encyclopedia of disability* (Vol. 3, pp. 1175–1177). Thousand Oaks, CA: Sage.

Kielhofner, G. (2009). *Conceptual foundations of occupational therapy practice* (4th ed.). Philadelphia: F. A. Davis.

Kramer, P., & Hinojosa, J. (1995). Epiphany of human occupation. In C. B. Royeen (Ed.), *The practice of the future: Putting occupation back into therapy* (AOTA Self-Study Series, pp. 8.1–8.17). Bethesda, MD: American Occupational Therapy Association.

Kramer, P., & Hinojosa, J. (1999). Domain of concern of occupational therapy: Relevance to pediatric practice. In J. Hinojosa & P. Kramer (Eds.), *Frames of reference for pediatric occupational therapy* (pp. 9–26). Baltimore: Lippincott Williams & Wilkins.

Kramer, P., Luebben, A., & Hinojosa, J. (2010). Contemporary legitimate tools of pediatric occupational therapy. In P. Kramer & J. Hinojosa (Eds.), *Frames of reference for pediatric occupational therapy* (3rd ed., pp. 50–66). Baltimore: Lippincott Williams & Wilkins.

Latham, C. A. T. (2008). Occupation: Philosophy and concepts. In M. V. Radomski & C. A. T. Latham (Eds.), *Occupational therapy for physical dysfunction* (6th ed., pp. 340–357). Philadelphia: Lippincott Williams & Wilkins.

Luebben, A., Hinojosa, J., & Kramer, P. (2010). Domain of concern of occupational therapy: Relevance to pediatric practice. In P. Kramer & J. Hinojosa (Eds.), *Frames of reference for pediatric occupational therapy* (3rd ed., pp. 31–49). Baltimore: Lippincott Williams & Wilkins.

Marx, P. (2012, October 8). Up life's ladder: Golden years. *The New Yorker,* pp. 72–75.

Maslow, A. H. (1971). *The farther reaches of human nature.* New York: Viking.

Maslow, A. H., Frager, R., & Fadiman, J. (1970). *Motivation and personality* (Vol. 2, 2nd ed.). New York: Harper & Row.

Mosey, A. C. (1981). *Occupational therapy: Configuration of a profession.* New York: Raven Press.

Mosey, A. C. (1985). A monistic or a pluralistic approach to professional identity [Eleanor Clarke Slagle Lecture]. *American Journal of Occupational Therapy, 39,* 504–509. http://dx.doi.org/10.5014/ajot.39.8.504

Mosey, A. C. (1986). *Psychosocial components of occupational therapy.* New York: Raven Press.

Mosey, A. C. (1996). *Applied scientific inquiry in the health professions: An epistemological orientation.* Bethesda, MD: American Occupational Therapy Association.

Nelson, D. L. (1988). Occupation: Form and performance. *American Journal of Occupational Therapy, 42,* 633–641. http://dx.doi.org/10.5014/ajot.42.10.633

Nelson, D. L. (1997). Why the profession of occupational therapy will flourish in the 21st century [1996 Eleanor Clarke Slagle Lecture]. *American Journal of Occupational Therapy, 51,* 11–24. http://dx.doi.org/10.5014/ajot.51.1.11

Nelson, D. L., & Jepson-Thomas, J. (2003). Occupational form, occupational performance, and a conceptual framework for therapeutic occupation. In P. Kramer, J. Hinojosa, & C. B. Royeen (Eds.), *Perspectives in human occupation: Participation in life* (pp. 87–155). Philadelphia: Lippincott Williams & Wilkins.

Peloquin, S. M. (1991). Occupational therapy service: Individual and collective understandings of the founders, Part 2. *American Journal of Occupational Therapy, 45,* 733–744. http://dx.doi.org/10.5014/ajot.45.8.733

Pierce, D. (2001). Untangling occupation and activity. *American Journal of Occupational Therapy, 55,* 138–146. http://dx.doi.org/10.5014/ajot.55.2.138

Reed, K., & Sanderson, S. (1999). *Concepts of occupational therapy.* Philadelphia: Lippincott Williams & Wilkins.

Strauss, A. L. (2001). *Professions, work, and careers.* New Brunswick, NJ: Transaction.

World Health Organization. (2001). *International classification of functioning, disability and health (ICF).* Geneva: Author.

CHAPTER 2.

PERSPECTIVES ON OCCUPATION AND ACTIVITIES

Marie-Louise Blount, AM, OT, FAOTA; Wesley Blount; and Jim Hinojosa, PhD, OT, BCP, FAOTA

Highlights

✧ Activities and lifestyle performance: Gail Fidler
✧ Legitimate tools: Anne C. Mosey
✧ Occupational behavior: Mary Reilly
✧ Model of Human Occupation: Gary Kielhofner
✧ Occupational science: University of Southern California's Department of Occupational Science and Occupational Therapy
✧ Activities health: Simme Cynkin
✧ Person–Environment–Occupation Model: Mary Law
✧ Occupation: Charles Christiansen and Carolyn Baum
✧ Occupational form and occupational performance: David Nelson
✧ Ecology of Human Performance: Winnie Dunn
✧ Occupational adaptation: Janette Schkade and Sally Schultz
✧ Theories of learning: SCOPE–IT and CO–OP
✧ Occupation analysis and the synthesis of ideas
✧ Considering perspectives.

Key Terms

✧ Activity
✧ Activity analysis
✧ Activity process
✧ Adaptations
✧ Assistive technology
✧ Canadian Occupational Performance Measure
✧ Client
✧ Comparative effectiveness
✧ Conscious purpose
✧ CO–OP
✧ Doing
✧ Ecology of Human Performance
✧ Extrinsic motivation
✧ Feedback
✧ Frames of reference
✧ Habituation
✧ Holistic view of practice

- ✧ Interests
- ✧ Interpersonal process
- ✧ Intrinsic motivation
- ✧ Legitimate tools
- ✧ Life Style Performance Model
- ✧ Model of Human Occupation
- ✧ Model of Occupational Adaptation
- ✧ Occupation
- ✧ Occupational activities
- ✧ Occupation Analysis framework
- ✧ Occupational behavior
- ✧ Occupational dysfunction
- ✧ Occupational form
- ✧ Occupational function
- ✧ Occupational performance
- ✧ Occupational readiness
- ✧ Occupational science

- ✧ Occupational synthesis
- ✧ Occupations of daily living
- ✧ Open system
- ✧ Performance
- ✧ Person–Environment–Occupation model
- ✧ Physical modalities
- ✧ Play
- ✧ Purposeful activity
- ✧ SCOPE–IT
- ✧ Sociocultural dimension
- ✧ Systems theory
- ✧ Task
- ✧ Treatment
- ✧ Unconscious purpose
- ✧ Values
- ✧ Volition

As much as occupational therapy has always been defined by the use of occupation and purposeful activity, very little has been done to pull together the concepts of *purposeful activities* and *occupation* that theorists use to define the profession. Needless to say, many differing theoretical approaches have grown and transformed as the profession has grown and changed over the years. As theorists have added to the body of knowledge from different perspectives, these differing approaches have led to multiple realities regarding the ways in which occupational therapy is seen, with each relevant term taking on a different meaning with each new theorist. At the same time, to carve out unique vantage points, theorists frequently ignore others' definitions or subtly redefine the scope of another's work.

This chapter serves as an overview of the work of major theorists and thinkers in occupational therapy, including details of their important contributions and summaries of their major concepts. We believe understanding these major concepts can guide current understanding and future directions of the profession's theoretical underpinnings.

The broadening range of occupational therapy's areas of practice has necessitated a continual need to expand the definitions that make up the very notion of the profession. What began as a limited range of arts and crafts activities has grown to include the rehabilitation of soldiers; pediatric therapy and the role of play; examination of self-care; and, recently, spirituality and nonactive occupations of different

kinds. Each expansion has brought with it a reexamination of the very notion of what constitutes purposeful activities and occupation, and delicate nuances have separated terms that often seem similar, such as *occupation* and *purposeful activities*.

It would be difficult under any circumstances to create an overview of the development of theoretical terms in occupational therapy, which may explain why few attempts have been made to bring together the various contributions of the professions' important theorists and comprehensively examine them. Since the publication of this book's first edition, however, several books and articles (e.g., Christensen & Baum, 1991; Schkade & Schultz, 2003) have presented similar historically based approaches to developing theories or practice models.

Several new theorists, added to this edition, have entered the fray with new conceptual approaches to the profession, definitions, and theoretical approaches underpinning the therapeutic models. Some of the theorists we originally discussed have refined their approaches, and occupational science has grown in ways that may be beyond the scope of occupational therapy. What has become clearer in the years since the first edition is that theory in occupational therapy has become a synthesis of ideas relating to activity and performance.

Our goal here is not to pick "winners and losers" among theoretical concept; it is to look at key points of each important work to develop a sense of common themes and terms while noting the continual dynamic aspects that will affect future developments.

We believe that nothing can substitute for reading the works of each of these distinguished contributors in their original form. Each theorist has, in some way, attempted to draw, respectfully, on earlier work to ground his or her approach; each definition of *activity* is, in some way, a refinement of past work.

What we present here is an overview of the major theorists and their important contributions to the concepts of occupation and purposeful activities. Any attempt at defining terms must reflect the continual change and synthesis that persists in developing theoretical approaches. Some of the theoretical approaches we discuss are included primarily for their historical importance to the field rather than for their current applications, but, when taken together, they show the progression of thinking about occupational therapy practice.

Activities and Lifestyle Performance: Gail Fidler

As an occupational therapist, association leader, educator, and scholar, Gail Fidler (Figure 2.1) had a powerful influence on the profession's knowledge and understanding of purposeful activities, which continues after her death (Gillette, 2005). Fidler's views and opinions about purposeful activities came from her conviction that doing activities is vitally important and therefore meaningful to people. In occupational therapy, activities have powerful therapeutic merit. From Fidler's (1996)

Figure 2.1. Gail Fidler.

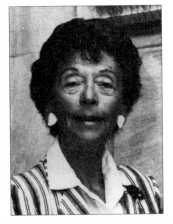

Source. Wilma L. West Library, American Occupational Therapy Foundation, Bethesda, MD. Used with permission.

perspective, *purposeful activities* and *occupation* are synonymous terms for the same construct.

Fidler recognized that if society is to value occupational therapy and the use of activities as authentic therapeutic modalities, occupational therapy practitioners need a conceptual rationale for using activities. In 1948, observing that the occupational therapy literature discussed only the appeal, interest factors, and popularity of activities, Fidler argued that occupational therapists needed a scientific method of empirically examining activities and analyzing their value. She proposed an *activity analysis* as one approach, giving practitioners a means to examine activities by dividing them into component parts. Understanding an activity's component parts provides the information that a practitioner needs to match a specific activity to a client's need and treatment objectives (Fidler, 1948). This original activity analysis is the foundation for many activity analyses used today. Subsequently, Fidler (1969) turned her attention to the therapeutic value of active involvement in doing activities in task groups.

In 1954, with her husband, Jay Fidler, Fidler published a book titled *Introduction to Psychiatric Occupational Therapy*. This text included extensive discussion of the use of activities in psychiatric settings and provided a conceptual rationale for using purposeful activities for all occupational therapy practitioners. Analyzing the component parts of an activity provides the information that practitioners require to correlate the client's needs, interests, and abilities. Moreover, occupational therapy impels the client to develop skills through an action-oriented learning experience (Fidler & Fidler, 1954).

Fidler and Fidler introduced occupational therapy practitioners to the psychodynamic properties of activities. Some aspects of the activity to be examined were related to then-contemporary psychodynamic beliefs, including motion, procedures, materials, creativity, symbols, hostile and aggressive components, control, predictability, narcissism, sexual identification, dependence, reality testing, and group relatedness. Fidler and Fidler also stressed the importance of human and nonhuman environments in understanding and performing activities.

In a 1978 article titled "Doing and Becoming: Purposeful Action and Self-Actualization," Fidler and Fidler provided a theoretical rationale for purposeful activities. They selected the word *doing*, saying that "doing is viewed as enabling the development and integration of the sensory, motor, cognitive, and psychological systems; serving as a socializing agent; and verifying one's efficacy as a competent, contributing member of one's society" (p. 305). Knowledge about activities allows an occupational therapy practitioner to select a particular activity that matches the client's therapeutic needs, learning readiness, intact functions, and values. The practitioner then plans and implements an action-learning experience to allow the client to develop skills (Fidler & Fidler, 1978). Purposeful activities provide opportunities and means for a person to achieve mastery and competence because all activities have social relevance; each person has individual activity interests, which have personal meaning and a place in the social construct; and these activities can remediate dysfunction and have therapeutic value (Fidler, 1981).

In the introduction to *Activities: Reality and Symbol*, Fidler and Beth Velde (1999) summarized the elements that define activity, and in 2002, Velde and Fidler put forward the *Life Style Performance Model* to provide a comprehensive picture of a person's activities, abilities, needs, interests, capacities, and self-expectation of his or her human and non-human world. This model highlights the interrelatedness of person, environment, activity profile, and quality of life. The model describes four activity domains: (1) activities concerned with self-care and self-maintenance, (2) personally referenced pleasure and intrinsic gratification, (3) societal contribution, and (4) interpersonal engagement.

The role of a practitioner in this model is to work with a client toward a healthy activity pattern. Quality of life is considered to be extremely important, and the practitioner needs to have a *holistic view of practice,* that is, getting direction from the client. In this respect, the Life Style Performance Model closely resembles the work of Mary Law's (1998) Person–Environment–Occupation (PEO) model. As with Law (see the section, "Person–Environment–Occupation Model: Mary Law"), the client interview is paramount, the client's needs are foremost, and the measures for successful intervention are on the personal rather than the scientific level. The role of purposeful activity is individual and personalized.

Focusing on the benefits of therapeutic intervention for the person is obviously an important part of practice; however, one also needs to recognize the difficulty of objective study of the roles and effectiveness of different activities within these client-centered

performance models. Fidler's synthesis of the ideas she developed with her collaborators shows both how theoretical thinking evolves over time and that inclusive theories adapt well as new concepts arise.

Legitimate Tools: Anne C. Mosey

A student of Fidler, Anne C. Mosey has gone on to become a key scholar and thought leader in the field. In 1968, Mosey proposed that occupational therapy practitioners should develop and use *frames of reference* to guide their evaluation and interventions. Frames of reference provide practitioners with an organized theoretical knowledge base for practice. Practitioners use a variety of means to carry out or implement their theoretically based interventions, which Mosey (1981) labeled the profession's *legitimate tools*—the means that a professional uses to accomplish a goal, including activities, actions, instruments, modalities, methods, and processes (Mosey, 1981).

The perspective of a profession having legitimate tools acknowledges that although many different professions use the same therapeutic modalities, no one profession "owns" them. Professions may share tools, but each profession uses them in unique ways that are authorized by society. This dynamic view of a profession's legitimate tools means that a profession's tools change as the profession evolves. Moreover, this view recognizes that the use of a tool is directed by the theoretical perspective that the practitioner has selected to address the client's needs.

Before her classification of legitimate tools, Mosey (1973) had identified the unique therapeutic value of activities in assisting people with mental illness to become part of their communities and to engage in their daily lives. In this text, *Activities Therapy,* Mosey described the power of doing an activity as a means for a person to learn new skills and behaviors. She underscored the potential of learning through doing; purposeful "activities are used to provide familiar life situations in which participants are assisted in identifying faulty patterns of behavior and the ideas, feelings, and values that support these faulty patterns" (Mosey, 1973, p. 2).

Activities provide practitioners with a means to understand the person and a method to assist him or her in participating in the tasks at hand. Important aspects of using activities therapeutically are, among others, that they involve the here and now, they are action oriented, and they involve learning through doing. Mosey also emphasized the notions of satisfaction and enjoyment of the activity and the therapeutic benefit to the client.

In 1986, Mosey proposed that occupational therapy practitioners have six primary legitimate tools: (1) nonhuman environment, (2) conscious use of self, (3) the teaching–learning process, (4) purposeful activities, (5) activity groups, and (6) activity analysis and synthesis. In her extensive discussion of purposeful activities as a legitimate tool, Mosey described the characteristics important for evaluation and intervention in occupational therapy. Practitioners develop expertise and skills in using these therapeutic tools as part of their basic professional education and ongoing postprofessional education (Mosey, 1986, 1996).

According to Mosey (1986), *purposeful activities* are a "doing process that requires the use of thought and energy and are directed toward an intended or desired end result" (p. 227). Mosey specified that people who are engaged in purposeful activities are aware of the reason for doing them and do them of their own free will without being coerced. In addition, she proposed that purposeful activities have the following characteristics:

- People who are engaged in purposeful activities are aware of the reason for doing them;
- People participate in purposeful activities of their own free will and are not being coerced;
- Purposeful activities have a planned end result that is not necessarily a material product;
- Purposeful activities have the potential to be symbolic;
- Purposeful activities are universal in that they exist as part of the human experience of interacting with one's environments, and people participate in them throughout their daily lives;
- Purposeful activities are ordinary in nature;
- Purposeful activities are essential to the development of humans in all aspects of their development; and
- Purposeful activities are made up of elements that can be identified, holistic, able to be manipulated, promoting differential responses, able to be graded, facilitating communication, having a focusing organizing effect, emphasizing doing, frequently involving the nonhuman environment, varying on a continuum from conscious to not conscious/unconscious, varying on a continuum from simulated to natural. (p. 241)

Mosey (1986) included purposeful activities as one of occupational therapy's major legitimate tools until 1996, when she proposed a new taxonomy of occupational therapy's legitimate tools. This revised taxonomy of legitimate tools consisted of *interpersonal process* (i.e., relating between people), *activity process* (i.e., participation in a task or action to get something done), and *physical modalities* (i.e., "those procedures and interventions that are systematically applied to modify specific client factors when neurological, musculoskeletal, or skin conditions are present that may be limiting occupational performance"; American Occupational Therapy Association, 2012, p. S78; Mosey, 1996). It did not include purposeful activity itself as a separate legitimate tool, instead including it as a subcomponent of other tools. This categorization may reflect the trend in occupational therapy toward moving away from using specific purposeful activities and instead focusing on the foundation for participation in occupations.

Mosey (personal communication, 2001) then revised her list of legitimate tools to include seven tools:

1. *Conscious use of self:* Preplanned verbal and nonverbal responses to a person
2. *Activities:* Tasks or interactions in which people typically engage
3. *Activity groups:* Types of primary groups that involve participation in activities or discussion of anticipated or current involvement in activities
4. *Stimulus–response interactions:* Specific sensory input with a predictable motor response
5. *Atmospheric elements:* Aspects of the physical environment that can be modified
6. *Assistive technology:* Devices, equipment, or systems specifically designed or adapted to prevent or remediate dysfunction or to maintain or improve function
7. *Physical agent modalities:* Properties of temperature, light, sound, water, and electricity that produce selected effects on soft tissue.

This taxonomy continues to recognize that occupational therapy practitioners may use frames of reference or other theoretically based guidelines for intervention that do not emphasize the importance of purposeful activities. Many guidelines for intervention address a specific component deficit. Other guidelines for intervention may use activities but are less concerned with the purposefulness of the activity to the client. In these situations, the purpose is defined by the practitioner who has identified explicit outcomes for the client.

Occupational Behavior: Mary Reilly

A seminal and critical writer and thinker in occupational therapy, Mary Reilly had not devoted all of her attention to issues of activity and occupation, but her ideas, eventually subsumed under the term *occupational behavior* (Reilly, 1966), gave attention to the role of activity as an underlying theme.

Among Reilly's concerns was the impetus to study and investigate the profession to clearly establish its contributions to science. Reilly (1960) therefore suggested that a major area for occupational therapy research should be the nature and meaning of activity. The presumption that people require activity to attain and maintain health is fundamental to the profession's beliefs in Reilly's (1960) opinion: "We are becoming more aware of the fact that the interests of man emerge in the gratification of his senses" (p. 208). Indeed, she stressed that investigation of the need to engage in activity should move beyond traditional occupational therapy's reliance on arts and crafts and into analysis of such activities as the appropriate level for the investigation (Reilly, 1960). She emphasized the physical, sensory, and psychic rewards inherent in activity and spoke against the idea that various approaches to the use of activity (e.g., separating dance from recreation from crafts) serve as the best approach to the application of therapeutic activity.

In her Eleanor Clarke Slagle Lecture, Reilly (1962) further affirmed the centrality of work to human existence. Her thesis in this presentation was that human productivity provides the most life satisfaction and that occupational therapy applies this principle to the maintenance and restoration of health. Occupational therapy intervention (*treatment,* in her words) requires that the practitioner

investigate and address problems people have in coping with "play, work, and school" (Reilly, 1962, p. 7). She also expressed in this presentation her rejection of the word *activity* to describe how occupational therapy practitioners engage patients, because she had become wary of the increasing use of terms such as *activity therapy* in treatment settings that moved occupational therapy away from seeking to enhance individual human productivity.

As Reilly's (1966) approach to the study of occupational therapy came to be called *occupational behavior,* which Reilly defined as engaging in meaningful occupations along a play–work developmental continuum, she referred back to the core ideas of early occupational therapy thinkers: that a satisfying life required a balanced approach to work, rest, and play. Occupational therapy, appropriately applied, would establish a setting in which all of these aspects of life could be addressed. In describing a model program that addresses all of these factors, Reilly included exercise programs, required work activities, and learning recreational skills and included some group activities and social skills.

Reilly's interest in occupation and related activities later developed into a special concentration on the occupation of play as it applied to both children and adults (Reilly, 1974). She investigated, along with her students, the development of occupational behaviors during play and play's relationship to people's exploration of their environments, their development of competence, and their fulfillment of the drive to achieve. After a long and influential career, Reilly passed away in 2012.

Reilly's striving to understand the nature and functions of human occupation and to apply this knowledge to occupational therapy intervention led to the development of the Model of Human Occupation (MoHO) and eventually to the field of study called *occupational science.*

Model of Human Occupation: Gary Kielhofner

As students of Reilly, Gary Kielhofner (Figure 2.2) and Janice Burke took the theory of occupational behavior and expanded both its external framework and its organizing principles. Kielhofner continued to refine this theoretical approach as a *MoHO* (Forsyth & Kielhofner, 2003; Kielhofner, 1995,

Figure 2.2. Gary Kielhofner.

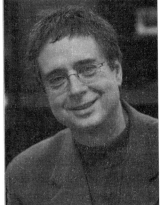

Source. R. Taylor. Used with permission.

2008, 2009; Kielhofner & Burke, 1980) until his passing in 2010, and he used the model to observe and explain most aspects of theory related to occupational therapy. Indeed, one of the central tenets of the model is that human occupation can be used for therapeutic benefit, which also advocates a balanced lifestyle that includes both work and leisure (thus expanding on Reilly's [1974] notion of play).

In Kielhofner's (1985) view, "Occupation is a multifaceted phenomenon that involves the simultaneous operation of biological, psychological, social, and ecological factors" (p. xvii). By using broad, inclusive definitions of terms, such as *occupation,* Kielhofner opened up the multitude of possibilities inherent in human behavior.

Kielhofner (1995) began his model by developing historical perspectives on human behavior within the context of *systems theory,* a holistic approach to examining the range of human potential. From this viewpoint, he posited that human beings are an example of an *open system,* that is, that human activity involves taking in information (or input), synthesizing the information, and then creating output. The important quality of an open system, he argued, is the opportunity for *feedback,* responses to the output that allow the person to make changes and, with the same input, create a different output.

Kielhofner and Burke (1980) saw several components and determinants within the person that affect human behavior. These included volition, habituation, and performance. *Volition* refers to the impulses that cause the person to value certain types of occupation, including personal causation (i.e., the knowledge of self), *values* (i.e., images of what is good, right, or important), and *interests* (i.e., the disposition to find particular occupations pleasurable). *Habituation,* in turn, refers to the normative definitions the person places on occupation, encompassing roles (i.e., publicly recognized positions, or society's input) and habits (i.e., the private regulation of behavior). *Performance* deals with the person's skills in performing occupations, containing communication, process, and perceptual–motor skills (Kielhofner, 1995).

After laying down the internal structures that make up individual behavior, Kielhofner (1985) then dealt with the external aspects of human occupation, including determining whether the person is functional or dysfunctional and thus in need of therapeutic intervention. Just as function in his view had three levels—exploration, competence, and achievement—Kielhofner (1985) saw dysfunction as having three corresponding levels—inefficiency, incompetence, and helplessness. He emphasized that both function and dysfunction should be seen as processes, not static states. For *occupational dysfunction* to exist, Kielhofner explained, the person in his or her social group does not meet expectations for productive and playful participation. Moreover, the person "does not fulfill the urge to explore and master" (Kielhofner, 1985, p. 64) his or her environment.

Using this model, Kielhofner (1992, 2009) developed ideas about the optimal use of therapy in treating dysfunction and worked to fit the model into larger contexts such as the conceptual foundations of occupational therapy. Indeed, the model was initiated with the specific goal of developing resources to guide and enhance practice (Forsyth & Kielhofner, 2003), and Kielhofner's later collaborations focused on the model's application to practice. He and his colleagues developed and tested many assessments (Model of Human Occupation Clearinghouse, 2013) that are currently widely used around the world.

Kielhofner did not engage in the debate regarding terms such as *activity* or *occupation*—he ignored it altogether. He used occupation as his central concept in developing theories regarding occupational therapy, but more fundamentally, he believed that the person's role in the complex process of human occupation defined what people and (following Kielhofner's model) practitioners do to improve human function. Similarly, in Kielhofner's (2008) last update to the model, he pointed out that the MoHO has always been a client-centered approach to occupational therapy. Kielhofner's detailed model, with its emphasis on human behavior, remains a key step toward establishing a psychological framework for the human need for occupation in daily life.

Occupational Science: University of Southern California's Department of Occupational Science and Occupational Therapy

Occupational science is the study of occupation and its role in human experience. Developed at the University of Southern California, occupational science seeks to broaden theories of occupation beyond the notion of therapeutic intervention. By examining all forms of occupation in various contexts, the discipline of occupational science offers new and complex insights into many aspects of the human experience. Not all of these insights necessarily apply directly to occupational therapy practice (e.g., work related to anthropology), but the emphasis on scientific method and considering insights from outside of the therapeutic setting in practice have given occupational science a key role in developing new ideas and concepts at a macro level.

Florence Clark (Figure 2.3) and colleagues (1991) defined *occupation* as "chunks of culturally and personally meaningful activity in which humans engage that can be named in the lexicon of culture"

Figure 2.3. Florence Clark.

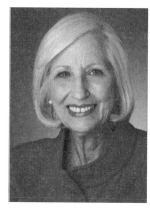

Source. F. Clark. Used with permission.

(p. 301). The study of occupation is grounded in a model of human subsystems that influences occupation. Similar to Kielhofner's and Burke's (1980) MoHO, it is based on an open systems model that includes feedback, which allows the person to make changes in occupational behavior.

Because of the focus on generalized concepts of occupation and not on specific uses of purposeful activities in therapeutic settings, occupational science writings can deal with the theoretical issues developed here often in ways tangential to larger questions. Interest in occupational science as a field of study related to occupational therapy has continued to grow, leading to additional graduate programs around the world, a scholarly journal, and many meetings to share new work. These works range from broad studies of occupations in different societies to looking at occupational roles and their therapeutic benefit.

Over time, occupational science has begun to fit more comfortably in the overall schematic of ideas around occupation, activity, and therapeutic intervention. In a sense, whereas many of those examining the field of occupational therapy have moved from the specific to the general, occupational science works from the outside in. It develops a generalized understanding of occupation in many aspects of society and culture and then works back to how using specific activities in specific settings can achieve certain societal outcomes or therapeutic goals. In this way, occupation can be seen more broadly than as just the use of therapeutic intervention in a rehabilitation setting. For instance, occupation and activity can be used in multiple settings, in a variety of ways, to reach more generalized goals, broadening the field and our understanding of occupation and activity in many aspects of life.

Purposeful activities are embedded within the occupational science definition of *occupation*. A person's participation in meaningful and socially valued activities is emphasized as the core of occupational therapy's moral philosophy (Zemke & Clark, 1996). This belief is generated from the fact that occupational therapy practitioners focus on the everyday things that people need to do. Some have felt the need to immerse themselves in the study of these occupations of daily living in which people engage during their lifetime. Henderson (1996) stated that confusion exists between the terms *occu-*

pation and *purposeful activity* because the vocabulary of occupational science has not been agreed on and the terms are used interchangeably. Similarly to Clark et al. (1991), Henderson described *occupation* as being chunks or units of culturally and personally meaningful activity within the stream of human behavior, with each level of occupation further subdivided into smaller units. Henderson believed that *occupation* and *purposeful activity* are equated in the field of occupational therapy; therefore, practitioners must seek to further understand their interrelationships to distinguish the levels of occupations in which people engage.

Purposeful activity is defined in relation to particular activities and accepted with the notion that adaptations can occur in people's activities. Humans have a self-reinforcing power to challenge themselves in an array of adaptive strategies to improve quality of life. This power is most relevant after a disability, when adaptation is required for people to again participate in occupations in which they previously engaged (Frank, 1996).

An important milestone for humans that is discussed in occupational science is play. *Play* has its importance in the ability to interact with our environment; children thus use it to cope with changes when they occur (Burke, 1996). Play is a purposeful vehicle for change, one that truly encompasses the traditional definition of *purposeful activity*. The literature on play and purposeful activity go hand in hand and are the root of much of what occupational therapy practitioners talk about in the therapeutic process. Play, as a purposeful activity, encompasses much of what occupational science is centered on. Play is an important occupation beginning in childhood and continuing throughout the lifespan. Through childhood play exploration, the child creates the act of doing in the activities that he or she carries out daily.

An example of how occupational science can play a wider role than simply therapeutic intervention, taking occupational therapy in new directions, is the development of a pilot study in California to see whether programs around occupation and activity can benefit a broad elderly population in a variety of settings (Clarke et al., 1997). A key aspect of the study was developing measurable criteria and a randomized approach that emphasized scientific, measurable data to evaluate effectiveness, providing concrete evidence of the use and value of a program of occupation and activity (Clark, Jackson, & Carlson, 2004).

Every aspect of occupational science, and all its areas of research, study, and theory, may not directly apply to the study and practice of occupational therapy. However, what once seemed a potential outlier has become an important generator of ideas that can grow and change the profession by looking at occupation and activity outside of the strictly therapeutic context and applying familiar concepts such as activity analysis to different populations and uses. In addition, the emphasis on scientific study and measurable results in occupational science offers a rigorous examination that adds to the bedrock of valuable information on how activity and occupation play a role in improved life outcomes. Understanding the concepts of occupational science can help broaden the thinking and understanding of practitioners, even for those focused intently on using activities primarily in therapeutic settings, by providing a greater and wider context.

Activities Health: Simme Cynkin

Simme Cynkin (1979; Cynkin & Robinson, 1990) provided perspective on the fundamental nature of activity as a therapeutic response to dysfunction. In this perspective, the fundamental value of activities to humans is the basis for occupational therapy. Activities are part of people's human existence, and Cynkin believed the very presence of activity in people's daily lives promotes their physical and mental well-being. This belief is discussed in four assumptions about activities:

1. Activities of many kinds are the essence of human existence, based on the interactions of the individual and the environment. Activities are centered on survival, subsistence, and coexistence.
2. Activities are a culmination of acceptable norms of behaviors that are defined by a sociocultural system of values and beliefs.
3. Acceptable and unacceptable variations exist in individual activities.
4. Engaging in meaningful activities leads to a satisfying way of life and personal fulfillment. (Cynkin, 1979; Cynkin & Robinson, 1990).

Cynkin and Robinson's (1990) assumptions are derived from a historical perspective: Activity has always defined human existence, and activities are basic to human survival. Drawing on the works of Jean Piaget and Mary Reilly, Cynkin and Robinson centralized human nature and a person's humanity around the performance of a variety of activities, both personal and interpersonal. To this foundation, they added the notion of differing sociocultural norms and differing values placed by various societies on particular activities.

Building on the notion that people can change, Cynkin and Robinson (1990) further argued that behavior related to activity can be changed and that behavioral changes can improve the person's functioning. Moreover, the person can learn to improve function, and this learning process can take place in a variety of ways, both direct and indirect.

The importance of these assumptions, and the framework Cynkin and Robinson (1990) developed from them, laid the foundation for the teaching of ideas behind occupational therapy. "Early occupational therapy was founded on the belief that being engaged in activities promotes mental and physical well-being and that, conversely, absence of activity leads . . . at worst to deterioration or loss of mental and physical functioning" (Cynkin & Robinson, 1990, p. 4). Although theorists such as Fidler (1948) had developed ways of analyzing activity, Cynkin (1979) provided an important additional link: that placing activity in a context of overall human behavior provides greater understanding of its therapeutic importance. Cynkin offered the strongest method possible to give the occupational therapy student not just the tools to assist in restoring function but also the philosophical structure that underlies the importance of activity in everyday life.

Person–Environment–Occupation Model: Mary Law

In conjunction with a variety of different collaborators, Mary Law (Figure 2.4) has focused on the relationship between the practitioner and the person receiving services, or client, to develop a client-centered approach to occupational therapy. In developing this approach, Law (1998) and her Canadian colleagues have continued to refine the theories developed in the *PEO model,* which

Figure 2.4. Mary Law.

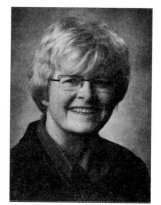

Source. M. Law. Used with permission.

defines the interrelationship of the person to his or her environment and both of these elements to the role of occupation. In defining each element, Law et al. (1994) differentiated among *activity, task,* and *occupation* as follows:

- *Activity* is the basic unit of a task. It is defined as a singular pursuit in which a person engages as part of his or her daily occupational experience. An example of an activity is the act of writing.
- *Task* is defined as a set of purposeful activities in which a person engages. An example of a task is the obligation to write a report.
- *Occupation* is defined as groups of activities in which a person engages over the life span. *Occupations* are defined as those clusters of activities and tasks in which the person engages to meet his or her intrinsic needs for self-maintenance, expression, and fulfillment. These are carried out within the context of individual roles and multiple environments.

Using the PEO model, Law and her team have looked across the literature to validate their approach (Peachey-Hill & Law, 2000) and worked to turn the model into a practical application for occupational therapy (Strong et al., 1999). In its application, this model becomes a way for the occupational therapy practitioner to take into account the multiplicity of factors affecting the client's performance, and a treatment plan is developed that takes into account not only the impact of different activities on the person but also how those activities are appropriate for the environment in which the person will make use of them.

All of this work is informed by the client-centered approach that Law and her team have developed alongside the model. This approach to occupational therapy brings together several strands of observation and research from occupational therapy and other disciplines. For example, Law and Mills (1998) cited the work of psychologist Carl Rogers (1951) as an early basis for the client-centered approach. Rogers emphasized the need for therapists to work with clients in developing solutions to problems rather than direct the course of therapy. Law and Mills (1998) also took into account the views of people with disabilities and their feelings about treatment.

The client-centered approach was developed in Canada as a series of guidelines for practice produced by the Canadian Association of Occupational Therapists (1991). Law et al. (1994) designed the *Canadian Occupational Performance Measure,* an assessment tool that measures "a client's self-perception of occupational performance" (p. 191). Although Law et al. subsequently referred to the pilot testing as covering a broad spectrum of clients and environments, the participants were mostly people older than age 60 years residing in inpatient geriatric facilities. Thus, this group of participants may have been better able to use the client-centered approach to assess their own conditions and treatment needs than a population less able to indicate self-awareness or occupational needs, such as children with developmental disabilities.

In fact, contributors to *Client-Centered Occupational Therapy* (Law, 1998) discussed in several chapters the various ways of interpreting the term *client.* The client comes to be seen as not only the person receiving therapy but also "someone who wishes to make a change through the process of therapy" (Pollock & McColl, 1998, p. 91), that is, possibly the caregiver or parent. A frequent example used in the works of these authors and Law is that of the patient with Alzheimer's disease who may be unable to communicate his or her needs. In this case, the client is considered to be the caregiving spouse (and the term *spouse* is the one most often used in this example), and as in the client-centered approach, the caregiver's role is what changes.

In the client-centered approach, then, the client defines the activity and occupation that provide therapeutic benefit, and the client's needs are foremost in the development of interventions created in partnership between the client and the practitioner. This approach may seem somewhat reflexive because an assessment model would seem to always require that the client's needs be part of the determination of appropriate therapy. What is important to Law and her colleagues, however, is that the assessment comes from the client and the value of the therapy is always best evaluated by the client; the practitioner serves as a facilitator who aids the client in identifying areas of concern and assists in developing a plan to address those areas (and, in theory, those areas alone).

One of the central concepts of client-centered practice is that occupational therapy service delivery is flexible and individualized, and the very flexibility and mutability of using occupation and activity make it difficult to determine a specific approach to using occupation as a means of therapy in the client-centered practice. Law and Mills (1998) acknowledged the lack of specific methodologies in client-centered therapy.

The focus of client-centered occupational therapy is on changing the overall approach to therapy from that of the medical model. In the medical model, practitioners are perceived as all-knowing and treatment is evaluated on generalized goals such as "independence at all costs" (Law, 1998, p. 71; see also Baum & Law, 1997). In the client-centered approach, the focus is on the client's finding meaning in everyday occupations and the development of active collaboration between the occupational therapy practitioner and client to resolve occupational performance problems (Baum & Law, 1997). Specific assessments and treatment plans are not spelled out because the client-centered approach makes those determinations part of the larger client–practitioner process of developing a relationship. As with Fidler (1996), the approach makes scientific and comparative evaluation of treatment methods challenging but refocuses the role of therapy on the benefits to the person.

Since the last edition of this book, Mary Law has begun collaborating with Winnie Dunn (see the section, "Ecology of Human Performance: Winnie Dunn") and Carolyn Baum (see next section) on ways to improve outcomes measurement when studying therapeutic interventions and effectiveness (Law, Baum, & Dunn, 2005). As Law et al. explained in the first chapter of *Measuring Occupational Performance: Supporting Best Practice in Occupational Therapy,*

The health system focuses on outcomes because of the need to be accountable, not only to the clients in need of services, but also to the government and/or the third party who is paying the bill. With a shift in focus toward primary and secondary prevention, it is also important to know if interventions are successful in reducing the impact of secondary problems. Medical outcomes are being defined as well-being and quality of life; improved occupational performance is a critical construct in measuring quality of life regardless of the measure that is used. (p. 10)

Law et al. (2005) went on to discuss the different frameworks—such as Ecology of Human Performance (EHP; Dunn, Brown, & McGuigan, 1994) and the MoHO—and the different measurement issues of each in an attempt to develop good measurement processes for research and to allow practitioners to develop a standard of comparison across frameworks. This perspective reflects a growing sense in U.S. health care that *comparative effectiveness*—the ability to evaluate different treatment options on the basis of the best outcomes for the client—is a key piece of improving health care delivery. Although this work is still in its early stages, developing good measurement tools and focusing on outcomes (as in occupational science, discussed previously) in a client-centered approach to care are key steps toward taking theories of practice into real-life, practical settings, identifying what works and what works well in improving occupational performance.

Occupation: Charles Christiansen and Carolyn Baum

The Canadian models also informed Charles Christiansen's (Figure 2.5) and Carolyn Baum's (Figure 2.6) attempts to bring together differing theories of activity and occupation to lay a theoretical framework for teaching practice. Although their organizing principle has shifted with each edition, Christiansen and Baum's texts have illustrated the evolving nature of how educators approach theoretical concepts in occupational therapy and the challenges in providing theoretical context to new students.

In *Occupational Therapy: Overcoming Human Performance Deficits*, Christiansen and Baum (1991)

Figure 2.5. Charles Christiansen.

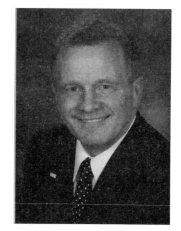

Source. C. Christiansen. Used with permission.

proposed an occupational performance hierarchy that centers on "*the activity,* which consists of specific goal-oriented behaviors . . . directed toward the performance of a task" (p. 28). The emphasis on activities as related to the performance of tasks creates the theoretical basis for occupational therapy as a way to treat dysfunction or disability. The work of previous authors serves in this context as a way to take ideas about activity and apply them to the practice of occupational therapy. By contrast, in *Occupational Therapy: Enabling Function and Well-Being,* Christiansen and Baum (1997) focused much more on the development of a definition of *occupation,* moving away from both activity and the notion of disability.

Revisions to the text allowed for the incorporation of newer ideas from different theorists but also underscored the difficulty of taking the differing approaches and blending them into a coherent whole. Like Kielhofner, Christiansen and Baum

Figure 2.6. Carolyn Baum.

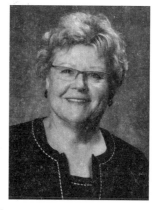

Source. C. Baum. Used with permission.

(1997) developed a model that is referred to at the start of each chapter, attempting to encompass all possible facets of human performance in an arrow-shaped form that points to well-being, and each chapter in the text is meant to present a part of this triangular model. Using the ideas developed by Law and colleagues (Gill & Brockett, 1987; Law, 1998; Law et al., 1994; Law & Mills, 1998), Christiansen and Baum (1997) emphasized the client-centered approach, with a resulting de-emphasis on specific practice solutions to problems and greater emphasis on the client's needs and perceptions. This de-emphasis on specific treatments for dysfunction also incorporated the occupational science focus on wellness and healthy occupational performance.

In *Occupational Therapy: Performance, Participation and Well-Being,* Christiansen, Baum, and Bass-Haugen (2005) moved toward an almost entirely theoretical approach to discussing occupational therapy. Occupational performance now sits at the center of a four-concentric-circle model balancing well-being and quality of life, and the book's essays generally cover different theoretical approaches to various aspects of the field. Although Law's PEO model was still central to the understanding of occupation, Christiansen et al. examined and discussed a wide range of theoretical concepts in detail, and even when discussing practical concepts, such as interventions, their greater focus was on rationale over specific applications.

Although the book is a fascinating compendium of deep thinking about the role of occupational therapy, whether its heavy emphasis on theory is ultimately beneficial to entry-level students remains to be seen. The ongoing evolution of the text, though, illustrates how a developing theoretical consensus continues to shape the way in which the field is taught.

Occupational Form and Occupational Performance: David Nelson

David Nelson was particularly interested in the term *occupation* and its meaning for occupational therapy practitioners. In his 1996 Eleanor Clarke Slagle Lecture, he related this interest to part of a historical tradition and set of beliefs of practitioners: "The human being can attain . . . health and quality of life by actively doing things that are personally meaningful and purposeful, in other words, through occupation" (Nelson, 1997, p. 11). His principal contribution to this perspective has been semantic and includes developing a nomenclature to delimit the use of the term *occupation* by practitioners. His terms apply to the therapeutic discipline of occupational therapy.

Nelson (1994) divided the term *occupation* into his terms for its essential aspects, occupational form and occupational performance. *Occupational form* has to do with the objects and circumstances that make the occupation possible. Forms can be a game, a building in which an occupation takes place, a piece of equipment, a piece of music, or another person, to name just a few. Forms are essential to the occupation.

Occupational performance, however, is what the person does to accomplish the occupation. Nelson (1994) stated that performance, in this sense, must be voluntary: "The 'doing' is the occupational performance, and the 'something' to be done is the occupational form" (p. 11). Occupational performance, then, is playing the game, constructing the building, lifting the weight for exercise, playing the music, or teaching something to the other person.

Nelson (1994) viewed occupation as the relationship between an occupational form and an occupational performance. Occupations may be as variable as the people who are performing them. If the occupation is eating a meal, the occupational forms, at a simple level, may be breakfast, lunch, or dinner. The occupational performances may be as divergent as a baby eating some oatmeal and "feeding" the rest to the high chair tray and the floor or a diet-conscious 20-year-old woman picking carefully at the low-fat foods on her plate. Some variables that come into play include duration, certainty of outcome, and intricacy.

According to Nelson (1994), the term *occupational form* has a physical dimension and a sociocultural dimension. The *physical dimension* is measurable and includes objects, other physical characteristics of the occupation, and the temporal aspects of the occupation. The *sociocultural dimension* includes social and cultural practices, expectations, and settings. For example, for the occupation of playing music, a contemporary, atonal classical piece may be played on an electronic keyboard in a museum in Bucharest, Romania, which might define the piece's sociocultural dimension.

Nelson and Jepson-Thomas (2003) divided the sociocultural dimension into symbols, norms, roles, variations, and language. Therefore, for the person playing the keyboard in the previous example, some of the symbols are the notes on the musical score; a norm might be the loudness or softness of the sound; the pianist is enacting a role; variations in tempo or improvisations may also be present. The language, perhaps Romanian, may not be as relevant as the musical sounds. Change and social hierarchies have also been incorporated into the system (Nelson & Jepson-Thomas, 2003). Occupational form, as Nelson and Jepson-Thomas described it, is a very complex entity.

The person brings all of his or her abilities and characteristics to occupational performance (Nelson & Jepson-Thomas, 2003). Terms used by occupational therapy practitioners (e.g., *sensorimotor, cognitive, psychosocial*) describe the developmental structure. Meaning is also brought to the occupation by the person performing it. If the pianist in the previous musical example disliked atonal music, his concert might be very different from one for which he had selected his favorite piece.

Any given occupation may have more than one purpose. Not only may a given person have more than one purpose for performing an occupation, but also others may each have different purposes for performing the same occupation. Participating or engaging in an activity solely for the pleasure of doing it, such as reading a novel for enjoyment, is *intrinsic motivation. Extrinsic motivation,* however, is a purpose found outside the occupation itself, for example, reading a textbook to pass an exam. Conscious and unconscious purposes also exist. According to Nelson (1994), a *conscious purpose* occurs when a person is aware of what he or she is doing and why, and an *unconscious purpose* is one involved with a habitual occupation that a person performs routinely with little thought.

One step of an occupation has an impact on those that follow (Nelson, 1994). For example, purchasing fabric and using a pattern to cut out a jacket are steps that have an effect on the actual construction of the jacket. Changes also occur in the person performing an occupation, which are *adaptations.* In addition, Nelson and Jepson-Thomas (2003) defined *activities* as the building blocks of adaptation. They designated these portions of occupations as suboccupations or even sub-suboccupations.

The occupational therapy practitioner and student must have a structure and process in which to perceive occupation to move onto therapeutic application. Nelson (1994) termed that process *occupational synthesis,* designating an occupational experience that will have therapeutic impact. The recipient of service is a collaborator in the therapeutic process. Nelson and Jepson-Thomas (2003) stated that occupational synthesis is the job of the occupational therapy practitioner.

Nelson (1994) deliberately avoided the word *activity.* In his view and in the view of others, this term is not specific enough because it is sometimes applied to other than human enterprises and because it is not always purposeful. He pointed out that terms such as *molecular activity* and *solar activity* (Nelson, 1994) clearly do not refer to human enterprises and that *activity* can refer to any kind of liveliness (see also Darnell & Heater, 1994). In a recent article (Bauerschmidt & Nelson, 2011), Nelson and his cowriter examined the history of the use of the terms *occupation* and *activity* in occupational therapy publications and found that each term has had periods of predominant use, with *occupation* having the most recent predominance. Nelson's emphasis on an accurate nomenclature for the profession helps continue the development of a common language for theorists to explore and debate ideas.

Ecology of Human Performance: Winnie Dunn

Drawing on the interest in developing a comprehensive framework, Winnie Dunn (Figure 2.7), along with Catana Brown and Ann McGuigan, constructed the *EHP* (Dunn et al., 1994). Similar to the PEO model, the central focus of this group from the University of Kansas is on the environment and how the person fits into it. Drawing on Mosey's (1981) notion of frame of reference and Nelson's (1994) occupational forms, the Kansas group developed a framework of context to explain the way in which a person and the tasks the person does fit into an environment. *Tasks* are defined as objective sets of behaviors necessary to accomplish a goal (Dunn, Brown, & Youngstrom, 2003; Dunn et al., 1994).

Drawing on the work of environmental psychologists, the EHP thus makes context the center of the therapeutic evaluation and intervention. In this way,

Figure 2.7. Winifred Dunn.

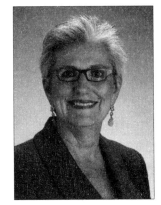

Source. W. Dunn. Used with permission.

it is similar to the notion of *lifestyle* advanced by Fidler (1996) and the holistic analysis envisioned in the *client-centered approach* (Law, 1998). A key difference, however, is the change in emphasis to the environment. As with Kielhofner (1985), Dunn and colleagues (1994, 2003) were less interested in defining *activity* vs. *occupation* and have instead focused more on the external framework into which the person and the therapeutic intervention fit in various situations.

Using the EHP framework, Dunn et al. (1994) then described five different potential relationships for therapeutic intervention as it relates to the person:

1. Therapeutic intervention can establish or restore (or remediate) the person's skills and abilities.
2. Intervention can also alter the context in which a person performs, selecting a context that enables him or her to perform with current skills and abilities.
3. The occupational therapy practitioner can also adapt the contextual features and task demands to design a more supportive context for a person's performance.
4. Intervention can prevent the occurrence or evolution of maladaptive performance in context.
5. The practitioner can create circumstances that promote more adaptable or complex performance in context.

Using these five therapeutic choices, the practitioner can evaluate the person in the appropriate context and design an intervention best suited to the person's needs within that context (Dunn et al., 1994).

By emphasizing the role of context and environment in making therapeutic assessments, the EHP

takes a different look at familiar concepts. In so doing, it exemplifies the value of synthesis within the profession, taking existing ideas and thinking about them in new and different ways. The EHP takes many things as given, such as the role of tasks in a person's life and the use of tasks to provide therapeutic benefit. These are ideas that other theorists continue to debate, but clearly the importance of making careful, individualized assessments has become a key part of the theoretical approach to practice, and the EHP offers yet another way to look at the environmental factors that can affect treatment. As mentioned before, Dunn has begun work with Mary Law and Carolyn Baum to develop an approach to measuring outcomes as a way to establish best practices in the field.

Occupational Adaptation: Janette Schkade and Sally Schultz

Synthesizing much of the work that came before them, Janette Schkade and Sally Schultz of Texas Woman's University developed the *Model of Occupational Adaptation (MOA)* as a holistic approach to contemporary practice (Schkade & Schultz, 1992). The MOA focuses on the interaction between the person and the occupational environment, which is the context in which occupations occur. *Occupations,* in their approach, are activities characterized by three properties: (1) active participation, (2) meaning to the person, and (3) a product that is the output of a process (Schkade & Schultz, 1992). In this model, the person's desire for mastery will cause him or her to develop an adaptive response to an occupational challenge. At the same time, a demand for mastery comes from within the occupational environment. In the interaction between the desire and the demand, the person will develop adaptive responses to gain mastery of the occupational challenge.

Schultz and Schkade (1992) then applied this model to occupational therapy practice. In practice, occupational adaptation is focused on *occupational function*—that is, the person's ability to function in the environment—rather than on the acquisition of particular functional skills. In practice, the occupational therapy practitioner works in a therapeutic climate with the patient to determine the goal of therapy. The practitioner then uses *occupational activities* (i.e., discrete activities that can promote occupational adaptation) and *occupational readiness* (i.e., skill-based activities and interventions to prepare for occupational activities, such as resistive exercise or use of assistive devices) to allow the client to develop relative mastery. In many cases, these activities are related to *occupations of daily living*, the unique patterns of occupations in which the person regularly engages.

In attempting to make the MOA universal, Schkade and Schultz (2003) synthesized many of the prior theoretical notions of activity and occupation to draw together a common perspective. The focus is on synthesizing ideas, not developing altogether new ones, and occupational adaptation as a theory adapts the material that has come before to develop a holistic methodology. Although Schkade and Schultz's focus on the adaptive process and the desire for mastery is differentiated from those of others, the notion of activity and occupation (and the client-centered approach) for therapeutic benefit fits comfortably into the theoretical underpinnings of the profession as it continues to develop. Schultz and others supporting this approach continue the work and related publications; Schkade passed away in 2008.

Theories of Learning: SCOPE–IT and CO–OP

Although it is possible to broaden definitions of *activity* and *occupation* to include almost all occupational therapy practice, the specific role of childhood development and the process of learning in children make for very specific differences in approach and treatment. Many of the theories discussed thus far focus primarily on adults, particularly older adults, but theories of occupation that deal with common adult tasks (e.g., activities of daily living, leisure, work) are not necessarily immediately applicable to children.

Two teams of international occupational therapy practitioners—one based in Canada and one in Australia—have begun to examine how theories of learning affect approaches to occupational therapy in children. Both teams have developed new, somewhat different frameworks for approaching childhood developmental issues, but they share a similar learning-based approach to activity and occupational therapy for children, examining how children learn and how the therapeutic experience can be a teaching and learning tool.

Jenny Ziviani, an associate professor at the University of Queensland (Brisbane, Australia), along with Sylvia Rodger, head of the Division of Occupational Therapy, has worked to develop a comprehensive view of childhood development and the role occupational therapy can play within it (Rodger & Ziviani, 2006). Developing comprehensive knowledge of children's activities demands that we reach beyond an understanding of the age appropriateness of a given object or activity. Likewise, understanding children's activity patterns requires more than decontextualized lists of children's daily activities and pie graphs of children's time use (Law, Petrenchik, Ziviani, & King, 2006). This view, then, is an adaptation of a client-centered approach, understanding that when a child is the primary recipient of therapeutic intervention, his or her needs are different from those of adults, and the role of parents and community may also be different.

More than with adults, the role of the occupational therapy practitioner with a child may be very similar to that of a teacher; thus, it becomes important to consider how children learn and what kind of strategies should be used to teach them skills. "Using appropriate instructional strategies may help overcome dependence on the part of the child, while also helping minimize the experience of failure" (Greber, Ziviani, & Rodger, 2007, p. 149). Out of these considerations of how children approach activity and occupation and how they learn, Anne Poulsen, along with Ziviani and others, developed *SCOPE–IT* (Synthesis of Child, Occupational Performance, and Environment in Time; Poulsen & Ziviani, 2004). In this model (which follows from notions developed by Kielhofner, 1992, 1995), environmental and temporal factors are examined to help identify strategies that will engage children in greater physical activity. Although SCOPE–IT, as such, is not a theory, its concerns with how to engage children in activity and strategies that acknowledge the role of both work and play serve as a natural development of the larger considerations about learning and childhood development that are under discussion.

Along with the Australians (Rodger & Ziviani, 2006), a group of Canadian occupational therapy practitioners based in Ontario have also been developing a theory of learning that serves as an approach to therapy with children. Led by educators at several universities, these practitioners draw on educational theories to provide context for approaches to therapy in children. The theories that provide guidance for a *cognitive,* or problem-solving, orientation arise from the fields of cognitive and educational psychology. In recent years, it has become evident that these theories are also entirely compatible with the evolution of theory that has taken place in the fields of motor learning and motor control (Missiuna, Mandich, Polatajko, & Malloy-Miller, 2001).

In Canada, concerns about developmental coordination disorder and approaches to childhood development have led to the development of the *CO–OP,* or the Cognitive Orientation to Daily Occupational Performance (Missiuna et al., 2001). The CO–OP is a practical model of a strategy for learning, especially around motor skills: "Through [a] process of guided discovery, the child, in collaboration with the therapist or adult, identifies specific strategies that facilitate performance of the task" (Taylor, Fayed, & Mandich, 2007, p. 125). Here again, the initial focus is on learning in children and how to break down and teach a task or skill, taking into account how children learn and the practitioner's role in facilitating learning of skills. And again, CO–OP is not a theoretical framework, but its practical approaches to teaching skills are grounded in notions of childhood development that serve as an important new theoretical framework.

In subsequent work, researchers have broadened the use of CO–OP across a variety of populations of both children and adults, particularly persons with nervous system disorders, such as brain injuries and stroke (Dawson et al., 2009; Skidmore et al., 2011). The study of CO–OP's use is focused on more than specific interventions or on just one aspect of treatment (for instance, physical vs. mental); rather, use of CO–OP focuses on strategies for encouraging learning and development, particularly making the client an active participant in the process (Hyland & Polatajko, 2012).

Occupation Analysis and the Synthesis of Ideas

Recently, a group of occupational therapy practitioners from Australia, led by Gjyn O'Toole, offered Occupation Analysis the framework as a way of examining occupations in a holistic way (Mackenzie & O'Toole, 2011). *Occupation Analysis framework* posits "six innate intrinsic elements and seven environmental contexts that influence performance of occupation" (Mackenzie & O'Toole, 2011, p. 3). It proposes to analyze occupation in a similar manner to activity analysis but viewing an activity as a component element of an occupation.

Like several approaches we have discussed, the Occupation Analysis framework attempts to be broadly inclusive in approaching the idea of occupation, and as with occupational science, tries to look at occupation beyond the notion of therapeutic intervention. It refers back to the basics of Fidler's ideas of analyzing activities to find their purpose and usefulness. Like Nelson, Occupation Analysis develops a practical nomenclature of terms. And, similar to Kielhofner, the overall goal is to develop a comprehensive model—or frame of reference, as Mosey suggests—of occupation that encompasses most every aspect of a person in society.

Because Occupation Analysis is so recent, it is probably too soon to fully evaluate its value and impact on the profession overall and to ascertain its full application as a tool for practitioners. However, the development of Occupation Analysis is itself a good summary of all that has come before and an indication of where things stand on a theoretical level within occupational therapy. It synthesizes several different ideas and approaches and attempts to be broadly comprehensive in examining the human experience and endeavor, with an eye toward understanding occupation and activity in more than just the therapeutic context.

Considering Perspectives

Since we first began examining perspectives on the nature and role of purposeful activities for the first edition of this book, we have tried to develop a similar comprehensive understanding of the theoretical underpinnings of the nature of occupation from a surveying vantage point. Here, we have aimed to lay the groundwork of important concepts as they have developed over time and taken note of new theories, while trying to tease out common ideas, approaches, and questions for further thought. A single complete, comprehensive definition of the whole of human occupation may be more than any theorist can encompass, but ideas about the nature of activity and occupation, and the ways in which activities can be used for therapeutic benefit, are grounded in the concepts developed over time by the key theorists we have included in this chapter. It is just as important, we believe, to see how these ideas and concepts can be translated into practical use for human benefit.

Some concepts that have been raised are a running thread through the works of theorists whose conclusions can vary widely from one another. Clearly, theorists have evolved a more personal, individualized approach to therapeutic intervention, one that in many cases may be hard to quantify but nevertheless makes paramount the person receiving treatment, respect for the person's environment, and treating the person with dignity. Although the nomenclature may differ, the role of purposeful activities—be they activities, tasks, or occupations—in therapeutic interventions remains a central focus of the theoretical writings.

At the same time, important unique ideas set these theorists apart from one another. For the practitioner, one strategy for processing and incorporating the work of various theorists is to study more than one but find one who best matches the area of practice in which the practitioner will focus. Reilly's focus on pediatrics, Law's focus on gerontology, and Kielhofner's focus on mental health all offer ways to use theoretical concepts in specific areas of practice. We think that Fidler, in defining ways to think about activity; Nelson, in deriving a nomenclature; and Cynkin, in developing a notion of how to teach activity theory, stand as important guides to how theorists in occupational therapy approach writing and thinking about these issues. It is also clear that occupational science brings in important concepts about establishing research that can show measurable results and broadens the idea of how occupation and purposeful activity can be of benefit to a variety of populations.

Summary

The terms presented here, and the ways in which they are defined, deal with important theoretical issues, but the questions raised are provocative and open to debate. One of the most central is, Who is defining these concepts? Others include, Who determines what is a meaningful outcome? What constitutes a purposeful activity? Whose purpose should it serve? How broadly do concepts like occupation need to be defined?

Most important, occupational therapy continues to grow and evolve, bringing out new ideas in a rapidly changing field. Although room exists for a variety of perspectives, it is necessary to constantly reexamine established thought in the face of newly developed concepts and theories. In dealing with the complexities of human occupation and purposeful activities, occupational therapy takes on tremendous challenges and offers substantial rewards. The search for understanding the role of occupation and purposeful activities in human existence is ongoing.

References

American Occupational Therapy Association. (2012). Physical agent modalities: A position paper. *American Journal of Occupational Therapy, 66*(Suppl.), S78–S80. http://dx.doi.org/10.5014.ajot.2012.66S78

Bauerschmidt, B., & Nelson, D. L. (2011). The terms *occupation* and *activity* over the history of official occupational therapy publications. *American Journal of Occupational Therapy, 65,* 338–344. http://dx.doi.org/10.5014/ajot.2011.000869

Baum, C., & Law, M. (1997). Occupational therapy practice: Focusing on occupational performance. *American Journal of Occupational Therapy, 51,* 277–288. http://dx.doi.org/10.5014/ajot.51.4.277

Burke, J. (1996). Variations in childhood: Play in the presence of chronic disability. In R. Zemke & F. Clark (Eds.), *Occupational science: The evolving discipline* (pp. 413–418). Philadelphia: F. A. Davis.

Canadian Association of Occupational Therapists. (1991). *Occupational therapy guidelines for client-centered practice.* Toronto, ON: CAOT Publications ACE.

Christiansen, C., & Baum, C. (Eds.). (1991). *Occupational therapy: Overcoming human performance deficits.* Thorofare, NJ: Slack.

Christiansen, C., & Baum, C. (Eds.). (1997). *Occupational therapy: Enabling function and well-being* (2nd ed.). Thorofare, NJ: Slack.

Christiansen, C., Baum, C. M., & Bass-Haugen, J. (2005). *Occupational therapy: Performance, participation, and well-being* (3rd ed.). Thorofare, NJ: Slack.

Clark, F., Azen, S. P., Zemke, R., Jackson, J., Carlson, M., Mandel, D., . . . Lipson, L. (1997). Occupational therapy for independent-living older adults: A randomized, controlled trial. *JAMA, 278,* 1321–1326. http://dx.doi.org/10.1001/jama.1997.03550160041036

Clark, F., Jackson, J., & Carlson, M. (2004). Occupational science, occupational therapy and evidence-based practice: What the Well Elderly Study has taught us. In M. Molineux (Ed.), *Occupation for occupational therapists* (pp. 200–218). Oxford, England: Blackwell.

Clark, F., Parham, D., Carlson, M., Frank, G., Jackson, J., Pierce, D., . . . Zemke, R. (1991). Occupational science: Academic innovation in the service of occupational therapy's future. *American Journal of Occupational Therapy, 45,* 300–310. http://dx.doi.org/10.5014/ajot.45.4.300

Cynkin, S. (1979). *Occupational therapy: Toward health through activities.* Boston: Little, Brown.

Cynkin, S., & Robinson, A. (1990). *Occupational therapy and activities health: Toward health through activities.* Boston: Little, Brown.

Darnell, J. L., & Heater, S. L. (1994). Occupational therapist or activity therapist—Which do you choose to be? *American Journal of Occupational Therapy, 48,* 467–468. http://dx.doi.org/10.5014/ajot.48.5.467

Dawson, D., Gaya, A., Hunt, A., Levine, B., Lemsky, C., & Polatajko, H. (2009). Using the Cognitive Orientation to Occupational Performance (CO–OP) with adults with executive dysfunction following traumatic brain injury. *Canadian Journal of Occupational Therapy, 76,* 115–128. http://dx.doi.org/10.1177/000841740907600209

Dunn, W., Brown, C., & McGuigan, A. (1994). The Ecology of Human Performance: A framework for considering the effect of context. *American Journal of Occupational Therapy, 48,* 595–607. http://dx.doi.org/10.5014/ajot.48.7.595

Dunn, W., Brown, C., & Youngstrom, M. J. (2003). Ecological model of occupation. In P. Kramer, J. Hinojosa, & C. B. Royeen (Eds.), *Perspectives in human occupation: Participation in life* (pp. 222–263). Philadelphia: Lippincott Williams & Wilkins.

Fidler, G. S. (1948). Psychological evaluation of occupational therapy activities. *American Journal of Occupational Therapy, 2,* 284–287.

Fidler, G. S. (1969). The task-oriented group as a context for treatment. *American Journal of Occupational Therapy, 23,* 43–48.

Fidler, G. S. (1981). From crafts to competence. *American Journal of Occupational Therapy, 35,* 567–573. http://dx.doi.org/10.5014/ajot.35.9.567

Fidler, G. S. (1996). Lifestyle performance: From profile to conceptual model. *American Journal of Occupational Therapy, 50,* 139–147. http://dx.doi.org/10.5014/ajot.50.2.139

Fidler, G. S., & Fidler, J. W. (1954). *Introduction to psychiatric occupational therapy.* New York: Macmillan.

Fidler, G. S., & Fidler, J. W. (1978). Doing and becoming: Purposeful action and self-actualization. *American Journal of Occupational Therapy, 32,* 305–310.

Fidler, G. S., & Velde, B. (1999). *Activities: Reality and symbol.* Thorofare, NJ: Slack.

Forsyth, K., & Kielhofner, G. (2003). Model of Human Occupation. In P. Kramer, J. Hinojosa, & C. B. Royeen (Eds.), *Perspectives in human occupation: Participation in life* (pp. 45–86). Philadelphia: Lippincott Williams & Wilkins.

Frank, G. (1996). The concept of adaptation as a foundation for occupational science research. In R. Zemke & F. Clark (Eds.), *Occupational science: The evolving discipline* (pp. 47–55). Philadelphia: F. A. Davis.

Gill, T., & Brockett, M. (1987). The guidelines for the client-centered practice of occupational therapy: The basis for practice in Canada. *Canadian Journal of Occupational Therapy, 54*(2), 53–54.

Gillette, N. P. (2005). A tribute to Gail S. Fidler, our esteemed mentor. *American Journal of Occupational Therapy, 59,* 609–610. http://dx.doi.org/10.5014/ajot.59.6.609

Greber, C., Ziviani, J., & Rodger, S. (2007). The four quadrant model of facilitated learning: A clinically based action research project. *Australian Occupational Therapy Journal, 54,* 149–152. http://dx.doi.org/10.1111/j.1440-1630.2006.00558.x

Henderson, A. (1996). The scope of occupational science. In R. Zemke & F. Clark (Eds.), *Occupational science: The evolving discipline* (pp. 419–424). Philadelphia: F. A. Davis.

Hyland, M., & Polatajko, H. (2012). Enabling children with developmental coordination disorder to self-regulate through the use of dynamic performance analysis: Evidence from the CO–OP approach. *Human Movement Science, 31,* 987–998. http://dx.doi.org/10.1016/j.humov.2011.09.003

Kielhofner, G. (Ed.). (1985). *A Model of Human Occupation: Theory and application.* Baltimore: Lippincott Williams & Wilkins.

Kielhofner, G. (1992). *Conceptual foundations of occupational therapy.* Philadelphia: F. A. Davis.

Kielhofner, G. (Ed.). (1995). *A Model of Human Occupation: Theory and application* (2nd ed.). Baltimore: Lippincott Williams & Wilkins.

Kielhofner, G. (Ed.). (2008). *A Model of Human Occupation: Theory and application* (4th ed.). Baltimore: Lippincott Williams & Wilkins.

Kielhofner, G. (2009). *Conceptual foundations of occupational therapy practice* (4th ed.). Philadelphia: F. A. Davis.

Kielhofner, G., & Burke, J. (1980). A Model of Human Occupation, Part one: Conceptual framework and content. *American Journal of Occupational Therapy, 34,* 572–581. http://dx.doi.org/10.5014/ajot.34.9.572

Law, M. (Ed.). (1998). *Client-centered occupational therapy.* Thorofare, NJ: Slack.

Law, M., Baptiste, S., Carswell, A., McColl, M. A., Polatajko, H., & Pollock, N. (1994). *Canadian Occupational Performance Measure* (2nd ed.). Toronto: Canadian Association of Occupational Therapists.

Law, M., Baum, C., & Dunn, W. (2005). *Measuring occupational performance: Supporting best practice in occupational therapy.* Thorofare, NJ: Slack.

Law, M., & Mills, J. (1998). Client-centered occupational therapy. In M. Law (Ed.), *Client-centered occupational therapy* (pp. 1–18). Thorofare, NJ: Slack.

Law, M., Petrenchik, T., Ziviani, J., & King, G. (2006). Participation of children in school and community. In S. Rodger & J. Ziviani (Eds.), *Occupational therapy with children* (pp. 67–90). Oxford, England: Blackwell.

Mackenzie, L., & O'Toole, G. (Eds.). (2011). *Occupation analysis in practice.* Oxford, UK: Blackwell.

Missiuna, C., Mandich, A. D., Polatajko, H. J., & Malloy-Miller, T. (2001). Cognitive Orientation to Daily Occupational Performance (CO–OP): Part I—Theoretical foundations. In C. Missiuna (Ed.), *Children with developmental coordination disorder: Strategies for success* (pp. 69–81). New York: Haworth.

Model of Human Occupation Clearinghouse. (2013). Department of Occupational Therapy, College of Applied Health Sciences, University of Illinois at Chicago. Retrieved from www.uic.edu/depts/moho/images/

Mosey, A. C. (1968). Recapitulation of ontogenesis: A theory for practice of occupational therapy. *American Journal of Occupational Therapy, 22,* 426–432.

Mosey, A. C. (1973). *Activities therapy.* New York: Raven Press.

Mosey, A. C. (1981). *Occupational therapy: Configuration of a profession.* New York: Raven Press.

Mosey, A. C. (1986). *Psychosocial components of occupational therapy.* New York: Raven Press.

Mosey, A. C. (1996). *Applied scientific inquiry in the health professions: An epistemological orientation* (2nd ed.). Bethesda, MD: American Occupational Therapy Association.

Nelson, D. L. (1994). Form and function. In C. B. Royeen (Ed.), *The practice of the future: Putting occupation back into therapy* (AOTA Self-Study Series Lesson 2). Bethesda, MD: American Occupational Therapy Association.

Nelson, D. L. (1997). Why the profession of occupational therapy will flourish in the century [1996 Eleanor Clarke Slagle Lecture]. *American Journal of Occupational Therapy, 51,* 11–24. http://dx.doi.org/10.5014/ajot.51.1.11

Nelson, D. L., & Jepson-Thomas, J. (2003). Occupational form, occupational performance, and a conceptual framework for therapeutic occupation. In P. Kramer, J. Hinojosa, & C. B. Royeen (Eds.), *Perspectives in human occupation: Participation in life* (pp. 87–155). Philadelphia: Lippincott Williams & Wilkins.

Peachey-Hill, C., & Law, M. (2000). Impact of environmental sensitivity on occupational performance. *Canadian Journal of Occupational Therapy–Revue Canadienne d'Ergotherapie, 67*(5), 304–313. http://dx.doi.org/10.1177/000841740006700503

Pollock, N., & McColl, M. (1998). Assessment in client-centered occupational therapy. In M. Law (Ed.), *Client-centered occupational therapy* (pp. 89–106). Thorofare, NJ: Slack.

Poulsen, A. A., & Ziviani, J. M. (2004). Health enhancing physical activity: Factors influencing engagement patterns in children. *Australian Occupational Therapy Journal, 51,* 69–79. http://dx.doi.org/10.1046/j.1440-1630.2004.00420.x

Reilly, M. (1960). Research potentiality of occupational therapy. *American Journal of Occupational Therapy, 14,* 206–209.

Reilly, M. (1962). Occupational therapy can be one of the great ideas of 20th century medicine. *American Journal of Occupational Therapy, 16,* 1–9.

Reilly, M. (1966). A psychiatric occupational therapy program as a teaching model. *American Journal of Occupational Therapy, 22,* 61–67.

Reilly, M. (Ed.). (1974). *Play as exploratory learning.* Beverly Hills, CA: Sage.

Rodger, S., & Ziviani, J. (Eds.). (2006). *Occupational therapy with children: Understanding children's occupations and enabling participation.* Oxford, England: Blackwell.

Rogers, C. R. (1951). *Client-centered therapy: Its current practice, implications and theory.* Boston: Houghton Mifflin.

Schkade, J. K., & Schultz, S. (1992). Occupational adaptation: Toward a holistic approach to contemporary practice, Part 1. *American Journal of Occupational Therapy, 46,* 829–837. http://dx.doi.org/10.5014/ajot.46.9.829

Schkade, J. K., & Schultz, S. (2003). Occupational adaptation. In P. Kramer, J. Hinojosa, & C. B. Royeen (Eds.), *Perspectives in human occupation: Participation in life* (pp. 181–221). Philadelphia: Lippincott Williams & Wilkins.

Schultz, S., & Schkade, J. K. (1992). Occupational adaptation: Toward a holistic approach to contemporary practice, part 2. *American Journal of Occupational Therapy, 46,* 917–926. http://dx.doi.org/10.5014/ajot.46.10.917

Skidmore, E. R., Holm, M. B., Whyte, E. M., Dew, M. A., Dawson, D., & Becker, J. T. (2011). The feasibility of cognitive strategy training in acute inpatient stroke rehabilitation: Case report. *Neuropsychological Rehabilitation, 21,* 208–223. http://dx.doi.org/10.1080/09602011.2011.552559

Strong, S., Rigby, P., Stewart, D., Law, M., Letts, L., & Cooper, B. (1999). Application of the Person–Environment–Occupation Model: A practical tool. *Canadian Journal of Occupational Therapy–Revue Canadienne d'Ergotherapie, 66*(3), 122–133. http://dx.doi.org/10.1177/000841749906600304

Taylor, S., Fayed, N., & Mandich, A. (2007). CO–OP intervention for young children with developmental coordination disorder. *OTJR: Occupation, Participation and Health, 27,* 124–130.

Velde, B. P., & Fidler, G. S. (2002). *Lifestyle performance: A model for engaging the power of occupation.* Thorofare, NJ: Slack

Zemke, R., & Clark, F. (Eds.). (1996). *Occupational science: The evolving discipline.* Philadelphia: F. A. Davis.

CHAPTER 3.

DIMENSIONS OF OCCUPATIONS ACROSS THE LIFESPAN

Ruth Segal, PhD, OTR

Highlights

- ✧ Occupations across the lifespan
- ✧ Evolution of occupation
- ✧ Early childhood (birth to 7 years)
- ✧ Middle childhood (ages 7 to 11 years)
- ✧ Adolescence (ages 12 to 18 years)
- ✧ Adulthood (ages 18 to 65 years)
- ✧ Older adulthood (ages 66 years or older)
- ✧ Occupations that involve eating.

Key Terms

- ✧ Activity
- ✧ Activity of eating
- ✧ Anorexia nervosa
- ✧ Balanced reciprocity
- ✧ Behavior
- ✧ Bulimia nervosa
- ✧ ChooseMyPlate
- ✧ Clean
- ✧ Cognition
- ✧ Competitive food giving
- ✧ Cultism
- ✧ Etiquette

- ✧ Family constitution
- ✧ Generalized reciprocity
- ✧ Meaning
- ✧ Negative reciprocity
- ✧ Occupations
- ✧ Older adulthood
- ✧ Patterns of behavior
- ✧ Pollution
- ✧ Purity
- ✧ Social cognition
- ✧ Social construction of childhood

*O*ccupations are complex constructs that consist of highly personal yet socioculturally embedded meanings. In Chapter 1, "Occupation, Activities, and Occupational Therapy," Hinojosa and Blount defined *occupations* from the person's perspective, writing that "*occupations* are activities that are personally meaningful to the person who voluntarily engages in them out of personal choice or sociocultural necessity" (p. 3). Clark et al. (1991), however, defined occupations from a cultural perspective, as "chunks of activities that are culturally defined" (p. 301). Taken together, these definitions suggest that occupation lies in the transaction between the person and his or her contexts or environments. Thus, the same set of activities may constitute different occupations and have different meanings in different situations or contexts. Driving, for example, may be a vocation, a hobby, or a chore, depending on the situation and the meaning assigned to it by the person who engages in the driving.

The meanings that people assign to occupations occur within "temporal, psychological, social, symbolic, cultural, ethnic and/or spiritual contexts" (American Occupational Therapy Association, 1997, p. 865). *Meaning* is the sense in which something is understood. People personally assign meaning through subjective interpretation (Strauss & Quinn, 1997). Such interpretations are the subject of study of certain academic disciplines such as philosophy, psychology, sociology, and anthropology. None of these disciplines uses occupation as the concept guiding research in the way that occupational therapy does. Yet, in occupational therapy, no longitudinal studies have described how occupations evolve and develop across the lifespan. Hence, this chapter represents my attempt to understand the phenomenon of occupation across the lifespan from my point of view.

In developing and writing this chapter, I made the following five assumptions:

1. The most important aspect of occupation is the meaning attached to it.
2. Meaning is context dependent.

Exercise 3.1. Activities in Your Own Life

Think of a set of activities in your life, and identify how they may become different occupations when the context in which you perform them changes.

---

3. The contexts of human life from birth to death are unpredictable, but their number and variety increase from infancy to adulthood and often decline again with old age.
4. Chronic illness and disability often limit a person's life contexts.
5. Poverty limits life contexts.

Building on these assumptions, I consider the purposeful *activity of eating*—getting the nourishment needed for survival and health—and explore its transformation into various occupations in three trajectories: (1) from birth to death, (2) in health and illness, and (3) in affluence and poverty.

Occupations Across the Lifespan

The assumption that the evolution of meaning is context dependent and, therefore, each person's life, in its particular context, will influence but not determine the meaning of activities makes it impossible to identify a sequence of occupations that is typical across the lifespan. Indeed, I suggest that at the present state of knowledge, no typical sequence can be identified because social norms and cultural practices limit and afford a person participation in various contexts. These norms and practices are based on age, ethnic background, socioeconomic status, profession, and many other social determinants. Although general descriptions of the evolution of occupations and the socially sanctioned activities that are involved in early childhood, middle childhood, adolescence, adulthood, and older adulthood are given in this chapter, these descriptions are not complete because the range of activities within each age category is wide.

This chapter briefly outlines contexts or socially sanctioned activities within each age group and elaborates on the use of food in each category. As much as possible, I base these examples on research rather than products of my own construction. I base my discussion of the evolutionary process or development on texts on human development, focusing on its social and psychological aspects.

Evolution of Occupation

Occupations evolve and transform as a person develops and matures. For occupations to become part of one's repertoire or lifestyle, they must be assigned meanings and must be interpreted in a cultural context. This characterization of occupation implies that a child cannot have occupations until he or she can assign meaning to phenomena or activities. Kramer and Hinojosa (1995) described the early emergence of occupations:

> When children are born, they are purely reflexive beings. Their behavior is dominated by sensory responses to their feeling state and their environment, and occupation is not yet evident. However, as children begin to respond to and interact with people and objects within their environment, they begin to develop rudimentary patterns of behavior. Responses to specific people or stimuli become almost predictable, and they develop into patterns. These patterns involve a variety of actions that have meanings to the children; thus, the children are stimulated to engage in selected activities. For example, infants begin to recognize their parents very early. When a parent walks into the room, the infant follows the parent with his or her eyes and begins to wave his or her arms and legs. This indicates that the child expects there to be some inter-action. This initial attachment to the person or object is the first phase of object relations (Spitz, 1965).
>
> Often, the infant's responses take the form of motor actions. When repeated, these actions become *patterns of behavior.* In this sense, *behavior* is used to mean the emotional responses and reactions of the child. The infant first relates to people in the environment and then begins to react and respond to objects. These behaviors often become activities. *Activity* is used in this context to mean constructive action that enhances development and results in a productive outcome, such as when a child learns to reach out for his or her mother when she walks near the crib. The child's repertoire of behaviors and activities expands and forms a multitude of patterns. As these patterns of behaviors and specific activities are repeated over time, they develop more and more meaning to the child and become occupations. Thus, *occupations* are defined in this context as natural patterns of daily activity that are meaningful to the

individual. When observing infants, one can see a particular child enjoying play with a rattle, whereas another child may ignore the rattle and spend time with a busy box. Personal preference in activities is evident at a very early age, which can then give rise to varying occupational patterns. (pp. 6–8)

Kramer and Hinojosa's (1995) overview of the evolution of occupations reflects the typical way in which human development is described. In other words, the focus is on the increasing abilities and variety of activities and the different meanings assigned to similar activities (i.e., occupations ascribed to people). After the developmental stage described by Kramer and Hinojosa in the preceding quotation, a different aspect of development begins that is not commonly accounted for, namely, the development of the variety of meanings that each person attaches to similar activities. These meanings, as suggested by Kramer and Hinojosa (1995); Hinojosa and Blount in Chapter 1, "Occupation, Activities, and Occupational Therapy"; and Strauss and Quinn (1997), develop as children's social world enlarges and with it their participation and experiences.

As Kramer and Hinojosa (1995) suggested, occupations in general do not occur during infancy. The importance of food throughout infancy can be discussed only in terms of health and survival. Although attachment is an important aspect of infancy that has been connected with feeding, feeding too can be discussed in terms of survival rather than in terms of infant occupations, consistent with Lowenberg's (1970, as cited in Kittler & Sucher, 2001) application of Abraham Maslow's hierarchy of needs (Maslow, 1954) to food consumption. The most basic human need is the physical need for survival; infants' motivation to feed is their physical survival. Infants are measured, and these measurements are compared with established growth charts that indicate whether their growth is age appropriate and whether their ratio of length and weight is within normal limits. If either of these measurements is not within normal limits, medical intervention, or at least an investigation into the infant's health and well-being, is needed.

The introduction of eating as a social and cultural phenomenon is important. All humans consume some form of milk at the beginning of life, but by early childhood, the diets of humankind are very diverse (Rozin, 2006, 2007; Torres & Park, 2013), suggesting that food is a vehicle for many nonbiological functions and meanings. For example, food and eating can be viewed as a system of communication (Counihan & Van Esterik, 2013; Douglas, 1982). Meals can demonstrate differences in status, social groupings, and relationships. Food also has symbolic social and economic meanings. Furthermore, giving and receiving food allows people to correctly exercise their roles. For the young, meals are important socialization tools because they teach what is acceptable and unacceptable. Mealtimes are also good for developing self-image and social roles. For sociologists, what underlies food and meal preparation, cookery, and consumption holds the most value (Wood, 1995).

Exercise 3.2. Food

How is food in your life part of a system of communication? What social and economic symbolic meanings does food have for you?

Early Childhood (Birth to 7 Years)

During early childhood, when children are between birth and age 7 years, they learn basic life skills. Childhood is a socially constructed status (Lee, 2001). In other words, social and cultural values, beliefs, and traditions shape what are considered to be the appropriate social interactions for children, including with whom and while doing what. They have changed with history and still differ among cultures and societies and also within societies (Lee, 2001; Lemert, 2011; Wyness, 2012).

Childhood is the period of life in which children are prepared for adulthood by the adults in society. The *social construction of childhood* refers to the patterns of activities and participation that are open to children or in which their participation is required. These activities are constructed on the basis of current scientific knowledge about children's physical, cognitive, psychosocial, and emotional development and are dependent on traditions, beliefs and customs, social status, and ethnic background, to name a few factors. These factors are also time dependent, and they change over time with changes in scientific knowledge and in society (Lee, 2001).

Figure 3.1. Mother exposes her child to new foods and foods with different textures.

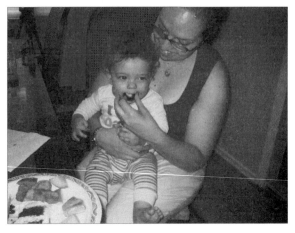

Source. M. Podvey. Used with permission.

The overall structure of childhood in the Western world is one of increasing exposure; as children progress through childhood, they are exposed to a greater variety of environments, activities, and occupations (Figure 3.1).

In early childhood, usually up to about age 7 years, children's cognitive, physical, emotional, and psychosocial needs are such that their social status does not include any major social responsibilities for others. During this period, however, their array of social interactions increases in variety, giving ample opportunities for the development of mapping in the brain. Children begin to interact more with other children and adults in a greater variety of contexts. Therefore, similar activities may be performed in a variety of social and cultural contexts and are thus constructed as different occupations. Participating in similar activities in different contexts evokes a variety of experiences that are connected with the occupations. For example, play can take the form of playing alone, with a caregiver, with siblings, with friends, at home, in the park, and at school. The variety of play situations and experiences creates connections in the brain that increase in their versatility and complexity. Participation in play allows children to develop preferences and assert choices.

During this period, children begin to eat in a variety of contexts and begin to differentiate between the different meanings of food and eating. For example, birthday parties are connected with certain foods such as birthday cake and party bags of sweets, which are generally considered unhealthy

Figure 3.2. Families with young children frequently dine in fast-food establishments.

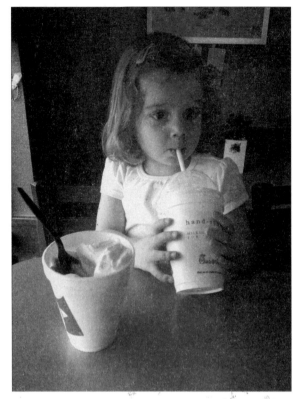

Source. A. Hofmann. Used with permission.

and would not be a part of the child's typical diet. Birthday parties also include savory food such as pizza or hot dogs. The context of eating at a birthday party includes singing a birthday song when the birthday cake is brought in with lighted candles on it and the particular types of room decorations.

Parents may take young children to restaurants that serve food appropriate for children (Babycenter, 2013). Around age 2 years, children become more involved in selecting or ordering food and table manners. These restaurants include self-service fast-food restaurants and full-service family restaurants (Figure 3.2). Going to school introduces another way of consuming food. School lunches are either brought from home or bought at school, and children socialize while eating their lunches. At this age, lunchtime is supervised closely by educators or other school employees.

During this phase of life, parents may provide a variety of food to promote consumption as a means of promoting and maintaining health. Further, children are exposed to foods from peers and preschool and school environments (Nicklaus, 2009).

The question of what constitutes *healthy food* is dependent on the dimensions of culture and time. Currently, in the United States, particular diets are commonly believed to lead to health and well-being. Therefore, the U.S. Department of Agriculture (n.d.) has released *ChooseMyPlate* (available at http://www.choosemyplate.gov/), which delineates the amount and type of foods that make up an individualized healthy diet. The information on this website is reported to be based on scientific data, although these data have been challenged (see Hess, Visschers, & Siegrist, 2012; Nestle, 2002; Nestle & Wilson, 2012) due to the influence of the U.S. food industry on the development of the diet. Such government initiatives are not unique to the United States and can be found in many Western countries.

Government policies and recommendations are an example of how social organizations affect individual food preferences and construct shared meanings. For example, consider the belief that fresh fruit and vegetables are good for one's health. Such a belief seems obvious to us, but it has not always been that way. In the Middle Ages, for example, cucumbers and melons were considered dangerous to human health (Albala, 2002).

Beliefs, Religion, and Culture

Another dimension of food and eating habits that begins in early childhood is the socialization of children into the eating habits identified with the family's particular beliefs, religion, and culture. Many food habits stem from religion; for example, religious groups may use food laws to differentiate themselves from others. These restrictions may come from holy books or from moral beliefs and attitudes. Additionally, some members of the religious group may follow relaxed food restrictions and some may follow stringent rules. For example, *cultism* describes eating patterns that seem bizarre under conventional wisdom. Cultist food practices satisfy followers' social and psychological needs but are often nutritionally deficient (Fieldhouse, 1986). The following sections summarize information about food and beliefs that Fieldhouse (1986) described in greater detail.

Prestige and status

Some foods confer high prestige and status on those who eat them; others imply prestige and status because of the human groups who usually eat them. The differences between the meals of medieval nobles and those of peasants symbolize the power that the nobles held over the food supply and, thus, over the peasants. Prestige can also be attached to the circumstances and ways in which food is served. Food can make social distinctions, overt or subtle, depending on the situation. For example, the Hindu caste system, which has strict rules regarding who can eat with whom, obviously outlines social distinctions.

Status through food behavior

Status through food behavior is conveyed in having the freedom to choose rare and costly items to impress others, select expensive restaurants for personal gratification, and prepare difficult and time-consuming dishes. To be denied any sort of choice in Western society is seen as negative. The ability to choose freely is tied to economic status, which is also tied to social status. When food choices are limited, people feel uncomfortable and are more likely to complain. Lack of choice also decreases self-esteem.

Exotic, complex, or expensive dishes convey a higher status. This higher status can derive from several factors, such as the location, the time or skill necessary to prepare the dishes, or the distance between the person who consumes the food and the person who prepares it. At dinner parties, the food served can be not only a sign of the host's status but also a sign of the status that the host ascribes to his or her guests.

Food and fashion

Fashion continually changes as people find current clothes trendy and stylish. Like fashion, food is associated with particular groups of people who enjoy high-status food. A food may have a high status only because high-status groups consume it. However, a food may have a high status but then become widely available to all classes, causing it to lose that status. Preferences for high-status food may develop without any regard to the food's actual taste. Humans are the only animal that will shun a nutritional food because of its lower status and replace it with a nutritionally mediocre one of higher status. The value of prestigious food lies in how much social recognition it will bring.

Status and food ownership

In some places in the world, food ownership brings some of the same prestige or status as food consumption. In some parts of Africa, for example, owning cattle conveys tremendous economic status; cows are kept as a sign of wealth and are rarely killed for food.

Food, friendship, and communication

Friendships and communication among friends offers centers around food oriented activities. The level of intimacy between people can often be gauged by the foods that they share. The act of eating together implies some degree of compatibility. Closeness may be acknowledged with elaborate food. In many places, it is common to keep some sort of food on hand for callers because to not offer food would be to lose social status. One exception is the Bemba people of Africa, who send people food to be consumed in private rather than shared together as a sign of respect.

Peer acceptance

Food is also an expression of the human need to belong or peer acceptance. The wish to eat what others eat may result in altered food patterns that may not be nutritionally sound. Teenagers are especially susceptible to this. Food choice in specific cases can be limited by social norms dictated by the choices of others.

Food as reward and punishment

Children learn what is acceptable and approved of in terms of food consumption through a system of reward and punishment. Rewards and punishments may be explicit or implicit and may be accompanied by reinforcing messages.

Gifts of food and sharing

Gifts of food and sharing food are symbols of social relationships, removed from the food's monetary value. Psychologically, people who were raised in an environment in which food was in abundance tend to develop a predisposition toward sharing, and those who were not raised in such an environment do not develop this trait. As a gift, food can symbolically express a wide range of emotions and sentiments. Three basic types of reciprocity for food exchanges exist. First, *generalized reciprocity* implies that there is no immediate expectation of return, no attempt to determine the gift's value, and no attempt to make gift giving "balance out." Second, *balanced reciprocity* occurs between social equals who have a personal relationship and takes into account the gift's value and implies some expectation of return. This return may be at a later date. Third, *negative reciprocity* involves immediate exchange and strict accounting of value in an impersonal exchange. Exchanges can also diffuse foods' status. Reciprocity-based food exchanges are common in situations in which environmental resources are limited. If reciprocity is not adopted, then *competitive food giving,* in which a person or group of people try to win influence and recognition by providing more complicated, expensive, or fancier food to a situation, can result.

Feasts and festivals

Feasts and festivals are held for many reasons and for many types of personal, cultural, or religious observances. Feast foods are usually scarce, high-quality, expensive, and difficult or time-consuming to prepare. Festivals are complex, colorful rituals found in nearly every society in some form. The main types of festival are ecofests (i.e., astronomical or seasonal events such as May Day), theofests (i.e., religious events such as Easter), secular festivals (i.e., national holidays), and personal festivals (i.e., major life events).

Rituals and sacrifices

Many pagan and religious rituals and sacrifices involve food. The need for ritualistic food may have contributed to the spread of some religions. In the past, rituals food offerings were usually animal. In many societies, these animal sacrifices have fallen out of favor and have been replaced by a recommendation for a moral sacrifice, such as one involving prayer or money. Sacrifices may be made for a variety of reasons, but they always imply an asymmetrical status relationship. The following motivations are the most common: to provide food for the gods, to propitiate an affronted deity, to effect communication with a deity through the eating of a victim, for maintenance or renewal of life, for purposes of divination, to confirm a covenant, to ward off evil, and in exchange for favors.

Sacraments

During some religious celebrations or dinners, members carry out sacraments that involve ceremonial foods and rites. Many cultures, especially ancient ones, have sacred foods that are often embodiments of the gods. Some cultures practice sacramental killing and eating of animals (Fieldhouse, 1986). Other cultures require special foods and may specify the methods used to prepare them (Kittler, Sucher, & Nelms, 2012).

Exercise 3.3. Meaning of Food

What meaning does food have in your life? As you reflect on your life, identify how each of the following categories relates to food in your family life and food in relation to others: prestige and status; status through food behavior; food and fashion; status and food ownership; food, friendship, and communication; peer acceptance; food as reward and punishment; feasts and festivals; rituals and sacrifice; and sacraments.

Social Situations

In early childhood, children begin to be exposed to a greater variety of social situations in which food is consumed. In addition, with their increased ability to perceive and interpret the world, they begin to observe and experience different types of foods and their social and cultural meanings. With these changes and developments, children begin to differentiate between different occupations that involve eating. For instance, they know the difference between a birthday party and a daily school lunch and between an ordinary family dinner and a holiday dinner. Not only are these differences evident in the type of food consumed, but they are also embedded in interactions with others and the accompanying experiences. This variety of experiences, in turn, helps develop many connections in the brain related to eating and linked to the related experiences and meanings that are unique to each child (Figure 3.3). These meanings are shared with other children and family members, because they participate in the same events.

Figure 3.3. It is important to provide a child with a variety of experiences to support developing multiple connections in the brain related to eating.

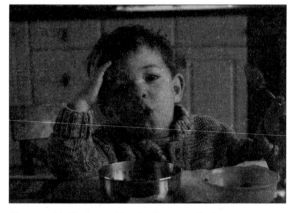

Source. M. Podvey. Used with permission.

Middle Childhood (Ages 7 to 11 Years)

During middle childhood, children gain greater exposure to social contexts and experience decreasing levels of supervision. For example, the interactions among children during lunchtime at school are less closely monitored. Peer groups become increasingly important, and empathy and other prosocial behaviors are learned. During this time, children become more aware of themselves and others. They learn to control the expression of their feelings and become more selective in choosing friends. Their self-awareness increases, and their self-esteem tends to decrease.

Children's peer groups become sensitive to customs and principles of society. Children become more aware of their own familial situation in comparison with that of others. Children's well-being continues to depend on the quality of parenting and the social setting rather than on the *family constitution,* which is the configuration of the family (e.g., whether the parents are of the same or different gender, whether the family is single parent or two parent, and whether or not the parents are the biological parents).

School-age children are considered more capable and independent, so they are allowed to venture out into the world more. A key part of their development is *social cognition,* that is, understanding other people and groups. During the school years, children gain a better understanding of human behavior. Children can see the origins and future implications of an action, and their understanding of personality traits increases. They also begin to learn about society's customs and principles.

Family Dinners

In terms of food consumption, family dinners, if they occur, become a greater social and educational affair during middle childhood because the child's ability to participate in conversations improves. At home, family dinners are an important means of socialization. Dinner conversations are used to convey rules of conversation, resolve conflicts, and establish and challenge social roles (Grieshaber, 1997; Ochs, Taylor, Rudolph, & Smith, 1992; Segal, 1999; Vuchinich, 1987). Although the family dinner is considered an important occupation, even to the point of becoming the space and time in which family members become a family (DeVault, 1991), the nature of interactions during such dinners may be unpleasant when conflicts occur. These experiences may lead people to attach negative meanings to this particular occupation. In the following sections, I give examples of depictions of family dinners in some older films and a new television series and discuss their implications.

Interpretation of Dining Space in Films and a Television Show

The act of eating together reveals the quality of relationships and social interactions. Until the 1950s, the site of this act was almost always the home. Family dining represented family unity. However, modern life has seen a shift from dining in the home to dining in restaurants, particularly fast-food establishments, as reflected in many American films (Figure 3.4). Furthermore, these films show that the bonding and sense of wholeness once experienced at home can now be experienced at fast-food restaurants and that dining at home is a source of conflict and distress.

These films redefine social order and the boundaries between order (or *purity*) and disorder (or *pollution*) in dining. In addition, technology, advertising, changing family structure, and various other factors have led to the rise of fast food and its central place in U.S. society. The films discussed

Figure 3.4. Tsu-Hsin and Ray dine together at a restaurant.

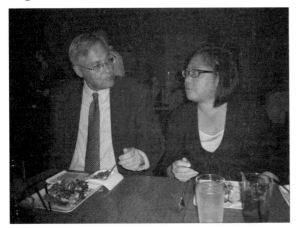

Source. J. Hinojosa. Used with permission.

here reveal fast food's new place in U.S. society and illustrate the shift in dining from the private to the public domain. However, the TV show, which began in 2010, also includes segments that illustrate the importance of family meals at home.

Mystic Pizza (Levinson & Petrie, 1988) is a film that follows three young women (sisters Kat and Daisy and their friend Jojo) who work together at Mystic Pizza as they prepare for adulthood. The pizzeria is depicted as the place where the girls bond over meals. The owner of the pizzeria, Leona, is a motherly figure to them. No meals are ever shown being eaten at home, except for one tense meal at the home of Daisy's boyfriend, Charlie. The characters seem to eat most of their meals at Mystic Pizza. All bonding between characters in the movie takes place inside the restaurant: The restaurant is where Jojo holds her wedding reception, where Kat finds out that Leona has agreed to help with her Yale tuition, and where Daisy reconciles her difficult relationship with her mother.

In *Ordinary People* (Schwary & Redford, 1980), home dining is the source of conflict, whereas McDonald's is the only place where the main character can find any nurturing. The film is about the lives of Beth and Calvin and their son Conrad after the death of their other son Buck. Buck died in a boating accident while out with Conrad, and the guilt drove Conrad to attempt suicide. Beth finds herself unable to deal with the disorder in her family and responds by behaving coldly toward Conrad. This behavior is often evidenced in din-

ing scenes. When Conrad reunites at McDonald's with a girl he met in the hospital, and later when he takes another girl there on a date, the viewer sees scenes of peaceful, communal dining.

The family dining scenes in *Better Off Dead* (Friesen, Jaffe, Meyer, & Holland, 1985) satirize the concept of family mealtime bonding. The mother of the family, Jenny, prepares horrible food that her family does not want to eat. The father, Al, spends meals complaining to or about his teenage son, Lane. The other son, Badger, spends mealtimes cutting coupons from cereal boxes or sitting in his bedroom playing with a toy. Lane eats alone, leaves meals early, or is forced into eating with the family by his mother. The film also satirizes the "polluted reality" of fast-food restaurants while also showing them as the only place where Lane can dine with someone and make a connection.

Bluebloods (Green & Burgess, 2010) is a television drama series about an Irish-American family of police officers in New York City. The Reagan family always eats Sunday dinner together. At that time, the family members discuss the events of the week. Sunday dinner time and space is used to talk, argue, fight, plan vacations, and just enjoy each other's company. It is the time when the family experiences itself as a family. The importance of the family Sunday dinner is purposely emphasized by the show writers, and each dinner is carefully planned, including the menu.

Location changes in films

Film media draws from current socially accepted practices to highlight changes in how and where people eat. These changes establish new boundaries for people who watch a film and may change their ideas about family dining. The lack of successful family dining in these movies indicates a notion of alienation among family members and illustrates how dining is changing in response to technological and social change. The activity of eating is based on what society classifies as edible and nonedible, and the location of eating is often determined by order and disorder. In the three films, home is shown as a place of disorder, whereas restaurants provide order and a sense of unity of experience. These restaurant eating scenes reproduce old ideals of family dining and update them for modern times.

Structural changes and landscape of power in films

Eating and dining have changed in response to societal changes and the influence of major corporations that control the food industry. Changes in societal structure may be the cause of the changes in dining because they shape habits and the meaning of food. Families integrate the power of these changes into daily life. Capitalism, marketing, giant food conglomerates, fast-food chains, and technological advances have all led to the rise of dining in fast-food restaurants rather than family dining at home.

Family structure in films

Along with social structure, family structure and its meaning have also changed. With more mothers working, school-age children involved in after-school activities, and teenagers working part-time or playing sports, family dining is harder to coordinate and the cultural importance of family dining has decreased. These films depict these changes (Ferry, 2003).

Interpretation of dining in television

As with films, television has changed the way that people perceive and experience eating. Beyond the content of the shows, television ads communicate acceptable models for eating, encourage snacking at nonmeal times, and reinforce positive emotions linked to food (Harris, Bargh, & Brownell, 2009). Television's content and its advertising influence people's preferences, values, and habits.

Exercise 3.4. Dining in Films and Television Shows

Select a film or television show that you have seen with a storyline that involves a family's daily life. Reflect on how family dining was represented. How have films and television shows influenced your thoughts about dining?

Adolescence (Ages 12 to 18 Years)

People typically think of adolescence as the time for developing self-identity. This process is related to interactions with family members and friends. It is a time

when those relationships evolve into their adult forms. By late adolescence, adolescents are comfortable with relationships with the other sex, their sexual identity has developed, and their communication with same-sex friends and parents has progressed. Adolescent children struggle for independence from their parents in terms of values, behaviors, and life in general.

One of the issues around food that may begin at this phase of human development is that of eating disorders (e.g., anorexia nervosa, bulimia, overeating). These disorders have many psychological explanations. When one talks about an eating disorder as an occupation whose meaning lies within the person (i.e., psychological explanations), one needs to address the social and cultural environments that contribute to the meaning of thinness and the ways to achieve it.

Eating Disorders in Sociological and Historical Contexts

The evolution of eating disorders can be followed in both sociological and historical contexts. Whether eating disorders are a modern development or if they came about over the past 100 years or so is not known. The increased awareness of eating disorders in recent decades signals an increase in both medical knowledge and their incidence. Mennell, Murcott, and van Otterloo (1992) suggested that this increased awareness is the result of long-term changes in society, civilization, and attitudes toward appetites. In the Middle Ages, nutrition was not distributed evenly among social classes, and having an abundance of food was a way for the upper class to show its importance. As time went by, the abundance of food reached the lower classes as well, and the food quality then became what set the higher classes apart from the lower ones. In addition, during the 19th century, the concept of moderation became popular and imposed some restrictions on diets. The 20th century brought an expectation of dietary self-control that stressed a person's control over food.

Anorexia nervosa, an eating disorder in which people have a pathological fear of becoming fat and engage in excessive dieting, was first diagnosed in the 19th century. Much of the research on eating disorders has focused on medical and psychological factors rather than social factors. The fact, however, that anorexia nervosa affects particular demographic groups (most typically, young, White, affluent women) cannot be ignored (Lock et al., 2010). Throughout the 20th century, the ideal body type for a woman has become thinner and thinner. The pressure to be thin and the importance attached to thinness are rooted in the behavior and personality traits associated with a thin physique, such as success and power, whereas being overweight carries a negative stigma.

The fact that the lower and working classes only acquired the means and abilities to afford enough food to become overweight in the past 100 years may be why the upper classes, who had typically been plump, now find themselves stressing slimness. Therefore, it is not surprising that women are more obsessed than ever with food and calorie intake, with most women reporting that they would like to be thinner (Vartanian, 2012).

Correlations between eating habits that are deemed socially acceptable and those of eating disorders suggest that eating disorders are extreme manifestations of eating habits that are deemed acceptable. Research has also noted that the pressure to be thin is widely felt among men and women (Brewis & Wutich, 2012; Dittmar, 2009; Smolak, 2012). For women, however, increased pressure to be thin fits into their pattern of female socialization (Brown & Dittmar, 2005). Modern women are placed in a tough situation, faced with opportunities for success and power but often raised with traditional female values of compliance and passivity. Women born in the late 20th century were the first to feel this pressure (Mennell et al., 1992).

Women have historically tried to change their bodies to meet cultural beauty standards. Advertising tells American women that they are not thin enough. Although the average American model is 5'1" and weighs 117 pounds, the average American women is 5'4" and 140 pounds (Loken & Peck, 2005). Models in movies and magazines compare happiness to being thin.

Buote, Wilson, Strahan, Gazzola, and Papps (2011) conducted eight studies using a variety of content analysis, surveys, and experimental methods to examine women and men's ideal appearance. One of their major findings was that women had higher personal standards for themselves for obtaining an ideal then they did for other women.

Separate Social Contexts

In relation to other aspects of food and eating, adolescents may begin eating in separate social contexts (e.g., going on dates, going out in groups). Typically, considering their budgets, fast-food chains at the mall or food at movie theaters might be popular choices. Adolescents are also left alone at home; therefore, at this stage, in addition to refining the skills around eating and eating appropriately whose development began in middle childhood, cooking food and providing for one's own nourishment and that of younger siblings may begin.

Adulthood (Ages 18 to 65 Years)

Adulthood is different from childhood not only because the adult becomes a legally independent member of society but also because society does not establish a single path for transitioning from early adulthood to older adulthood. In fact, since the late 20th century, adulthood has been marked by decreased predictability about the way life will evolve (Lee, 2001). Human development texts identify three general foci of adult life: having (1) a family, (2) a career, and (3) friendships and intimacy (and here, I discuss friendships and intimacy in relation to dining out). The way in which adults attend to these foci is determined by social and cultural forces. During adulthood, issues such as gender, socioeconomic status, race, ethnicity, religion, and sexual orientation become more apparent in the options open to people and the choices they make. Although these issues affect children and adolescents as well, the way in which they encounter and address these issues is largely dependent on how their parents construct their exposures to them.

Family

For adults, having a family typically means raising children. The family constitution and legal status may vary from marriage to cohabitation to single parenthood. Parents may be of different sexes or the same sex and may be either biological or nonbiological parents of the children. In each case, the role of parenting is an important aspect of the lives of many adults.

As parents, adults are responsible for the physical, psychological, and social well-being and development of their children. One of these responsibilities is to socialize their children to the different occupations of eating in context. They are responsible for introducing culturally relevant foods to their children as a way to socialize them into that culture. These foods may be fairly simple things such as the kind of breakfast being served. Choices can be to follow the traditional meaning of *breakfast* in terms of the types of food served (see next section) or to break with tradition by following new scientific information about foods that are good or bad for one's health (e.g., high levels of cholesterol and the consumption of eggs). Foods eaten at breakfast, as a family and at family meals, are socially and culturally determined. In the following sections, I discuss the practices, habits, and routines that are associated with this fundamental occupation.

Food for breakfast

The most flexible versions of breakfast are probably the Central and North European buffets of breads, pastries, cheeses, and cold meats, or their Middle Eastern equivalents of bread, yoghurt, fruit, and preserves. Substantial breakfasts include the modern British fry-up and the North American version, with numerous variations on the theme of eggs, bacon, sausage, and pancakes and waffles with maple syrup. Traditional Indian breakfasts include dal, rice, breads, samosas, and fruit. Comforting bowls of hot cereal mixtures are popular, from the Scottish oatmeal porridge to the rice porridges eaten across much of Asia, of which congee is the best known. Minimal approaches to breakfast include croissants and *café au lait* in France, chocolate and churros in Spain, and many variations of muesli for those who think that cereal, nuts, and dried fruit are key to good health (Davidson, 1999, p. 104).

The type of food consumed imparts information and signifies meaning. For example, a television advertisement showing a frying pan with two eggs and bacon while the announcer says "breakfast for dinner" suggests that eating eggs in the United States is related to breakfast. In Israel, however, eggs are commonly eaten for the evening meal, which is *supper* rather than *dinner*. Even within the United States, a great variety of foods is consumed by different ethnic groups in different geographic locations and according to many other delineations. The variety is so great that Kittler et al. (2012) devoted a whole book to describing it.

Food and the family

Issues of food and family are closely related to those of nutrition and responsibility, and different cultures can have different understandings of what is healthy. Parents share the responsibility of balancing diet and health for themselves and their families. The roles of fathers and mothers can vary depending on family configuration and other factors, including cultural expectations, available time, available money, and environmental influences and upbringing. When deciding on a family diet, they make food choices on the basis of their desire to be good parents.

When parents are middle-aged adults, balancing diet and eating habits can be complicated by being the middle generation of their extended families. Immediate family ties are often strong at this time, as are those between middle-aged adults and their elderly parents. When adult children have children of their own, a new link between generations is formed. During this stage of life, parents keep in touch with family members who no longer live at home, celebrate achievements, and get the family together. Decisions about what to eat and how to celebrate are often compromised among various family members' expectations.

Media, including advertising and the Internet, is a valuable source of information about nutrition and health. The influence of these media depends on the parent's beliefs and resources. Mass media advertising also influences parent's decisions about which food to purchase (Nestle, 2013). Research has shown that mass media messages can influence dietary patterns and decisions, such as those about salmonella, mad cow disease, listeria, and botulism (Funk, Gilad, Watkins, & Jansen, 2009). Informal nutritional education can be just as influential and important as formal nutritional education.

Family meals

Holidays and dining are important times for family members and friends to socialize and enjoy each other's company. One way of keeping the extended family together is through a holiday get-together such as Thanksgiving or Christmas. The preparation of holiday meals may consist of following old traditions and bringing in new ones. For example, parents who did not like certain foods as children may introduce new dishes to make the experience of a festive dinner a better one for their own children. Engaging in festive family meals is an important feature of the con-

Figure 3.5. A child learns manners and appropriate social behaviors when given opportunities to dine out with the family.

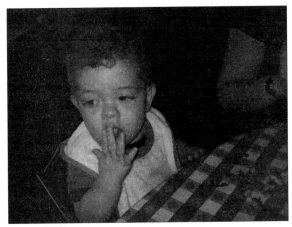

Source. M. Podvey. Used with permission.

struction of a family out of its individual members. Without getting together, regardless of the quality of experiences, interactions and attachments would not occur (DeVault, 1991; Gillis, 1996; Hasselkus, 2002; Kantor & Lehr, 1975).

Another context of eating mentioned previously is the socialization of children into dining out (Figure 3.5). Dining out is an experience that has become much more common in the United States and other places with the emergence of fast-food and other affordable restaurants. Dining out as a context for eating is large and diversified in every aspect: The cost of a meal can be close to a dollar or up to a few hundred dollars; the type of food served represents many combinations of varied tastes and cultural, social, and religious factors; the nature of service can range from self-service to specialized wait staff. With all these variations come different behavioral expectations, experiences, and meanings.

Parents are responsible for socializing their children into the dining-out contexts that are relevant to their social and cultural backgrounds. For example, some cultures whose food is spicy begin introducing spicy food to children around age 10 or 11 (Davidson, 1999). This introduction may not be a socializing aspect of eating in cultures whose food is not spicy, so people may acquire the taste for it only in later life. Another aspect of dining out is *etiquette,* or good manners. The appropriate way to behave in a self-service restaurant such as a fast-food chain differs from that in a self-service restaurant that presents food buffet style. Eat-

ing utensils and their use are also related to the type of restaurant (e.g., chopsticks or knife and fork, one set of utensils or several sets). These observable elements can give information about the types of food served and how expensive they might be. Observing a person holding and using a knife and a fork can give a broad idea of his or her country of origin: People in the United States do not tend to hold the knife in their right hand and the fork in their left hand while eating, whereas people from Europe do. These habits and pieces of information are imparted to children by their parents to support them in their adult life.

Career

Career is another important aspect of adult life. Careers can be a source of income and be used as a social ladder because they generate income and develop social connections. A career often necessitates special forms of eating. For example, the daily lunch at work can take the form of eating food brought from home, buying a meal and eating it in the office, or going out to a restaurant. The variety of restaurants open for lunch affords a choice that signals differentiation among the levels of employees or business people. The type and price of food consumed can serve as a good indicator of the socioeconomic level of the person eating.

Another type of eating in the context of a career can be eating at workplace parties and during special occasions. These events may be associated with holidays, office celebrations, and personal celebrations for birthdays, marriages, and new babies. These events may occur in the office with either catered food or a potluck, in a restaurant, or perhaps in someone's home. Each event and location requires unique behaviors and manners attached to a unique set of experiences and meanings.

Careers can also involve business meals, including breakfast, lunch, or dinner, and once again the type of food and location may vary greatly. On these occasions, the focus of the conversation is business rather than social and the food and location may serve to impress the invited party.

Friendships and Intimacy (and Dining Out)

Adults take on many roles to fulfill their need for friendships and intimacy, each of which demands a type of personal sacrifice. Young adults, usually free of overriding commitments, often create broad networks of friends in various settings and among various groups. Once marriage occurs, however, the wide friendship network frequently shrinks because of the time needed to establish a marriage and a home on top of other obligations. Focus on raising a family, however, does not exclude an important occupation that is related to maintaining friendships and intimacy, namely, dining out. Dining out is not as simple as merely eating at a location away from home.

Dining out is not only about the food consumed but also about the experience itself (Campbell-Smith, 1967; Warde & Martens, 2000). Finkelstein (1989) applied a more sociological, structuralist view to this concept in her book *Dining Out: A Sociology of Modern Manners*. She wrote that dining out has much to do with self-presentation and social relationships.

Restaurants have a cultural reputation as being a site of well-being, excitement, and pleasure, which is why elements other than the food are important. For example, the restaurant's décor and the cost and nature of the service may serve as indications of its patrons' socioeconomic status. Finkelstein (1989), moreover, suggested that things such as cost and status are more important than the nature and quality of the food because cost and status are objective factors that are easier for people to agree on than food.

The objective factors of dining out allow for standardization of meal experiences. By making these objective factors part of restaurants, patrons know what the experience should be like; therefore, they go to a particular restaurant for the particular experience they are looking for at that particular time (Finkelstein, 1989). For example, when taking children out to dine in the United States, the typically appropriate restaurant (other than fast-food chains) would be inexpensive and relatively casual and have a children's menu. In France, however, it is not uncommon to see children in upscale restaurants that may also have a children's menu. Another example is parents' decision to dine at an expensive restaurant on their anniversary with the hope of having an experience that is different from their family's typical dining-out experience.

Older Adulthood (Ages 66 Years or Older)

Older adulthood is sometimes described in terms of increased frailty and health concerns. In sociologi-

cal terms, older adulthood is often defined by the changes in older people's roles and occupations. Some of these changes occur as a result of the biological and physiological changes that occur with aging. Some are the result of life circumstances, such as grown children. Some arise from the organization of society. In general, the way people change their lives with aging greatly depends on their previous lifestyle and their social, cultural, and economic situation.

In terms of eating, changes would similarly depend on social status, economic situation, cultural background, and established eating habits. The need to control some aspect of diet may increase as people get older, according to the belief that what people consume affects their health. Most of these changes in food intake occur before one reaches older adulthood and depend on one's personal health considerations, which may include conditions such as diabetes, high blood pressure, or heart disease. Such changes in diet are dominated by scientific findings and common beliefs about the healthful qualities of particular foods.

Occupations That Involve Eating

The earlier description of and discussion about the different occupations that involve eating was not meant to be exhaustive but illustrative. My purpose was to demonstrate that the basic human need for food leads all humans to engage in the basic *activity of eating*. This activity consists of placing food into one's mouth, chewing, swallowing, and digesting. Humans, however, are animals who construct social meanings; therefore, the activity of eating can be performed and experienced in different contexts and in different forms, amounting to the creation of multiple occupations that involve eating. Occupations are phenomena that lie within the person, because only the person can interpret and assign meaning to activities and events. Humans are social animals, and the interpretations and meanings that they assign to occupations are closely related to their life experiences. These life experiences are greatly shaped by temporal, psychological, social, symbolic, cultural, ethnic, and spiritual meanings.

In addition to parents, both society and culture shape children's experiences by sanctioning what

Figure 3.6. Eating various foods gives a child new experiences that he or she can transfer to other contexts and situations.

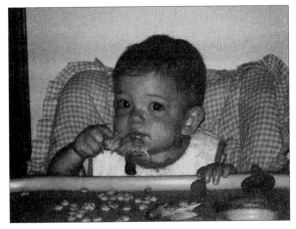

Source. M. Podvey. Used with permission.

environments are appropriate for children and at what ages. As children get older and gain increasing experience with the same activity in different contexts, their understanding becomes richer. In other words, eating in various contexts teaches children that hunger can be satisfied with different kinds of food and in different situations (Figure 3.6). They also learn that foods other than the food served at home are available and that they will like some of these foods better than those regularly served at home. In addition, they learn that different contexts correspond to different experiences and meanings (e.g., birthday parties, holiday meals).

As children grow up, not only do they frequent more environments, but they also spend more of their time with peers in environments away from their families. At this point, activities that are carried out with peers acquire meanings without parental influence shaping the experiences. Such experiences and meanings, translated into connections in the brain, contribute to people's uniqueness. Each child or adolescent has a life context fairly similar to that

Exercise 3.5. Food Study

In the preceding description, I used the terms *social* and *cultural* because these are the main areas of academic study that look at food in relation to context. Explore the literature about food to assess the influence of context on food.

of his or her parents, yet each participates in new and different contexts that are shared with peers. All of these lead to shared experiences across generations (with parents) and across cohorts (with peers), allowing the social scientist to study the similarities and differences among such groups.

As adults, people are more consciously aware of their contexts, their limitations, and how these relate to lifestyle and experiences. Adults have the power, as sanctioned by society, to raise and socialize their children as long as they do not violate certain boundaries as defined by law (e.g., child abuse and neglect, avoiding schooling, child labor). Parents can shape their children's contexts, thus constructing experiences and meanings for various childhood activities.

Examples of such shaping include embracing one's cultural heritage through the types of food served at home, thus supporting the development of tastes for ethnic food. Parents may also decide that they want to do just the opposite, serving nonethnic food with the hope of assimilating their children into the larger society.

Alternatively, parents may serve food that is not related to a particular culture but that is deemed at that time to be healthy and most appropriate for the child's development and well-being. In this case, children are socialized into the concept of food as a means of maintaining health rather than a means of cultural identification.

In either case, these experiences are mapped in children's brains as they learn to identify the foods with meanings presented at home. These different meanings associated with eating present different occupations—for example, eating as a marker of cultural identity in which the taste of food is essential in contrast to eating as a means of maintaining health in which the taste of food is not essential.

The sources of parents' decisions about how to socialize their children, although coming from within themselves, are influenced by their life experiences. For example, if parents' social life involves participation in occupations with great cultural emphasis, then they would very likely emphasize food in its cultural forms.

Summary

Occupations have meaning attached to them by the person who engages in them. Using the purposeful activities associated with eating, I explored the importance of these occupations across the lifespan. Eating is a social and cultural phenomenon that evolves and changes as the person grows and matures. Culture and life experiences determine its form and importance to the person. The family and social environment influence the life experiences that a person has around food, and meanings are assigned to the occupation of eating that are closely related to life experiences and shaped by temporal, psychological, social, symbolic, cultural, ethnic, and spiritual meanings.

Acknowledgment

A special thanks is extended to Kaitlin R. Jessing-Butz, who assisted in the preparation of the manuscript of this chapter.

References

Albala, K. (2002). *Eating right in the Renaissance.* Berkeley: University of California Press.

American Occupational Therapy Association. (1997). Statement—Fundamental concepts of occupational therapy: Occupation, purposeful activity, and function. *American Journal of Occupational Therapy, 51,* 864–866. http://dx.doi.org/10.5014/ajot.51.10.864

Babycenter. (2013). *How to dine out with kids . . . and enjoy it! (ages 2 to 4).* Retrieved from http://www.babycenter.com/0_how-to-dine-out-with-kids-and-enjoy-it-ages-2-to-4_63913.bc?page=2

Brewis, A. A., & Wutich, A. (2012). Explicit versus implicit fat-stigma. *American Journal of Human Biology, 24*(3), 332–338. http://dx.doi.org/10.1002/ajhb.22233

Brown, A., & Dittmar, H. (2005). Think "thin" and feel bad: The role of appearance schema activation, attention level, and thin–ideal internalization for young women's responses to ultra-thin media ideals. *Journal of Social and Clinical Psychology, 24,* 1088–1113.

Buote, V. M., Wilson, A. E., Strahan, E. J., Gazzola, S. B., & Papps, F. (2011). Setting the bar: Divergent sociocultural norms for women's and men's ideal appearance in real-world contexts. *Body Image, 8*(4), 322–334. http://dx.doi.org/10.1016/j.bodyim.2011.06.002

Campbell-Smith, G. (1967). *The marketing of the meal experience.* London: Surrey University Press.

Clark, F. A., Parham, D., Carlson, M. E., Frank, G., Jackson, J., Pierce, D.,... Zemke, R. (1991). Occupational science: Academic innovation in the service of occupational therapy's future. *American Journal of Occupational Therapy, 45,* 300–310. http://dx.doi.org/10.5014/ajot.45.4.300

Counihan, C., & Van Esterik, P. (2013). Why food? Why culture? Why now? Introduction to the third edition. In C. Counihan & P. Van Esterik (Eds.), *Food and culture: A reader* (pp. 1–15). New York: Routledge.

Davidson, A. (1999). *The Oxford companion to food.* New York: Oxford University Press.

DeVault, M. J. (1991). *Feeding the family: The social organization of caring as gendered work.* Chicago: University of Chicago Press.

Dittmar, H. (2009). How do "body perfect" ideals in the media have a negative impact on body image and behaviors? Factors and processes related to self and identity. *Journal of Social and Clinical Psychology, 28,* 1–8. Retrieved from http://ezproxy.library.nyu.edu/docview/224859660?accountid=12768. http://dx.doi.org/10.1521/jscp.2009.28.1.1

Douglas, M. (1982). *In the active voice.* Boston: Routledge & Kegan Paul.

Ferry, J. F. (2003). *Food in film: A culinary performance of communication.* New York: Routledge.

Fieldhouse, P. (1986). *Food and nutrition: Customs and culture.* Dover, NH: Croom Helm.

Finkelstein, J. (1989). *Dining out: A sociology of modern manners.* New York: New York University Press.

Friesen, G., Jaffe, M., Meyer, A. (Producers), & Holland, S. S. (Director). (1985). *Better off dead* [Motion picture]. Los Angeles: Warner Brothers.

Funk, S., Gilad, E., Watkins, C., & Jansen, V. A. A. (2009). The spread of awareness and its impact on epidemic outbreaks. *Proceedings of the National Academy of Sciences, 106,* 6872–6877.

Gillis, J. (1996). Making time for family: The invention of family time(s) and the reinvention of family history. *Journal of Family History, 21,* 4–21. http://dx.doi.org/10.1177/036319909602100102

Green, R., & Burgess, M. (Creators). (2010). *Bluebloods.* Studio City, CA: CBS Productions.

Grieshaber, S. (1997). Mealtime rituals: Power and resistance in the construction of mealtime rules. *British Journal of Sociology, 48,* 649–666. http://dx.doi.org/10.2307/591601

Harris, J. L., Bargh, J. A., & Brownell, K. D. (2009). Priming effects of television food advertising on eating behavior. *Health Psychology, 28*(4), 404–413. http://dx.doi.org/10.1037/a0014399

Hasselkus, B. R. (2002). *The meaning of everyday occupation.* Thorofare, NJ: Slack.

Hess, R., Visschers, V. H. M., & Siegrist, M. (2012). Effectiveness and efficiency of different shapes of food guides. *Journal of Nutrition Education and Behavior, 44,* 442–447. http://dx.doi.org/10.1016/j.jneb.2011.09.005

Kantor, D., & Lehr, W. (1975). *Inside the family: Toward a theory of family process.* San Francisco: Jossey-Bass.

Kittler, P. G., & Sucher, K. P. (2001). *Food and culture* (3rd ed.). Belmont, CA: Wadsworth Thompson Learning.

Kittler, P. G., Sucher, K., & Nelms, M. (2012). *Food and culture* (6th ed.). Belmont, CA: Wadsworth.

Kramer, P., & Hinojosa, J. (1995). Epiphany of human occupation. In C. B. Royeen (Ed.), *Human occupation* (AOTA Self-Study Series). Bethesda, MD: American Occupational Therapy Association.

Lee, N. (2001). *Childhood and society: Growing up in an age of uncertainty.* Philadelphia: Open University Press.

Lemert, C. C. (2011). *Social things: An introduction to the sociological life.* Lanham, MD: Rowman & Littlefield.

Levinson, M. (Producer), & Petrie, D. (Director). (1988). *Mystic pizza* [Motion picture]. Los Angeles: Samuel Goldwyn.

Lock, J., Le Grange, D., Agras, W., Moye, A., Bryson, S. W., & Jo, B. (2010). Randomized clinical trial comparing family-based treatment with adolescent-focused individual therapy for adolescents with anorexia nervosa. *Archives of General Psychiatry, 67*(10), 1025–1032. http://dx.doi.org/10.1001/archgenpsychiatry.2010.128

Loken, B., & Peck, J. (2005). The effects of instructional frame on female adolescents' evaluations of larger sized female models in print advertising. *Journal of Applied Social Psychology, 35*(4), 850–868. http://dx.doi.org/10.1111/j.1559-1816.2005.tb02149.x

Lowenberg, M. E. (1970). Sociocultural basis of food habits. *Food Technology, 24,* 27–32.

Maslow, A. H. (1954). *Motivation and personality.* New York: Harper.

Mennell, S., Murcott, A., & van Otterloo, A. H. (1992). *The sociology of food: Eating, diet, and culture.* Thousand Oaks, CA: Sage.

Nestle, M. (2002). *Food politics: How the food industry influences nutrition and health.* Berkeley: University of California Press.

Nestle, M., & Wilson, T. (2012). Food industry and political influences on American nutrition. In N. J. Temple, T. Wilson, & J. D. R. Jacobs (Eds.), *Nutritional health* (pp. 477–490). New York: Humana Press.

Nestle, M. (2013). *Food politics: How the food industry influences nutrition and health.* Berkeley: University of California Press.

Nicklaus, S. (2009). Development of food variety in children. *Appetite, 52*(1), 253–255. http://dx.doi.org/10.1016/j.appet.2008.09.018

Ochs, E., Taylor, C., Rudolph, D., & Smith, R. (1992). Storytelling as a theory-building activity. *Discourse Processes, 15,* 37–72. http://dx.doi.org/10.1080/01638539209544801

Rozin, P. (2006). The integration of biological, social, cultural, and psychological influences on food choice. In R. Shepherd & M. Raats (Eds.), *The psychology of food choice* (pp. 19–39). Wallingford, UK: CABI.

Rozin, P. (2007). Food and eating. In S. Kitayama & D. Cohen (Eds.), *Handbook of cultural psychology* (pp. 391–416). New York: Guilford Press.

Schwary, R. L. (Producer), & Redford, R. (Director). (1980). *Ordinary people* [Motion picture]. Los Angeles: Paramount.

Segal, R. (1999). Doing for others: Occupations within families with children with special needs. *Journal of Occupational Science, 6,* 53–60. http://dx.doi.org/10.1080/14427591.1999.9686451

Smolak, L. (2012). *Appearance in childhood and adolescence.* Retrieved from http://www.oxfordhandbooks.com/view/10.1093/oxfordhb/9780199580521.001.0001/oxfordhb-9780199580521-e-13

Spitz, R. A. (1965). *The first year of life: A psychoanalytic study of normal and deviant development of object relations.* New York: International Universities Press.

Strauss, C., & Quinn, N. (1997). *A cognitive theory of cultural meaning.* New York: Cambridge University Press.

Torres, D. P. M., & Park, Y. W. (2013). Human milk. In Y. W. Park & G. F. W. Haenlein (Eds.), *Milk and dairy products in human nutrition: Production, composition and health* (pp. 659–677). Oxford, UK: John Wiley & Sons.

U.S. Department of Agriculture. (n.d.). *Choosemyplate.* Retrieved from http://www.choosemyplate.gov

Vartanian, L. R. (2012). Self-discrepancy theory and body image. In T. F. Cash (Ed.), *Encyclopedia of body image and human appearance* (Vol. 2, pp. 711–717). London: Elsevier.

Vuchinich, S. (1987). Starting and stopping spontaneous family conflicts. *Journal of Marriage and the Family, 49,* 591–601. http://dx.doi.org/10.2307/352204

Warde, A., & Martens, L. (2000). *Eating out: Social differentiation, consumption and pleasure.* New York: Cambridge University Press.

Wood, R. C. (1995). *The sociology of the meal.* Edinburgh, Scotland: Edinburgh University Press.

Wyness, M. G. (2012). *Childhood and society* (2nd ed.). Basingstoke, UK: Palgrave MacMillan.

CHAPTER 4.

OCCUPATION AND ACTIVITY ANALYSIS

Karen A. Buckley, MA, OTR, and Sally E. Poole, OTD, OT/L, CHT

Highlights

✧ History of activity analysis
✧ Occupational therapy's perspectives on activity and occupation analysis
✧ Occupation analysis process
✧ Occupation analysis
✧ Multicomponent activity analysis
✧ Occupation analysis summary
✧ Occupation and activity analysis within a frame of reference.

Key Terms

✧ Activity analysis
✧ Acuity
✧ Adequate response
✧ Arts and crafts movement
✧ Attention span
✧ Auditory processing
✧ Axial alignment
✧ Basic learning
✧ Basic skills
✧ Bilateral integration
✧ Body scheme
✧ Body strength
✧ Categorization
✧ Complex skills
✧ Concentric muscle contraction
✧ Concept formation
✧ Coping skills

✧ Copying
✧ Crafts
✧ Crossing the midline
✧ Cylindrical grasp pattern
✧ Depth perception
✧ Distract
✧ Eccentric muscle contraction
✧ Endurance
✧ Episodic memory
✧ Extremity strength
✧ Figure–ground perception
✧ Fine motor coordination and dexterity
✧ Fine motor skill
✧ Form constancy
✧ Frame of reference
✧ Function–dysfunction continuum
✧ Generalization

- ✧ Grasp patterns
- ✧ Gustatory processing
- ✧ Habits
- ✧ Hook grasp pattern
- ✧ Hypermobility
- ✧ Hypomobility
- ✧ In context
- ✧ Initiation of activity
- ✧ Interpersonal skills
- ✧ Isometric muscle contraction
- ✧ Kinesthesia
- ✧ Kinetic analysis
- ✧ Knowledge
- ✧ Laterality
- ✧ Lateral pinch grasp pattern
- ✧ Learning
- ✧ Level of arousal
- ✧ Memory
- ✧ Midline sagittal plane
- ✧ Mobility
- ✧ Motor control
- ✧ Neurodevelopmental treatment approach
- ✧ Occupation analysis
- ✧ Occupation-as-means
- ✧ Occupation-based activity analysis
- ✧ Ocular–motor control
- ✧ Olfactory processing
- ✧ Oral–motor skill
- ✧ Orientation
- ✧ Position in space
- ✧ Postural alignment
- ✧ Postural control
- ✧ Postural praxis
- ✧ Praxis
- ✧ Prehension

- ✧ Procedural memory
- ✧ Proprioceptive processing
- ✧ Range of motion
- ✧ Reciprocal patterns
- ✧ Recognition
- ✧ Rehearsing
- ✧ Restricted activity analysis
- ✧ Reverse a sequence
- ✧ Right–left discrimination
- ✧ Scanning
- ✧ Self-control
- ✧ Semantic memory
- ✧ Sensory modulation
- ✧ Sensory processing
- ✧ Sequencing
- ✧ Skills
- ✧ Social skills
- ✧ Spatial operations
- ✧ Spatial relations
- ✧ Spherical grasp pattern
- ✧ Stereognosis
- ✧ Symmetrical performance
- ✧ Tactile processing
- ✧ Tasks
- ✧ Termination of activity
- ✧ Theory-based activity analysis
- ✧ Time management
- ✧ Tip-to-tip pinch grasp pattern
- ✧ Topographical orientation
- ✧ Vestibular input
- ✧ Visual fixation
- ✧ Visual–motor integration
- ✧ Visual reception
- ✧ Visual tracking

This chapter presents a brief historical overview of the importance of activity and occupation in the health and well-being of a person. We begin by reviewing the evolution of activity and occupation analysis. We then explain the three parts of a systematic approach for occupational therapy practitioners to use in both activity and occupation analysis. Finally, we provide a sample form (Appendix 4.A., "Occupation Analysis Form") and a completed occupation analysis form (Appendix 4.B., "Occupation Analysis Form: Repot a Plant").

History of Activity Analysis

Ancient History

As early as 2600 BC, historical records document the concept that people must use both mind and body to maintain *health* and *well-being*. The ancient Chinese, Persians, and Greeks understood that a mutually dependent relationship existed between physical and mental health and well-being. Egyptians and Greeks saw diversion and recreation as treatment of the sick.

Later, the Romans recommended activity for those with mental illness (Hopkins & Smith, 1978).

1700s and 1800s

Many centuries later in Europe and the United States, the use of activity and occupation was described as a treatment modality for people with mental and physical illness. In 1798, Benjamin Rush, the first American psychiatrist, advocated the use of domestic occupations for their therapeutic value. Weaving, spinning, and sewing were occupations that he considered therapeutic because of their personal interest to the patients of the era and because of their social and cultural relevance (Dunton & Licht, 1957). In the 18th and 19th centuries in the United States, people accepted the use of occupations in the care of patients with mental illness. In 1892, Edward N. Bush, superintendent of a psychiatric hospital in Maryland, wrote, "The benefits of occupation are manifold. Primarily, even the most simple and routine tasks keep the mind occupied, awaken new trains of thought and interests, and divert the patient from the delusions or hallucinations which harass and annoy him" (as cited in Dunton & Licht, 1957, p. 9).

In addition to the use of occupations in psychiatric treatment in the 18th and 19th centuries, early documentation has shown that people used occupations to build muscles and improve joint range. In 1780 in France, Clément-Joseph Tissot, a physician in the French cavalry, described the beneficial use of arts and crafts and recreational activities to mediate the physical effects of chronic illness (as cited in Dunton & Licht, 1957). Tissot named "shuttlecock, tennis, football, and dancing" (as cited in Dunton & Licht, 1957, p. 9) as activities to promote range of motion for all joints of the upper and lower extremities. In this early literature about occupations and activities, little description is available about the precise methodology used to select activities that addressed specific problems. Instead, activities appear to have been selected for their cultural, social, recreational, and diversional characteristics and, one assumes, meaningfulness to the person.

Early 1900s to World War I

In the early 1900s, occupational therapy practitioners embraced the arts and crafts movement that was a backlash against the social ills perceived to have resulted from the Industrial Revolution (Reed, 1986). The *arts and crafts movement* promoted a simpler life in which activities were performed at a slower pace than required by factory production, the process was as important as the end product, the creative spirit was valued, and manual learning was valued rather than intellectual learning alone (Reed, 1986). Before World War II, little literature indicated that practitioners selected activities on the basis of anything other than intuition (Creighton, 1992; Reed, 1986).

At the end of World War I, two factors had a strong influence on occupational practitioners' use of activities and related occupations. First, the end of the arts and crafts movement in the United States and Europe meant that many activities were not valued in the same way. Second, practitioners found themselves treating patients who were exhibiting both physical and psychological trauma. Practitioners began selecting activities on the basis of the patient's particular deficits and needs. They first carefully analyzed each patient's deficits and, using a problem-solving approach, determined which specific activity would be appropriate to address the deficit. Practitioners used activities because of their characteristics, but no formal analysis was part of the practitioner's treatment routine. Practitioners and physicians, however, began to look beyond the profession of occupational therapy to gain knowledge about activity analysis.

In this early development of the occupational therapy profession, activity selection and subsequent intervention were influenced by at least two men outside the profession: Frank Gilbreth and Jules Amar (Creighton, 1992). Gilbreth, an engineer by training, studied jobs to identify the most productive and least fatiguing methods of job performance. His work, which industry accepted, examined the worker, environment, and motion. While visiting European hospitals to study physicians and how they worked, he became acquainted with the research of Amar, a French physiologist. Amar had been commissioned by the French government to study how to prepare wounded soldiers for reentry into the workforce, which he did by measuring the physiological requirements of many jobs. His work influenced Gilbreth by making him aware of the possibilities of applying motion studies to the reeducation of returning wounded veterans.

Gilbreth presented his work at the 1917 annual meeting of the National Society for the Promotion of Occupational Therapy, which led to the eventual inclusion of this concept of activity analysis into the field of occupational therapy. Activity analysis was incorporated into occupational therapy textbooks as early as 1919 (Creighton, 1992).

1920s to World War II

The years between World War I and World War II saw the establishment of the American Occupational Therapy Association (AOTA), formerly the National Society for the Promotion of Occupational Therapy, and further development of the profession in general. AOTA encouraged practitioners to establish departments and to publish papers to help them do so. In addition, AOTA published papers to assist practitioners with the appropriate selection of activities. *Crafts,* which are culturally defined handiwork or construction, were the treatment activities of choice, although they included both work-related and recreational activities (Creighton, 1992). In 1922 and 1928, AOTA published papers promoting the analysis of crafts for psychiatric occupational therapy and for physical restoration.

World War II propelled women out of the home and into the workforce and propelled occupational therapy practitioners from traditional roles into new, real-life circumstances. As a result of improvement in medical and surgical care, veterans were surviving severe physical injuries and living with permanent disability. Practitioners began to specialize in the practice area of physical disabilities. Again, occupational therapy practitioners referred to Gilbreth's work, now being carried on by his wife Lillian, who proposed that engineers and rehabilitation professionals work together to assist soldiers with disabilities (Creighton, 1992). At the same time, the U.S. Army developed its own manual of therapeutic activities (U.S. Department of War, 1944) that detailed activities to use to improve joint range of motion and strengthening of all extremities. The military, in fact, "divided" the body so that occupational therapy practitioners worked with the upper body and physical therapists worked with the lower body (Hinojosa, 1996). Many policies and procedures laid down by the military for occupational therapy practitioners are still followed today.

Post–War to Mid-Century

Soon after World War II, Sidney Licht, who at the time was president of the American Congress of Rehabilitation Medicine and the editor of *Physical Medicine Library,* published an article in 1947 advocating the use of a more precise method for analyzing activity for occupational therapy practitioners working in the area of physical disabilities. He believed that craft analysis looked at "psychomotor values, economic factors, tempo, or other inherent characteristics" (Licht, 1947, p. 75). He coined the term *kinetic analysis,* however, to refer to when the tools or activities were to be analyzed for the motions involved. Many of Licht's ideas continue to influence practice in the area of physical disabilities. Contemporary occupational therapy practitioners who are concerned about muscle contractions, joint range of motion, precision and accuracy of intervention, ergonomics of body mechanics, and control variants continue to use the criteria for examining motion that Licht originally proposed for kinetic analysis.

Occupational therapy practitioners working in physical medicine appear to have become interested in activity analysis before those working in mental health. In 1948, Gail Fidler proposed that practitioners working in psychiatric occupational therapy use scientific analysis of activities:

> While the functioning of a personality is certainly not as quantifiable as a muscle, the use of activity for the psychiatric patient should be more scientifically allied with the principles of dynamic psychiatry and treatment objectives than it is at the present. (p. 284)

Fidler also proposed an outline for activity analysis to help occupational therapy practitioners meet the goals or aims of treatment so that occupational therapy in psychiatry could, in fact, be elevated from diversion to the level of therapy.

Late 20th Century and Early 21st Century

Activity analysis had remained rudimentary in occupational therapy and focused almost exclusively on the product rather than the process of analysis. Gradually, the process of analysis has become more important than the end product.

For example, Mosey (1981) proposed that *activity analysis* is the process of closely examining an activity to distinguish its component parts. This careful examination allows a skilled occupational therapy practitioner to select the most therapeutic and appropriate activities from those available and ensures that the selected activities are relevant and correspond to the client's needs.

Activity analysis also plays an important part of deductive reasoning in whatever *frame of reference* (i.e., theoretically based guideline for intervention) or approach occupational therapy practitioners use with clients. Mosey (1986) suggested two goals for activity analysis that would serve to firmly establish the process as a legitimate tool of the profession. The first goal is to enable the practitioner to learn more about the activity's inherent properties, the personal goals of the client, and the range of skills the client needs to perform the activity.

After the practitioner has an understanding of the client and his or her personal goals and present performance skills, he or she then selects an appropriate frame of reference to initiate intervention. Under these conditions, the occupational therapist can do a *restricted activity analysis,* that is, focus on the *function–dysfunction continuum* (i.e., focused and limited analysis) of the specific frame of reference. The activity analysis is restricted, because the practitioner only examines specified factors that are identified by a particular frame of reference and that relate to the client's ability to complete a specific task. This focus is the second goal for activity analysis. The intent is to identify whether the activity is well suited to promote change in the underlying skills or abilities deemed to be the focus of intervention. This approach to activity analysis is directly related to the postulates regarding change that were identified in the selected frame of reference.

Activity analysis enables occupational therapy practitioners to determine an activity's therapeutic properties so that they can make an appropriate match between the client's interests and abilities and the activity that will meet the client's health needs (Mosey, 1986) and established intervention goals. Activity analysis can be approached from many perspectives, depending on the reason for the analysis and the specific focus of interest. Trombly and Scott (1977) proposed that performance areas be analyzed first. Cynkin and Robinson

(1990) proposed that practitioners begin an activity analysis with the performance context. Chapter 6, "Activity Synthesis as a Means to Structure Occupation," states that activity analysis assesses the person, activity, and context. For example, a practitioner who works in a hand therapy practice would begin by analyzing activity-based motor and sensory skills; hence, activities used in the clinic would be selected on the basis of how they address specific deficits. An activity analysis should also consider the person's present, past, and future occupations.

In 2003, Crepeau described three levels of activity analysis: (1) activity analysis, (2) theory-based activity analysis, and (3) occupation-based activity analysis. An *activity analysis* investigates the demands of the activity and the hypothetical influence of context and personal meaning. *Theory-based activity analysis,* not unlike Mosey's (1981) restricted analysis, asks the occupational therapy practitioner to determine the therapeutic use of an activity on the basis of practice theory. Crepeau (2003) stated that activity analysis and theory-based activity analysis are done in the abstract. Only *occupation-based activity analysis* studies the person "engaging in occupations within [that person's] unique physical, cultural, and social environment" (p. 192).

We believe that the three-part "Occupation Analysis Process" as presented in this chapter can be used for any of these three analyses. However, when all three parts of our occupation analysis are completed, they will satisfy the description of an occupation-based activity analysis.

Occupational Therapy's Perspectives on Activity and Occupation Analysis

Traditionally, occupational therapy students focused on learning how to do activity analysis and learning the aspects of dividing an activity into its component parts. These students learned to analyze an activity by focusing on the performance of the activity's individual *tasks,* that is, the steps necessary to complete the activity. This process of microanalysis often led the student and, subsequently, the practitioner to not consider the whole activity, the context in which the person usually performs it, and the important occupation with which the activity is associated. Occupational therapy students learning how to do activity analysis need to be able to identify more than just the fact that the skill is present; they need to know to what degree this skill is used in the context of the activity being performed. Therefore, today, it is more common for the student and practitioner to focus on occupation analysis. What is the distinction?

Activity analysis is a neutral examination of an activity divided into its component parts. When a practitioner does an activity analysis, he or she is interested in breaking down the components to understand the decontextualized activity (Crepeau, Schell, Gillen, & Scaffa, 2014). For example, a practitioner might be interested in knowing what is required to saw a board. He or she examines the sensory, physical, cognitive, and social requirements of completing the activity itself. Activity analysis is neutral because it is not specific to a particular person or situation; it is only concerned with an examination of the activity itself. Thus, the occupational therapy practitioner is able to decide whether he or she can use an activity as part of an intervention.

Occupation analysis is concerned with understanding the activity in context. In other words, the occupational therapy practitioner examines the performance of an activity in relation to roles of the client and in the client's natural environment. This analysis is from the client's unique perspective. The practitioner centers the occupation analysis on how a person with his or her unique experiences and abilities performs the activity in his or her natural environment, or *in context*. The occupation analysis recognizes that personal attributes, environment, previous experiences, personal beliefs and values, and other factors determine a person's performance of an activity. This perspective also recognizes that activities and tasks together form an occupation when the person performing them assigns meaning to them.

The following example illustrates the difference between activity and occupation analysis. Occupational therapy students were assigned the analysis of buying a greeting card. One student bought a birthday card for her grandfather. She explained the meaning of the activity: "Before I began college my mother purchased birthday cards for my grandfather. Only once I began living on my own and started earning some money from part-time jobs did I take over this responsibility. Therefore I now view participation in this activity as a sign of my adulthood and independence" (Snow, 2013, p. 13). In addition, she related the purchase to fulfilling one of her responsibilities of her role as granddaughter. Another student's analysis of the same task was completely different because it had little meaning to him. He explained that he does not buy cards but sends personal text messages instead. For this student, buying a card was an activity analysis, not an occupation analysis.

Occupation Analysis Process

The occupation analysis process includes examining both activities and the contexts in which a person performs them. This process is drawn from various sources within the occupational therapy literature, including *Uniform Terminology for Occupational Therapy* (3rd ed.; AOTA, 1994), *Occupational Therapy Practice Framework: Domain and Process* (2nd ed.; AOTA, 2008), *Occupational Therapy Practice Framework: Domain and Process* (3rd ed.; AOTA, 2014), and *International Classification of Functioning, Disability and Health* (*ICF*; World Health Organization [WHO], 2001). In addition, many of the ideas presented have become common knowledge within occupational therapy; therefore, it is impossible to determine with whom these ideas or concepts originated (Allen, 1987; Ayres, 1983; Kremer, Nelson, & Duncombe, 1984; Llorens, 1973, 1986; Mosey, 1981; Neistadt, McAuley, Zecha, & Shannon, 1993; Nelson, 1996; Pedretti & Wade, 1996). The occupational analysis outline includes an activity description, the personal context, and client factors; a multicomponent analysis; and a summary that relates the activity to the person (see Appendix 4.A, "Occupation Analysis Form").

Occupation Analysis

This section describes the occupation, personal context, client factors, and context that influence the person's ability to perform it, including both internal and external characteristics.

Description of the Occupation and Its Related Activities

The occupational therapy practitioner begins the occupation analysis by describing the occupation and how a person would perform it under usual circumstances. In this section, the occupation is named and the specific sequence of steps required to perform it is described. Each step is identified in the order in which it is performed to complete the full occupation and describe it in detail. In addition, the following considerations are made concerning the time needed to complete the occupation or perform individual steps:

- Can the person complete the occupation in one session?
- Can the person perform the occupation over time?
- Does the activity naturally divide into segments so that a person can perform it over time?
- Do the steps in the activity require that it be performed over a period of time?

The required objects, materials, tools, equipment, and their properties; physical space demands and environment; and safety precautions and contraindications are also identified.

Personal Context, Client Factors, and Context

While conducting an evaluation, the occupational therapist appraises the activity relative to personal context, including demographic data collected from the occupational profile; its meaning, value, and relevance to the person's present, past, and future roles and occupations; and client factors (values, beliefs, and spirituality). The therapist also appraises the activity relative to the context (e.g., social, cultural, temporal, virtual) in which the client will perform it. For example, does the person perform the occupation alone or with others, and how does culture affect performance? When the occupational therapy practitioner is using occupation analysis as part of an intervention, he or she should keep the whole person in mind, that is, how and why the activity is relevant to the person.

The occupational therapy practitioner identifies ideas or beliefs that are important to the person. Which of the following features could influence the person's participation or engagement in an activity?

- The person's inferred personal value for the occupation

- The person's underlying meaning associated with the occupation
- The person's perceived purpose of the occupation
- The occupation's ability to meet a desired need
- The occupation's ability to promote independence or self-reliance
- The occupation's ability to address a personal challenge or facilitate desired change
- The occupation's potential to facilitate exploration of life's meaning.

The practitioner can use the analysis to identify whether the occupation incorporates skills that can be associated with a desired role.

Multicomponent Activity Analysis

In this section, we describe the multicomponent activity analysis, including physical signs that influence the person's ability to perform the activity.

Required Knowledge, Abilities, and Skills

A key consideration of the analysis is the practitioner's understanding of the knowledge, abilities, and skills required for a person to complete the activity. The *ICF* (WHO, 2001) concerns people's ability to participate in activities and society. Its taxonomy is divided into two broad categories: (1) functioning and disability and (2) contextual factors. According to the *ICF*, functioning and disability include two components: (1) body function and structures and (2) activities and participation. Contextual factors include personal factors and environmental factors that influence performance of the activity and the level of participation. The broad categories of required action and performance skills (AOTA, 2014; WHO, 2001) serve as a framework for the occupation analysis presented in this chapter. We do not use the *ICF* taxonomy in its entirety; rather, we limit its use to categories that we determined were most relevant to the process of occupation analysis.

The *ICF* (WHO, 2001) taxonomy provides a broad structure for the analysis and the basis for identifying basic requirements of an activity. The occupational therapy practitioner identifies whether a specific skill is necessary during the performance of the activity (requiring a yes or no answer). A "yes" response indicates that the performance skill will need to be focused on in the subsequent sections of the analysis form. On the basis of the client's performance (AOTA, 1994), the practitioner determines the level of influence that each element has on the client's ability to do the activity. Eventually, the practitioner must understand how impairment affects or challenges the client's performance of the activity. Another reason for analyzing an activity is to identify its potential for providing stimulation or opportunities to use specific skills as part of intervention. A 5-point scale can be used to rate the influence of each element:

- 0 = *Component has no effect or influence on the ability to do the activity.*
- 1 = *Component has only a minimal effect or influence on the ability to do the activity.* The activity would not substantially stimulate or address the performance component element.
- 2 = *Component has a moderate effect or influence on the ability to complete the activity.* If a client has a deficit, compensation may have to be made for the client to perform the activity. The activity would present a challenge to the performance component element.
- 3 = *Component has a substantial effect or influence on the ability to complete the activity.* The activity would be extremely difficult to complete if the client has a deficit in this performance component. The activity would present a substantial stimulation or opportunity to address the performance component element.
- 4 = *Component has a major effect or influence on the completion of the activity.* A performance component deficit in this area would seriously influence the person's ability to do the activity. Such a person would be very likely not to be able to complete the activity. The activity would present

a major stimulation or opportunity to address this performance component element.

The observation section is used to describe special circumstances or concerns and provides space to include any other comments a practitioner has relative to performance.

In the next section, we define each skill and provide several questions that an occupational therapy practitioner would consider when assessing the role the skill plays in completing the activity. These questions are not definitive but rather a starting point when considering each skill or action. After considering each question, the practitioner rates the skill's or action's influence and writes observational notes (Exhibit 4.1).

Learning and Applying Knowledge (Sensory–Perceptual Skills)

Occupational therapy practitioners also analyze activities in relation to their sensory processing demands. *Sensory processing* is the internal mechanism a person uses to process and respond to sensory input. A person's central nervous system processes sensory information and integrates this information, so he or she can make an adaptive response. Sensory processing may influence the client's ability to reach a calm state of alertness, affecting his or her ability to engage in and complete an activity. Each activity presents unique sensory processing requirements. Therefore, the ability to organize and integrate multiple sensory processes during performance (i.e., for *adequate response*) of an activity is critical.

Knowledge is what is learned. *Learning* is based on thinking, solving problems, and making decisions. Learning is also influenced by sensory experiences. Activities are about applying knowledge for

---

Exhibit 4.1. Practitioner's Observational Notes

Skill:	
Level of influence	Observations
☐ 0	
☐ 1	
☐ 2	
☐ 3	
☐ 4	

a meaningful outcome. The first step to examining this aspect of the activity is to consider what the activity requires the person to do. This screening gives the practitioner guidance about which components need to be analyzed further. Answering the following questions guides practitioners to the next step of the analysis:

- Does the activity require watching (using the sense of seeing intentionally to experience visual stimuli, such as watching a sporting event or children playing)? Visual reception is the underlying prerequisite.
- Does the activity require listening (using the sense of hearing intentionally to experience auditory stimuli, such as listening to music or a lecture)? Auditory processing is the underlying prerequisite.
- Does the activity require other purposeful sensing (using the body's other basic senses intentionally to experience stimuli, such as touching and feeling textures, tasting sweets, or smelling flowers)? Tactile, proprioceptive, vestibular input, olfactory, and gustatory senses may need to be examined.

Sensory processing

Questions to ask about sensory processing include

- Does the activity require the person to make changes on the basis of sensory input?
- Does continuity of performance depend on the ability to proceed on the basis of sensory input?
- Is the ability to end performance based on sensory processing (e.g., physical discomfort, a problem with the activity)?
- What degree of sensory modulation is required?
- Will an adverse response influence performance (e.g., defensiveness)?
- Will a diminished response influence the activity?

Visual reception

Visual reception involves decoding stimuli through the eyes, including peripheral vision, acuity, and awareness of color and pattern. Questions to ask include

- Does the activity require the person to fixate on a stationary object (*visual fixation*)?
- Does the activity require slow, smooth movements of the eyes to maintain fixation on a moving object (*visual tracking*)?

- Must the person rapidly change fixation from one object in the visual field to another (*scanning*; e.g., locating a misplaced utensil during cooking, locating a dropped object while performing a sport)?
- What degree of discrimination of fine detail (i.e., *acuity*) is required to do the activity?
- Does the activity require changes in focus such as from near to far?

Auditory processing

Auditory processing involves interpreting and localizing sounds and discriminating among background sounds. Questions to ask include

- Does the activity require the person to listen to sounds and interpret their meaning (e.g., musical notes, verbal instructions, verbal communication, warning sounds [e.g., alarm buzzers])? Are there functional sounds that assist the person with monitoring the environment (e.g., water running, frying, opening sounds, traffic, closing sounds)?
- Does the activity produce loud or harsh sounds during its performance (e.g., hammering, power tools)? Could these sounds be stressful to the person?
- Does the activity environment require the person to discriminate or suppress background sounds?
- Does the person use or rely on sound while moving (e.g., search for a source of sound and move toward it)?

Tactile processing

Tactile processing involves interpreting light touch, pressure, temperature, pain, and vibration through skin contact and receptors. Questions to ask include

- Does the activity require the person to hold objects gently, or is a degree of pressure important?
- Are the materials used at room temperature, or do they require heat or cooling?
- Does the activity require the person to appreciate or tolerate vibration (e.g., electric tools)?
- Does the activity require tactile discrimination?
- Are body parts always within the visual field? When must a person rely on tactile input?
- Could the tactile properties of the activity be perceived as noxious (e.g., eliciting defensiveness)?
- Is the ability to localize tactile input part of the task?

Proprioceptive processing

Proprioceptive processing involves interpreting stimuli originating in muscles, joints, and other internal tissues that give information about the position of one body part in relation to another. Questions to ask include

- Does the activity distract (separate) or compress joints and tissues?
- Is weight bearing part of the activity (lower extremities or upper extremities)?
- What is the degree of pushing, pulling, or lifting that occurs during the activity?
- Do movements and position of the extremities occur outside the visual field (reaching in or out)?

Vestibular input

Vestibular input—interpreting stimuli from the inner ear receptors regarding head position—contributes to appropriate righting and equilibrium reactions, automatic postural responses, and maintaining posture and movement during activity performance. Questions to ask include

- Does the activity require quick movements of the head or body?
- Does the activity require postural maintenance or change in relation to gravity or acceleration and deceleration forces (e.g., sit to stand, sudden change in forward movement, vertical or horizontal changes)?
- Does the activity require muscular co-contraction?
- Does the activity require coordinated eye movements?
- Does the activity require postural background movements (e.g., adequate extension; ability to dissociate head, neck, and arm movements)?

Olfactory processing

Olfactory processing involves interpreting odors. Questions to ask include

- Does the activity involve odors that might be interpreted as noxious?
- Does the activity involve odors that might be alerting (e.g., burning) or calming?
- How might the scents affect one who is overresponsive to odors?

Gustatory processing

Gustatory processing involves interpreting tastes. Questions to ask include

- Does the person need to interpret taste to enhance or contribute to performance?
- Does the taste or texture elicit an overresponsive reaction?

Basic Learning

Basic learning encompasses the skill areas of copying and rehearsing. Answering the following questions guides the occupational therapy practitioner to the next step of the analysis:

- Does the activity require *copying* (imitating or mimicking as a basic component of learning, such as copying a gesture, a sound, or the letters of an alphabet)? Prerequisites to be examined are recognition, form constancy, spatial relations, and position in space.
- Does the activity require *rehearsing* (repeating a sequence of events or symbols as a basic component of learning, such as counting by 10s or practicing the recitation of a poem)? Sequencing is the prerequisite skill.

Recognition

Recognition involves identifying familiar faces, objects, and/or other previously presented material, which requires recall of salient features. One question to ask is

- Does the person have to recognize people, body parts, and objects to engage in the activity?

Form constancy

Form constancy involves recognizing forms and objects as being the same in various environments, positions, and sizes. Questions to ask include

- Does the activity occur in two dimensions or three?
- Does the activity require the person to respond to changing representations of objects?
- Do the materials change form (e.g., laundry hanging on a line or folded)?
- Does the size of the tools, utensils, or letters change?

Spatial relations

Spatial relations involve determining the position of objects relative to one another. Questions to ask include

- Does the activity require the use of spatial concepts (manipulation, take apart, put together)?
- Does the activity require the person to estimate sizes?
- Does the activity require the person to judge distances or estimate size?
- Does the activity require orientation of shapes, sizes, or designs?
- Does the activity require attention to detail in positioning?

Position in space

Position in space refers to determining the spatial relationship of figures and objects to the self and other forms and objects. Questions to ask include

- Does the activity require the person to determine front, back, top, bottom, beside, behind, under, or over?
- Does the activity require that the person understand the relationship between action and his or her body?

Sequencing

Sequencing involves placing information, concepts, and actions in order. Questions to ask include

- Does the activity require the person to arrange items or perform steps in a serial order?
- Does the activity require an understanding of before and after?
- Does the activity require the person to *reverse a sequence* (i.e., going from forward to backward and vice versa; e.g., put on clothing or take it off, put a toy together or take it apart)?
- Does the activity allow the person to have personal choice in the manner of sequencing (e.g., morning care, dressing, showering)?

Acquiring Skills

Engaging in an activity creates situations in which people gain skills. *Skills* are the sets of actions that a person has learned and is able to apply in given situations.

Skills are often divided into basic and complex skills. *Basic skills* are elementary and purposeful actions, such as learning to manipulate eating utensils, a pencil, or a simple tool. *Complex skills* are integrated sets of actions to follow rules and to sequence and coordinate movements, such as learning to play games such as football or to use a building tool. Answering these questions provides guidelines to the occupational therapy practitioner for the next step of the analysis:

- Occupational therapy practitioners must often assess a person's cognitive abilities before determining his or her capacity to learn or apply knowledge. Does the activity require the participant to focus intentionally on specific stimuli, such as filtering out distracting noises? Level of arousal, orientation, sensory modulation, and attention span must be considered.
- Does the person have adequate skills to support the efficient completion of the activity? Consider motor control, praxis, body scheme, ocular motor control, oral–motor skill, fine motor coordination and dexterity, visual–motor integration, crossing the midline, right–left discrimination, laterality, and bilateral integration.
- When engaged in the activity, what thinking processes does the activity require the person to use (formulating and manipulating ideas, concepts, and images—whether goal oriented or not—either alone or with others, such as creating fiction, providing a theorem, playing with ideas, brainstorming, meditating, pondering, speculating, reflecting)? Consider memory, categorization, concept formation, spatial operations, learning, and generalization.
- Solving problems requires that a person find solutions to problems or challenges to complete the activity. Simple problems involve a single issue or question. Solving complex problems requires the person doing the activity to consider multiple and interrelated issues or several related problems. To solve problems related to activities, a person must identify and analyze issues, develop solutions, evaluate potential effects of the solutions, and execute the chosen solution. Therefore, learning and memory must be examined.
- Making decisions requires choosing among options, implementing the choice, and evaluating the effects of that choice. Consider memory, concept formation, categorization, and generalization.

Level of arousal

Level of arousal includes demonstrating alertness and responsiveness to environmental stimuli. Questions to ask include

- Does the time of day influence the person's arousal level?
- What arousal level is needed to provide an adequate length of time to complete the activity?
- Do fatigue and pain factors affect arousal level and the ability to attend to the task?

Orientation

Orientation includes identifying the person, place, time, or situation. In orientation to person, questions to ask include

- Does the activity relate to the person's lifestyle?
- Is the activity associated with a role that is meaningful to the person?
- Could the activity be influenced by the person's routines (e.g., clean the bathroom on Tuesday, clean the bathroom when it needs cleaning)?

In orientation to place, one question to ask is

- Does the activity require the person to know where he or she is?

In orientation to time, one question to ask is

- Does the person need to know the exact time, date, or time of year to engage in the activity?

In orientation to situation, questions to ask include

- What is the relationship between the activity and the person's environment and roles?
- Does the person need to understand the circumstances in which the activity is performed?
- Does the person understand time restrictions or demands placed on performance?

Sensory modulation

Sensory modulation involves the ability to respond appropriately to incoming stimuli. Questions to ask include

- Does the person overrespond to sensory stimuli (e.g., showing sensory defensiveness, becoming overly stressed by stimuli)?
- Does the person underrespond to sensory stimuli (e.g., does not appear to register stimuli, is slow to respond)?
- Does the person seek out sensory stimuli (e.g., rocking, excessive mouthing of objects, spinning)?

Attention span

Attention span refers to the ability to focus on a task over time. Questions to ask include

- How long must the person attend?
- Will the person be required to selectively attend (e.g., focus on specific stimuli) or disregard irrelevant stimuli?
- Does the activity demand sustained attention?
- Does the activity require the person to shift attention (e.g., frying eggs, making toast, pouring coffee while cooking)?

Motor control

Motor control involves using functional and versatile movement patterns. Questions to ask include

- Does the activity require repetition? If so, what kind (e.g., putting a puzzle together, catching a ball)?
- Do numerous joints need to be controlled during a complex activity?
- Does the activity require the person to inhibit movements to be most efficient (e.g., using scissors)?
- Does the activity require constant or variable changes in speed, tempo, or rhythm (e.g., dealing cards, playing jacks)?
- Is the pace of the activity externally or internally controlled?
- Does the activity require manipulation and control of tools or utensils (e.g., the person must control the tool and the limb)?

Praxis

Praxis involves conceiving and planning a motor act in response to an environmental demand. Questions to ask include

- Does the activity require the person to assume a novel position (*postural praxis;* e.g., yoga, martial arts, dance routines for the novice)?
- Does the activity require the person to plan movements that are not habitual?
- Does the activity involve the use of new tools or utensils?
- Does engagement require the person to have a plan?
- Is the activity new and unusual for the person?

Body scheme

Body scheme refers to having an internal awareness of the body and the relationship of body parts to each other. This component is closely related to kinesthesia and proprioception because it requires integration of sensation from muscles and joints. Questions to ask include

- Does the activity require that the person have an appreciation for his or her body and be able to sense how the different parts work together (e.g., playing basketball)?
- Does the activity require the person to have an internal awareness of body actions that must happen in a specific sequence (e.g., ballroom dancing)?

Ocular–motor control

Ocular–motor control refers to the ability to move the eyes to focus on and follow objects. One question to ask is

- Is the person able to fixate on a stationary object and track a moving object with smooth pursuits?

Oral–motor skill

Oral–motor skill refers to use of muscles in and around the mouth. One question to ask is

- Is the person able to coordinate tongue, lips, and jaw for the purposes of clear speech or feeding?

Fine motor coordination and dexterity

Fine motor coordination and dexterity involve using small muscle groups for controlled movements, particularly in-hand object manipulation. Questions to ask include

- What degree of isolated finger use is required?
- Which grasp patterns are used during different functions?
  - *Hook:* Fingers alone, without use of the thumb and palm (e.g., holding a briefcase)
  - *Cylindrical:* Fingers and thumb close and flex around the object, which is stabilized against the palm of the hand (e.g., holding a hammer)
  - *Spherical:* Hold a ball
  - *Three-jaw chuck:* Thumb against pads of index and middle finger (e.g., grasping a block)
  - *Lateral pinch:* Thumb against lateral side of the index (e.g., holding a key)
  - *Tip-to-tip pinch:* Thumb tip to index or middle finger (e.g., picking up a grain of rice).
- Is speed a necessary element of the activity?

Visual–motor integration

Visual–motor integration refers to the ability to coordinate the interaction of information from the eyes and body movement. One question to ask is

- What degree of eye–hand or eye–foot coordination is required (e.g., tracing, copying, pencil tasks, balance beam)?

Crossing the midline

Crossing the midline involves moving the limbs and eyes across the *midline sagittal plane* (i.e., plane that divides the body into right and left halves) of the body. Questions to ask include

- Does the activity require the person to scan the environment to find tools and utensils? If so, how frequently?
- Does the activity require that the person cross the midline of the body with his or her arms or legs (e.g., dressing)?

Right–left discrimination

Right–left discrimination refers to differentiating one side of the body, space, object, or other person from the other. Questions to ask include

- What degree of bilateral coordination is required to do the activity?
- Does the person need to be able to use or apply right–left concepts?

- Does the activity require that the person be able to follow verbal or written directions that require actions to the left, right, or both sides of the body?
- Does the activity involve tools that require bilateral coordination, such as the use of one hand as a stabilizer or assist while the other hand operates the tool?
- Does the activity require the person to differentiate right and left on another person (e.g., following demonstrated instruction as in martial arts, dancing)?

Laterality

Laterality refers to using a preferred or dominant hand or foot. Questions to ask include

- Does the activity require a high degree of skill in which the person needs to use a preferred hand or foot (e.g., cooking, sewing, writing)?
- Does hand or foot preference influence how smoothly or effortlessly the person performs the activity?

Bilateral integration

Bilateral integration refers to coordinating both sides of the body. Bilateral integration is considered a prerequisite for gross and fine motor coordination and affects acquisition of skills. Questions to ask include

- How frequently do both sides of the body have to cooperate during the activity?
- Does one side of the body need to stabilize while the other side acts?
- Does the activity require crossing the midline in a rotatory, asymmetrical pattern (e.g., golf, baseball swing)?
- Does the activity require that the person use both sides of the body in the same manner (*symmetrical performance;* e.g., pushing, pulling)?
- Does the activity require *reciprocal patterns,* that is, a corresponding action with the other extremity (e.g., bike riding, swimming, running, martial arts)?

Memory

Memory entails recoding information after a brief or long period. Questions to ask include

- What are the activity's memory requirements, for example, immediate (1 minute), short-term (>1 minute, <1 hour), or long-term (>1 hour)?
- If the activity requires long-term memory, what sensory processing skills are needed?
- What information related to personal experience (*episodic memory*) is needed for the activity?
- What factual knowledge of the world (*semantic memory*) is needed for the activity?
- What knowledge of the world or how to do something (*procedural memory*) is needed for the activity?
- Is the long-term memory modality specific (e.g., visual, auditory, verbal)?

Categorization

Categorization refers to identifying similarities and differences among pieces of environmental information. Questions to ask include

- Does the activity require the person to group objects or information according to characteristics (e.g., visual features, tactile features, similarities, differences)?
- Does the activity require mental grouping (e.g., playing cards, different name brands to be purchased, price differences, nutritional contents)?
- Does the activity require construction in which the person must understand how parts relate to a whole or how to break the whole down into its parts?

Concept formation

Concept formation refers to organizing a variety of information to form thoughts and ideas. This component is related to the ability to categorize. Questions to ask include

- Does the activity require synthesis of ideas (e.g., formulation of a hypothesis about the how or why)?
- Does the activity require abstract thought processes?
- Does the activity require symbolic thinking?
- Does the activity require the person to question himself or herself or evaluate performance?

Spatial operations

Spatial operations involve mentally manipulating the position of objects in various relationships. Questions to ask include

- Does the activity require the person to mentally visualize different perspectives (e.g., two-dimensional diagrams, three-dimensional objects)?
- Does the activity involve mental visualization of performance?
- Does the activity require that the person visualize how the object or activity should look on completion (e.g., clothing on a hanger or self, how a table will be set for a dinner party, how a cake will look after baking)?

Learning

Learning refers to acquiring new concepts and behaviors. Questions to ask include

- Does the activity provide a structured or unstructured learning experience?
- Does the activity provide feedback about performance?
- What type of learning is expected (e.g., motor, verbal, emotional, attitudinal)?

Generalization

Generalization refers to applying previously learned concepts and behaviors to a variety of new situations. Questions to ask include

- Can the activity be performed in different contexts (e.g., bathing at bedside, sponge bathing at sink, tub bathing)?
- Does the activity provide opportunities to apply learned skills to a new situation?

General Activity Demands

Completing an activity requires that people carry out simple or complex and coordinated actions. These actions are related to mental, physical, and social factors. Some actions produce a single simple activity that is clearly defined or time limited, such as initiating or terminating the activity. Single complex tasks need to be carried out in sequence or simultaneously, such as arranging the furniture in one's home or completing an assignment for school. Moreover, activities are influenced by the people who participate in them. Consideration of the following information guides practitioners to the next step of the analysis:

- A person's mental and physical status influences how he or she carries out simple or complex activities. Prerequisite components to be examined are initiation of activity, time management, termination of activity, coping skills, and self-control.
- Some activities are composed of multiple tasks that need to be carried out in sequence or simultaneously, such as preparing a multicourse meal, with each course requiring initiation and management of time. Space to prepare a salad, main course, and side dishes must be organized, and several tasks may occur together or sequentially. The salad ingredients and vegetables are washed together, and a sequence of peeling and chopping vegetables and salad ingredients must occur to complete the activity. Prerequisite components to be examined are initiation of activity, time management, termination of activity, coping skills, and self-control.
- Simple, complex and multiple activities may be carried out independently or within a group setting. When they occur independently, prerequisite components to be examined are initiation of activity, time management, termination of activity, coping skills, and self-control. When tasks occur in a group, also examine social skills and interpersonal skills.

Initiation of activity

Initiation of activity refers to starting a physical or mental activity. Questions to ask include

- Does the activity require the person to self-start?
- Does the person have to plan the start (e.g., alarm clock)?
- Is the activity motivated by personal meaning and relevance?
- How would the person's mental health status affect the performance of this activity?

Time management

Time management involves anticipating, planning, and using parcels of time as they relate to completion of activities. Questions to ask include

- Is the activity performed in one session or multiple sessions?
- Are there set time constraints for portions of the activity (e.g., bake at 350° for 30 minutes)?

- Is the activity part of a personal routine that has self-imposed time restrictions (e.g., morning care consisting of 10 minutes each for showering, dressing, and grooming)?
- Does the activity allow for choices about the use of time (e.g., a craft project in which the detailing could require additional time because of increased interest or skill level)?
- Does the activity require organization and setting realistic priorities to complete it?

Termination of activity

Termination of activity refers to stopping an activity at an appropriate time. Questions to ask include

- What is the person's control over engaging in and disengaging from the activity?
- Is the activity time limited?
- Is the activity rote or repetitive?

Coping skills

Coping skills involve identifying and managing stress and related factors. Questions to ask include

- Is this activity new for the person or is it part of an established personal routine?
- Are parts of the activity automatic and therefore less stressful (e.g., habitual)?
- Does the activity environment influence the perceived stress?
- Does the activity provide an appropriate level of challenge without promoting undue stress?
- Does the activity require exactness, or is there a range of acceptable performance?
- Is performance of the activity externally or internally controlled?

Self-control

Self-control involves modifying one's own behavior in response to environmental needs, demands, and constraints; personal aspirations; and feedback from others. Questions to ask include

- Should mishaps in the activity or environment be expected?
- Does the outcome of the activity lead to attainment of goals?
- Do the activity demands require the person to modify performance in response to changes in the environment?

- Will the person be required to respond to feedback about performance (e.g., criticism or praise)?
- To what degree does the activity challenge physical, social, or cognitive ability?

Social skills

Social skills involve interacting while using manners, personal space, eye contact, gestures, active listening, and self-expression appropriate to one's environment and satisfying to oneself and others. Questions to ask include

- In what type of social environment does the activity occur?
- Does the activity require cooperative behavior?
- What are the accepted personal boundaries of the activity (e.g., while playing sports, playing at a card table)?
- Does the social environment present expectations concerning appropriate interaction and communication (e.g., with authority figures, peers)?
- Does the activity require the person to initiate and sustain appropriate communication?
- Does the activity require the person to initiate or answer questions or make suggestions?

Interpersonal skills

Interpersonal skills involve using verbal and nonverbal communication to interact in a variety of settings. Questions to ask include

- Does the activity require independence, cooperation, or competition?
- What degree of verbal interaction or casual conversation is required?
- Does the activity require active verbal and nonverbal participation?
- Does the activity require expression of emotions?
- Does the activity require specific nonverbal behavior (e.g., appropriate sitting posture, signs of active listening, changes in facial expression, use of appropriate gestures)?
- Does the activity require the person to assume an unfamiliar interaction style?
- Does the activity require the person to recognize and respond to others' nonverbal behavior?

Mobility

Mobility involves changing body positions or location by transferring from one place to another;

by carrying, moving, or manipulating objects; by walking, running, or climbing; and by using various forms of transportation. Changing and maintaining body position may occur during performance of the activity. An assessment of mobility begins with an examination of muscle tone. Prerequisite performance components to be examined are postural alignment, postural control, depth perception, and body strength. The following questions guide the occupational therapy practitioner to the next step of the analysis:

- Does the activity require changes in body positions?
- Does the activity require sufficient muscle tone to allow movement into or against the forces of gravity?
- When completing specific tasks, must one get into or out of a particular body position?
- Does the activity require moving from one location to another, such as getting up from a chair to lie down on a bed and getting into and out of kneeling or squatting positions?
- Does the activity require the person to transfer from one surface to another?
- What degree of control does the person need to move from one surface to another?

Postural alignment

Postural alignment refers to maintaining the biomechanical integrity among body parts. Questions to ask include

- What degree of *axial alignment* (i.e., vertical orientation of the head, neck, and spine) does the activity require?
- Does the pelvic position change during performance of the activity (e.g., when taking off shoes)?
- Does the activity require frequent changes in alignment (e.g., when reading while seated, playing racquetball)?
- What postures are needed to optimally perform the activity?

Postural control

Postural control involves using righting and equilibrium reactions to maintain balance during functional movements. Questions to ask include

- Does the activity have the potential for a sudden displacement of the center of gravity?
- Do changes in the base of support occur while engaging in the activity?
- Does head position change frequently?
- Must the person stabilize against the forces of gravity when engaged in the activity (i.e., lean forward, lean back, lean to the side)?
- Does the activity require the person to anticipate postural adjustments?

Depth perception

Depth perception involves determining the relative distance between objects, figures, or landmarks and the observer and changes in planes and surfaces. Questions to ask include

- Does the person have to reach distances to acquire objects or complete the activity?
- Does the person need to place body parts in relation to changing elements of the environment (e.g., step up or down)?

Body strength

Body strength refers to the degree of muscle power required to complete the activity. Questions to ask include

- How does gravity influence the performance of the activity?
- Does the activity provide resistance to movement of the body?
- Does the activity require *concentric* (i.e., shortening contraction), *eccentric* (i.e., lengthening contraction), or *isometric muscle contraction* (i.e., contraction without length change)?

Carrying, Moving, and Handling Objects

Completing many activities requires that a person be able to handle, move, and manipulate objects with his or her upper extremities and hands. Movements may be gross or fine or a combination of both. Sometimes, the actions demand intricate, coordinated finger movements. Other actions require lower-extremity strength and control. Answering the following questions guides practitioners to the next step of the analysis:

- Are any of the following upper-extremity movements done while performing the activity: pulling, pushing, reaching, throwing, or catching? Prerequisite components to be examined are range of motion, extremity strength, and endurance.
- Must the person move and manipulate objects with his or her upper extremities? Prerequisite skills for upper-extremity control are range of motion, extremity strength, endurance, stereognosis, kinesthesia, and figure–ground perception.
- Must the person carry or transport objects while walking? Prerequisite skills are range of motion, extremity strength, endurance, and topographical orientation.
- What type of grasp or prehension patterns are needed to carry, move, or handle the object?

Range of motion

Range of motion refers to actively moving body parts through an arc of motion. Questions to ask include

- What movements are required of the head, neck, and trunk during the activity?
- What degree of range of motion is required of the extremities during the activity (most critical to performance)?
- Which joints are positioned statically, and which joints are active?
- Does the activity require the person to control movements at multiple joints?
- Where are rotational movements required?
- Are there any soft-tissue conditions that would affect range of motion, such as *hypermobility* (i.e., joints that stretch farther than normal) or *hypomobility* (i.e., a decrease in the normal movement of joints)?

Extremity strength

Extremity strength refers to the grade of muscle strength required in the extremities to complete the activity. Questions to ask include

- How does gravity influence the performance of the activity?
- Does the activity require concentric, eccentric, or isometric muscle contraction?

Endurance

Endurance involves sustained cardiac, pulmonary, and musculoskeletal exertion over time. Questions to ask include

- What is the duration of the activity (time)?
- How repetitive is the activity?
- Are portions of the activity resistive?
- Does fatigue occur as a result of the activity?

Stereognosis

Stereognosis involves identifying objects through proprioception, cognition, and the sense of touch. Questions to ask include

- Does the activity require the hands or feet to identify or manipulate objects without reliance on vision (e.g., reaching into a pocket to find a coin, reaching into a drawer)?
- Do aspects of the activity require visual vigilance that may call for the person to find, manipulate, or reach for objects outside the visual field (e.g., sewing on a machine)?

Kinesthesia

Kinesthesia involves identifying the *amount* and direction of movement. Questions to ask include

- Does the activity require movements to be coordinated over multiple joints?
- Does the activity require visual attention so that the person must rely on the ability to move without the aid of vision (e.g., swinging a bat at a baseball, playing tennis, playing basketball)?
- Does the activity require the person to change directions of movements (e.g., fingers during typing)?

Grasp patterns

Grasp patterns are the gross movements of the hand involving the fingers and thumb used to hold objects. Questions to ask include

- What specific grasp patterns (i.e., hook, cylindrical, spherical, three-jaw chuck, lateral pinch, tip-to-tip pinch) are used to complete the activity?
- Does the person demonstrate age-appropriate grasp patterns?

Prehension patterns

Prehension involves refined movements of the thumb, index, and middle finger to pinch and grasp. Questions to ask include

- What specific pinch patterns (i.e., three-jaw chuck, lateral pinch, tip-to-tip pinch) are required to complete the activity?
- Does the person demonstrate age-appropriate prehension patterns?

Fine motor skill

Fine motor skill refers to the ability to use small hand muscles and joints to perform refined actions. Questions to ask include

- What kind of fine motor actions (e.g., manual dexterity, control) does the activity require?
- Does the activity require in-hand manipulation of small objects or small tool use?
- Does the activity require small, joint-isolated movements (e.g., movement of the thumb into the palm of the hand)?

Figure–ground perception

Figure–ground perception involves differentiating between foreground and background forms and objects. Questions to ask include

- Does the activity require the person to distinguish an object or image from a complex background (e.g., word-search games, finding hidden objects)?
- Does the activity require the person to discriminate among two- or three-dimensional figures to complete tasks?
- Does the activity require the person to locate objects from a cluster of objects (e.g., food in a refrigerator, clothes in a closet, an item in a junk drawer)?

Topographical orientation

Topographical orientation refers to determining the location of objects and settings and the route to the location. Questions to ask include

- Does the activity require the person to follow a familiar route or negotiate unfamiliar surroundings?

- Does the activity require the person to retrace routes from spatial memory?
- Does the activity rely on the person's ability to identify visual landmarks?

Occupation Analysis Summary

The summary serves as a tool for the occupational therapy practitioner to reflect on and analyze the information culled from the analysis. This section is particularly useful when the practitioner is using the analysis to determine whether the activity is appropriate for intervention (*occupation-as-means*) strategy—meaning, the goal of intervention is the person's ability to engage in the occupation. When the analysis is complete, consider the following three questions in relation to the client:

1. *Is the goal of the occupation or activity relevant to the person?* As presented in Chapter 1, "Occupation, Activities, and Occupational Therapy," it is critical to determine whether the activity will allow the person to be an active participant based on his or her present abilities and whether the activity can provide a challenge that will improve skills and abilities during the intervention process. The practitioner decides whether the activity will contribute to the development of competence and mastery of the environment. Information gained from the occupational profile provides the foundation for the person's personal meaning and value of potential activities, guides the practitioner's exploration and analysis of potential therapeutic activities, and provides the context in which the activity will take place (Henderson et al., 1991).
2. *Is the occupation part of the person's habits, routines, or rituals?* An analysis for a particular person does not occur in isolation. An occupational therapy practitioner should give consideration to the process of engaging in the selected activity. Does the activity encompass basic, automatic behaviors (*habits*) and routines? Does the sequence provide structure for engagement in occupations? Has the person assigned symbolic meaning to the activity or portions of the occupation?
3. *Is the activity of interest to the person, and does it provide an opportunity for self-expression or*

enhance self-efficacy? The occupational therapy practitioner considers whether engagement in the activity enables the person to explore his or her interests and needs. When using an intervention, the person's capacities and potential for change are also weighed (Evans, 1987). Consider the following:

- How does the activity stimulate the person?
- Is it repetitive?
- Does it offer opportunities for self-expression?
- Does it offer an appropriate degree of challenge (e.g., cognitive, motor)?
- What are possible attractions to participating in the activity?
- What are the positive feelings associated with the activity (e.g., physical challenge, fellowship with others, intellectual challenge, demonstration of capacity or creativity)?
- Does the activity facilitate development of self-efficacy or a sense of competence?

Exercise 4.1. Example of an Occupation Analysis

Review Appendix 4.B. How does the occupation analysis document the activity of repotting a plant? How would an occupational therapy practitioner use this information?

Exercise 4.2. Analysis of a Daily Life Activity

Consider the activity of frying an egg for breakfast or folding clothes. Think about the way in which you normally do the activity. Follow the process outlined in this section. The purpose of this assignment is to appreciate that everything you do is potentially a therapeutic activity. Through the analysis, you learn the component pieces outside the context of the real world of activities. In practice, occupational therapy practitioners perform activity analysis with consideration of the client's real activities, the context in which they are performed, and the meanings that the activities have for the client.

Occupation and Activity Analysis Within a Frame of Reference

Activity analysis is a tool that occupational therapy practitioners use to determine an activity's thera-

peutic potential. As such, this analysis provides the means for understanding the client and his or her ability to perform specific purposeful activities. Up to this point, activity analysis has been described as a process to examine or analyze specific activities. When occupation analysis, however, is used within the context of a frame of reference, a guideline for practice, or a conceptual framework, the framework provides the guidelines for the activity analysis. For example, if the practitioner is working with a client with left hemiparesis, the client most likely has intact language skills. After screening the client, the practitioner determines that the client's postural control, sitting and standing balance are fair and that he has problems with upper-extremity motor control. On the basis of this information, the practitioner determines that the *neurodevelopmental treatment approach* (i.e., frame of reference that involves direct handling and guidance to optimize function) is most appropriate to restore postural control and balance. Given that the client wants to dress himself, the practitioner evaluates his performance of upper-body dressing, which is best done by having the client attempt to dress. The practitioner then does an occupation analysis of the way the client performs the activity, with special attention given to his neuromotor functioning.

Before observing the client attempting various activities, the occupational therapy practitioner does an activity analysis of the typical performance of the various purposeful activities involved in upper-body dressing, which involves knowing the skills necessary for upper-body dressing. For example, a button-down shirt presents different challenges than a pullover shirt. In the case of the client with left hemiparesis for whom the neurodevelopmental treatment approach has been selected to guide intervention, the practitioner attends to the motor and sensory demands of the trunk and upper extremities during dressing. The practitioner uses the frame of reference to guide the focus needed as the client attempts to complete the occupation.

Summary

The ability to analyze an occupation or activity competently is a critical piece of an occupational therapy practitioner's repertoire. Without the ability to analyze activities, the practitioner is left to use trial and error to plan and carry out interventions with clients. In this chapter, we described the development of activity and occupation analysis over the years. No doubt, further developments will occur as the profession evolves. The ability, however, to analyze an activity in the context of the person and his or her life enables both the client and the practitioner to reach agreement on goals for the client. The chapter includes a comprehensive outline to approach an activity or occupation analysis for the occupational therapy student and practitioner. Although the analysis may seem tedious and difficult to the beginning student, it is a process that gradually becomes integrated into clinical reasoning as an occupational therapy practitioner considers activities as therapeutic intervention tools. Experienced clinicians integrate activity and occupation analysis into the evaluation and treatment process so smoothly that it may not be obvious to the novice practitioner.

Acknowledgment

We thank Sunny M. Dawson, a graduate student at New York University, Class of 2014, for providing the activity analysis of her personal experience of repotting a jade plant.

References

Allen, C. K. (1987). Activity: Occupational therapy's treatment method [1987 Eleanor Clarke Slagle Lecture]. *American Journal of Occupational Therapy, 41,* 563–575. http://dx.doi.org/10.5014/ajot.41.9.563

American Occupational Therapy Association. (1994). Uniform terminology for occupational therapy (3rd ed.). *American Journal of Occupational Therapy, 48,* 1047–1054. http://dx.doi.org/10.5014/ajot.48.11.1047

American Occupational Therapy Association. (2008). Occupational therapy practice framework: Domain and process (2nd ed.). *American Journal of Occupational Therapy, 62,* 625–683. http://dx.doi.org/10.5014/ajot.62.6.625

American Occupational Therapy Association. (2014). Occupational therapy practice framework: Domain and process (3rd ed.). *American Journal of Occupational Therapy, 68*(Suppl.1), S1–S48. http://dx.doi.org/10.5014/ajot.2014.682006

Ayres, A. J. (1983). *Sensory integration and the child.* Los Angeles: Western Psychological Services.

Creighton, C. (1992). The origin and evolution of activity analysis. *American Journal of Occupational Therapy, 46,* 45–48. http://dx.doi.org/10.5014/ajot.46.1.45

Crepeau, E. B. (2003). Analyzing occupation and activity: A way of thinking about occupational performance. In E. B. Crepeau, E. S. Cohen, & B. A. Boyt Schell (Eds.), *Willard and Spackman's occupational therapy* (10th ed., pp. 189–198). Philadelphia: Lippincott Williams & Wilkins.

Crepeau, E. B., Schell, B. A. B., Gillen, G., & Scaffa, M. E. (2014). Analyzing occupations and activity. In B. A. B. Schell, G. Gillen, & M. E. Scaffa (Eds.), *Willard and Spackman's occupational therapy* (12th ed., pp. 234–248). Philadelphia: Wolters Kluwer Health/Lippincott Williams & Wilkins.

Cynkin, S., & Robinson, A. M. (1990). *Occupational therapy and activities health: Toward health through activity.* Boston: Little, Brown.

Dunton, W. R., & Licht, S. (1957). *Occupational therapy principles and practice.* Springfield, IL: Charles C Thomas.

Evans, K. A. (1987). Definition of occupation as the core concept of occupational therapy. *American Journal of Occupational Therapy, 41,* 627–628. http://dx.doi.org/10.5014/ajot.41.10.627

Fidler, G. S. (1948). Psychological evaluation of occupational therapy activities. *American Journal of Occupational Therapy, 2,* 284–287.

Henderson, A., Cermak, S., Coster, W., Murray, E., Trombly, C., & Tickle-Degnen, L. (1991). Occupational science is multidimensional. *American Journal of Occupational Therapy, 45,* 370–372. http://dx.doi.org/10.5014/ajot.45.4.370

Hinojosa, J. (1996). Practice makes perfect. *OT Practice, 1,* 34–38.

Hopkins, H. L., & Smith, H. D. (1978). *Willard and Spackman's occupational therapy* (5th ed.). Philadelphia: Lippincott.

Kremer, E. R., Nelson, D. L., & Duncombe, L. W. (1984). Effects of selected activities on affective meaning in psychiatric patients. *American Journal of Occupational Therapy, 38,* 522–528. http://dx.doi.org/10.5014/ajot.38.8.522

Licht, S. (1947). Kinetic analysis of crafts and occupations. *Occupational Therapy and Rehabilitation, 26,* 75–78.

Llorens, L. A. (1973). Activity analysis for cognitive–perceptual–motor dysfunction. *American Journal of Occupational Therapy, 27,* 453–456.

Llorens, L. A. (1986). Activity analysis: Agreement among factors in a sensory processing model. *American Journal of Occupational Therapy, 40,* 103–110. http://dx.doi.org/10.5014/ajot.40.2.103

Mosey, A. C. (1981). *Occupational therapy: Configuration of a profession.* New York: Raven.

Mosey, A. C. (1986). *Psychosocial components of occupational therapy*. New York: Raven Press.

Neistadt, M. E., McAuley, D., Zecha, D., & Shannon, R. (1993). An analysis of a board game as a treatment activity. *American Journal of Occupational Therapy, 47,* 154–160. http://dx.doi.org/10.5014/ajot.47.2.154

Nelson, D. L. (1996). Therapeutic occupation: A definition. *American Journal of Occupational Therapy, 50,* 775–782. http://dx.doi.org/10.5014/ajot.50.10.775

Pedretti, L. W., & Wade, I. (1996). Therapeutic modalities. In L. W. Pedretti (Ed.), *Occupational therapy practice skills for physical dysfunction* (pp. 293–317). St. Louis: Mosby.

Reed, K. L. (1986). Tools of practice: Heritage or baggage? [1986 Eleanor Clarke Slagle Lecture]. *American Journal of Occupational Therapy, 40,* 597–605. http://dx.doi.org/10.5014/ajot.40.9.597

Snow, D. (2013). *Activity analysis.* Unpublished manuscript, New York University.

Trombly, C. A., & Scott, A. D. (1977). *Occupational therapy for physical dysfunction*. Baltimore: Williams & Wilkins.

U.S. Department of War. (1944). *Occupational therapy.* Washington, DC: U.S. Government Printing Office.

World Health Organization. (2001). *International classification of functioning, disability and health.* Geneva: Author.

Appendix 4.A. Occupation Analysis Form

Part 1: Occupation Analysis

Description of the occupation:

Sequence (steps) of occupation. (*Note.* Include as many steps as necessary.)

1.

2.

3.

Time needed to complete the occupation or perform individual steps:

Required objects, materials, tools, equipment, and their properties:

Physical context (environment and space demands):

Safety precautions and contraindications:

Personal context, client factors, and context include

- Personal information (e.g., age, gender, socioeconomic status, education):
- The activity's meaning, value, and relevance to the person's present, past, and future roles and occupations:
  - Present:
  - Past:
  - Future:
- Client factors (values, beliefs, spirituality):
- Context (social, cultural, temporal, and virtual conditions within and around the person that influence performance)
  - Social:
  - Cultural:
  - Temporal (time):
  - Virtual:

Part 2: Activity Analysis

Required Knowledge, Abilities, and Skills

Check "yes" or "no" to indicate whether the activity requires watching, listening, or other purposeful sensing. Next, rate each element's influence according to the following scale:

- 0 = *Component has no effect or influence on the ability to do the activity.*
- 1 = *Component has only a minimal effect or influence on the ability to do the activity.* The activity would not substantially stimulate or address the performance component element.

Note. Courtesy of Karen A. Buckley, MA, OT/L, and Sally E. Poole, OTD, OT/L, CHT. Used with permission.

(Continued)

- 2 = *Component has a moderate effect or influence on the ability to complete the activity.* If a client has a deficit, compensation may have to be made for the client to perform the activity. The activity would present a challenge to the performance component element.
- 3 = *Component has a substantial effect or influence on the ability to complete the activity.* The activity would be extremely difficult to complete if the client has a deficit in this performance component. The activity would present a substantial stimulation or opportunity to address the performance component element.
- 4 = *Component has a major effect or influence on the completion of the activity.* A performance component deficit in this area would seriously influence the person's ability to do the activity. Such a person would be very likely not to be able to complete the activity. The activity would present a major stimulation or opportunity to address this performance component element.

Learning and Applying Knowledge (Sensory–Perceptual Skills)

Activity requires	Yes	No	Focus on
Watching			Visual reception, sensory processing
Listening			Auditory processing, sensory processing
Other purposeful sensing			Tactile, proprioceptive, olfactory, gustatory, and sensory processing, and vestibular input

Sensory processing—Internal mechanism used by the person to process and respond to sensory input

Level of influence	Observations:
☐ 0 ☐ 1 ☐ 2 ☐ 3 ☐ 4	

Visual reception—Decoding stimuli through the eyes, including peripheral vision, acuity, and awareness of color and pattern

Level of influence	Observations:
☐ 0 ☐ 1 ☐ 2 ☐ 3 ☐ 4	

Auditory processing—Interpreting and localizing sounds and discriminating among background sounds

Level of influence	Observations:
☐ 0 ☐ 1 ☐ 2 ☐ 3 ☐ 4	

Tactile processing—Interpreting light touch, pressure, temperature, pain, and vibration through skin contact or receptor

Level of influence	Observations:
☐ 0 ☐ 1 ☐ 2 ☐ 3 ☐ 4	

(Continued)

Proprioceptive processing—Interpreting stimuli originating in muscles, joints, and other internal tissues that give information about the position of one body part in relation to another

Level of influence	Observations:
☐ 0 ☐ 1 ☐ 2 ☐ 3 ☐ 4	

Vestibular input—Interpreting stimuli from the inner-ear receptor regarding head position

Level of influence	Observations:
☐ 0 ☐ 1 ☐ 2 ☐ 3 ☐ 4	

Olfactory processing—Interpreting odors

Level of influence	Observations:
☐ 0 ☐ 1 ☐ 2 ☐ 3 ☐ 4	

Gustatory processing—Interpreting tastes

Level of influence	Observations:
☐ 0 ☐ 1 ☐ 2 ☐ 3 ☐ 4	

Basic Learning

Activity requires	Yes	No	Focus on
Copying			Recognition, form constancy, spatial relations, position in space
Rehearsing			Sequencing

Recognition—Ability to identify familiar faces, objects, and other previously presented material

Level of influence	Observations:
☐ 0 ☐ 1 ☐ 2 ☐ 3 ☐ 4	

Form constancy—Recognizing forms and objects as the same in various environments, positions, and sizes

Level of influence	Observations:
☐ 0 ☐ 1 ☐ 2 ☐ 3 ☐ 4	

(Continued)

Spatial relations—Determining the position of objects relative to each other	
Level of influence ☐ 0 ☐ 1 ☐ 2 ☐ 3 ☐ 4	Observations:

Position in space—Determining the spatial relationship of figures and objects to self and other forms and objects	
Level of influence ☐ 0 ☐ 1 ☐ 2 ☐ 3 ☐ 4	Observations:

Sequencing—Placing information, concepts, and actions in order	
Level of influence ☐ 0 ☐ 1 ☐ 2 ☐ 3 ☐ 4	Observations:

Acquiring Skills

Activity requires	Yes	No	Focus on
Basic skills			Motor control, praxis, body scheme, ocular–motor control, oral–motor skill, fine motor coordination and dexterity, visual–motor integration crossing the midline, right–left discrimination, laterality, bilateral integration
Complex skills			
Applying knowledge			Level of arousal, orientation, sensory modulation, attention span
Thinking			Memory, categorization, concept formation, spatial operations, learning, generalization
Solving problems—simple			Learning, memory
Solving problems—complex			
Making decisions			Memory, concept formation, categorization, generalization

Level of arousal—Demonstrating alertness and responsiveness to environmental stimuli	
Level of influence ☐ 0 ☐ 1 ☐ 2 ☐ 3 ☐ 4	Observations:

(Continued)

Orientation—Ability to identify person, place, time, and situation

Level of influence	Observations:
□ 0	
□ 1	
□ 2	
□ 3	
□ 4	

Sensory modulation—Ability to generate responses that are appropriately graded in relation to incoming sensory stimuli

Level of influence	Observations:
□ 0	
□ 1	
□ 2	
□ 3	
□ 4	

Attention span—Focusing on a task over time

Level of influence	Observations:
□ 0	
□ 1	
□ 2	
□ 3	
□ 4	

Motor control—Use of functional and versatile movement patterns

Level of influence	Observations:
□ 0	
□ 1	
□ 2	
□ 3	
□ 4	

Praxis—Conceiving and planning a new motor act in response to an environmental demand

Level of influence	Observations:
□ 0	
□ 1	
□ 2	
□ 3	
□ 4	

Body scheme—Internal awareness of the body and the relationship of body parts to each other

Level of influence	Observations:
□ 0	
□ 1	
□ 2	
□ 3	
□ 4	

Ocular–motor control—Ability to move eyes to focus and follow objects

Level of influence	Observations:
□ 0	
□ 1	
□ 2	
□ 3	
□ 4	

(Continued)

Oral–motor skill—Use of muscles in and around the mouth

Level of influence □ 0 □ 1 □ 2 □ 3 □ 4	Observations:

Fine motor coordination and dexterity—Using small muscle groups for controlled movements, particularly in-hand object manipulation

Level of influence □ 0 □ 1 □ 2 □ 3 □ 4	Observations:

Visual–motor integration—Coordinating the interaction of information from the eyes and body movement

Level of influence □ 0 □ 1 □ 2 □ 3 □ 4	Observations:

Crossing the midline—Moving the limbs and eyes across the midline sagittal plane of the body

Level of influence □ 0 □ 1 □ 2 □ 3 □ 4	Observations:

Right–left discrimination—Differentiating one side from the other

Level of influence □ 0 □ 1 □ 2 □ 3 □ 4	Observations:

Laterality—Use of a preferred or dominant hand or foot

Level of influence □ 0 □ 1 □ 2 □ 3 □ 4	Observations:

Bilateral integration—Coordinating both sides of the body

Level of influence □ 0 □ 1 □ 2 □ 3 □ 4	Observations:

(Continued)

Memory—Recoding information after a brief or long period of time	
Level of influence ☐ 0 ☐ 1 ☐ 2 ☐ 3 ☐ 4	Observations:

Categorization—Identifying similarities and differences among pieces of environmental information	
Level of influence ☐ 0 ☐ 1 ☐ 2 ☐ 3 ☐ 4	Observations:

Concept formation—Involves organizing a variety of information to form thoughts and ideas	
Level of influence ☐ 0 ☐ 1 ☐ 2 ☐ 3 ☐ 4	Observations:

Spatial operations—Mentally manipulating the position of objects in various relationships	
Level of influence ☐ 0 ☐ 1 ☐ 2 ☐ 3 ☐ 4	Observations:

Learning—Acquiring new concepts and behaviors	
Level of influence ☐ 0 ☐ 1 ☐ 2 ☐ 3 ☐ 4	Observations:

Generalization—Applying previously learned concepts and behaviors to a variety of new situations	
Level of influence ☐ 0 ☐ 1 ☐ 2 ☐ 3 ☐ 4	Observations:

General Activity Demands

Activity requires	Yes	No	Focus on
Simple task			Initiation of activity, time management, termination of activity, coping skills, self-control
Complex task			
Multiple tasks			
Independent performance			
Group performance			Social skills, interpersonal skills

(Continued)

Initiation of activity—Starting a physical or mental activity

Level of influence	Observations:
☐ 0 ☐ 1 ☐ 2 ☐ 3 ☐ 4	

Time management—Ability to manage parcels of time as they relate to the performance of tasks or activities

Level of influence	Observations:
☐ 0 ☐ 1 ☐ 2 ☐ 3 ☐ 4	

Termination of activity—Stopping an activity at an appropriate time

Level of influence	Observations:
☐ 0 ☐ 1 ☐ 2 ☐ 3 ☐ 4	

Coping skills—Identifying and managing stress-related factors such as anger, disappointment, or frustration

Level of influence	Observations:
☐ 0 ☐ 1 ☐ 2 ☐ 3 ☐ 4	

Self-control—Modifying one's own behavior in response to environmental needs, demands, constraints, personal aspirations, and feedback from others

Level of influence	Observations:
☐ 0 ☐ 1 ☐ 2 ☐ 3 ☐ 4	

Social skills—Involves interacting by using manners, personal space, eye contact, gestures, active listening, and self-expression appropriate to the situation

Level of influence	Observations:
☐ 0 ☐ 1 ☐ 2 ☐ 3 ☐ 4	

Interpersonal skills—Involves using verbal and nonverbal communication skills appropriately

Level of influence	Observations:
☐ 0 ☐ 1 ☐ 2 ☐ 3 ☐ 4	

(Continued)

Mobility

Activity requires	Yes	No	Focus on
Changing and maintaining body position			Postural alignment, postural control, depth perception, body strength
Transferring oneself			

Postural alignment—Maintaining biomechanical integrity among body parts	
Level of influence ☐ 0 ☐ 1 ☐ 2 ☐ 3 ☐ 4	Observations:

Postural control—Using righting and equilibrium reactions to maintain balance during functional movements	
Level of influence ☐ 0 ☐ 1 ☐ 2 ☐ 3 ☐ 4	Observations:

Depth perception—Involves determining the relative distance between objects, figures, or landmarks and the observer and changes in planes and surfaces	
Level of influence ☐ 0 ☐ 1 ☐ 2 ☐ 3 ☐ 4	Observations:

Body strength—Degree of gross muscle power when body movement is resisted or is against gravity	
Level of influence ☐ 0 ☐ 1 ☐ 2 ☐ 3 ☐ 4	Observations:

Carrying, Moving, and Handling Objects

Activity requires	Yes	No	Focus on
Lifting			Range of motion, extremity strength, endurance
Carrying			
Fine hand use			Range of motion, extremity strength, endurance, stereognosis, kinesthesia, figure–ground perception, grasp patterns, prehension patterns, fine motor skills
Hand and arm use			
Moving objects with lower extremities			Range of motion, extremity strength, endurance
Walking and moving			Range of motion, extremity strength, endurance, topographical orientation

(Continued)

Range of motion— Moving body parts through an arc of motion	
Level of influence ☐ 0 ☐ 1 ☐ 2 ☐ 3 ☐ 4	Observations:

Extremity strength—Grade of muscle strength when body movement is resisted or is against gravity	
Level of influence ☐ 0 ☐ 1 ☐ 2 ☐ 3 ☐ 4	Observations:

Endurance—Sustained cardiac, pulmonary, and musculoskeletal exertion over time	
Level of influence ☐ 0 ☐ 1 ☐ 2 ☐ 3 ☐ 4	Observations:

Stereognosis—Identifying objects through proprioception, cognition, and sense of touch	
Level of influence ☐ 0 ☐ 1 ☐ 2 ☐ 3 ☐ 4	Observations:

Kinesthesia—Identifying the excursion and direction of movement	
Level of influence ☐ 0 ☐ 1 ☐ 2 ☐ 3 ☐ 4	Observations:

Grasp patterns—Identifying the type(s) of grasp required to perform the activity	
Level of influence ☐ 0 ☐ 1 ☐ 2 ☐ 3 ☐ 4	Observations:

Prehension patterns—Identifying the type(s) of pinch required to perform this activity	
Level of influence ☐ 0 ☐ 1 ☐ 2 ☐ 3 ☐ 4	Observations:

(Continued)

Fine motor skill—Ability to use small hand muscles and joints to perform refined actions	
Level of influence ☐ 0 ☐ 1 ☐ 2 ☐ 3 ☐ 4	Observations:

Figure–ground perception—Differentiating between foreground and background forms and objects	
Level of influence ☐ 0 ☐ 1 ☐ 2 ☐ 3 ☐ 4	Observations:

Topographical orientation—Determining the location of objects and settings and the route to the location	
Level of influence ☐ 0 ☐ 1 ☐ 2 ☐ 3 ☐ 4	Observations:

Part 3: Occupation Analysis Summary

Once you have completed the analysis, consider the following:

1. Is the goal of the occupation or activity relevant to the person?

2. Is the occupation part of the person's habits, routines, or rituals?

3. Is the activity of interest to the person, and does it provide an opportunity for self-expression or enhance self-efficacy?

Appendix 4.B. Occupation Analysis Form: Repot a Plant

Part 1: Occupation Analysis

Description of the occupation:

My occupation is repotting a plant. I chose to repot a 6-inch jade plant from a small plastic container into a larger plastic container. This activity is personally relevant, allowing me to engage in a meaningful leisure activity and fulfill a valued role as a gardener. This activity is also functionally relevant to promote the growth of the plant. Although I have past experience repotting plants outdoors, I had to make adjustments to perform this activity within the context of a small New York City apartment that has no outdoor space.

Sequence (steps) of occupation:

Assuming I've set up my workspace (jade plant in its current pot, new pot, hand shovel, and cup of water placed on top of a piece of spread-out newspaper; open bag of soil placed on the newspaper on my left-hand side) and seated myself in a comfortable side-sitting position on the floor, I follow these steps (with the time taken included):

1. I visually compare the size of the new pot with its current pot and decide I need to fill my new pot roughly two-thirds full of soil. (3 seconds)
2. I grasp the shovel's handle with my right hand, and crossing my midline, dig into the bag of soil using my left hand to make the opening of the bag as wide as possible. (3 seconds)
3. I bring the shovel full of soil toward the new pot, moving my left hand to grip the side of new pot and stabilize it while I fill it with the soil from my shovel. (4 seconds)
4. I repeat Steps 2 and 3 two more times until I have my new pot roughly two-thirds full. (14 seconds)
5. I put down the shovel and with my right hand smooth and pat down the soil. (3 seconds)
6. I reach for and grasp the original pot with my right hand and set it on top of the soil in the new pot to see if I need more soil. The soil level in the current pot is level with the lip of the new pot, so I decide I do not need to add more soil. (4 seconds)
7. I take the jade plant out with my right hand, holding it about 1 foot above the ground, gently pinch the stem with my left thumb and index finger, and squeeze the container a couple times while leaning the plant to the side. (3 seconds)
8. Supporting the stem and some of the attached soil with my left hand, I use my right hand to remove the container completely and set it down. (2 seconds)
9. I hold the plant horizontally in my left hand and use my right fingers to pinch and remove about one-third of the soil from the bottom of the plant, being careful not to damage any hanging roots and letting the residual dirt drop into the original pot below. (18 seconds)
10. I place the jade plant into the new pot and then use both hands to center it. (5 seconds)
11. Holding the centered plant with my left hand, I pick up the shovel with my right, reach across my midline, scoop a large amount of soil, bring it back to the new pot, and gently let it slide down and fill in the gaps while I rotate the new pot counterclockwise. I rotate in this direction and reach for five more scoops of soil until the entire round is full and the plant is standing independently. Some soil spills during this step. (37 seconds)
12. I put the shovel down and use index and middle fingers from both hands to pack the soil down in and around the jade plant. (8 seconds)
13. I pick up the shovel again with my right hand and retrieve one more large scoop of soil. (3 seconds)

Note. Courtesy of Sunny Dawson, Occupational Therapy Student. Used with permission.

(Continued)

14. I turn the container counterclockwise with my left hand and slowly add in the soil until it reaches about a 1/2 inch below the lip of the new pot all the way around. (8 seconds)
15. I use both hands to pack down the soil, making sure the plant is standing upright and the soil is even across the pot. (10 seconds)
16. To remove any air pockets, I lift the pot with both hands a few inches from the ground and let it thump on the floor. I repeat this two more times. (4 seconds)
17. I use my right hand to reach for and grip the cup of water, bring it close to the new pot, and pour about a 1/2 cup across the entire surface of the soil. I use my left hand to stabilize the pot. (4 seconds)

Time needed to complete the occupation or perform individual steps:
Two minutes, 19 seconds, is the time it took me to repot my jade plant. A larger pot that requires a greater amount of soil would increase the time it takes to retrieve soil from the bag, assuming a similar sized hand shovel was used.

Required objects, materials, tools, equipment, and their properties:
I used the following objects to complete this activity:

- One full-page newspaper sheet measuring 24 inches wide by 23 3/4 inches long, laid on the floor to serve as my repotting stage and catch any falling soil
- One newly opened bag of potting soil weighing 3.7 pounds, packaged in a plastic bag, with components of hypnum peat, compost, aged pine bark, sand, and perlite
- One hand shovel measuring 9 inches long, made up of a 4-inch wooden handle and 5-inch steel trowel that comes to a sharp point
- A plastic cup holding about 1 cup of room-temperature water
- One 6-inch jade plant (*Crassula ovata*), a common houseplant that has thick stems and round, green, waxy leaves potted in a dark green plastic pot measuring 3 inches tall and 3 inches in diameter with three evenly spaced drainage holes in the bottom
- One empty dark green plastic pot measuring 3 3/4 inches tall and 4 1/2 inches in diameter with eight evenly spaced drainage holes in the bottom, approximately 3 times the volume of the smaller container.

Physical context (environment and space demands):
Repotting a plant can be done indoors or outdoors and requires a surface to set your materials. Given the constraints of my apartment (no outdoor space, no free tabletop surface) and the small size of the plant, I completed this activity inside on the wooden floor of my living room. This space provided adequate room for me to spread out the newspaper, place the materials on top of the paper, and position myself in a side-sitting position directly in front of my workspace. Sitting provided enough vertical height over the plant I chose to repot.

Safety precautions and contraindications:
I am aware of the sharp point of the hand shovel and grasp it only by the wooden handle. I set it down flat and position the trowel's point away from my body when it is not in use. The jade plant does not have thorns, but others should be cautious when handling a plant that has thorns or spines on the leaves or stems. Gardener's gloves should be used in that case to prevent cuts or pricks.

Personal context, client factors, and context:
- Personal information (e.g., age, gender, socioeconomic, education):
  I am a 26-year-old female, currently enrolled in a full-time graduate occupational therapy program. I grew up in a middle-class family in Hawaii. I live in a two-bedroom apartment in Brooklyn shared among myself, my boyfriend, and another roommate. I spend my free time attending concerts, trying

(Continued)

new restaurants, and exploring New York City attractions. I am in the slow process of decorating and furnishing our apartment.

- **The activity's meaning, value, and relevance to the person's present, past, and future roles and occupations:**
  - *Present:*

    Just having a few houseplants has allowed me to participate in the role of gardener. Repotting my plants is a productive leisure activity that makes me feel more connected to the natural world. Because I am currently in the stages of decorating my apartment, this activity is very meaningful because I hope to cover my windowsills in houseplants. It is springtime now, and seeing the trees and blossoms out in my neighborhood and around New York University has contributed to my enthusiasm for acquiring more flora. Lately, when I've bought plants, I've needed to repot them into larger containers to promote growth come summertime. One of my roommates also likes to smoke a cigarette on occasion (with the window open, thankfully), so I hope that the plants will help remove any residual toxins from the air.

  - *Past:*

    Previously, I was an active gardener in my California apartment with an outdoor patio where I kept many potted plants, including flowers, herbs, and vegetables. I also relate this activity to growing up as a daughter of a gardener. My mother had a huge influence on the meaning and value I attach to growing and surrounding myself with plants. My former roommate would tell our visitors that I had the green thumb, so I identified greatly with the role of gardener.

  - *Future:*

    In the future, I would like to continue participating in my role as a gardener and expand my current collection of houseplants. This activity will also lend itself to my role as a friend, when I am able to use the cuttings to propagate my plants as gifts. This activity will also contribute to my role as a partner to my boyfriend, an aspiring chef, because I hope to grow more herbs and vegetables to cook with in the future. I would also like to get a few tomato and basil plants and try to grow them on the roof of my apartment. In the distant future, I would love to do this on a grander scale (in an outdoor garden) to provide for my future family, especially because my boyfriend is an aspiring chef and cooking with fresh ingredients is ideal.

- **Client factors (values, beliefs, spirituality):**

  I believe that having plants in my living space makes me a happier and healthier person. I appreciate the aesthetics of plants and flowers and also their air-filtering purposes. Thus, I value the activities that are involved in taking care of plants and flowers, including the task of repotting a plant. Not only is it functional—in terms of the health and growth of the plant—but I also value it as a leisure activity. I find it visually stimulating, relaxing, and I like getting my hands dirty and feeling the textures of the soil (hence, why I choose not to wear gloves). I also find it adds to my self-efficacy and feelings of productivity because it is done in a short amount of time. However, I only find the activity necessary when the plant has outgrown its current pot, and I want it to continue to grow. For some plants, I am content with their current size and would not choose to repot them.

- **Context (social, cultural, temporal, and virtual conditions within and around the person that influence performance):**
  - *Social:*

    This activity—repotting a single plant—is usually completed alone. If there are multiple plants to be repotted or if the plant is particularly heavy, you may enlist the help of others. If performed with others, they might expect you to follow their preferred method or sequence, they may prefer a specific brand of soil, or they could expect the use of additional tools. My social environment involves two

(Continued)

roommates and friends I've made in my neighborhood and at school. I performed this activity alone while both of my roommates were at work.

o *Cultural:*

I grew up in Hawaii, a very tropical, lush environment. We had a large yard with many garden spaces and trees and also kept some plants indoors. As a child, some of my chores included watering the houseplants, weeding the garden, and picking the fresh fruits and vegetables. I enjoyed helping my mom in the gardens and came to value the role of gardener early on. Eating locally and taking care of the natural environment is also a huge part of the Hawaiian culture. This background contributed to my desire to surround myself with plants, especially because my neighborhood has very little green space.

o *Temporal (time):*

Temporal conditions contributed to my participation in this activity. It is now spring; the weather has finally warmed, and all the trees and flowers are beginning to grow leaves and bloom. Spring is the best time to repot plants in anticipation of the growth period that happens during the long, hot summer days. I am more personally motivated by the warmer weather because my plants are more likely to survive. I made a point to perform this activity on a specific day of the week (the day I water all my other plants) to preserve my watering routine and work this jade plant into that scheme. I also like participating in the role of caregiver and, at this stage in my life, plants are the easiest living thing to care for (as opposed to a pet or a child).

o *Virtual:*

Virtual conditions did not influence my completion of this activity.

Part 2: Activity Analysis

Required Actions, Knowledge, Abilities, and Skills

Check "yes" or "no" to indicate whether the activity requires watching, listening, or other purposeful sensing. Next, rate each element's influence according to the following scale:

- *0 = Component has no effect or influence on the ability to do the activity.*
- *1 = Component has only a minimal effect or influence on the ability to do the activity.* The activity would not substantially stimulate or address the performance component element.
- *2 = Component has a moderate effect or influence on the ability to complete the activity.* If a client has a deficit, compensation may have to be made for the client to perform the activity. The activity would present a challenge to the performance component element.
- *3 = Component has a substantial effect or influence on the ability to complete the activity.* The activity would be extremely difficult to complete if the client has a deficit in this performance component. The activity would present a substantial stimulation or opportunity to address the performance component element.
- *4 = Component has a major effect or influence on the completion of the activity.* A performance component deficit in this area would seriously influence the person's ability to do the activity. Such a person would be very likely not to be able to complete the activity. The activity would present a major stimulation or opportunity to address this performance component element.

Learning and Applying Knowledge (Sensory–Perceptual Skills)

Activity requires	Yes	No	Focus on
Watching	X		Visual reception, sensory processing
Listening		X	Auditory, sensory processing
Other purposeful sensing	X		Tactile, proprioceptive, olfactory, gustatory, and sensory processing, and vestibular input

(Continued)

Sensory processing—Internal mechanism used by the person to process and respond to sensory input	
Level of influence ☐ 0 ☐ 1 ☐ 2 ☐ 3 X 4	Observations: • I need to coordinate the following sensory inputs efficiently to complete this activity: visual, tactile, proprioceptive, and vestibular. • I used visual input to estimate how much soil I needed for my new pot. • I relied on proprioceptive input in lifting and handling the objects appropriately and efficiently. • I used vision, touch, and proprioception carefully to remove the plant from its pot. • I depended on my proprioceptive and tactile input when packing down soil to know whether I needed to pack more or move on to the next step. • If someone has an adverse tactile response to dirt, completion of this activity (without gloves) would be difficult. • Diminished vision would affect the time it took to complete this activity, but one could probably still perform it relying primarily on touch. • Diminished tactile input would affect all grasps, pinches, and the pressure needed to hold objects or pack down soil.

Visual reception—Decoding stimuli through the eyes, including peripheral vision, acuity, and awareness of color and pattern	
Level of influence ☐ 0 ☐ 1 ☐ 2 X 3 ☐ 4	Observations: • The activity required I fixate on each of my materials as I used them. • I used visual tracking to follow the shovel into and out of the soil bag and when I emptied the soil into the pot. • I had to quickly scan my workspace when I needed to use my shovel and when I needed to grasp the plant in its original container, the water cup, and so forth. • I needed to be able to discriminate fine details such as the level of soil in my pot, where I should pinch my plant, the roots of the plant, and the water level in the new pot as I poured. • I needed to visually determine the center of the new pot and stand my plant in an upright supported position. • I did not need to focus from near to far because all the materials I needed were within my reach.

Auditory processing—Interpreting and localizing sounds and discriminating among background sounds	
Level of influence X 0 ☐ 1 ☐ 2 ☐ 3 ☐ 4	Observations: • I did not need to listen or interpret sounds to complete the activity. • There were only a couple of sounds I produced during the activity, but they had no effect on completing the task. They included rustling of the bag as I retrieved soil and a few thuds when I purposely dropped the plant in its new pot to the ground to remove air pockets. • I did not need to suppress any background sound because it was quiet in my apartment.

(Continued)

Tactile processing—Interpreting light touch, pressure, temperature, pain, and vibration through skin contact or receptor	

Level of influence
☐ 0
☐ 1
☐ 2
☐ 3
X 4
	Observations:
	• I held different objects with varying degrees of pressure:
	   o Gentle when handling the plant itself
	   o Some pressure to grasp the empty new pot
	   o Greater amount of pressure to grasp the heavier shovel, plant in its pot, and water cup.
	• I needed to squeeze the original pot a couple of times to remove it from the plant. It was a small, young plant so it did not take much pressure to loosen it from the pot.
	• I depended on tactile input from my left hand to stabilize and keep the plant upright in its new pot while I retrieved soil with the shovel in my right hand.
	• I also relied on tactile input when packing down the soil—once it was fairly solid, I stopped packing it down.
	• I used tactile input to differentiate between soil and roots when I was removing excess soil from the bottom of the plant.
	• All materials were room temperature.
	• Some might not enjoy this activity if they do not like handling soil or getting their hands dirty.

Proprioceptive processing—Interpreting stimuli originating in muscles, joints, and other internal tissues that give information about the position of one body part in relation to another	
Level of influence ☐ 0 ☐ 1 ☐ 2 ☐ 3 X 4	Observations: • I am weight-bearing on my pelvis in my side-seated position. • The shovel and added soil place weight on my right upper extremity, and when I hold the plant in my hand, it places weight on my left upper extremity. • The only movement that occurs outside of my visual field is when I reach into the depths of the soil bag, I cannot see the entire way down and must judge by proprioceptive input if I am retrieving enough soil. • I repeatedly lift the shovel with and without added soil, the plant, and the water cup. • I compress the joints in my hands and wrist when I apply pressure to pack down the soil in and around the plant. • I need to be able to coordinate the proprioceptive input to make my movements efficient.

Vestibular input—Interpreting stimuli from the inner ear receptor regarding head position	
Level of influence ☐ 0 ☐ 1 ☐ 2 X 3 ☐ 4	Observations: • I found myself making quick and subtle head movements depending on where my gaze focused—I turned my head to the left whenever I reached for soil—and the action being performed. • In my side-sitting position, it was important for me to maintain an upright posture to be engaged in the activity and manipulate the objects with my upper extremities. • When I leaned the plant to the side to remove the pot, I moved my torso, head, and neck simultaneously, almost mimicking the action of the plant. • There were no sudden movements or changes in movement necessary. • I needed to coordinate my hand–eye movements the entire time.

Olfactory processing—Interpreting odors	
Level of influence ☐ 0 X 1 ☐ 2 ☐ 3 ☐ 4	Observations: • I did not attend to any smells during my activity, though the soil does have some earthy fragrance to it. Neither the soil nor the plant were fragrant enough to warrant a reaction. • In other circumstances, the plant or soil might be fragrant and have either a desirable (i.e., sweet-smelling flower) or off-putting (i.e., if the soil has rotted components or manure) effect.

(Continued)

Gustatory processing—Interpreting tastes	
Level of influence X 0 ☐ 1 ☐ 2 ☐ 3 ☐ 4	Observation: • I did not use taste when I performed this activity.

Basic Learning

Activity requires	Yes	No	Focus on
Copying	X		Recognition, form constancy, spatial relations, position in space
Rehearsing	X		Sequencing

Recognition—Ability to identify familiar faces, objects, and other previously presented material	
Level of influence ☐ 0 ☐ 1 X 2 ☐ 3 ☐ 4	Observation: • I recognized all components and objects involved in my activity: newspaper, soil, shovel, jade plant, pots, water.

Form constancy—Recognizing forms and objects as the same in various environments, positions, and sizes	
Level of influence ☐ 0 ☐ 1 X 2 ☐ 3 ☐ 4	Observations: • The activity occurs in three dimensions. • I needed to make sure the new pot was bigger than the original pot. (They were made of the same material and were the same color.) • I needed to respond to the change in level of soil in the new pot as I filled it. • I was also aware of the change in form I initiated when removing excess soil from the plant. • I needed to recognize that when I poured the water, it would pool but eventually disappear into the soil surrounding the plant.

Spatial relations—Determining the position of objects relative to each other	

Level of influence
☐ 0
☐ 1
☐ 2
☐ 3
X 4
	Observations:
	• Almost all objects (except the bag of soil and the discarded original pot) had some sort of relationship to the plant or the new pot, not limited to the following:
	  • new pot and shovel when filling it with soil
	  • new pot and plant when judging soil level and positioning
	  • plant and shovel when filling in gaps with more soil
	  • water cup and new pot and plant.
	• I also made sure the newspaper spread out was large enough to encompass all my tools and materials in case of spills.
	• I had to estimate visually the space in the new pot that I needed to fill with soil.
	• This activity required I pay attention to detail when pinching and handling the plant, positioning it in the center of the new pot, filling the gaps in the new pot with soil, and watering the plant without disturbing it.

(Continued)

Position in space—Determining the spatial relationship of figures and objects to self and other forms and objects	
Level of influence ☐ 0 ☐ 1 ☐ 2 ☐ 3 X 4	Observations: • I needed to initially position myself within reaching distance to all of my tools and supplies. • I needed to determine the sides, top, and bottom of the pots, plant, shovel, and soil bag to manipulate them effectively. I am always holding or stabilizing an object or tool throughout the entire activity. • I needed to understand the relationship of the shovel and my hand when retrieving soil, as well as the position of the plant when I needed to remove the original pot and the excess soil. • I needed to understand the relationship of the plant to its new pot to center it efficiently and fill the gaps with additional soil.

Sequencing—Placing information, concepts, and actions in order	
Level of influence ☐ 0 ☐ 1 ☐ 2 X 3 ☐ 4	Observation: • I performed this activity in a specific sequence I had planned in advance. There might be slight variations in this sequence or added steps, but most of the actions must be followed in the order I did them.

Acquiring Skills

Activity requires	Yes	No	Focus on
Basic skills	X		Motor control, praxis, body scheme, ocular–motor control, oral–motor skill, fine motor coordination and dexterity, visual–motor integration crossing the midline, right–left discrimination, laterality, bilateral integration
Complex skills	X		
Applying knowledge	X		Level of arousal, orientation, sensory modulation, attention span
Thinking	X		Memory, categorization, concept formation, spatial operations, learning, generalization,
Solving problems—simple	X		Learning, memory
Solving problems—complex	X		
Making decisions	X		Memory, concept formation, categorization, generalization

Level of arousal—Demonstrating alertness and responsiveness to environmental stimuli	
Level of influence ☐ 0 ☐ 1 ☐ 2 X 3 ☐ 4	Observations: • Time of day did affect my arousal level—I performed this activity midday just before lunch so I was very awake and alert. I would not choose to perform it very early in the morning or late at night when I am most tired. • This activity requires an alert and focused arousal level to efficiently manipulate the tools, not spill the soil or water, and handle the plant without dropping or damaging it. • I did not fatigue or experience pain, but someone with arthritis in their hands might be distracted from the task.

(Continued)

Orientation—Ability to identify person, place, time, and situation	
Level of influence ☐ 0 ☐ 1 ☐ 2 ☐ 3 X 4	Observations: • Person: This activity directly related to my appreciation for flora and desire to decorate my apartment with plants. It is associated with my role as a gardener, but I view it more in terms of a caretaker role because I am limited to indoor houseplants. I chose to perform this activity on the same day that I water all my plants, to maintain a routine. • Place: I performed the activity in my own apartment and was aware of where I was. I could also perform it in a friend's apartment or outdoor space and still be relatively comfortable. • Time: I did not attend to the time of day. I was aware that it is spring and is an optimal time for repotting a plant (before the summer growth period). I was also aware of the day of the week, because I planned the activity to coincide with my weekly watering routine. • Situation: I needed to be oriented to the activity to be prepared with the appropriate supplies and recall the necessary steps. I needed to understand that the activity should be done fairly quickly so the plant doesn't experience shock.

Sensory modulation—Ability to generate responses that are appropriately graded in relation to incoming sensory stimuli	
Level of influence ☐ 0 X 1 ☐ 2 ☐ 3 ☐ 4	Observations: • Because I performed this activity in my apartment, I did not need to modulate too much external stimuli—it was quiet and I am used to muffled sounds outside my windows, I am visually familiar with the layout, and there were no smells or tastes that interfered. • I anticipated working with soil and getting my hands and fingernails dirty, so I did not need to attend very much to its tactile sensations.

Attention span—Focusing on a task over time	
Level of influence ☐ 0 ☐ 1 ☐ 2 X 3 ☐ 4	Observations: • The activity does not take very long, but I attended to each action for the entire duration. • I needed sustained attention to fill the pot with soil without spilling, handle the plant and pots without damaging them, and pour the water without spilling or overwatering. • Once I had the plant stabilized with my left hand in its new pot, I shifted my attention to grabbing the shovel and retrieving more soil with my right hand.

Motor control—Use of functional and versatile movement patterns	
Level of influence ☐ 0 ☐ 1 ☐ 2 ☐ 3 X 4	Observations: • This activity required that I repeat the action of retrieving soil from the bag with my shovel and emptying the soil into a pot. I also repeated the movement of applying pressure to the soil to pack it down. • I needed to control finger, wrist, elbow, and shoulder joints to do most of the actions required by this activity, including grasping the shovel. • The pace of this activity is controlled internally. I kept a steady pace throughout the entire activity, not speeding up or slowing down and not stopping to take a break.

Praxis—Conceiving and planning a new motor act in response to an environmental demand	
Level of influence ☐ 0 ☐ 1 ☐ 2 X 3 ☐ 4	Observations: • I had to plan movements that are familiar but not habitual, such as digging for soil with a shovel, removing the pot from the plant, and packing down the soil. • I am familiar with using a shovel, but it is not a tool I use often. • I had a planned sequence that I followed during the activity and knew I would need to repeat actions (retrieving soil), but I did not plan a specific number of retrievals in advance.

(Continued)

Body scheme—Internal awareness of the body and the relationship of body parts to each other	
Level of influence ☐ 0 ☐ 1 ☐ 2 X 3 ☐ 4	Observations: • I needed a great appreciation of the upper extremities and how they worked together to initiate both gross and especially fine motor movements. • I maintained an internal awareness of my lower body position, but it was static as I leaned and moved my torso during the activity. It served as a large and comfortable base of support, allowing me to focus most attention on the actions required of my upper extremities.

Ocular–motor control—Ability to move eyes to focus and follow objects	
Level of influence ☐ 0 ☐ 1 ☐ 2 X 3 ☐ 4	Observations: • I relied heavily on my ocular motor abilities to focus on the tools and objects I was handling. • I only used near focus because the activity was very close to my body.

Oral–motor skill—Use of muscles in and around the mouth	
Level of influence X 0 ☐ 1 ☐ 2 ☐ 3 ☐ 4	Observation: • I did not need oral–motor abilities to complete this activity.

Fine motor coordination and dexterity—Using small muscle groups for controlled movements, particularly in-hand object manipulation	
Level of influence ☐ 0 ☐ 1 ☐ 2 ☐ 3 X 4	Observations: • I used intrinsic and extrinsic hand muscles when I manipulated the plant, the pots, the shovel, and the water cup. • I used a few different pinch and grasp patterns to effectively hold the plant, remove the pot, stabilize the pots, hold the shovel, and stabilize the soil bag. These patterns included tip-to-tip pinch, cylindrical grasp, palmar prehension grasp, and three-jaw chuck. • I also needed to pronate forearms when packing down soil and supinate my left forearm to remove the plant from its original pot. • I relied on the synergies of my wrist flexors and extensors to hold my hand steady when I removed the pot from the plant. • Speed is a factor. I did not want to leave the plant out of a container for more than a minute for fear of shock and potential death.

Visual–motor integration—Coordinating the interaction of information from the eyes and body movement	
Level of influence ☐ 0 ☐ 1 ☐ 2 X 3 ☐ 4	Observation: • I needed to have a high level of hand–eye coordination when performing this activity, from holding the shovel and digging for soil to manipulating the plant and pots.

(Continued)

Crossing the midline—Moving the limbs and eyes across the midline sagittal plane of the body

Level of influence	Observations:
☐ 0 ☐ 1 X 2 ☐ 3 ☐ 4	• I scanned my environment often to pick up and set down objects as I needed to use them. • I sat in a side-sitting position with my left lower leg crossing the midline. • My arms came close to the midline but never crossed, whereas my right forearm and hand crossed my midline often, especially because I placed the soil bag to my left and chose to retrieve it with my right dominant hand. • I tended to operate a little to the left of center when removing the original pot and excess soil, and thus crossed the midline with my right hand and wrist and not with my left. • When placing the plant in its new pot and packing down soil, both hands worked very near to the midline but did not cross it.

Right–left discrimination—Differentiating one side from the other

Level of influence	Observations:
☐ 0 ☐ 1 ☐ 2 ☐ 3 X 4	• A high level of bilateral integration is necessary to complete this activity efficiently. • I used tools and did the most manipulation with my right dominant hand but still needed my left hand for stability purposes. • I did not have to follow verbal or written instructions or differentiate between left and right on another person.

Laterality—Use of a preferred or dominant hand or foot

Level of influence	Observations:
☐ 0 ☐ 1 ☐ 2 X 3 ☐ 4	• I am right-hand dominant, and I favored my right hand to grasp and use the shovel, remove the original pot from the plant, remove excess soil, and pour the water. • Using my right hand to perform most of the action while my left stabilized made completing the activity easier than if I were to reverse their responsibilities.

Bilateral integration—Coordinating both sides of the body

Level of influence	Observations:

☐ 0
☐ 1
☐ 2
☐ 3
X 4
	• The majority of my activity required bilateral integration, especially during the following tasks:
	  o Using one hand to retrieve soil while the other hand stabilized the bag
	  o Using one hand to empty the soil into the pot while the other hand stabilized the pot
	  o Holding the plant with one hand and removing its original pot with the other hand
	  o Holding the plant with one hand and removing excess soil with the other hand
	  o Stabilizing the plant in its new pot while retrieving soil with the other
	  o Coordinating both hands to pack down the soil symmetrically and simultaneously
	  o Coordinating both hands to pick up and drop the plant symmetrically and simultaneously.

Memory—Recoding information after a brief or long period of time

Level of influence	Observations:
☐ 0 ☐ 1 ☐ 2 X 3 ☐ 4	• I used long-term memory (mostly visual) from past experience to recall the tools I needed and the sequence I should perform. • It is important to have some knowledge of this procedure to provide the plant with an easy transition. Therefore, I filled the new pot with soil before removing the plant from its old pot. Additionally, it would not be optimal to water the plant in the middle of this sequence. • Regarding factual knowledge, I knew that most plants grow in soil, need adequate room for roots in the pot, and require water.

(Continued)

Categorization—Identifying similarities and differences among pieces of environmental information	
Level of influence □ 0 X 1 □ 2 □ 3 □ 4	Observations: • I had two similar looking pots and categorized them separately based on their size. • I deconstructed the plant (removed it from its smaller pot and removed some of the attached soil) and reconstructed it in the larger pot (added more new soil).

Concept formation—Involves organizing a variety of information to form thoughts and ideas	
Level of influence □ 0 X 1 □ 2 □ 3 □ 4	Observations: • Repotting a plant did not require me to think abstractly. • I did make sure to get the loose plant into its new pot quickly because I understood the concept of shock as it applies to plants.

Spatial operations—Mentally manipulating the position of objects in various relationships	
Level of influence □ 0 □ 1 X 2 □ 3 □ 4	Observations: • I needed to visualize the three-dimensional perspective of the new pot when I was determining how much soil I needed. • I had a mental image of the end product to guide my actions, specifically when centering the plant and making sure it stood at the right level in the pot.

Learning—Acquiring new concepts and behaviors	
Level of influence □ 0 □ 1 X 2 □ 3 □ 4	Observations: • Repotting a plant is a structured learning experience because it required me to follow a sequence using specific objects within a certain time. • This activity had me using both hands to actively manipulate the objects, providing mostly tactile and proprioceptive feedback. • Having done this activity before, it was not a new concept, but because each plant presents differently, I had to stay focused to manipulate it without causing damage. • Sensorimotor learning occurred as I determined how much pressure I needed to hold the stem, decided what movements my upper extremities needed to make to remove the plant from its pot, and visually gauged how much soil and water would be appropriate.

Generalization—Applying previously learned concepts and behaviors to a variety of new situations	
Level of influence □ 0 □ 1 □ 2 X 3 □ 4	Observations: • I used past experience of repotting many different plants to complete this activity. • There is an endless amount of flora, but I anticipated that the plant would sit in soil, have roots, have a stem, have leaves, and need water at the end of the process. • I can generalize this skill to other flora I acquire.

General Activity Demands

Activity requires	Yes	No	Focus on
Simple task	X		Initiation of activity, time management, termination of activity, coping skills, self-control
Complex task	X		
Multiple tasks	X		
Independent performance	X		
Group performance		X	Social skills, interpersonal skills

(Continued)

Initiation of activity—Starting a physical or mental activity	
Level of influence ☐ 0 ☐ 1 X 2 ☐ 3 ☐ 4	Observations: • Once I set up my workspace with all the necessary objects and sat on the floor, the activity began. • This activity is self-started, but I did plan on performing it when I knew I had some free time. • This activity was extremely relevant as I bought the plant that morning and was eager to promote its growth and display it on my windowsill. • This would be a good activity to perform during times of stress, but it could also place a burden on those who do not find it meaningful.

Time management—Ability to manage parcels of time as they relate to the performance of tasks or activities	
Level of influence ☐ 0 ☐ 1 X 2 ☐ 3 ☐ 4	Observations: • I performed this activity in one session, and it requires following a sequence. • There are no set time restraints for performing this activity; however, it is optimal for the life of the plant to do this within a few minutes so the plant does not experience shock. • The activity is not a part of my routine, because it should be performed only when the plant needs more room to grow (a couple times a year), and it requires some preparation so it can be done efficiently.

Termination of activity—Stopping an activity at an appropriate time	
Level of influence ☐ 0 ☐ 1 X 2 ☐ 3 ☐ 4	Observations: • The activity is limited by the size of the pot; it ended when I watered the plant in its new pot. • I knew that I should stop watering when I saw water pooling on the surface of the soil.

Coping skills—Identifying and managing stress-related factors such as anger, disappointment, or frustration	
Level of influence ☐ 0 X 1 ☐ 2 ☐ 3 ☐ 4	Observations: • This activity did not cause me stress because I am familiar with the procedure and see it as a form of leisure, though one I do not take part in on a regular basis. • I performed this activity in a quiet, private setting so the environment did not have any effect on stress. • There was a range of acceptable performance that could still accomplish the end goal, and I was not upset with myself when I spilled small amounts of soil here and there. • The activity might be stressful for someone who has never performed it before, someone who does not like getting their hands dirty, or someone who strives for complete perfection—he or she might be upset with spilling dirt or not having a perfectly centered plant.

Self-control—Modifying one's own behavior in response to environmental needs, demands, constraints, personal aspirations, and feedback from others	
Level of influence ☐ 0 X 1 ☐ 2 ☐ 3 ☐ 4	Observations: • Some dirt spilled from my shovel when I filled in the sides around the plant, but it was a negligible amount and did not affect my performance satisfaction. • Had I been spilling a significant amount, I would have to modify the position of the shovel relative to the pot or retrieve a smaller, more manageable amount of soil. • I relied on my own feedback and judgment about my performance and I was satisfied. • The outcome (jade plant in a new pot) did lead to my goal of promoting growth for the plant.

(Continued)

Social skills—Involves interacting by using manners, personal space, eye contact, gestures, active listening, and self-expression appropriate to the situation

Level of influence	Observation:
X 0 ☐ 1 ☐ 2 ☐ 3 ☐ 4	• I performed this activity alone in my apartment and did not interact with anyone.

Interpersonal skills—Involves using verbal and nonverbal communication skills appropriately

Level of influence	Observations:
X 0 ☐ 1 ☐ 2 ☐ 3 ☐ 4	• I performed this activity independently. • I did not speak or interact with anyone while completing this activity.

Mobility

Activity requires	Yes	No	Focus on
Changing and maintaining body position	X		Postural alignment, postural control, depth perception, body strength
Transferring oneself		X	

Postural alignment—Maintaining biomechanical integrity among body parts

Level of influence	Observations:
☐ 0 ☐ 1 X 2 ☐ 3 ☐ 4	• I maintained a side-seated posture throughout the duration of the activity. • Once seated, I did not change my pelvic position. • The activity required me to make slight adjustments in alignment when I leaned forward, to the side, twisted my torso, or reached my hands through space. • It would still be possible for someone with postural alignment problems to complete this activity by wearing a brace or positioning the materials at a level that does not require trunk flexion.

Postural control—Using righting and equilibrium reactions to maintain balance during functional movements

Level of influence	Observations:
☐ 0 ☐ 1 X 2 ☐ 3 ☐ 4	• I maintained a static base of support throughout the activity in a side-sitting position. • I used some slight head righting and equilibrium reactions to maintain my balance when I leaned forward and to the side, but given my large base of support, I did not worry about or anticipate losing my balance. • I stabilized my trunk against gravity when I leaned forward to pack down the soil and water the plant and when I leaned to the side to retrieve soil. • I had to maintain posture to actively use my upper extremities and focus visually.

Depth perception—Involves determining the relative distance between objects, figures, or landmarks and the observer and changes in planes and surfaces

Level of influence	Observations:
☐ 0 ☐ 1 ☐ 2 X 3 ☐ 4	• I visually estimated the amount of soil I needed for the new pot given its dimensions and depth. • I had to understand the depth of the soil bag to retrieve an adequate scoop. • I reached for the objects from the floor in front of me, including the plant, pots, soil, shovel, and water cup. • I had to bring objects close together using both hands separately: watering the newly potted plant, bringing the shovel to the soil bag, and moving the plant into its new pot. • My lower body remained static, but I moved my torso in the sagittal plane and my upper extremities in sagittal, coronal, and transverse planes.

(Continued)

Body strength—Degree of gross muscle power when body movement is resisted or is against gravity	
Level of influence □ 0 □ 1 X 2 □ 3 □ 4	Observations: • Trunk and neck control allowed me to stay upright and lean over my workspace. • I needed moderate strength in my upper extremity to hold the weight of the objects and move them through space. • Lifting the objects required concentric contraction of upper-extremity muscles, whereas setting them down required eccentric upper-extremity muscle contraction and holding them in space for a moment or two required isometric upper-extremity muscle contraction.

Carrying, Moving, and Handling Objects

Activity requires	Yes	No	Focus on
Lifting	X		Range of motion, extremity strength, endurance
Carrying	X		
Fine hand use	X		Range of motion, extremity strength, endurance, stereognosis, kinesthesia, figure–ground perception, grasp patterns, prehension patterns, fine motor skill
Hand and arm use	X		
Moving objects with lower extremities		X	Range of motion, extremity strength, endurance
Walking and moving		X	Range of motion, extremity strength, endurance, topographical orientation

Range of motion—Moving body parts through an arc of motion	

Level of influence
□ 0
□ 1
□ 2
X 3
□ 4
	Observations:
	• I rotated my head and neck slightly to shift my visual focus between the soil bag placed on the left and the plant and pots placed on the floor in front of me.
	• My head stayed in a relatively static, slightly flexed position as I concentrated on the objects on the floor in front of me.
	• I moved between 0° and 45° of trunk flexion depending on what component I was working on. I found myself in the most trunk flexion when patting down the soil and making sure the plant was centered.
	• Regarding the upper extremity, I needed to be able to move through the following ranges:
	  ○ 0° to 45° shoulder abduction when filling the pot with soil
	  ○ 45° to 90° elbow flexion to reach for and manipulate the objects in space
	  ○ 0° to 45° of scapular plane motion to work with the objects in front of me
	  ○ 0° to 30° wrist extension when grasping and manipulating the pots and water cup
	  ○ 0° to 90° forearm supination and pronation when removing the plant from its original pot
	  ○ 0° to 90° forearm pronation when emptying the soil from my shovel and when patting down the soil in the pot.
	• Other movements of the upper extremity:
	  ○ Some shoulder adduction when reaching across the midline to retrieve soil and when patting down the soil in the pot
	  ○ Scapular protraction to manipulate the objects in front of me
	  ○ Finger flexion to grasp and pinch the objects
	  ○ Finger extension to pat down the soil
	  ○ Thumb flexion to pinch, grasp the shovel and pots, and stabilize the plant.
	• All lower extremity and hip joints remained static and served as my base of support: side-sitting position, hips flexed to 90°; left leg abducted to 30° with left knee flexed to 150° and right leg abducted to 60° with right knee flexed to 150°; feet neutral.
	• Someone with upper-extremity issues, especially any hand, wrist, or elbow mobility or range-of-motion limitations, would have trouble completing the activity.

(Continued)

Extremity strength—Grade of muscle strength when body movement is resisted or is against gravity	
Level of influence □ 0 □ 1 □ 2 X 3 □ 4	Observations: • Most of the actions I used to complete this activity are against gravity and with a small amount of resistance (the weight of the shovel, pots, plants, water cup); thus a muscle strength grade of 4, or good (perhaps a 3+ because of the low weights of the objects) would be needed to successfully complete this activity. • This activity required that I concentrically contract my upper-extremity muscles when retrieving the soil, lifting the plant pots, and lifting the water. • I used isometric contractions to hold the plant in space for a few seconds while I removed extra soil from the bottom and when I poured the water. • I used eccentric contractions of the upper extremity when lowering the pots, plant, water, and shovel to the floor.

Endurance—Sustained cardiac, pulmonary, and musculoskeletal exertion over time	
Level of influence □ 0 □ 1 X 2 □ 3 □ 4	Observations: • This activity required a minimal level of endurance; however, there were some repetitive actions that could be fatiguing for someone with muscle weakness. • I needed some endurance to retrieve an adequate amount of soil for the new pot. I repeated the action of scooping soil with my shovel seven times total. • I needed to be able to lift the shovel by itself and when it was filled with soil and move it through space. • I did not get fatigued because the activity lasted only a couple of minutes and the weight of the shovel, plant, pots, and soil is relatively low.

Stereognosis—Identifying objects through proprioception, cognition, and sense of touch	
Level of influence □ 0 X 1 □ 2 □ 3 □ 4	Observations: • I used stereognosis when I stabilized the plant in its new pot with my left hand and focused my visual attention to retrieving more soil with my right hand. • I could not see to the bottom of the soil bag and relied on my proprioceptive and tactile input (specifically weight) when retrieving soil.

Kinesthesia—Identifying the excursion and direction of movement	
Level of influence □ 0 □ 1 □ 2 X 3 □ 4	Observations: • I coordinated my thumb, finger, wrist, radioulnar, elbow, and shoulder joints to manipulate the plant pots, cup of water, shovel, and soil bag. • I coordinated all finger joints when I removed soil from the bottom of the plant, moving between flexion and extension at different rates for each finger. • I chose to position myself in side-sitting position, which initially required me to coordinate all lower body joints into a comfortable and stable position. • I made subtle changes between torso flexion, extension, and rotation throughout the entire activity.

Grasp patterns—Identifying the type(s) of grasp required to perform the activity	
Level of influence □ 0 □ 1 □ 2 □ 3 X 4	Observations: • I used a palmar prehension grasp with both hands when dropping and thumping the new pot on the ground. • I used a power grasp to hold the shovel. • I used a cylindrical grasp to manipulate the circular plant pots and the cup of water.

Prehension patterns—Identifying the type(s) of pinch required to perform this activity	
Level of influence □ 0 □ 1 X 2 □ 3 □ 4	Observations: • I used pad-to-pad pinch to hold the stem of the plant as I removed it from its original pot. • I used the three-jaw chuck to hold the plant (in its original pot) as I judged how much soil I needed in the new pot.

(Continued)

Fine motor skill—Ability to use small hand muscles and joints to perform refined actions	
Level of influence ☐ 0 ☐ 1 ☐ 2 ☐ 3 X 4	Observations: • Given the small size of the pots I was working with and the small size of the plant, I needed to use fine motor skills to do the following actions: o Manipulate the stem of the plant o Remove soil from the bottom of the plant o Center and stabilize the plant in its new pot o Pack down the soil with my fingers.

Figure–ground perception—Differentiating between foreground and background forms and objects	
Level of influence X 0 ☐ 1 ☐ 2 ☐ 3 ☐ 4	Observation: • I did not need to use figure–ground perception when I repotted my plant because I had five very distinguishable tools and objects placed directly in front of me.

Topographical orientation—Determining the location of objects and settings and the route to the location	
Level of influence X 0 ☐ 1 ☐ 2 ☐ 3 ☐ 4	Observation: • I did not use topographical orientation during this activity because I was seated on the floor of my apartment for the entire duration.

Part 3: Occupation Analysis Summary

1. *Is the goal of the occupation or activity relevant to the person?*
   Gardening in many forms has been an interest of mine since I was a young girl helping my mother in her garden. My interest in gardening continues into my adulthood.

2. *Is the occupation part of the person's habits, routines, or rituals?*
   This activity is a part of a seasonal ritual that I do during the spring. Each year, when the weather warms, I start noticing the natural life around me and I start planning what I want to grow during the summer. This year is a little different because I do not have the capacity to grow a bunch of vegetables (although I do hope to have a couple of tomato and basil plants on my roof), so I have been mostly researching hardy houseplants that need only a few hours of sunlight. Once I acquire my set of plants, I like to repot them to promote growth.

3. *Is the activity of interest to the person, and does it provide an opportunity for self-expression or enhance self-efficacy?*
   This activity facilitates a great amount of self-expression. I have a choice in which plants I acquire, and I take into account the look and personality of each plant, in addition to its hardiness and functional benefits. I would love to own a Venus flytrap, not because I have flies, but because I think it represents my adventurous side. The actual task of repotting a plant—what size or color pot I use, if I mix and match plants in the same pot, the soil I use—also allows me to express myself through my choice of materials. For instance, to perform this activity, I just bought a larger plastic container for my jade plant because I am on a budget and would rather spend money elsewhere than on an expensive terra cotta pot.

   I attribute a lot of meaning and value to this activity, so it greatly enhances my self-efficacy. I feel that I can participate in my desired role as a gardener and caretaker by being able to repot my plants. It makes me feel productive and relaxed at the same time. The activity is not strenuous, but working with plants makes me feel healthier and more connected to nature. It also contributes to my relationship with my mom, who still lives in Hawaii. I ask her for gardening advice and tips, and we swap stories about our experiences with different plants. When I become a mother, I want to be able to share this "green" bond with my own children. Knowing how to repot a plant is an important element to gardening that also fosters an appreciation for nature.

CHAPTER 5.

THE OCCUPATIONAL PROFILE

Judy Urban Wilson, MA, OTR

Highlights

✧ Occupational profile
✧ Occupational therapy evaluation
✧ Intervention and the occupational profile
✧ Outcomes and the occupational profile.

Key Terms

✧ Analysis of occupational performance
✧ Context
✧ Data collection
✧ Domain of concern of occupational therapy
✧ Ethnographer
✧ External contexts
✧ Health
✧ Internal contexts
✧ Interview
✧ Occupational Performance History Interview–II

✧ Occupational profile
✧ Occupational therapy evaluation
✧ Occupational therapy intervention
✧ Outcome measures
✧ Participant observation
✧ Task
✧ Time
✧ Self-care
✧ Space

What we do, and what we think about what we do, encompasses who we are. We act and we react. Sometimes we take a line of action by choice, and at other times we act because we believe we can do nothing else. These daily actions are the occupations that define us to ourselves and also in the eyes of others.

Health, a state of physical, mental, and social well-being, assumes access to and participation in occupations. What cuts people off from occupations consequently impairs health, and disconnection from occupations puts one's sense of self at risk. Many conditions can threaten full engagement in meaningful occupations. Changes in body structure, paucity of available occupations, or a change in the context in which we must act out our occupations impede our full occupational engagement, leaving us in poor health. We need to regain a full and meaningful set of occupations to restore our healthy identity.

The *Occupational Therapy Practice Framework: Domain and Process* (the *Framework;* American Occupational Therapy Association [AOTA], 2014) places the occupational profile, defined subsequently, as a central pillar of clinical practice. This chapter explores how occupation connects to practice across the broad domain of occupational therapy. Good use of the occupational profile depends on thoughtful data collection. The occupational therapist uses interviewing skills in a client-centered interview and participant observation to determine the client's occupational profile. The occupational therapist needs to gain a focused understanding of a client's occupational profile to understand his or her life and therapeutic needs. The occupational profile interacts with the evaluation, interventions, and outcomes of the intervention process, shaping the future occupational profile. Attending to the occupational profile throughout the intervention process ensures that intervention is clearly occupational.

This chapter aims to capture what it means for therapy to be occupational in practice. I endeavor to keep it practical, showing that the long heritage of occupational therapy is present in the daily work of the practitioner. I cannot cite references for each idea because my thoughts are rooted in a wealth of occupational therapy literature that has brought me to where I am now. My ideas are not new; rather, they are basic to occupational therapy.

What I hope to offer readers is a series of reflections on occupation from the clinic floor. Keeping my attention on the occupational profile, the focal point of this chapter, reminds me of who we are professionally and propels me to continue growing as an occupational therapist.

Occupational Profile

The occupational profile is crucial for occupational therapy practitioners facilitating the achievement of occupational therapy objectives, which involve "the therapeutic use of everyday life activities (occupations) with individuals or groups" to enhance or enable participation (AOTA, 2014, p. S1). Because the key feature of an occupation is the meaning it holds for the person performing it, the specifics of occupation vary from person to person. Occupational therapy assists in linking a person to those occupations that define him or her. If the objective of occupational therapy is to engage people in occupations, the occupational therapist's first responsibility is to identify the client's occupations.

The *occupational profile* is a summary of the set of activities, routines, and roles that describes a client at any one point in time. This definition is the moving target an occupational therapist applies when identifying the occupational profile for a case in a practice setting. In practice, this means an imperfect collection of data gathered by the occupational therapist to try to capture the individual client's living occupational profile.

An ongoing discussion in the occupational therapy literature concerns how to define *occupations, roles, activities,* and *lifestyles* (e.g., AOTA, 1997; Hasselkus, 2006; Kielhofner, 1983, 1985, 1992, 2008; Kramer, Hinojosa, & Royeen, 2003; Nelson, 1996; Trombly, 1995). All these terms are used to express human actions and what they mean in the context of people's lives. In practice, the occupational therapy practitioner needs to identify and analyze these actions in relation to each client.

AOTA (2014) has defined an *occupational profile* as a "summary of client's occupational history and experiences, patterns of daily living, interests, values, and needs" (p. S14). This definition encompasses a lot of information. In fact, it describes an entire life. Biography, however, is not the goal of the

Figure 5.1. For Mark, building a campfire is an ordinary, yet meaningful, skill for fulfilling his occupation of father, husband, and adventurer.

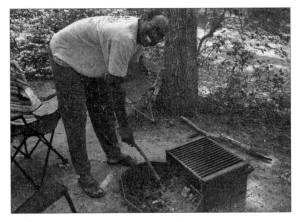

Source. J. Urban Wilson. Used with permission.

occupational profile. Accordingly, the occupational profile focuses on the mundane aspects of living rather than solely on the big events. The story of an accident or a list of a person's life accomplishments is only relevant to the occupational profile because of the impact it has on the person's daily activities and roles, not because of the events themselves (Figure 5.1). In the evaluation, the therapist seeks to uncover specific features of the client's story by looking for descriptions of activities performed, patterns of behavior, and where and with whom activities are performed. Furthermore, the therapist ascertains what makes these activities meaningful or important to the client, thus identifying the client's occupations.

When a person seeks or is scheduled to receive occupational therapy, he or she may have a variety of problems or areas of concern. Not all of the person's occupations, however, are impaired, changed, or threatened. Upon beginning to evaluate the client, the occupational therapist must focus on identifying the client's specific problems or areas to be addressed during therapy. The therapist uses the occupational profile to clarify the person's needs, values, and priorities.

Temporal Context

Developing a person's occupational profile requires the occupational therapist to focus on the temporal context, in this case, on current or recent occupa-

tions. These occupations are the ones most relevant to the client's present sense of self and current circumstances. If illness or injury has caused an unfavorable change in occupations, then the occupations performed just before the change are the most critical part of the profile. These recent occupations most accurately reflect the client's values, goals, ambitions, and aspirations.

A client's existing current occupations are especially critical to explore when they form a negative sense of self, such as in an abusive parent or a person who views himself or herself as "a helpless invalid." In addition, if the client performs activities because of physical, cognitive, psychosocial, or environmental limitations, then the therapist must consider how these limitations influence the client's ability to engage in occupations. For example, in the future, will the client need to perform most occupations from a wheelchair? If the client desires a change in these occupations, targeting them becomes a central goal of treatment. In sum, when an occupational therapy practitioner plans treatment, it is important that he or she knows the client's current occupations because they are the starting points for the creation of any therapeutic change.

Although the occupational profile focuses on present or recent occupations, some understanding of past and future occupations is also important. Past occupations helped shape those of the present and are a source of experience from which the client can continue to draw. It is also important to appreciate the client's vision of future occupations and to understand the importance and value of a particular occupation to the person, because such knowledge is essential for planning interventions. These past occupations and future aspirations are valuable sources for adjustments or renewals in a client's occupations as he or she moves forward.

Exercise 5.1. Personal Occupational Profile

What occupations make up your own occupational profile? Which occupations are the most important to you? Why? Pick one occupation, and list all the activities that it includes. Where do you perform these activities? With whom do you perform these activities? What is unique about how you do these activities?

Figure 5.2. How Morgan and Jojo perform their co-occupation of cousins is specific to this moment in time and will continually change over the years.

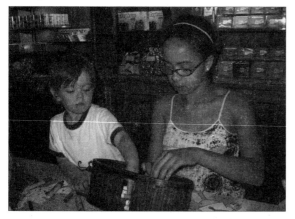

Source. J. Urban Wilson. Used with permission.

One challenge for the occupational therapist is to determine whether current, past, or future potential occupations are the most important and relevant to understanding the person. Measures such as the *Occupational Performance History Interview–II* (Kielhofner et al., 2004), which explores a person's past and current occupations, can be used to meet this challenge.

Time is a defining dimension of any occupational profile, yet the occupational profile is not simply a résumé-like document that builds over time; rather, it is a continually morphing entity. The past, present, and future shape a person's roles and routines. A person's occupational profile changes as he or she matures and in response to life events (Figure 5.2). A child stops playing with toy trucks and becomes interested in baseball. A student graduates and becomes a worker. A worker retires. A woman gives birth. An aunt becomes ill, and her niece takes her in. These transitions change a person's occupational profile.

In some cases, the occupational therapy practitioner works with a client in response to a particular event that changed the client's occupational profile. The client may have had an injury or illness that altered patterns of daily life and daily activities. In other cases, the client may have an unsatisfying or destructive occupational profile that he or she wants to change. Whether change is sought because of a sudden event or as a result of longstanding limi-

tations, the practitioner needs to learn about the client's previous and present occupational profiles as well as his or her needs and desires for a future occupational profile. Read Case Examples 5.1, 5.2, 5.3, and 5.4, and consider which time period in these clients' occupational profiles should have the strongest focus for treatment planning.

Exercise 5.2. Temporal Context of Personal Occupational Profile

Reflect again on your own occupational profile. When has it changed? What are past occupations in which you no longer engage? What impact does this change have on your present occupations? What occupations do you aspire to have in the future? Do these aspirations shape any of your present occupations?

Data Collection

The process of *data collection* to complete an occupational profile is time-consuming and extensive. It begins at the moment of meeting the client and continues throughout the occupational therapy intervention. The process generally starts with an interview. The client, however, usually does not share much of the most important data with the occupational therapist until rapport is established, which is accomplished through further interviewing and participant observation. Thus, the intervention plan changes as the intervention progresses.

Interview

The *interview*, which entails asking the client or the client's caretakers very detailed questions about

---

Case Example 5.1. Maria: Broken Radius

Maria is an 11-year-old girl who broke her radius playing soccer in her local league. She is in 6th grade and applying to a specialized science school starting in 7th grade. She has several neighborhood friends with whom she plays on weekends. She lives with her mother and little brother. Her father disappeared 2 years ago.

Case Example 5.2. Maureen: Major Depression

Maureen is an 87-year-old woman diagnosed with major depression who has been referred to a psychiatric day treatment program. She has been a widow for 30 years. She retired 2 years ago from her work as a secretary. After retirement, she moved away from the place where she had lived her entire life, leaving friends and her sisters, to move in with her daughter and son-in-law in a neighboring state. She now watches a little TV, knits, and tries to help her daughter around the house. She reports that her relationship with her daughter has become very strained.

Case Example 5.3. Alex: Severe Developmental Delays

Alex is a 4-year-old boy with severe developmental delays. He lives with his two parents, 1-year-old brother, and 6-year-old sister. His siblings play with him on the mat in the playroom. He has an adapted highchair in which his parents feed him. They transport him in an adapted stroller. His mother hopes to start him in the town's mainstream school system next year.

Case Example 5.4. Daniel: Chronic Obstructive Pulmonary Disease

Daniel is a 65-year-old man with chronic obstructive pulmonary disease (COPD) who worked as an elementary school janitor for many years. Ten years ago, he was no longer able to manage his work. He was diagnosed with COPD. Five years ago, he was placed on oxygen. He is divorced, with an adult son who lives out of state with Daniel's grandchildren. Over the past 10 years, he has stopped his frequent visits to the local pub where he played pool. He is starting to have trouble with his self-care: His clothes are unkempt, and he appears unwashed.

his or her occupations, is usually the first step of data collection; therefore, good interviewing skills are vital for the occupational therapist. The key to good interviewing skills lies not in the questions asked but in effective listening. From listening closely to what the client says, the therapist decides on and adapts his or her line of questioning. Once a dialogue has been established, the therapist seeks to clarify details and introduces new topics to explore other areas. The therapist probes for clarification and understanding as he or she listens to what the client says (Figure 5.3).

People are not accustomed to being asked questions about exactly how they do every *task,* or complete a specific aspect of an activity in their day. When asked what they do in the morning, many people answer that they get up and go to work. The occupational therapist, however, wants to know when they get up, what kind of bed they slept in, who is in the bed, where they go next, whether they wear slippers, and whether they brush their teeth or drink their coffee first. The therapist must therefore ask precise and probing questions.

Questions are influenced by the client's particular context. For example, a therapist treating a client with a broken finger will ask more about how the client holds the toothbrush and squeezes the toothpaste and less about what kind of slippers he or she wears. For the client with depression, however, the therapist will be less concerned about how the client grips the toothbrush but may focus instead on the time or the regularity of the tooth-

Figure 5.3. Occupational therapist Ruth interviews Karlo to obtain the occupational profile.

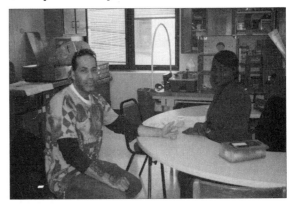

Source. J. Urban Wilson. Used with permission.

Interview a friend or family member (not an occupational therapy practitioner or occupational therapy student). Find out about the person's daily routines, responsibilities, and work and leisure activities.

brushing routine. The therapist uses clinical judgment and knowledge about the client's condition to shape the interview.

Rarely is the occupational therapist the first health professional in contact with a client. In previous health care environments, clients get used to answering questions about their symptoms; they do not expect to be asked about what they enjoy doing in their free time, what community groups they are involved in, and what responsibilities they have at home. It takes extra effort for the occupational therapist to refocus the conversation, often having to ask questions in multiple ways to find out about the client's activities and occupations.

Sometimes, simply asking the client a question is ineffective. The client may be a young child, be confused, or be unable to communicate. In these cases, the practitioner can usually ask family members for information because the family has much more extensive experience with the person and can flesh out the therapist's observations. In some cases, the family members may also be considered to be clients; therefore, the therapist may work closely with them to develop intervention priorities. For example, a mother may want to be able to fit her daughter into a car seat to ease transportation to school. In another family, the older son may worry about his elderly mother wandering into the kitchen and turning on the stove.

Sometimes, a client cannot speak for himself or herself, and no family members or friends are available to provide information. This scenario includes both clients who are unable to communicate and those who are resistive to intervention because of confusion or depression (see Case Example 5.5). In these cases, a standard interview will be unproductive. The occupational therapist must become a puzzle solver, piecing together a hypothesized profile. This profile is constantly updated from the general social data available, from pieces of conversations with the client who can communicate,

and from the client's reactions to activities. Success, however, relies on the waning of the client's resistance as rapport builds during the intervention process. For the client unable to communicate, success relies on the client's response to the practitioner and the activities presented.

Participant Observation

In some sense, the occupational therapy practitioner works as an _ethnographer,_ or a qualitative researcher who studies cultural phenomena. The first ethnographic method used to learn about the client and his or her life is the interview, and the second is _participant observation_—a research technique in which the researcher engages in activities with people to learn about them and their lives. In occupational therapy, as rapport is being established and the intervention has begun, the practitioner learns more about the client while engaging

---

Case Example 5.5. Ling Mei: Stroke

Ling Mei is an elderly Chinese woman, found on the streets of Chinatown, who had suffered a severe stroke. In the inpatient rehabilitation unit, Ling Mei claimed that she was fine and asked that someone take her to the statue of Confucius, where she could sit and panhandle. She told them, "I'll be fine." She had had substantial frontal lobe damage impeding awareness and potentially impeding cognitive skills. Her illiteracy and resistance to formal testing hampered the accuracy of the neuropsychological evaluation. The occupational profile became especially critical when the occupational therapist needed to report to the team whether the client was ready to be discharged safely into the community.

Could Ling Mei resume her previous activities adequately without social support? What skills should the therapist consider to be city survival skills? What occupations would you guess recently made up Ling Mei's profile? What activities would you try with her to see how she responds?

in activities with him or her. However, an essential difference exists between the ethnographer and the occupational therapy practitioner: The ethnographer values not influencing the research participants, whereas the practitioner enters the interaction with the purpose of working with the client to create change by gaining an understanding of the client.

The occupational therapy practitioner and the client work together to develop and implement a plan for service delivery. As the practitioner and the client jointly engage in the activities within the intervention, they interact, and rapport continues to build. Even when rapport is difficult to develop, interactions between the practitioner and the client provide information that broadens the practitioner's picture of the client. The practitioner uses activities pertinent to the client, often within the client's personal context. These interactions are the practitioner's "fieldwork" from which observations are made (Figure 5.4).

Participant observation provides new details about the client's performance in context that support or contrast with what the therapist learned in the interview. As the client chats with the occupational therapy practitioner, he or she shares information that triggers new ideas and new questions from the practitioner, leading to an increasingly rich occupational profile. A level of intimacy develops between client and practitioner, and as this relationship grows, the client may reach a point at which he or she shares sensitive personal information (Case Example 5.6).

As the occupational therapy practitioner enters the client's world, the client learns about the perspective and principles of occupational therapy through the shared experience of the intervention. As a client comes to a greater understanding of occupational therapy, he or she becomes more self-directed in the process. A client may see himself or herself successfully completing more activities and may identify which activities he or she wants to work on next in pursuit of a valued occupation. The client may bring up an old hobby or a long-held aspiration as he or she perceives that occupational therapy may be able to help him or her achieve such goals. Some clients take on more of a partnership role during intervention and are able to identify occupational issues not previously mentioned as they come to understand the potential of the occupational therapy process. Others need more direction to link the intervention process to their occupations.

Data collection for the occupational profile is an ongoing component of the evaluation. As the process moves into the intervention phase, the intervention planning begins to flow more directly from the new data emerging in the profile. The occupational therapist in collaboration with the occupational therapy assistant thus uses the occupational profile as an intervention tool. As the therapist learns about the client's past and present occupations, as well as future aspirations, he or she works with the client to identify occupations that are still attainable or that are especially self-affirming for the client. The occupational therapy practitioner emphasizes the occupations that help the client see his or her capabilities and encourages the client to actively choose which occupations he or she wishes to set as goals. Such a discussion between the client and the therapist is the first step in empowering the client to make changes for a healthier and richer occupational profile.

As with all ethnographers, the occupational therapist brings his or her own worldview to the process. Of course, the therapist uses clinical reasoning, understanding of medical and psychological conditions, and a growing understanding of the client to inform his or her decisions about what to ask and how to develop the interventions. The therapist, however, also brings a more

Figure 5.4. Observing Catie and Molly play reveals more details about their occupations than any interview could.

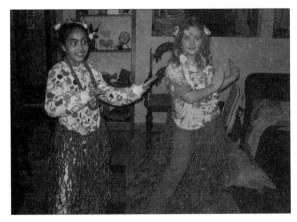

Source. J. Urban Wilson. Used with permission.

Case Example 5.6. Martha: Major Depression and Borderline Personality Disorder

Martha, age 40 years, was diagnosed with major depression with borderline personality disorder and referred to an outpatient psychiatric treatment program. At the initial interview with the occupational therapist (along with the chart review), Martha shared that since her "meltdown" she has been cutting herself, and as a result, she is on leave from her job as a music teacher in the local school system. Her husband is also a local teacher. She has two daughters, one in college and one doing well in high school.

Martha reported that when she was growing up, her mother had been domineering and emotionally abusive and forced her and her sisters to be performers all their lives. Martha had been sexually assaulted as a child and harbored a lot of anger toward her mother for never stopping or addressing the abuse. She describes herself as shy. Presently, Martha cannot tolerate crowds and is extremely uncomfortable around other people. The therapist observed that her social interactions were stunted.

The initial treatment plan included relaxation techniques for social situations and to help manage anger in relation to her mother; building self-esteem, beginning with emphasizing her successes, such as her two daughters; coping strategies for interacting with her mother; and graded resumption of social activities, with the eventual goal of returning to work. Returning to work was especially difficult because Martha lived in a small town and everyone knew why Martha was on leave. She eventually did return to work. Another big success was attending a concert given by her favorite singer.

After more than 1 year in treatment, Martha began to make small comments about her husband to her therapist. For example, she complained about cleaning the mouse cages that her husband brought home from his classroom. In addition, the therapist detected fear in Martha's voice at the mention of bringing financial problems to her husband During a program family event, the therapist noted that Martha was hyperattentive to her husband and that her husband seemed aloof. Furthermore, the therapist noted that others in the program complimented Martha on the town-wide children's concerts she once led, about which she seemed proud but reserved and reluctant.

Martha's confidence was growing, which allowed her to answer as the therapist began to question her more about her marriage. Slowly, the therapist learned that Martha's husband was neglectful and emotionally abusive and forced her into an introverted role in relation to his own high achievement. The treatment plan changed to focus on Martha's development of occupations outside the confines of her marriage.

Over time, Martha began jogging daily; she resumed playing the organ in church; she made new friends; she took on a caretaker role with her mother, who had suffered a stroke; she played piano for the town Christmas show; and she restarted the town-wide children's concerts. (*Note.* This case was contributed by Kathy Urban, MA, RN. Used with permission.)

Why could Martha discuss her marriage later in treatment while engaged in a cooking activity and not in the beginning? How did this change the treatment plan? How did the revelation about her marriage change the meaning of her past occupation as performer? How might the revelation about her marriage affect her social relationships? What did the therapist observe about Martha's occupations through interaction during activities with Martha?

personal and subjective perspective to the process. What questions are asked, what is considered relevant, and what actions are noticed all depend on what the therapist brings to the interaction. The therapist is influenced by the chosen theories and frames of reference, medical knowledge about the diagnosis and prognosis, his or her experience with other clients, and his or her personal experiences and prejudices (Urban 1998a, 1998b). It is important that therapists understand their own worldview and consider how it affects the interaction.

Exercise 5.4. Martha's Occupational Profile

In the case of Martha (Case Example 5.6), how did the therapist use the occupational profile as a tool? Think about which occupations the therapist reinforced as part of the treatment plan. Which past occupations opened new occupations for Martha?

How Context Affects the Occupational Profile

An activity out of context loses its meaning. *Context,* which refers to the various elements (physical and social) that are within and surround a person, shapes a person's performance of activities and occupations, and it can be internal or external to the client. *Internal contexts* involve the person's physical, social, and virtual realities, including his or her personal and spiritual beliefs. *External contexts* include time and space. *Time* is the time of day or the person's age. *Space* is the physical context relevant to the activity. When developing a client's occupational profile, the therapist needs to consider the contexts relevant to each activity and occupation. The context of many occupations is what individualizes them so that they have meaning to the person (Figure 5.5). The context shapes how the tasks are performed, where they take place, and how important they are.

For example, eating is strongly influenced by contextual factors. Having lunch at a restaurant is very different from having a picnic in the park. Likewise, a birthday dinner out is different from dinner at home. Eating is thus heavily influenced by internal and external contextual factors.

Self-care, which is engaging in activities that maintain oneself, is an occupation found in everyone's profile. Self-care, however, takes different forms for each person. One woman may need to wear nylons to work every day, whereas another may wear them only to church on Sundays. One woman may wear sneakers every day, whereas another may have been raised to believe that sneakers are unfeminine. One may dress in the bedroom, another in the bathroom. One elderly woman may feel that at her age, she has earned the right to have her children help her put on her shoes, whereas another would go barefoot before admitting that she could not do it herself. The elements affecting the single task of dressing are limitless. Under-

Figure 5.5. Depending on the individual and the context of the activity, washing a car can be a paid occupation, a chore within the occupation of car owner or driver, or a wet part of the occupation of play.

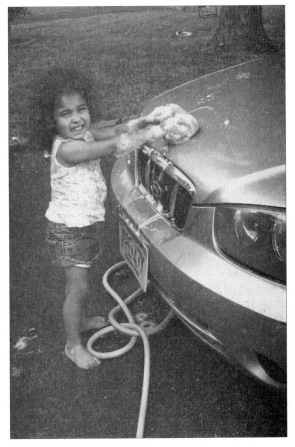

Source. J. Urban Wilson. Used with permission.

standing the specific contexts relevant to each person provides the critical data that give shape to the occupational profile.

Context also influences the process of obtaining the occupational profile. Issues of class, social norms, and the personal experiences of both the client and the therapist shape and inform the therapeutic relationship and in turn affect what information is shared. As therapists learn more about the context, they may adjust their approach. Sometimes a clearer occupational profile will emerge as the therapeutic relationship develops.

Ultimately, the therapist must respect the gaps in the occupational profile and acknowledge that the profile will never be complete. He or she needs to identify the occupations, with their contexts, that the client is willing to address at any given time.

Less obvious is the effect of the occupational profile itself on context. To consider this point of view, one must recognize that people are active forces in their contexts. People's occupations bring them to particular places and link them to particular people. Through their occupations, people have the power to change their physical and social environments.

Exercise 5.5. Context of Personal Occupational Profile

Think about one of your occupations, for example, the occupations of a student (e.g., writing a paper). Reflect on what contexts shape how you perform that occupation. What are the personal meanings of these contexts to you? Include cultural, physical, social, personal, spiritual, temporal, and virtual contexts. How do the details of your occupation differ from that of someone else you know?

Occupational Therapy Evaluation

Occupational therapy evaluation, which is a comprehensive process of obtaining and interpreting the data necessary to understand the person, has two components: the occupational profile and the *analysis of occupational performance,* which is a step in the evaluation of a client where his or her actual performance of an activity is assessed to identify assets, problems, or potential problems. Although the occupational profile is the starting point, these two aspects of the evaluation process are not sequential. The process of evaluation is a continuous interplay between the occupational profile and the analysis of occupational performance (AOTA, 2014).

The occupational profile identifies which occupations need to be evaluated for occupational performance. It pinpoints which occupations are priorities for intervention and what configuration of activities currently defines that occupation for the client. The therapist can then evaluate the client's performance in these activities. As the therapist analyzes the client's performance of the specified occupations, he or she observes the individual details of the client's task execution, which further flesh out the profile (Case Example 5.7).

Note that people may have difficulty describing their habits and routines, because these behaviors are so ingrained in their lives that they do not think about them anymore. Therefore, as the client performs a task, or tries to perform a task, the therapist sees what the client is able to do and how it is completed or attempted.

With new details observed while performing the analysis of the client's occupational performance,

---

Case Example 5.7. Enrique: Traumatic Brain Injury

Enrique is a 22-year-old man with a traumatic brain injury who was recently discharged from an inpatient rehabilitation hospital and referred for outpatient services. In the occupational therapist's initial interview, Enrique said he is having no problems. He lives with his mother, and every morning he gets up and gets his daughter ready for school. He spends his day helping around the house and taking care of his daughter. Enrique is eager to return to work but is concerned that he may not be able to return to construction work because his leg bothers him sometimes.

The therapist's formal testing showed severe disorganization, memory deficits with instructions, and inefficiency and multiple errors in task performance. The therapist decided to ask Enrique's mother about his daily routine. His mother reported that he sleeps late every day and cannot pick out his own clothes, even though he had always been a meticulous dresser. She takes care of his daughter. She does not let him out alone because he gets lost. She worries when she goes to work because Enrique once left the stove on, and she is afraid that he will wander off.

What information for the evaluation do the discrepancies in the reports provide? What suspicions do you think the therapist had that made her ask the mother for the same information she had asked of the client? What occupations does Enrique value? Which occupations are problematic? How does the additional information change the occupational focus of the intervention plan?

the therapist can then ask more questions, which further clarify the occupational profile, and in turn refocus the direction of the evaluation of occupational performance. Likewise, as the therapist identifies specific skill deficits through the analysis of occupational performance, he or she is able to anticipate what areas of occupations may be problematic and concentrate the questions there. For example, for a client with limited elbow flexion of the nondominant arm, the therapist will delve more deeply into the areas of applying make-up rather than painting fingernails or golfing rather than reading.

Observing a person's occupational performance, particularly in context, is an intimate act. As these activities are shared, the dialogue between the therapist and the client begins to develop. This dialogue is when the therapist learns the most about the client's occupational profile (Figure 5.6).

Figure 5.6. Sabrina brings her client, Antonia, into the community to evaluate her occupational performance in the same physical context that she will use after discharge.

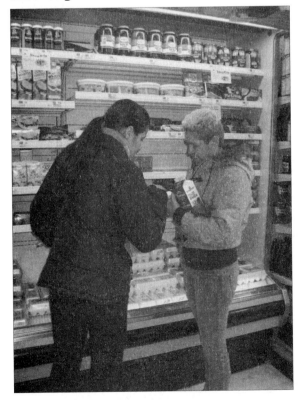

Source. J. Urban Wilson. Used with permission.

With a new injury or illness affecting occupational performance, the occupational therapy evaluation may be the first time clients are attempting some of the tasks important to their occupations. This situation makes the clients vulnerable because what they can and cannot do have changed. As they confront familiar tasks with new difficulties, the priorities and values in their occupational profiles shift. Moreover, this shift is emotionally charged. Clients often struggle down a tumultuous road toward new self-perceptions, which are tied directly to their occupational profile. They work to gain a vision of themselves in the future, a vision they use to set their goals and give meaning to the present (Morris, 1994). This metamorphosis spans the evaluation and intervention stages.

Intervention and the Occupational Profile

Occupational therapy intervention refers to theoretically based skilled actions used by the practitioner to facilitate positive change. Although constant adjustment of the occupational profile is most extreme with an acute injury or illness, occupational therapy intervention signifies a point of change for all clients. Even in healthy populations, if a person seeks an occupational therapy consultation, he or she is looking for ways to improve performance or decrease risk factors in occupations. As change occurs, the client's present occupational profile and vision of future occupations also change.

The occupational profile influences intervention by identifying the client's needs and priorities for intervention (Figure 5.7). Even, as is often the case, when clients' articulated goals are too general to use as intervention goals (e.g., "I want to go home," "I want to be like I used to be," "I want to walk," and "I want to get better"), the occupational profile gives the occupational therapy practitioner data with which to interpret these goals and form interventions. For example, in reviewing the client's array of occupations, the practitioner may find answers to questions such as where did the person walk in the past, what activities are necessary to survive at home, and which occupations are presently worse than before (see Case Example 5.8).

The occupational profile is also important in choosing types of interventions. It identifies what

Figure 5.7. The specifics of Carmen's occupational profile emerge through occupation-based interventions, which allow occupational therapist Michelle to best choose how she uses occupations as a treatment modality to address shoulder pain.

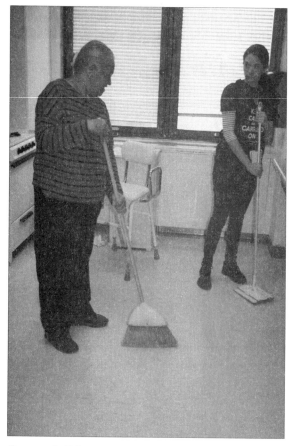

Source. J. Urban Wilson. Used with permission.

Case Example 5.8. George: Spinal Cord Injury

George, age 27 years, recently experienced a T–4 spinal cord injury and has a complete paraplegia. He hopes to walk and return to rock climbing and camping. He feels despair at times, convinced that he cannot even shave or feed himself. Sometimes, he just wants to indulge in his role as son and let his mother baby him, bathing him and combing his hair. At other times, he feels empowered, such as during his first time propelling himself in a wheelchair around the hospital unit.

George's occupational profile in relation to the present and the future is like his occupational performance in the evaluation and in ongoing treatment. Sometimes his only goal is to go home as soon as possible, with his mother and sister caring for him. Sometimes he can only address his occupations within the hospital stay, such as his self-care, his exercises, and his leadership role among other patients, but cannot discuss going home. At other times, he has many questions for the occupational therapist, asking about public transportation accessibility and information on wheelchair sports.

Which activities will the occupational therapist encourage? How can George's intervention plan capture his changing occupational profile and his changing focus? Which occupations are most urgent in intervention planning as his inpatient stay nears an end? How can his present occupations help build up his ability to support longer term occupations?

activities are important for the client and is also a source of ideas for the purposeful activities implemented in the intervention plan. The occupational therapy practitioner seeks purposeful activities that draw on the client's interests to be engaging and motivating for the client (Figure 5.8). Participating in purposeful activities builds the foundation on which the client's occupations can emerge.

The occupational profile also aids the occupational therapy practitioner in choosing a method to approach a goal. Knowing how the client has adapted his or her occupations at previous stages of life can help in the selection of an approach to which the client will be receptive. Where will the client be open to making changes? Would the cli-

ent rather scale back the performance of an occupation or completely redesign how to fulfill a role?

The occupational profile links the dynamic interrelationship among assessment, intervention planning, and intervention implementation (AOTA, 2014). The client's awareness of what he or she can and cannot do increases. The occupational therapy practitioner exposes the client to new experiences that may open possibilities in the client's eyes. The client travels through different emotional responses to the changes. In addition, the client–practitioner relationship is forged, and new revelations and understanding about the occupational profile emerge in the process.

Figure 5.8. From a detailed occupational profile of Charles, occupational therapist Raechel can target the critical skills Charles needs to return home. An important self-care activity, which is purposeful for Charles, is managing his own medications.

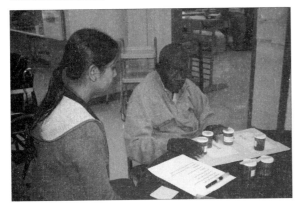

Source. J. Urban Wilson. Used with permission.

Exercise 5.6. Lifestyle Redesign

Read the story of Penny in Florence Clark's (1993) "Occupation Embedded in a Real Life: Interweaving Occupational Science and Occupational Therapy" (p. 1067). Consider these questions: Which occupations from childhood helped Penny reform her occupations after the "Big A"? Which occupations does Penny value most? What occupations did she modify to fulfill her roles? What are new occupations she has taken on to fulfill old roles?

Often when dealing with a premature child, in addition to the child's needs, parents' fears and anxiety complicate developing the child's occupational profile. In Case Example 5.9, Destiny's premature birth results in a complex evaluation.

Outcomes and the Occupational Profile

Beginning during the evaluation process, the occupational profile is a tool used to set specific *outcome measures,* which are the results of an activity, plan, process, or program. The *Framework* (2nd ed.) defined the *domain of concern of occupational therapy*

Case Example 5.9. Destiny: Premature Infant

Destiny was born 10 weeks prematurely. After 8 weeks in the neonatal intensive care unit, she was taking her meals by breast and bottle, so she was ready for discharge home. Her family (mom, dad, and two brothers, ages 5 and 3 years) were very excited to welcome her home. Now, 2 months later, Destiny is referred to occupational therapy because she has dropped below the first percentile weight for her age. The doctor ruled out metabolic causes and is concerned about her feeding skills. During evaluation, the occupational therapist identified concerns with her coordination and endurance with eating; she eats very small meals frequently, waking before getting enough sleep, in an exhausting and inefficient cycle. She has a very weak cry and fusses little. The evaluation also found Destiny's "quiet" behavior included minimal attempts to explore her environment visually or tactilely. Her mother is very concerned but is also very distracted by the demands of her other children.

Occupational therapist Elsie R. Vergara (2002) describes infants' primary occupations as play, social interaction, procuring (getting attention to have needs met), and feeding. Additionally, the *Framework* (AOTA, 2014) identifies sleep as an occupational activity. Which aspects of these occupations will be the focus of the intervention plan? How could the child's sleeping patterns be reflected in the goals? Looking at the family as the client, consider how Destiny's occupations intertwine with her parents' and her brothers' occupational profiles. Which aspects of their profiles need to be developed during interventions? How could the therapist include the family in treatment strategies using play and social interaction?

as "achieving health, well-being, and participation in life through engagement in occupation" (AOTA, 2008, p. 3). The *Framework* supports the idea that the desired outcome of occupational therapy interventions is engagement in occupations that promote health, wellness, and participation (AOTA, 2014).

The occupational profile identifies which of the client's occupations are desired, valued, and needed, providing details about the occupations in which the client seeks to participate and commits to engage in more fully. In designing the intervention plan, the practitioner uses the occupational profile to determine which occupational areas to target. The outcome measures thus flow directly from the occupational issues that surfaced in the profile, because the profile identifies the values, roles, personal meanings, and unique contexts of the occupations in the client's life (Figure 5.9). Successful outcomes represent meaningful change for the client. The direction taken by the outcome measures, however, varies greatly.

The outcome measure can be a resumption of impaired occupations, or it can be a change in or redefinition of the occupations. Activities that are health risks or that are unattainable for the client after a bodily change need to undergo alteration. For example, the outcome measures may target a

Figure 5.9. Outcome measures pull directly from the occupations valued by the individual person, such as participating in the co-occupation of daughter and mother.

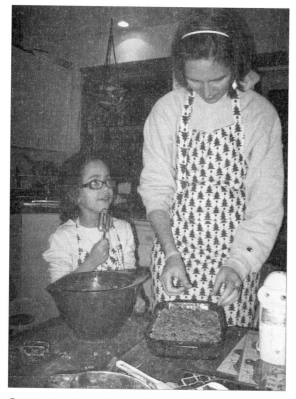

Source. J. Urban Wilson. Used with permission.

change in leisure skills for a person with a drug addiction or aim to redefine work for a person after a severe brain injury. Because the profile identifies the client's valued roles, it guides the client and the occupational therapy practitioner in channeling the activity changes to achieve role competence.

In some cases, the client may identify in the profile certain occupational performances with which he or she is disappointed. The therapist sets the outcome measure at satisfactory performance of that occupation, such as independence with work skills after a hand injury or resuming independent living at home after a stroke. In other cases, the client may be dissatisfied with his or her occupational engagement, and so the therapist may set the outcome measure to be a change in actions. Here, the profile identifies the components of the occupational challenge. For example, a client who describes a series of job losses because of fights with his coworkers illustrates a profile that is not satisfactory to the client at present. The outcome measure is the change in engagement that allows the client to maintain a job.

The therapist may choose to look at the occupational profile with the client as a conscientious part of jointly evaluating outcomes. This process allows the client to express satisfaction with changes or dissatisfaction with lack of changes. This process may also reveal a change in the client's perceptions and whether he or she has achieved great or little change in performance.

The ultimate goal of occupational therapy is for the client to spontaneously engage in occupations that he or she values. The client's quality of life is determined by the client's perceptions of his or her life and is strongly influenced by his or her ability to engage in meaningful occupations. The occupational profile's temporal context is most critical in setting outcome measures. To determine outcome measures, the occupational therapy practitioner considers the client's future, anticipated occupations, and past and present occupations. During intervention, the practitioner also guides a realistic development of that future occupational vision, and outcome measures are reworked throughout the intervention process as the client and practitioner reconfigure the occupational profile. The outcome is therefore both a product of the occupational profile and a transformative factor in the occupational profile.

The outcome measures arise from the occupational profile, and the client and therapist set goals while exploring the occupational profile together. This is not to say, however, that a successful outcome is a return to a fixed occupational profile. Remember that the occupational profile is a fluid entity. Indeed, throughout the occupational therapy intervention, the profile continues to transform. The client factors may have changed, the interventions may have changed the makeup of the activities, and the intervention may have modified the context or environment of the occupations. Even when body function has returned to normal and the occupations are performed in the same context as they were previously, the meaning of these occupations to the client has changed because of his or her experiences during the occupational therapy intervention. The outcome measures stemmed from the occupational profile; nevertheless, the outcome itself is part of the new occupational profile.

Exercise 5.7. Outcomes From the Occupational Profile

Review several of the case examples presented in this chapter. Identify appropriate outcome measures for each.

Summary

The occupational therapy profile is a useful tool to gain information about a client's occupations, and it is critical for planning and implementing occupational therapy interventions. The occupational profile provides a structured process for obtaining information about a client's set of activities, routines, and roles. Using the information obtained from the occupational profile, the occupational therapy practitioner is able to determine meaningful therapeutic goals that reflect the client's values and needs.

References

American Occupational Therapy Association. (1997). Statement—Fundamental concepts of occupational therapy: Occupation, purposeful activity, and function. *American Journal of Occupational Therapy, 51,* 864–866. http://dx.doi.org/10.5014/ajot.51.10.864

American Occupational Therapy Association. (2008). Occupational therapy practice framework: Domain and process (2nd ed.). *American Journal of Occupational Therapy, 62,* 625–683. http://dx.doi.org/10.5014/ajot.62.6.625

American Occupational Therapy Association. (2014). Occupational therapy practice framework: Domain and process (3rd ed.). *American Journal of Occupational Therapy, 68*(Suppl. 1), S1–S48. http://dx.doi.org/10.5014/ajot.2014.682006

Clark, F. (1993). Occupation embedded in a real life: Interweaving occupational science and occupational therapy [1993 Eleanor Clarke Slagle Lecture]. *American Journal of Occupational Therapy, 47,* 1067–1078. http://dx.doi.org/10.5014/ajot.47.12.1067

Hasselkus, B. R. (2006). The world of everyday occupation: Real people, real lives [Eleanor Clarke Slagle Lecture]. *American Journal of Occupational Therapy, 60,* 627–640. http://dx.doi.org/10.5014/ajot.60.6.627

Kielhofner, G. (1983). Occupation. In H. L. Hopkins & H. D. Smith (Eds.), *Willard and Spackman's occupational therapy* (6th ed., pp. 31–41). Philadelphia: J. B. Lippincott.

Kielhofner, G. (Ed.). (1985). *A model of human occupation: Theory and application.* Baltimore: Lippincott Williams & Wilkins.

Kielhofner, G. (1992). *Conceptual foundations of occupational therapy.* Philadelphia: F. A. Davis.

Kielhofner, G. (2008). *Model of Human Occupation: Theory and application* (4th ed.). Philadelphia: F. A. Davis.

Kielhofner, G., Mallinson, T., Crawford, C., Nowak, M., Rigby, M., Henry, A., & Walens, D. (2004). *Occupational Performance History Interview–II (OPHI–II), version 2.1.* Chicago: MOHO Clearinghouse.

Kramer, P., Hinojosa, J., & Royeen, C. B. (Eds.). (2003). *Perspectives in human occupation: Participation in life.* Philadelphia: Lippincott Williams & Wilkins.

Morris, J. (1994). Spinal injury and psychotherapy in treatment philosophy. In G. M. Yarkony (Ed.), *Spinal cord injury: Medical management and rehabilitation* (pp. 223–229). Gaithersburg, MD: Aspen.

Nelson, D. L. (1996). Therapeutic occupation: A definition. *American Journal of Occupational Therapy, 50,* 775–782. http://dx.doi.org/10.5014/ajot.50.10.775

Trombly, C. A. (1995). Occupation: Purposefulness and meaningfulness as therapeutic mechanisms [Eleanor Clarke Slagle Lecture]. *American Journal of Occupational Therapy, 49,* 960–972. http://dx.doi.org/10.5014/ajot.49.10.960

Urban, J. (1998a). *A critical analysis of "cultural sensitivity" in health care practice* (Unpublished master's thesis). Hunter College of the City University of New York.

Urban, J. (1998b, June). *Cultural issues in occupational therapy.* Paper presented at the 12th International Congress of the World Federation of Occupational Therapists, Montreal, Canada.

Vergara, E. R. (2002). Enhancing occupational performance in infants in the NICU. *OT Practice, 7,* 8–13.

CHAPTER 6.

ACTIVITY SYNTHESIS AS A MEANS TO STRUCTURE OCCUPATION

Paula Kramer, PhD, OTR, FAOTA, and Jim Hinojosa, PhD, OT, BCP, FAOTA

Highlights

- ✧ Synthesis in everyday life
- ✧ Occupational synthesis: A critical end product
- ✧ Importance of activity and occupational synthesis to intervention
- ✧ Other uses of activity and occupational synthesis in intervention
- ✧ Activity and occupational synthesis for health promotion
- ✧ Artful practice and synthesis
- ✧ Development of artful practice.

Key Terms

- ✧ Acquisitional frame of reference
- ✧ Acquisitional theory
- ✧ Activity modification
- ✧ Activity synthesis
- ✧ Adaptation
- ✧ ADL board
- ✧ Artful practice
- ✧ Client-centered approach
- ✧ Clinical reasoning process
- ✧ Context
- ✧ Developmental perspective
- ✧ Frames of reference
- ✧ Grading
- ✧ Grading the activity down
- ✧ Grading the activity up

- ✧ Guidelines for intervention
- ✧ Human environment
- ✧ Just-right fit
- ✧ Layered adaptation
- ✧ Models of practice
- ✧ Neurodevelopmental treatment
- ✧ Nonhuman environment
- ✧ Occupational adaptation
- ✧ Occupational analysis
- ✧ Occupational performance
- ✧ Occupational synthesis
- ✧ Performance
- ✧ Purposeful activities
- ✧ Scaling the activity
- ✧ Theoretical orientations

All thought, in its early stages, begins as action. The actions which you have been wading through have been ideas . . . but they had to be established as a foundation before we could begin to think in earnest.

—White, 1977, p. 11

Activity synthesis appears simple to the person viewing it, but it is actually a complex process. This chapter reviews the complexities of activity synthesis used by occupational therapy practitioners as a means to effectively engage clients in occupations and to meet therapeutic goals. The occupational therapy practitioner synthesizes activities directed by a theoretical focus. It is the theoretical focus that directs the activity synthesis and the process of adapting, grading, and modifying activities.

After discussing these basic components of activity synthesis, we discuss the complex process of creating new activities through the use of activity synthesis as the process moves toward occupational synthesis. The ways in which the practitioner uses activities to teach and refine skills are presented along with the role that activity synthesis can play in health promotion. The chapter ends with a discussion of the importance of artful practice when using activity synthesis, because it is foundational to occupational synthesis, and it takes art for the practitioner to create a revised activity that is meaningful to the client. Throughout the chapter, we take into account the complexities of this seemingly simple process and explain how the practitioner masters these complexities.

Synthesis in Everyday Life

The magician's sleight of hand is smooth and sinuous, creating only the illusion of reality. The audience members watch in awe, trying to reconcile the reality that they know exists with what they think they are seeing. It seems so simple, yet creating the illusion is very complex (Hunt, 1997). In many ways, the magician's act mirrors the activity synthesis carried out by an occupational therapy practitioner. *Activity synthesis* is the act of changing or modifying a specific activity so that the person can engage in it successfully. Make no mistake, the practitioner does not perform magic. Rather, he or

she puts so much thought and skill into developing and creating activities that the client's experience with the activities in therapy becomes seamless, much akin to observing the misleading simplicity of a magician's illusions.

Activity synthesis occurs in everyday life. People adapt, adjust, and make up activities all the time to meet the demands of day-to-day living. For example, many young children do not like to have clothes put on over their heads because it occludes their eyes. When a parent turns this task into a game, for example, by saying, "Where did Johnny go?" while putting the shirt over the child's head, the child will often laugh rather than be frightened. This parent has just synthesized the activity by modifying it to prompt the child's engagement with the task, thus leading to a successful outcome. Similarly, if a person becomes tired while performing a task standing up, he or she will try to find a way to do the same task sitting down. This synthesis could be as simple as pulling up a chair, or it might require moving the activity to a counter or table at a different height so that the task can be done sitting down (Figures 6.1A and 6.1B).

Because activity synthesis occurs every day, people think that devising an activity is something that is easy or natural, yet it is actually very complex. Because it looks so easy and is so common, people generally do not conceptualize the development of activities as synthesis in any special way. Occupational therapy practitioners, however, view activities and their synthesis in a complex and theoretical manner that centers on people's occupational preferences. Because the domain of concern of occupational therapy focuses on human occupation, practitioners synthesize activities as a means to advance a client's ability to participate in meaningful activities. Despite activity synthesis being central to the art and practice of occupational therapy, very little has been written specifically about this aspect of intervention. In this chapter, we delve into the myriad concerns and reasoning processes involved in activity synthesis in occupational therapy.

Synthesizing activities is something that people take for granted—they often modify, adapt, or alter activities seemingly without even thinking. However, even though it is viewed as part of a natural process by many people, it does require either some conscious thought or an "intuitive sense" of what

Figure 6.1. When tired from standing (A), a person finds a way to adapt the task to a seated position (B).

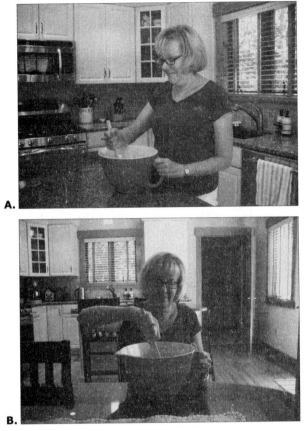

A.

B.

Source. P. Kramer. Used with permission.

changes need to be made to the activity. In other words, on some level, it requires a deeper understanding of why a task is not working the way it was originally supposed to and why it is important to make modifications to successfully complete the task.

Occupational Synthesis: A Critical End Product

Occupational synthesis is critical to the practice of occupational therapy. What is occupational synthesis? *Occupational synthesis* is a process that takes place within the client, in which the client internalizes the activity synthesis that has been performed by the occupational therapy practitioner. Occupational synthesis is a process that happens internally (and sometimes unconsciously) within the client as a result of the therapeutic process.

At the initiation of occupational therapy services, the client (or his or her significant others) conveys to the practitioner his or her meaningful occupations. It is critical that the practitioner uses this knowledge within the intervention process for activity synthesis. Once the client is involved in the occupational therapy process, he or she can work with the practitioner to begin engaging in tasks and activities that improve functional performance. At this point, the client either already has developed a sense of which of those activities contribute to personally meaningful occupations or will develop that understanding through the therapy process.

The identified meaningful occupations are critical to the client, that is, they are occupations that he or she truly wants to continue to do when occupational therapy is finished or they are essential to the maintenance of functional performance. For example, a client who injured her shoulder has been working on shoulder range of motion during occupational therapy, which is about to end. To help her maintain the gains she made during therapy, she and her occupational practitioner decide to rearrange her closet and put some of her favorite sweaters on a higher shelf in her closet. This rearrangement of her clothes forces her to reach up, thereby maintaining the range of motion in her shoulder and becoming part of her occupational synthesis. The ongoing use of the activity and its adoption into the client's routine signal that it has been incorporated into her daily life and occupations, which is essential for occupational synthesis to be effective.

The occupational therapy practitioner facilitates occupational synthesis by determining the occupations that are meaningful to the client and then working toward synthesizing appropriate therapeutic activities. In addition, to successfully carry out this synthesis process, the practitioner must gain an understanding of who the client is as a person. The practitioner needs to examine all the available data to develop interventions that will meet the occupational needs of the client. This process requires a *client-centered approach,* in which the practitioner explores the value of the occupation to the client and his or her personal choices in terms of occupations. Furthermore, the practitioner's professional judgment is critical, especially when a client cannot articulate meaningful occupations.

When an occupational therapy practitioner is unable to obtain useful information from the client about his or her occupational needs or desires, other sources of information must be found. These sources include talking with the client's caregivers and significant others, reviewing evaluation data, and considering the client's occupational profile in terms of contextual and temporal needs. The practitioner must then use trial and error by presenting various tasks, activities, and approaches to discover what motivates the client.

Note that practitioners should not make assumptions about a client's motivation, nor should they just choose occupations for the client. When a client values an occupation, he or she is more likely to engage in the activities related to the occupation. When a client is not motivated, however, the practitioner must use his or her clinical judgment to explore the situation. Is the client unmotivated because of the tasks and activities being presented, or does the client lack motivation in general? After trial and error with various tasks, if nothing seems to spark the client's engagement and motivation, another approach needs to be considered. The practitioner should select a theoretical perspective that addresses motivation to guide the intervention. Such perspectives include the Model of Human Occupation (Forsyth & Kielhofner, 2003; Kielhofner, 2008) and the Canadian Model of Occupational Performance (Law et al., 1990).

To use occupational synthesis effectively for the client who can articulate his or her occupational needs and goals, the occupational therapy practitioner should consider the following questions:

- Why is this activity important to the client?
- How does this activity relate to the client's occupations?
- What role does this occupation play in the client's life?
- How does this occupation need to be synthesized to fit into the client's life?
- How will this occupational synthesis fit into the context of the client's life?
- How will the synthesized activity help the client engage in meaningful occupations overall, within the client's life?

Determining the answers to these questions allows the practitioner to understand the activity and its relationship to the client's occupations.

The occupational therapy practitioner should also consider context when the synthesis of activities is related to intervention, because the ultimate goal is for the client to be able to perform the activity in the real world, not just in the simulated environment of the occupational therapy practice setting. *Context* involves the physical environment, social environment, and elements that are within and surround a client (i.e., cultural, personal, temporal, and virtual; American Occupational Therapy Association [AOTA], 2014; Christiansen, Baum, & Bass-Haugen, 2005; Dunn, Brown, & McGuigan, 1994). Context determines the demands on the person in many ways, so it is critical for the practitioner to choose tasks and activities with the person's context in mind. Understanding the context of the person is also part of the evaluation process and needs to be taken into account throughout the planning of therapy sessions, before even considering occupational synthesis. Clearly, context is critical to develop meaningful occupational synthesis for the client.

Theory

This section discusses the relationship between occupational therapy and theory. Although people naturally modify activities in a relatively unconscious manner, they do not generally adapt them in an organized fashion. No theoretical rationale exists for the adaptation of an activity, and people instead rely on what appears to be common sense. In doing so, people tend to look for a simple change in the activity that will bring about success rather than looking critically at the activity as a whole. Occupational therapy practitioners, however, use activity synthesis in an organized manner, determined by the frame of reference or theoretical perspective they are using to guide their intervention.

Returning to the metaphor of the magician, the magician creates the illusion by using principles of physics, visual misdirection, and knowledge of how people perceive situations. Thus, the magician uses the distraction of attractive people on the stage, so the viewer will not focus on specific actions the magician does as part of the act. The occupational therapy practitioner uses theory as a basis for what he or she does in a way that allows the client to focus on the simplicity of changing an activity to meet his or her goals.

Practitioners are guided by theory to plan the synthesis of an activity to meet therapeutic goals.

For example, a practitioner may use an *acquisitional theory* that is based on teaching and rewarding the learned behavior, such as Piaget's (1963) theory, to synthesize activities because he or she understands that the child actively seeks knowledge. The practitioner presents activities consistent with the child's stage of development and is sensitive to the child's cognitive level. For example, with a child younger than age 2 years, the practitioner would synthesize an activity based on the sensorimotor aspects of an activity rather than a Lego®-building activity, which is at a much higher level. Thus, the theory, or in some cases theories, provide the practitioner with the means of synthesis and an understanding of what is expected to happen.

Occupational therapy intervention is always based on theoretical perspectives, such as *models of practice* (i.e., uses one or more theories to devise a method for translating theory into practice; Hinojosa, Kramer, & Luebben, 2010), *theoretical orientations* (i.e., the theory underlying a model of practice or a frame of reference or a theoretical perspective), *guidelines for intervention* (i.e., specific information about how to put theoretical information into practice), or *frames of reference* (i.e., theoretically based sets of guidelines for intervention).

Many occupational therapy practitioners synthesize activities using established theoretical perspectives, paradigms, or frames of reference. Some examples are the Model of Human Occupation (MOHO; Forsyth & Kielhofner, 2003; Kielhofner, 2008), Ecological Model of Occupation (Dunn, Brown, & Youngstrom, 2003), Person–Environment–Occupation–Performance (PEOP; Baum & Christiansen, 2005), Cognitive Orientation to Daily Occupational Performance (Missiuna, Mandich, Polatajko, & Malloy-Miller, 2001), Bobath Approach (Levit, 2008), and sensory integration (Schaaf et al., 2009).

The theoretical perspective directs practitioners on how to modify the specific activity during the intervention. Thus, activity synthesis takes place within a theoretical framework guiding the intervention. Then, using the creative process within a theoretical framework, the practitioner devises or synthesizes activities that will meet the client's needs. If the client has no interest in the activity or does not see it as meaningful to his or her life, he or she will probably go through the actions with no personal investment. Moreover, the client may not

be self-motivated to participate in the activity at all, and its therapeutic value is thus minimized.

Whenever possible, the occupational therapy practitioner should use a client-centered approach (AOTA, 2014) to ensure that the therapeutic activities are meaningful to and elicit a positive response from the client. For the intervention to be successful, the synthesis of activities must always take the client's needs and wants into account. Some theoretical perspectives, like the MOHO and the Life Style Performance Model (Fidler, 1996), explicitly address the client's personal motivation (Fidler & Velde, 2002; Kielhofner, 2008); most others, such as the Ecological Model of Human Occupation and the PEOP Model, address the meaningfulness of the activity to the client. The practitioner should select a theoretical perspective that meets the needs of the client and also incorporates a client-centered approach.

In those models that focus on the importance of the activity to the client, the occupational therapy practitioner provides activities and options for the client as a means of intervention. The client then incorporates some of these activities into personally meaningful occupations. The occupational synthesis begins as collaboration between the practitioner and the client and then ultimately takes place within the client as he or she chooses those occupations to continue as part of everyday life. Note that the perspective we propose is not consistent with that proposed by Nelson and Jepson-Thomas (2003). They defined *occupational synthesis* as what the practitioner does—they did not use the term *activity* at all. We believe that the practitioner works with the client to develop an activity synthesis, whereas occupational synthesis ultimately occurs within the client.

Activity Analysis and Synthesis

Activity synthesis is based on the occupational therapy practitioner's comprehensive understanding of the activity and occupation. Initial understanding of the activity and occupation is based on the activity analysis. Activity analysis has been a basic competency for all practitioners since the 1940s (Creighton, 1992; Fidler, 1948; Mosey, 1981). As discussed in detail in Chapter 4, "Activity Analysis," activity analysis provides the practitioner with an understanding of the activity and its components. Activity synthesis uses this knowledge of the component elements to reconstruct or design a therapeutic activity. Although activity analysis and synthesis are usually discussed as two separate but associated processes that are used together, they provide the practitioner with the means to understand and successfully use purposeful activities for the client's benefit.

Interestingly, in occupational therapy professional education, much time is spent on activity analysis, and very little time is spent on activity synthesis. Hence, students and practitioners get the impression that activity analysis is more important to the intervention process than activity synthesis. However, if one observes children in a playground for a short period of time, one can see that adaptation and synthesis continuously occurs in play (Figure 6.2). This points to the need for synthesis.

The assumption in the focus on activity analysis is that once the practitioner understands the step or stage of a task that is problematic to the client, intervention can take place and the client will then work toward the successful completion of the task. This notion, however, that synthesis is not as important as analysis is not accurate; in fact, a constant interplay exists between analysis and synthesis. Nelson (1997) characterized *occupational analysis* as "what occupational therapists do" (p. 15), thus noting the importance of synthesis being interconnected with analysis rather than separate from it. Synthesis is considered to be an intellectual process and part of the clinical reasoning and decision-making aspects of practice (Mosey, 1996; Nelson & Jepson-Thomas, 2003).

Activity Synthesis as a Precursor to Occupational Synthesis

Generally, activity synthesis takes place prior to occupational synthesis and sets the stage for the client to be able to achieve occupational synthesis. How do occupational therapy practitioners use activity synthesis as part of their intervention? Where does activity synthesis fit into the overall intervention process? As presented in this chapter, activity synthesis involves and encompasses a complex reasoning process guided by theory that directs practitioners in the therapeutic use of activities. From a practitioner's perspective, activity synthesis begins with conceptualizing the activities

Figure 6.2. Playing in a playground on a wooden swing set requires children to learn to adapt to various challenges. Adaptation is an important part of synthesis.

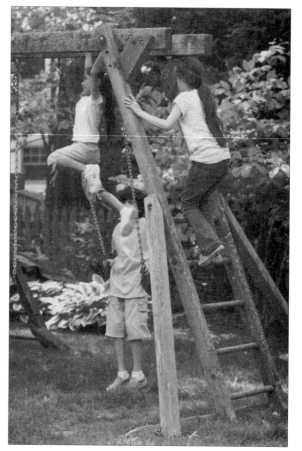

Source. Courtesy of the Public Health Image Library, Centers for Disease Control and Prevention. Photo by C. Martin.

that the client wants or needs to perform. Responsibility rests with the client and the practitioner to determine the importance of these actions, to think them through carefully, and to use this knowledge as the foundation for activity synthesis. This activity analysis ensures that the practitioner understands the components of the activity in the context of the client's performance of that activity.

Before analysis or synthesis can take place, the practitioner needs to understand the client and his or her life situation, which involves understanding the client's personal goals, desires, capacities, and limitations. Personal goals and desires may depend on context, and in some cases, they may be those of the family or society and may depend on certain life circumstances. Much of this information can be obtained from the occupational profile. Goals and desires then need to be explored within the context of capacities and limitations. Although one may have the desire to achieve something, the capacity for that achievement may not be present. Activities can be synthesized effectively only when the practitioner has a clear understanding of the client, his or her life, and all the contextual factors that affect the client (Figure 6.3).

Once the practitioner has selected the appropriate activity, he or she completes an activity analysis, taking into consideration the client's strengths and areas of concern. The activity analysis gives the practitioner a rudimentary understanding of the tasks that might be adapted or changed. With this information, the practitioner can begin to create modifications to the activity that meet the client's needs. The practitioner synthesizes an activity that is consistent with the theoretical perspective, model, or frame of reference that has been selected to guide his or her interventions with the client. The theoretical perspective determines how and in what ways an activity is synthesized in the therapeutic situation. By putting together the practitioner's professional knowledge, the expected outcomes of the therapeutic process, and the client's (or family's) mutually agreed-on goals, synthesis begins.

Figure 6.3. Learning to master the throwing and catching of a Frisbee is challenging. The adolescent must learn to modify his response for accuracy.

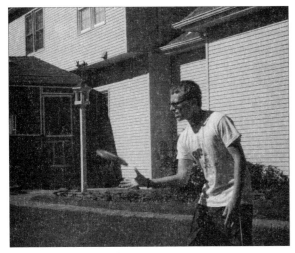

Source. P. Kramer. Used with permission.

Identifying and defining potential goals for the intervention require negotiation and collaboration between the client and the practitioner. This process goes two ways, and each person involved brings his or her own perspective: The practitioner brings a clinical understanding of the client's condition from a medical and psychosocial perspective and an understanding of the potential sequelae of the disease, and the client brings his or her unique sense of self and an understanding of his or her own aspirations, along with the drive to achieve the goal. Together, the practitioner and client develop goals that define the course of treatment and outcomes of the intervention. Ideally, the goals should relate to the occupations that the client currently wants to carry out or will engage in at some point in the future and should be oriented to the ability to participate in life and society. If the activities that are synthesized are meaningful to the client, he or she will be able to incorporate them into daily life as part of an occupational synthesis.

Process of Activity Synthesis in Occupational Therapy

In occupational therapy, when the activity analysis is complete and the theoretical perspective has been considered, the activity synthesis begins. This process starts with defining the key elements of the activity because one can only adapt an activity so much until it becomes a different activity.

For example, is it still baking if no oven or heat is involved? Is it still baseball without a ball and bat? When these key elements are no longer present, the activity is not the same. Once the activities are created and presented to the client, the occupational therapy practitioner observes the client's performance and continually reanalyzes it to adapt and resynthesize the activity to meet the client's changing needs and to move toward the end goal. The process is ongoing and dynamic.

Sometimes the activity needs to be reconstructed or synthesized in a different way to allow the client to be successful. The dynamic nature of this process confirms that analyzing the activity is not enough—understanding how one can construct or synthesize an activity is equally important for occupational therapy practitioners.

It is important to remember that synthesis involves more than just the activity itself; it involves the personal meaning of the activity. As discussed earlier, occupational therapy practitioners view synthesis in the context of the person as an occupational being. They ask,

- Who is the person involved in the intervention process?
- What occupations are important to this person?
- How do specific purposeful activities relate to these occupations?
- Does the accomplishment of a purposeful activity build on or allow this person to engage in meaningful occupations at his or her current stage of life or in the future?

The creative process of synthesis requires a thorough understanding of the activity, as well as a visualization of the goal and the desired end product.

All activities used by occupational therapy practitioners are viewed within the context of the occupations that are critical to the client. Practitioners use an organized conceptual approach to activity synthesis, based on the understanding of the occupation and its component activities. They view each activity as a whole, and an activity analysis is done to break it down into component parts. The final step in the process is to synthesize or recreate the activity with change, modification, or adaptation to allow the client to achieve success in the task.

Traditional activity synthesis requires that the chosen activity be reconstructed, incorporating the client's therapeutic goals, areas of strength and limitations, and the therapeutic relationship. The activity is reconfigured in ways that allow the client to approach it with minimal fear of failure and with greater potential for success. At this point, the activity synthesis can be used for various purposes: as an evaluative tool to see how the client responds to the modifications or as part of the intervention process. More specifically, activity synthesis can be used to evaluate occupational performance within a context, teach a new skill, refine a skill, or maintain a client's functional status or performance ability. These applications of activity synthesis are discussed later in this chapter.

Activity synthesis is based on the practitioner's skills and abilities, his or her understanding the theoretically based guidelines (e.g., models of practice, theoretical orientations, guidelines for intervention, or frames of reference) that the practitioner

has determined to be the most appropriate for the client, the client's needs, and the context in which the activity will occur. Activity synthesis is guided by the theoretical framework throughout the process. Thus, activities are used, adapted, modified, or created within the parameters of the chosen theoretically based guidelines (see Case Example 6.1).

Activity synthesis is a complex process of adapting and grading activities, modifying activities, and creating new activities based on theory, which are discussed in the following sections. Although we address each process individually as though it were distinct from the others, in practice, one or more processes may be used in combination; they overlap and are not mutually exclusive. As with learning any process, it is important that each component be appreciated and understood in relation to the others. By understanding the components of activity synthesis, one can attain a distinct knowledge of the whole process of synthesis.

Adapting and grading activities

Adapting and grading activities are critical to activity synthesis. *Adaptation* involves a change to the environment or the activity, not a change to the person. Adaptation of activities, therefore, involves changing the environment in which the activity occurs or the activity rather than working to bring about change in the person doing the activity. When a client is having difficulty with a task or activity, the activity is adapted for the client.

Adaptation begins with an activity analysis that considers the capabilities of the client, the activity, and the context in which it will be done. After analyzing the activity or completing the activity analysis, the occupational therapy practitioner uses the theoretical perspective to decide how the activity should be adapted or changed to meet the client's abilities, allowing the client to perform the activity in a specific context.

For instance, using a simple rehabilitation frame of reference, the therapist can, for example, modify the activity by having the client grip an implement (e.g., spoon with a built-up handle), change his or her position when engaging in a task, or sit down during an activity for energy conservation. If the therapist selects a different theoretical perspective, more of an adaptation would be involved, which is a more complicated process in which the defining features of the

Case Example 6.1. Alejandro: Two Frames of Reference to Address Difficulties With Fine Motor Coordination

Alejandro, age 6 years, is referred to occupational therapy for a fine motor coordination problem. After a comprehensive evaluation, the occupational therapist assigns Alejandro to an occupational therapy assistant to implement a program to develop hand and fine motor coordination by working with manipulative tools that strengthen muscles. Thus, a sensorimotor frame of reference is chosen. The therapist selects this frame of reference because she has determined that Alejandro has poor muscle strength and limited experience with fine motor activities. The intervention is carried out within the context of Alejandro's classroom because that is his natural context at school.

After meeting Alejandro, reviewing the recommendations, and discussing the frame of reference with the therapist, the occupational therapy assistant uses activity analysis and synthesis to develop activities for Alejandro. These activities involve Alejandro using an adapted pencil for writing and paper with raised lines that will give him increased sensory feedback. Another activity is spending playtime using building blocks such as Legos. In addition, the assistant observes the computer-based activities used in the classroom. After careful analysis of these computer-based activities, the assistant decides to replace Alejandro's keyboard with one that provides more resistance. The keyboard is also raised so that Alejandro must use more shoulder motion while working on the computer.

If a different frame of reference—one based on play (thus, the context is outside the classroom) and theories of psychosocial development—had been chosen to address Alejandro's fine motor problems, the following different approach

would have been used. The focus is on Alejandro's personal interests, analyzing purposeful activities, and synthesizing activities in response. For instance, the occupational therapy assistant observes that Alejandro enjoys the game Connect Four.® The objective of this game is to pick up small checkers and put them into a vertical form to line up four in a row. An understanding of theories of psychosocial development suggests that a 6-year-old boy can relate to others in a cooperative manner. Therefore, the occupational therapy assistant involves Alejandro in creating a way to play Connect Four while working on his fine motor skills.

After adapting the game to address some of Alejandro's fine motor needs, the assistant plays the game with Alejandro. Together, they then decide to place the checkers under various heavy objects around the room, forcing Alejandro to develop his strength by lifting the objects. In addition, before putting the checker in the vertical form, Alejandro and the assistant attempt to each balance prone over a small ball, using the nondominant hand to balance and support their weight. Guided by the psychosocial development frame of reference, the assistant synthesized an activity to engage Alejandro in terms of his stage of development and to be therapeutically valuable for his particular motor needs.

After this initial activity helps Alejandro develop more strength, the assistant uses cooperative play again to work on another, more demanding fine motor task with Legos.® The assistant then engages another child in cooperative play with Alejandro to develop both his psychosocial and fine motor skills while the children work together on a building project.

activity are changed. An example of an adaption is using the Ecological Model of Human Development in which the environment of the task is significantly changed, or the utensils used in the task are changed completely. Theoretical perspectives thus guide the adaptation and modification process.

Grading is a common way to adapt an activity. Although it is a basic principle in learning theory,

occupational therapy practitioners almost universally use grading. For this reason, it is critical to think about grading and how it is used in the context of specific theories that guide intervention. *Grading* can involve simplifying the activity, making the activity more complex, modifying the sequence or physical nature of the activity, or modifying the amount of time taken to complete the activity. Simplifying the activity (also known as *grading the activity down*) entails making the activity easier for the client in some way.

For example, for a child who is learning how to undress himself or herself (an *acquisitional frame of reference*, which is a theory-based intervention based on teaching and learning), grading might involve having the parent roll down the sock from the heel and then having the child pull it off or open the child's pants fastenings and then having the child remove the pants. In this case, the parent does part of the task and allows the child to do

---

Exercise 6.1. Adaptation

Think about an activity that you adapted to make your life easier. Reflect on the adaptation and the answers to the following questions:

- How did you deduce the appropriate adaptations?
- How did knowing your capabilities and having a goal in mind influence the way you approached the adaptation?
- What theoretical orientation did you use? (You may not have consciously been thinking of a theory, but whatever made you change the activity in the way you did is probably a theoretical orientation.)
- Can you make a different adaptation to the same activity using a different theoretical orientation?
- Did the adaptation of the activity affect the overall occupation?

Exercise 6.2. Adapting an Activity From a Biomechanical Perspective

Observe children playing on a playground or in a schoolyard. Select one activity in which they are engaged and answer the following questions:

- What is the overall occupation in which the child is engaged?
- What are 3 activities that are component activities of this occupation?
- Using a biomechanical perspective (i.e., increasing strength, endurance, and range of motion), how could you adapt one of these activities so that a child in a wheelchair could participate?

Exercise 6.3. Adapting an Activity Using a Sensory Integration Frame of Reference

Observe a child in a therapy session in which the practitioner is using a sensory integration frame of reference.

- What is the overall occupation in which the child is engaged?
- What are 3 activities that are component activities of this occupation?
- Using a sensory integration frame of reference, how could you adapt a playground activity for a child with tactile defensiveness?

---

the remainder. Once the child has accomplished a certain segment of the task, the task can be made slightly more difficult, thus *grading the activity up*.

Another way of grading a dressing task down while still using an acquisitional frame of reference is to buy the child pants with an elastic waist rather than those with a fastening at the waist or use pullover shirts rather than ones with buttons. Grading a task down allows the client to feel successful and gain confidence so that he or she becomes willing to try more difficult tasks, develop skills, or build on a previously acquired level of skill.

Whether adapting or grading, theoretical perspectives often require that the physical nature of an activity be changed by modifying the materials used in a task. From a *developmental perspective*, which involves changing an activity so that it is easier for the client to complete successfully, if a child has difficulty building with wooden blocks because

---

Exercise 6.4. Grading an Activity

Select an activity at which you are very competent but that one of your classmates cannot perform. For example, if you are good at playing chess or the piano or at baking, then select a student who does not know the rules of chess, how to play the piano, or how to bake. Develop and carry out one teaching session with your classmate that involves grading in some way. How did you grade the activity so that the other person would have a positive learning experience? How would you have graded the activity for a different person?

they are hard for him to grasp and lift, then smaller foam blocks can be provided that are lighter and easier to handle. This adaptation is grading the activity down so that the child can participate in block building despite having limited strength and grasping ability.

Modifying activities

Activity modification does not involve changing the activity but rather changing the way the activity is done. It can be seen as a specific type of grading that focuses on the activity itself. The purpose and goal of the activity remain the same, but the sequence or time requirements of the tasks encompassed in the activity may be altered. Modifying the sequence of tasks involves changing the order in which tasks are done so that the person can engage in the task more successfully. This approach is frequently used for energy conservation.

For example, to avoid energy depletion caused by repeatedly walking up and down stairs or back and forth across a room, the client can change the order in which he or she performs activities of daily living (ADL) tasks to minimize the walking involved in the task. Modifying the activity may also mean moving the venue of the activity, for example, from the kitchen counter, where the client has to stand to complete the activity, to the kitchen table, where the client can complete the task while sitting down. Another type of activity modification may involve *scaling the activity* (i.e., breaking the activity into smaller parts that are required to complete the activity as a whole), such as finishing part of a puzzle (e.g., the outer edges of the puzzle or one section) rather than the whole puzzle.

Performance (i.e., the actual doing) of tasks involves a time factor. To be functional, tasks have to be done either within a specified amount of time or at a certain time of the day or year. For example, a child spending a half-hour putting on a shirt would not be considered functional. In the therapeutic environment, the timing of a task can be modified or the time requirements of a task or activity can be changed: A client can take longer to complete a task without repercussions, or dressing can be done in the middle of the day rather than in the morning. Once a client has mastered an activity within an extended timeframe, the time allotted can be decreased.

Exercise 6.5. Altering the Sequence of Tasks

Think about the way in which you accomplish the self-care occupation of getting ready for work or school in the morning. List the tasks that you do to accomplish each activity (e.g., personal hygiene, selecting clothes, dressing). Select one activity. Consider how you would change the sequence of the task if you had to get ready in a shorter period of time one morning.

For example, when working with a child who is learning to put on a pullover shirt, at first, the child might be allowed to take as much time as he or she needs. Slowly, a time requirement would be added. After the child has mastered putting on the pullover shirt in a reasonable amount of time, he or she might be asked to put on a shirt with buttons in the same amount of time, even though this shirt is more difficult to put on. In this way, the task of putting on a shirt is made more challenging by the use of *layered adaptation,* which involves placing increasing demands in the activity as the client attains greater skill to improve performance. Each successive task is more complex than the previous one, with time becoming a more important component of the task at each stage.

Exercise 6.6. Altering the Timing of Tasks

Select an activity at which you are very skilled. Determine how much time it takes you to do the activity from beginning to end. Divide the time in half and do the activity. How is your performance affected? Now, double the time it takes to do the activity. How is your performance affected?

Creating new activities

The most complex type of activity synthesis is creating new activities. This synthesis occurs after the therapist evaluates a client and determines the areas that require intervention. In response to the evaluation, the practitioner creates an activity specifically for the client. Two types of activity can be created: (1) one that arises from the responsibility of the practitioner to present a specific level of challenge to the client and thus promote growth and (2) one based on the client's occupational needs and desires to move to a certain level of performance. Note that creating an activity is different from adapting and grading or modifying an existing activity because an entirely new activity emerges from the process.

Some theoretical perspectives and frames of reference, such as *neurodevelopmental treatment* and sensory integration, almost define the role of the occupational therapy practitioner as the creator of activities, placing responsibility for defining the activities on the practitioner. The role of the practitioner is based on the client's therapeutic needs and interests, and the goal of the frame of reference is to promote future growth and skills. From these perspectives, client collaboration is secondary to client need and is derived from engagement in the task. If the client does not engage, the practitioner must create new activities to entice him or her. Therefore, the practitioner's understanding of the client, creativity, and ability to engage the client are paramount in these perspectives.

In other theoretical perspectives and frames of reference, such as occupational *adaptation* and *occupational performance,* the creation of activities comes from the client and is based on perceived occupational needs rather than therapeutic needs. This synthesis requires the practitioner to have skill, creativity, and an in-depth understanding of the client. The resultant activity is based on an understanding of the client's interests, problematic areas, and goals. It is not based on activity analysis but is client centered and has a *"just-right" fit,* perfectly related to the client's needs and abilities.

In this type of synthesis, the nonhuman environment plays a very important role. The practitioner, therefore, must gain an understanding of both the *human* (i.e., the people in the environment who are important to the client) and the *nonhuman environment* (i.e., important things surrounding the person that are not live human beings) of the client's occupations to create activities that will engage the client. For example, if the client has a special pet and the practitioner can involve the care of that pet in an aspect of the intervention, then the client will be more likely to engage in the intervention (Figure 6.4; see also Case Example 6.2).

Figure 6.4. Sometimes a pet encourages participation in an activity.

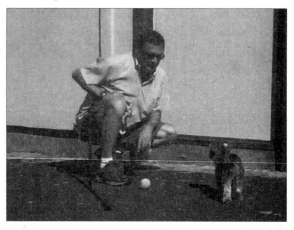

Source. J. Hinojosa. Used with permission.

Exercise 6.7. Creating a New Activity

Identify a skill, such as grasping a fork and using it for self-feeding, that needs to be developed. Determine a goal you have that is related to the development of that skill. After selecting the skill, look around your home and develop an original activity in which you could engage that would develop the skill.

Exercise 6.8. Creating New Activities With Defined Developmental Goals

You have been hired to work in a new occupational therapy practice with limited space and materials. All that you have in the treatment environment are 2 chairs and 1 small table. In the supply closet, you have access to masking tape, a box of colored 1-inch blocks, and 2 boxes of 12 (unsharpened) pencils each. You have 2 children scheduled for the day: Alex, a 21-month-old boy with developmental delays who functions at about a 9-month developmental level, and Maria, a 3-year-old girl with cerebral palsy athetoid type. Outline goals for a treatment session for Alex and Maria, and develop an activity using only the materials, supplies, and environment described.

Case Example 6.2. Elizabeth: Multiple Sclerosis

Elizabeth, age 62 years, has multiple sclerosis, is confined to a wheelchair, and resides in a nursing home. Before she came to the nursing home, she raised several dogs who were very important to her. The nursing home has a pet therapy dog, and the occupational therapist found that Elizabeth was much more likely to come to group activities when the therapy dog was present. This understanding of Elizabeth's interest in pets allowed the therapist to design appropriate and meaningful activities for her.

Exercise 6.9. Creating New Activities on the Basis of the Client's Needs

Scott is a 12-year-old child with attention deficit hyperactivity disorder. He wants to join the local Little League team but needs to develop basic skills in baseball and self-control. Create an activity that will move Scott toward his goal of playing on the team.

Importance of Activity and Occupational Synthesis to Intervention

Both activity and occupational synthesis are critical to the intervention process. People sometimes adapt to the way they do a task with little problem. For example, if a person is accustomed to preparing a meal standing at the kitchen counter and then develops limited standing tolerance, he or she can move meal preparation to the kitchen table to complete the task sitting down. This modification is likely to be acceptable. However, it is often difficult for people to modify the way they do particular tasks, especially when they have done those tasks for many years. Even if completing the task in the usual manner becomes very difficult, change may still be hard to accept because the modification alters the value or enjoyment they derive from the original task.

For example, when cleaning the home becomes too difficult, some obvious options include accepting assistance from others, cleaning one room each day until all are done, or doing minimal cleaning. Some of these options may be more acceptable than oth-

---

Case Example 6.3. Carmela: Adapting Activity

Carmela, age 78 years, had collected porcelain figurines over the years, and she liked to clean them periodically. These objects, however, were displayed on high shelves and could be reached only by standing on a ladder. Carmela conducted her own analysis of the task: As a senior citizen, she was aware that climbing on a ladder was no longer an acceptable option because she would risk falling and injuring herself. She considered hiring someone to do the task for her, but her collection was personally valuable to her and she did not like the thought of other people handling the objects, fearing they might break them.

Carmela eventually decided to hire someone to help her, but she was very clear in defining this person's role in the task. The helper was to climb the ladder to retrieve the objects from the shelf, and Carmela would then wash them and direct how they were to be put back in place. This modification of the activity allowed Carmela to have control over the task and to handle the things that were precious to her while avoiding the aspects of the activity that were difficult and potentially dangerous. Carmela synthesized the revised activity in a way that is both acceptable and safe for her.

---

ers. For some people, getting assistance with cleaning is perfectly acceptable, whereas for others it is not a suitable alternative because cleaning has been one of their life's occupations and a source of enjoyment and pride. For others, doing minimal cleaning may not be acceptable because of their personal beliefs or their desired standard of living. Case Example 6.3 illustrates how a client successfully adapted an activity to make it easier in a way that retains the value of the occupation.

Other Uses of Activity and Occupational Synthesis in Intervention

Up to this point, we have discussed activity synthesis as an intervention process used to bring about change in the client and how it relates to occupational synthesis. We have stressed the use of theoretical grounding in this process. Indeed, occupational therapy practitioners typically think about activity synthesis as a tool for treating a client. It is generally a medium that is used to improve function once a deficit has been identified.

Activity synthesis can, however, be used creatively in many more ways. As discussed previously, it can be used as a tool with which to evaluate client performance. We also noted earlier in the chapter that activity synthesis may be used to teach a new skill, refine a skill, or maintain functional status or performance abilities. The next sections present the use of activity synthesis for these various purposes. Note that occupational synthesis is an end product and does not occur at this point in the process.

Evaluating Performance

Activity synthesis can assist the therapist in evaluating a client's performance within a certain context. For example, the therapist may first see whether a child can close a zipper on a doll or on an *ADL board,* which is a piece of equipment used for practicing specific tasks related to ADL skills and includes things like buttons, zippers, and ties. The therapist may then observe the child's ability to close a zipper on his or her own coat. It may be easy for a child to close a zipper on an ADL board or on a doll, but it is critical for the child to be able to also close a zipper on his or her own coat.

The therapist uses the synthesized activity to evaluate the child's performance within two different contexts and by doing so can determine whether intervention is necessary and how to proceed with it. Even if the child can close a zipper on an ADL board, if the child is unable to zip a zipper on his or her own coat, then intervention would be warranted, because this performance is required in daily life (see Case Example 6.4).

Teaching New Skills

Using learning theories, a practitioner can use synthesis to teach new skills. This type of intervention is what an occupational therapy practitioner typically thinks of as activity synthesis. How does one devise a meaningful activity that will assist the client in developing new skills? Expanding on a previous

---

Case Example 6.4. Steve: Developing Social Skills

A therapist works with **Steve, age 12 years,** on developing social skills. In a group, Steve role-plays purchasing a shirt in a department store. During the role-playing, the therapist observes how Steve handles himself, whether his verbalizations are appropriate, and his ability to count out money to pay for the item. On the basis of Steve's ability to perform well in the role-playing situation, the therapist takes Steve into an actual store and observes his abilities in a real context rather than a simulated situation. The therapist uses these observations to give feedback to Steve and develop a plan for intervention. The therapist can also point out to Steve the differences between his performance in the simulated situation and in the real-life activity to help set mutually acceptable goals for performance.

---

example, when teaching a child to fasten clothes, practitioners may first work on the skill in isolation with a doll and then make it more complex by applying the skill to the child's own clothes. In this situation, the practitioner is identifying the skills that need to be developed and creating activities that will promote the development of that new skill (see Case Example 6.5).

Case Example 6.5. Latisha: Money Management

Latisha has difficulties with money management skills. She does not watch how much money she gives the store clerk and does not count her change. The therapist uses an acquisitional frame of reference and sets up a simulated store. Latisha must pay for everything she wants from the store, and the therapist works with her on money management within this context. Periodically, the therapist takes on the role of consumer and has Latisha take on the role of cashier. Through this activity, the therapist can begin to teach Latisha the basic skills necessary for developing the ability to manage her money.

Refining Skills

The practitioner can use activity synthesis to refine a skill, again using learning theories. Once the client has attained a basic skill level, the practitioner can enhance and embellish the activity to make the required skill level more complex. For example, when working on the development of communication skills with a client with psychosocial dysfunction, the practitioner might first work on having the client say "good morning" to others in a protected environment, such as a therapy group. Then they may work on asking people how they are and finally move to conducting an entire conversation. Although the activity synthesis might begin in a protected environment, eventually the skills would need to be tested in the real world to determine their viability (see Case Example 6.6).

As skill increases, the practitioner continually resynthesizes the activity to increase the demands on the client and refine the skills necessary for application in the real world. In essence, by grading up the task, the practitioner is synthesizing the activity to meet new goals.

Maintaining Functional Status or Performance Abilities

Synthesis can be used to maintain a person's functional status or performance ability. For example, if a client has been working on strengthening her hands and has achieved an acceptable level of strength, then it would be incumbent on the occupational therapy practitioner to work with her to synthesize activities that would maintain that level of strength after completion of intervention. The practitioner would first need to understand her meaningful occupations and then within this understanding synthesize activities that would be of sufficient interest to her so that she would want to continue doing them to maintain her hand strength (see also Case Example 6.7).

If the activities devised by the occupational therapy practitioner hold no interest for the client, the client will have little incentive to do them. Therefore, synthesized activities should incorporate purposeful and meaningful occupations for the client to maximize their success. For example, squeezing Theraputty™ may not be a meaningful occupation for a particular person, but molding clay into animals that could be given as gifts might be more purposeful, enjoyable, and rewarding. In this case, activity synthesis is based on a fundamental assumption of the profession, that is, engagement in occupations keeps people healthy, rather than on a theoretical perspective.

Another fundamental assumption of occupational therapy is that people are more likely to engage in activities that are meaningful to them; in other words, these activities are *purposeful*. Therefore, primary goals of the occupational therapy process are

---

Case Example 6.6. Jonathan: Developing Social Skills

Jonathan is developing social skills through role-playing in a group. He then tries the skills he has acquired in a real situation. The therapist works with Jonathan on refining his behavior in the real-world environment. Is he dressed appropriately to go out shopping? Does he make eye contact with store personnel? Can he ask questions appropriately if he needs to find an item to purchase? Can he handle money responsibly?

Case Example 6.7. Alicia: Maintaining Functional Status

Alicia has had difficulty with range of motion in her shoulder. She has received occupational therapy intervention and has been responsive to therapy. She can now raise her arms to 180° of shoulder flexion. The therapist initially suggested that Alicia do certain exercises to maintain function and ability, but Alicia did not follow through on the exercise program. During a subsequent home visit, the therapist suggested that Alicia place the dishes that she uses most often on the second shelf of her cabinets so that she will have to reach for them. Alicia agreed because it was more meaningful to her than doing specific exercises, even though she understood their value. Thus, the maintenance of her shoulder range became a part of her everyday life (Figure 6.5).

Figure 6.5. Dishes are placed on the second shelf to maintain shoulder range of motion.

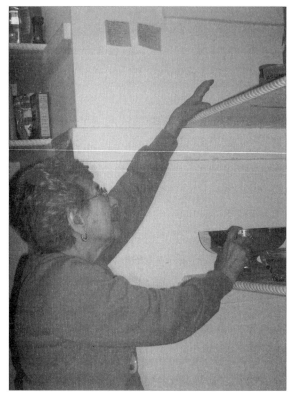

Source. P. Kramer. Used with permission.

not only to assist people in finding meaningful occupations but also to help them maintain and restore function so that they can use the activity synthesis process to engage in meaningful occupations. When people can explore how they can continue to engage in their chosen occupations, occupational synthesis can occur. Knowing the client and what he or she will enjoy are critical to synthesizing an activity that will be successful for the client and result in occupational synthesis.

Activity and Occupational Synthesis for Health Promotion

Occupational therapy practitioners have a responsibility that goes beyond intervention, to promote health in the client through activity and occupational synthesis. Activity synthesis is an important tool in this process, in which the practitioner takes an active role with the client, collaborating on the development of activities to promote health. Syn-

thesis may be necessary to develop activities that will assist the client in meeting goals and optimizing lifestyle. With the knowledge the practitioner has gained about the client's desires and abilities, he or she can assist in the development of specific activities that maintain physical, mental, and social health. For example, through activity synthesis, the practitioner can customize activities that promote continued engagement in social activities that reinforce participation. Synthesis may take many forms. For example, the practitioner may encourage clients to participate in a community center or may customize a home exercise program to address specific needs and abilities. Successful activity synthesis is necessary for successful occupational synthesis to occur.

Artful Practice and Synthesis

In the synthesis of activities with the intent to move toward occupational synthesis, the practitioner needs to be artful in developing or choosing an activity that suits both the client's needs from a functional perspective and the client's interests from a personal perspective (see Case Example 6.8). If both needs and interests are not met, the activity will not be successful in achieving its goal.

The occupational therapy practitioner first takes time to learn about the client, focusing on who he or she is as a person and his or her strengths and limitations. Then the practitioner, with the client's input, identifies goals for the client and the intervention. This step may involve analyzing the client's performance in particular activities and identifying performance components that interfere with successful completion of the task. It may also involve some aspect of client education to increase the client's awareness of how performance can be improved or how performance in a particular area is affecting overall functioning. Activities are then synthesized with the client so that they are meaningful and beneficial to him or her. Gaining the client's input at this stage of the intervention is key. Unless the activity is viewed as meaningful to the client, it will not result in occupational synthesis.

Remember that synthesis is not concrete: It does not follow a step-by-step process and instead may be undertaken in many different ways. Several elements, however, should be present for synthesis to be

Case Example 6.8. Janay: Hand Weakness

Janay has a weakness in her hands. When first synthesizing activities for Janay, the therapist considered using modeling clay as a therapeutic intervention, but Janay showed no interest in working with clay. She enjoys baking, however, and has expressed an interest in learning to bake bread. Baking bread requires kneading the dough, which will strengthen Janay's hands. Thus, baking bread has therapeutic value and is also a meaningful and pleasurable activity for Janay. The successful meeting of the therapeutic and personal needs specific to Janay and her situation can potentially lead to a more successful intervention.

successful. These elements are developing an understanding of the client, including what is important to this person and his or her meaningful occupations; analyzing activities to determine how deficits interfere with performance; and selecting a theoretically based guideline for intervention. Additionally, together with the client, the practitioner uses creativity to identify or devise activities that will help the client overcome his or her deficits or develop the skills necessary for successful task performance.

Development of Artful Practice

Activity and occupational synthesis require artful practice on the part of the occupational therapy practitioner. *Artful practice* is the skill with which the practitioner engages the client in occupations and activities, so the therapeutic intervention is meaningful and enjoyable to the client. It is not something that can be taught easily. It is, in part, the product of experience because one does not start out as an artist. One must learn how to use and play with materials; study techniques; develop skill with the materials; and, finally, develop a personal style. It also involves an element of creativity. These factors are the prerequisites to becoming an artist. Once a person possesses the basic skills, he or she may be able to develop into an artist, but it will take time, practice, and experience.

Exercise 6.10. Synthesizing Activities Using a Frame of Reference

You have just been assigned to a new client, David. He has a right hemiplegia secondary to a cerebral vascular hemorrhage. Before this trauma, David was an engineer in the U.S. Navy. He had a very high-level position designing equipment for ships. His hobbies included building things for his family and home, using multimedia (e.g., woodwork, electricity, mechanical devices). Choose a frame of reference or a theoretical perspective and synthesize several activities for David using the chosen perspective and incorporating his personal interests and preferred occupations. Describe the activities and how they reflect both David's interests and the theoretical perspective you have chosen.

Exercise 6.11. Activity Synthesis in a Clinical Environment

Observe an intervention with a client. Identify the activities that have been synthesized for that client. Try to identify the theoretical perspective or perspectives that provide the foundation for this intervention. Have the activities been synthesized specifically for this particular client? Can you determine the client's investment in the intervention? Are you observing artful practice? Do you see how this activity can become part of the client's occupational synthesis?

The same is true of the occupational therapy practitioner. Initially, the practitioner starts out as a novice with a technical or procedural understanding of what is going on with the client. The practitioner develops into an expert with time and experience. He or she learns how to get to know the client quickly; how to collaborate easily with the client; and ultimately, how to use this information to synthesize meaningful occupations for the client. Once the practitioner possesses expert-level skills, he or she can use synthesis as an effective tool and become an artful practitioner.

The *clinical reasoning process,* which is the way in which the practitioner makes decisions on the basis of understanding theory, the disabilities or functional deficits, and the client and his or her particular needs, is part of the art of practice. The practitioner develops reasoning skills in different areas and during varying stages of professional development.

Some aspects of clinical reasoning include scientific reasoning, narrative reasoning, pragmatic reasoning, and ethical reasoning (Schell & Schell, 2007). These different types of reasoning are discussed in depth in Chapter 7, "Clinical Reasoning and Reflective Practice." Clinical reasoning skills develop as the practitioner matures and reflects on his or her cumulative experiences. Engaging in the practice of synthesis, however, involves more than just reasoning; it involves understanding the client, his or her life, and oneself as a practitioner.

Experience contributes to one's ability to be an artful practitioner, enhancing knowledge of different approaches, a range of techniques and responses, and greater interaction skills. Having a multitude of experiences with clients with various disabilities and cultures, and in various settings, expands one's repertoire. The knowledge gathered from experience provides the practitioner with options for both intervention and interaction. Such knowledge is not necessarily an expansion of theoretical knowledge but an expansion of practical knowledge and a greater understanding of the self and the human condition—all elements essential to successful and appropriate occupational synthesis. The practitioner needs to be reflective (Cohn, Schell, & Crepeau, 2010; Robertson, 2012; Schön, 1983) and have a clearer understanding of the role of activity and occupation in the client's life. He or she is then able to creatively match intervention with the client's needs. The art thus comes from within the practitioner, not from a greater understanding of theory (Schell & Schell, 2007). It is a personal and professional development, not exclusively an intellectual development.

Although the art of practice does not come from an understanding of theory, it does, however, occur within a theoretical context. The practitioner should choose a theoretical framework or frame of reference that will fit the setting, the client's needs, and the practitioner's own knowledge base. The choice of a theoretical approach and, therefore, the choice or synthesis of activities requires considering all of these things and should not be based on one area alone. Understanding the personal, organizational, and client's context is critical to effective practice.

The artful occupational therapy practitioner creates the circumstances in which occupational synthesis can take place within the client. The practitioner uses his or her knowledge of human occupation integrated with theoretically based guidelines for intervention to provide activities and opportunities that the client then uses for occupational synthesis. The definitive goal of occupational therapy is to provide interventions that will produce the desired changes so that service recipients can participate in occupations that are personally meaningful to them (Hinojosa, Kramer, Royeen, & Luebben, 2003). The practitioner facilitates opportunities for occupational synthesis to occur by providing interventions that are relevant and creative. Again, this synthesis requires a successful interaction between the practitioner and the client so that the practitioner can gain an understanding of activities that are meaningful to the client, and the client can give feedback to the practitioner on the effectiveness of specific activity syntheses.

Artful practice requires that the practitioner experience the treatment with the client, using his or her own life experience as an active agent of change to design and implement treatments (Weinstein, 1998). As proposed by Schön (1983), the art of professional practice is built on a professional's reflection in action. The practitioner reflects on what is happening during treatment to continually modify, adapt, or change the intervention process or activity. Beyond the theoretical perspective, the practitioner experiences what is happening and is prepared to change strategies spontaneously. This skill does not occur automatically; rather, it is based on both reflection and experience. In some cases, modifying the activity, the environment, or the interaction will help to make the intervention more effective for the client. In other situations, when the predicted changes do not occur, the practitioner decides to change the intervention. In these cases, the artful practitioner proposes new hypotheses and implements the revised intervention. These modifications ensure that occupational synthesis takes place and that interventions are also related to the client's future occupations.

When interventions are relevant, the client is able to transpose the tasks or activities easily into his or her real-life occupations. Relevant interventions are judged by two criteria. First, are they appropriate for addressing the client's deficits? Second, are they pertinent to the client's life situation (e.g., goals, values, culture, lifestyle) as defined by the client?

Occupational synthesis is more likely to take place when the occupational therapy program is relevant to the client. The practitioner begins this process by considering the following four questions to ensure that the client's life situation is being addressed:

1. Do I understand the client's occupations?
2. Do I respect the client's occupations and personal choices?
3. Do I understand the client's activity patterns, particularly in relation to his or her cultural background, and do I respond to them appropriately?
4. How do my client's occupations influence other people in his or her daily life?

After reflection on this first set of questions, Hinojosa (2003) identified five additional questions that an occupational therapy practitioner might ask to assess the relevance of his or her interventions with regard to the concept of occupation:

1. Are my interventions reflecting an understanding of the client's life situations and his or her culture?
2. Have I developed an understanding of my client's occupations through discussions with him or her?
3. Have I considered clear ethical reasoning when developing my interventions within the context of the client's goals, priorities, and capacities?
4. Are my interventions based on an understanding of how the client defines his or her occupations?
5. Do my interventions result in enabling the client to engage in occupations and increase his or her life satisfaction?

Developing meaningful intervention using synthesis is a complex process. The practitioner usually starts by developing an understanding of activity synthesis. At the same time, he or she is developing sound clinical reasoning skills and, over time, gaining experience to develop the art of practice. With experience, the practitioner comes to understand the client's critical role and his or her unique situation. This process is not necessarily linear, but it is one that takes time and experience to develop. Once this development has occurred, occupational synthesis can be facilitated and intervention becomes truly meaningful. The ultimate demonstration and most valuable outcome of occupational synthesis can be observed when the client engages in his or her chosen occupations in real life rather than in an artificial clinical situation.

Summary

Activity synthesis is a common phenomenon that occurs in everyday life. People have many occupations and activities that are meaningful to them, and they modify and change activities so that they can perform them successfully. Activity synthesis appears simple precisely because it is so commonplace, yet most people do not synthesize activities in an organized and systematic manner. True activity synthesis is a complex skill, but very little has been specifically written about it.

Occupational therapy practitioners approach activity synthesis from an organized theoretical perspective requiring an understanding of activity analysis, the underlying components, the context, and the client. Furthermore, activity synthesis is strongly influenced by the frame of reference chosen for intervention and the artfulness of the practitioner. Activity synthesis is a critical function of the practitioner and is used frequently in day-to-day interventions. If used successfully in the intervention process, activity synthesis should result in occupational synthesis within the client.

In this chapter, we proposed that the practitioner needs to understand the importance of activity synthesis and how to approach it in an organized and systematic manner. Through effective activity synthesis and an understanding of the client, the practitioner will be able to help the client develop true occupational synthesis. Then, through ongoing development, reflection, and experience, the practitioner becomes both skillful and artful in developing interventions that are meaningful for the client.

References

American Occupational Therapy Association. (2014). Occupational therapy practice framework: Domain and process (3rd ed.). *American Journal of Occupational Therapy, 68*(Suppl. 1), S1–S48. http://dx.doi.org/10.5014/ajot.2014.682006

Baum, C. M., & Christiansen, C. H. (2005). Person–Environment–Occupation–Performance: An occupation-based framework for practice. In C. H. Christiansen, C. M. Baum, & J. Bass-Haugen (Eds.), *Occupational therapy: Performance, participation, and well-being* (3rd ed., pp. 243–259). Thorofare, NJ: Slack.

Christiansen, C., Baum, C. M., & Bass-Haugen, J. (2005). *Occupational therapy: Performance, participation, and well-being* (3rd ed.). Thorofare, NJ: Slack.

Cohn, E. S., Schell, B. A. B., & Crepeau, E. B. (2010). Occupational therapy as a reflective practice. In N. Lyons (Ed.), *Handbook of reflective inquiry* (pp. 131–157). New York: Springer.

Creighton, C. (1992). The origin and evolution of activity analysis. *American Journal of Occupational Therapy, 46*, 45–48. http://dx.doi.org/10.5014/ajot.46.1.45

Dunn, W., Brown, C., & McGuigan, A. (1994). The Ecology of Human Performance: A framework for considering the effect of context. *American Journal of Occupational Therapy, 48*, 595–607. http://dx.doi.org/10.5014/ajot.48.7.595

Dunn, W., Brown, C., & Youngstrom, M. J. (2003). Ecological model of occupation. In P. Kramer, J. Hinojosa, & C. Royeen (Eds.), *Perspectives in human occupation: Participation in life* (pp. 222–263). Philadelphia: Lippincott Williams & Wilkins.

Fidler, G. S. (1948). Psychological evaluation of occupational therapy activities. *American Journal of Occupational Therapy, 2*, 284–287.

Fidler, G. S. (1996). Life-Style Performance: From profile to conceptual model. *American Journal of Occupational Therapy, 50*, 139–147. http://dx.doi.org/10.5014/ajot.50.2.139

Fidler, G. S., & Velde, B. (2002). *Lifestyle performance: A model for engaging the power of occupation*. Thorofare, NJ: Slack.

Forsyth, K., & Kielhofner, G. (2003). Model of Human Occupation. In P. Kramer & J. Hinojosa (Eds.), *The core concept of occupation* (pp. 45–86). Philadelphia: Lippincott Williams & Wilkins.

Hinojosa, J. (2003). Occupation and continuing competence: Part II. *OT Practice, 8*, 11–12.

Hinojosa, J., Kramer, P., & Luebben, A. J. (2010). The structure of a frame of reference. In P. Kramer & J. Hinojosa (Eds.), *Frames of reference for pediatric occupational therapy* (pp. 3–22). Philadelphia: Lippincott Williams & Wilkins.

Hinojosa, J., Kramer, P., Royeen, C. B., & Luebben, A. (2003). The core concept of occupation. In P. Kramer, J. Hinojosa, & C. B. Royeen (Eds.), *Perspectives in human occupation: Participation in life* (pp. 1–17). Philadelphia: Lippincott Williams & Wilkins.

Hunt, D. (1997). *The magician's tale*. New York: Putnam.

Kielhofner, G. (2008). *Model of Human Occupation: Theory and application* (4th ed.). Baltimore: Lippincott Williams & Wilkins.

Law, M., Baptiste, S., McColl, M., Opzoomer, A., Polatajko, H., & Pollock, N. (1990). The Canadian Occupational Performance Measure: An outcome measure for occupational therapy. *Canadian Journal of Occupational Therapy, 57*, 82–87. http://dx.doi.org/10.1177/000841749005700207

Levit, K. (2008). Optimizing motor behavior using the Bobath Approach. In M. V. Radomski & C. A. T. Latham (Eds.), *Occupational therapy for physical dysfunction* (6th ed., pp. 642–666). Philadelphia: Lippincott Williams & Wilkins.

Missiuna, C., Mandich, A. D., Polatajko, H. J., & Malloy-Miller, T. (2001). Cognitive orientation to Daily Occupational Performance (CO–OP): Part I—Theoretical foundations. *Physical and Occupational Therapy in Pediatrics, 20*, 69–81.

Mosey, A. C. (1981). *Occupational therapy: Configuration of a profession*. New York: Raven Press.

Mosey, A. C. (1996). *Applied scientific inquiry in the health professions: An epistemological orientation* (2nd ed.). Bethesda, MD: American Occupational Therapy Association.

Nelson, D. L. (1997). Why the profession of occupational therapy will flourish in the 21st century [1996 Eleanor Clarke Slagle Lecture]. *American Journal of Occupational Therapy, 51*, 11–24. http://dx.doi.org/10.5014/ajot.51.1.11

Nelson, D. L., & Jepson-Thomas, J. (2003). Occupational form, occupational performance, and a conceptual framework for therapeutic occupation. In P. Kramer, J. Hinojosa, & C. Royeen (Eds.), *Perspectives on human occupation* (pp. 87–155). Philadelphia: Lippincott Williams & Wilkins.

Piaget, J. (1963). *Psychology of intelligence*. Paterson, NJ: Littlefield, Adams.

Robertson, L. (2012). *Clinical reasoning in occupational therapy: Controversies in practice*. Oxford, England: Wiley-Blackwell.

Schaaf, R. C., Schoen, S. A., Smith-Roley, S., Lane, S. J., Koomar, J., & May-Benson, T. A. (2009). Frame of reference for sensory integration. In P. Kramer & J. Hinojosa (Eds.), *Frames of reference for pediatric occupational therapy* (3rd ed., pp. 99–186). Philadelphia: Lippincott Williams & Wilkins.

Schell, B. A. B., & Schell, J. W. (2007). *Clinical and professional reasoning in occupational therapy*. Philadelphia: Lippincott Williams & Wilkins.

Schön, D. A. (1983). *The reflective practitioner: How professionals think in action*. New York: Basic.

Weinstein, E. (1998). *The nature of artful practice in psychosocial occupational therapy* (Unpublished doctoral dissertation). New York University, School of Education.

White, T. H. (1977). *The book of Merlin*. Austin: University of Texas Press.

CHAPTER 7.

CLINICAL REASONING AND REFLECTIVE PRACTICE

Fran Babiss, PhD, OTR/L

Highlights

✧ Decision making
✧ Defining clinical reasoning and reflective practice
✧ Clinical reasoning and reflective practice: A brief history
✧ Clinical reasoning and experience
✧ Types of reasoning about occupation and related activities
✧ New directions in clinical reasoning
✧ Knowing more than we can say
✧ Four-quadrant model of facilitated learning
✧ Case studies: Clinical reasoning in action.

Key Terms

✧ Clinical reasoning
✧ Cognitive figure–ground
✧ Conditional reasoning
✧ Epistemology of practice
✧ Ethical reasoning
✧ Ethnographic study
✧ Four-Quadrant Model of Facilitated Learning
✧ Habit
✧ Holistically
✧ Intentionality
✧ Interactional reasoning
✧ Intuition
✧ Knowing-in-action
✧ Mental models

✧ Metacognition
✧ Monistic thinking
✧ Narrative
✧ Narrative reasoning
✧ Phenomenological
✧ Pluralistic
✧ Pragmatic reasoning
✧ Procedural reasoning
✧ Reductionistic thinking
✧ Reflection-in-action
✧ Reflective practice
✧ Symbolic meaning
✧ Tacit knowledge
✧ Technical rationality
✧ Three-track mind

An occupational therapy practitioner must engage in clinical reasoning and reflective practice to grow and mature as a professional. In this chapter, I expand on the need for clinical reasoning and reflective practice by first defining the terms. The history of the growth and development of the importance of clinical reasoning and reflective practice in the profession of occupational therapy are discussed, along with some of the widely accepted ways of describing and organizing clinical reasoning. Because the ideas about clinical reasoning in occupational therapy are based on the work of Schön (1983) and Dreyfus and Dreyfus (1986), I summarize their work to provide a basic understanding about the development of the categories of clinical reasoning in occupational therapy. I then describe ways of looking at the complexities of clinical reasoning as they relate to occupational therapy.

Decision Making

An occupational therapy practitioner whose work requires collaboration with the people he or she treats has an enormous responsibility, which involves many levels and areas of decision making. During an occupational therapy student's fieldwork, an inevitable moment comes in which this enormity becomes very tangible, often in the form of fears about saying or doing the wrong thing with a client. That "what if" is the starting point of clinical reasoning. It is an awareness of the power that each of us has to affect destiny through the choices we make. What we say or do is never guaranteed to have the outcome for which we strive, but we are responsible for taking action, and the practitioner's job is to develop the skill to make such choices.

I have had students ask me, "How did you know what to say to that client?" The answer to this question begins with an examination of the decision-making process that an occupational therapy practitioner refines as he or she interacts with a client. It is a complex process of reasoning and reflection. The practitioner reasons about occupations and their related activities to make decisions about what course of intervention to pursue with a specific client. Can we make the best decision? How do we know we have taken the right course, and essentially, how do we go about the process of deciding what activities to choose in working with others? Moreover, how do we know that we have chosen from viable and validated interventions?

We live in a time when consumers are asking, "Does your intervention really work?" The Joint Commission (2013) has begun to identify and promote top performers in health care on the basis of their use of evidence-based practices. The Agency for Healthcare Research and Quality (AHRQ; 2013) has synthesized processes from the military and aviation professions to standardize interventions and enhance teamwork and communication to improve patient safety and decrease errors in treatment. In spite of this effort, my belief is that no printed or electronic manual for treatment or intervention will ever replace an occupational therapy practitioner who is skilled in clinical reasoning and reflective practice. As Florence Clark (2012) said in her American Occupational Therapy Association (AOTA) presidential address, "We all know that tacit reasoning has an impact on the quality of our care just as much as external evidence does, even if it does not receive equal time and attention" (p. 649).

Most often, people do not function in a *metacognitive* mode. In other words, it is a rare occurrence to think about one's own thinking in an overarching manner. Therefore, it is a difficult task. Whether it is something you are aware of or something you develop over time, decision making and reasoning about occupation, and their related activities, are skills you will need to hone as a professional. You may not always make the right decision, but you can learn to make the best decision.

Exercise 7.1. Making a Decision

Take a few minutes to reflect on the way in which you decided to become an occupational therapy practitioner. Think about your age at the time of the decision. What was going on in your life? When you decided to become an occupational therapy practitioner, what other career choices did you consider, and why did you decide on occupational therapy? Can you tease out the cognitive and emotional mechanisms you used to settle on your chosen course? More important, can you remember what happened immediately after the point at which you made the decision?

Defining Clinical Reasoning and Reflective Practice

Defining *clinical reasoning* and *reflective practice* is not an easy task. Many years ago, when I was beginning my study of occupational therapy, I was told repeatedly that occupational therapy practitioners worked *holistically.* Not only do they pay attention to a person's physical or mental health concerns, but they also consider the interaction among body, mind, and spirit.

I still believe this holistic view to be true, and it contributes to the intricacy of my reasoning about occupations, activities, and purposeful activities. It also makes defining *clinical reasoning* and *reflective practice* very difficult. Part of this difficulty is because the labels used to define these terms are not always the same and the ideas behind them not necessarily uniform. Defining these terms is, however, a starting point, and the inherent difficulty supports the argument for looking at these concepts from a *pluralistic* standpoint (i.e., the belief that there is more than one basic principle; Mosey, 1985).

Clinical reasoning is complex (Mattingly & Fleming, 1994), and many definitions for it exist. Consistent with my views, Schell (2003b) described it as a process that is both complex and multifaceted. She went on to define *clinical reasoning* as "the process used by practitioners to plan, direct, perform, and reflect on client care" (p. 131). Reflective practice is a complex concept as well, and it is discussed in depth later in this chapter. Whereas Schell's definition of clinical reasoning indicates that clinical practices are used to choose interventions for and interactions with clients, *reflective practice* means that occupational therapy practitioners examine why particular interventions and interactions are chosen, whether the choices were appropriate, and what they will do the next time they encounter a similar situation. Schön (1983), considered the father of modern day reflective practice, described *reflective practice* as what occurs when a seasoned professional, acting on intuition, stops to take the time to contemplate what he or she is doing while in the midst of doing it.

Building on Exercise 7.1, think about what happened to you once you decided to become an occupational therapy practitioner. A decision is nothing more than what you think until you begin to take action based on that decision. This thought process is the planning stage of clinical reasoning. At first, deciding to become an occupational therapy practitioner seems no different from deciding to become a black belt in karate. The way in which you or anyone else knows that a decision has been made is by the behavior you engage in after having made the decision. This behavior is the performance stage of clinical reasoning.

The following example shows the complexity involved in reflective practice. An occupational therapist must use clinical reasoning to decide what action would be the most effective and appropriate for Mr. Ames. Mr. Ames and his occupational therapist determine that he will need 120° of forward shoulder flexion to permit him to return to his job stocking shelves in a warehouse, which is a clear course of action designed to assist him in a return of range of motion. Complexity enters in the form of deciding what to do to implement that increase in movement. In addition, how does the therapist know that Mr. Ames wants to return to work, and can he be provided an environment that closely approximates the conditions of his workplace? A dozen more questions can and should be asked before action can take place.

Clinical Reasoning and Reflective Practice: A Brief History

The history of a close examination of reflective practice and the clinical reasoning process began when Cohn (1991) traced the origin of the inquiry to Joan Rogers's (1983) Eleanor Clarke Slagle Lecture devoted to explicating clinical reasoning. This analysis was a natural development in the maturation of occupational therapy as a profession. Rogers concluded that occupational therapy practitioners need to examine their thinking more systematically for the purpose of making it accessible to the profession. She correctly connected an improvement in a practitioner's art of practice with a greater awareness about the ways in which he or she thinks about that practice.

On the basis of this beginning, Mattingly and Fleming (1994) and Mattingly and Gillette (1991) worked with the AOTA and the American Occupational Therapy Foundation to conduct an *ethnographic study* (i.e., a qualitative research design that explores cultural phenomena) to begin to explain the thinking that takes place when an occupational therapist solves treatment problems. Today, clinical reasoning has been incorporated into occupational therapy curricula to address the expanding knowledge required of practitioners. The need to move to evidence-based practice models has furthered the necessity of teaching students professional reasoning (Coster, 2008).

I have said that it was a natural development within the profession of occupational therapy to explore the concepts of clinical reasoning and reflective practice. In many ways, these concepts have become explicit knowledge, as evidenced by the inclusion of clinical reasoning in standards for accredited educational programs for occupational therapists and occupational therapy assistants (Accreditation Council for Occupational Therapy Education [ACOTE®], 2012). In addition, fieldwork experiences for occupational therapy practitioners are required to provide environments designed to promote clinical reasoning and reflective practice (ACOTE, 2012).

Including clinical reasoning and reflective practice in professional standards and direct experience is based on the following premise: With the ability to perform reasoning about occupation, occupational therapy practitioners should be able to solve treatment problems that exist outside of their experience or training and learn how to think about a profession, which improves the ability to engage meaningfully in that profession. Throughout their professional careers, practitioners continue to develop clinical reasoning skills and reflective practice.

Underlying Framework

The underlying framework for clinical reasoning and reflective practice in occupational therapy was developed largely by Schön (1983) and Dreyfus and Dreyfus (1986). The catalyst for much of the thinking about thinking in occupational therapy is based on the work of Schön. Dreyfus and Dreyfus contributed to the understanding of the movement of the practitioner from novice to expert. Therefore, this section summarizes the work of Schön and of Dreyfus and Dreyfus to give readers a better understanding of the development of the categories of clinical reasoning and reflective practice in occupational therapy.

Reflective Practitioner

Schön's (1983) work is credited as being the starting point for the exploration of the workings of clinical reasoning, as well as the reflective practitioner, in occupational therapy. He explored the development of professions and how they acquire their particular knowledge. He created an *epistemology of practice* (i.e., the study of knowledge) on the basis of the premise that most practicing professionals know more in practice than they can verbalize, as expressed in the beginning of this chapter, which represents the strongest argument for professionals to participate in the training of occupational therapy students as they think about choices made in practice. When asked how decisions are made during practice, the occupational therapy practitioner is sometimes at a loss to explain the process. Schön explored this inability to say what one knows.

The task for a professional is to develop an art of practice in spite of the multiple frames of reference that exist. Schön (1983) believed that the conflicts and difficulties that exist in solving professional problems are what allow a professional to grow in his or her ability to solve these problems artfully, and I agree. Pluralism is healthy for a profession (Mosey, 1985), and the art of practice can be developed regardless of the techniques chosen. It is true that professional occupational therapy practice includes an irreducible element of art, and it is also true that gifted engineers, teachers, scientists, architects, and managers sometimes display artistry in their day-to-day practice. If the art is not unchanging, known, and teachable, it appears, nonetheless, at least for some people to be learnable (Schön, 1983).

Schön (1983) labeled the simple application of learned techniques of practice as *technical rationality*. The movement to full professional status of an artful practitioner involves progressing from what Schön (1983) termed *knowing-in-action* to *reflection-in-action*. *Knowing-in-action* involves the concept of *tacit knowledge,* a term credited to Polanyi (1962) that describes a form of knowing without knowing how one knows.

For example, you may have no difficulty knowing that you like or dislike a certain work of art, but you might not be able to say what it is that makes you like or dislike it. In the same way, people often use language without the slightest understanding of its grammatical underpinnings. A sentence may be dissonant to a person's ears, but he or she would be challenged to provide the grammatical rule broken that is the cause of discomfort. Similarly, a practitioner may interact with or choose a purposeful activity with a client without being able to explain why a statement was made or an intervention chosen.

Much knowing-in-action is a function of experience as a practitioner. As the practitioner experiences situation after situation, a collection of data is created. After time and repetition, experience and action become separated, much in the same way that a person can daydream while driving home from work, yet find himself or herself at the front door without any difficulty. While writing this chapter, I asked many practitioners to pay attention to their thinking about what they did as they practiced, and some likened the experience to waking up. This response is not to say that many occupational therapy practitioners sleep in practice but that certain practices become so automatic that they disappear from our awareness and become tacit knowledge. Hence, the question from a student, "How did you know how to do that?" is an opportunity to explore knowing-in-action and make the tacit explicit. Then, a piece of the art of practice becomes learnable.

Danger lurks, though, in the habituation to tacit ways of applying clinical knowledge, which is addressed by the cliché "When all I have is a hammer, the whole world looks like a nail." In my practice, I have come to specialize in working with people diagnosed with borderline personality disorder. As a result, I often see the patterns associated with this disorder in many of the clients with whom I work.

This perspective creates a tunnel vision that negates the possibility of entertaining other possible explanations about the way in which a client functions, which was made explicit to me by an occupational therapy student who had worked in the school system for many years before pursuing a career in occupational therapy. During an occupational therapy activity, a client got up from the table and took a lap blanket from a chair, reseating herself wrapped with the blanket. After the group, the student and I were reflecting on the group, and I described the client's behavior as a need to direct the group's attention to her because the group was focused on another client. The student opined that

perhaps the client's behavior had been an indication of a need for tactile pressure because she was starved for sensory input. I will return to this example shortly.

Reflection-in-action is a characteristic of a professional who is practicing at the highest level of expertise. It is the ability to reason about what is going on as it is in the process. Schön (1983) saw reflection-in-action as the positive outcome when the professional is confronted by a situation that falls outside of the applied science of technical rationality, the experience of knowing-in-action, and catapulted into a world of problem solving in which he or she must entertain new thinking and actions. Schön (1983) remarked,

> Many practitioners, locked into a view of themselves as technical experts, find nothing in the world of practice to occasion reflection. They have become too skillful at techniques of selective inattention, junk categories, and situational control, techniques that they use to preserve the constancy of their knowledge-in-practice. For them, uncertainty is a threat; its admission is a sign of weakness. Others, more inclined toward and adept at reflection-in-action, nevertheless feel profoundly uneasy because they cannot say what they know how to do, cannot justify its quality or rigor. (p. 69)

At this point, it is helpful to return to the previous anecdote in which my student and I had such different explanations for the behavior of the client who wrapped herself in a blanket. In terms of reasoning about the incident, we each saw it through the lens we had been using, either sensory or psychological. Either conclusion could lead to differences in intervention, even interventions that could be counterproductive for the client. Schön (1983) described a virtual world in which the student and supervisor can imagine a situation without being in the situation.

Although this strategy works for the architect planning on paper or the psychotherapist analyzing the transference, it is not helpful in this situation because not enough information is available about the client. The answer to the problem of the need for attention versus the need for tactile pressure can be solved by reflection-in-practice, which involves continued observation of and interaction with the client. As it turned out, by asking questions and providing different input, we determined that the client needed both tactile input and others' attention, and the incident provided a learning experience in creating interventions that worked along both axes. Schön (1983) likened reflection-in-action to a form of research designed for learning new and different ways of thinking about phenomena. It challenges the practitioner to stretch the limits of his or her knowledge.

Many occupational therapy practitioners have used Schön's (1983) work to guide their own practice and to assist students in reflection for the purpose of professional growth. Duncombe (2008) depicted her own personal journeys in reflection as a path to using reflection with interning practitioners. She made use of a population of 57 students over the course of 115 affiliation experiences to gather material about how the students reflected on their practice. The information gathered by means of such questions as "How have you used occupation-based practice in this fieldwork?" was analyzed by using qualitative methods that allowed the faculty of Boston University to realize that they needed to explain and address occupation-based treatment in greater depth.

Schön (1983) acknowledged the value of experience in passing on the skill of being a reflective practitioner. The movement of a practitioner from novice to professional is another area of professional development that has a strong impact on reasoning about activity.

Clinical Reasoning and Experience

Suppose you were told that to become an expert occupational therapy practitioner you would have to rely on intuition? In other words, what you could learn by rules, regulations, and experience was not enough. If learning the rules and exceptions were enough, the problem of computer artificial intelligence would have been solved by now. Dreyfus and Dreyfus (1986), brothers who are professors of philosophy and industrial engineering, have explored the progression of people from novice to expert in different careers and skill acquisitions. Their inves-

tigations have provided a framework for understanding growth in the ability to reason about activities as a function of time and experience. The five stages that a person may pass through are (1) novice, (2) advanced beginner, (3) competence, (4) proficient, and (5) expert.

Stage 1: Novice

In the novice stage, the beginner who is learning a new skill is taught to recognize certain features and rules that are based on features of the task at hand. For example, when a novice dancer is learning to waltz, the order of the steps is the focus of the activity. The rules about the order of steps in the dance are what Dreyfus and Dreyfus (1986) referred to as "context free" (p. 21) because they can be recognized without a need to be aware of anything else that is happening. In fact, the novice dancer might not be able to learn the steps of the dance if she or he had to focus on anything other than their order. The novice could not account for the crowd on a dance floor or the dance style of a partner. It would not be possible for the novice to carry on a conversation while waltzing.

A novice occupational therapy practitioner beginning school 25 years ago was given rules for behavioral health practice in his or her introductory classes. At that time in the history of the profession, a student was often taught exact prescriptions of activities to be used with clients, much of them based on psychodynamic theories of the meaning of symbols. He or she was taught that male clients would prefer leather- and woodworking and female clients would be motivated by needlework crafts. When writing a paper for school, the student would follow these rules assiduously.

Stage 2: Advanced Beginner

At the advanced beginner stage, the learner of a new skill or profession is continuing to gather more context-free facts. The context the learner perceives is becoming larger because of the experience gained through practicing in concrete situations in the world. He or she is beginning to gather a "database" of past situations with which current experiences can be compared. Thus, the advanced beginner begins to use situational cues for reasoning and practice. The dancer begins to be able to look around the dance floor and negotiate and adjust steps to avoid colliding with others. Knowing the steps is not enough. To survive on the dance floor, one must learn to avoid others in the same space.

In the behavioral health clinic, it did not take long to gather a collection of situations in which the "gender" of a craft was often useless. From these experiences, occupational therapy practitioners learned that although preference for activities might still relate to generalizations about gender, asking a client what he or she enjoyed doing had more value and helped the practitioner to establish rapport with the client. The rules these practitioners had learned as novices did not serve them well in each real-world situation.

Stage 3: Competence

At the competence stage, the learner has amassed so many context-free rules and situational experiences that he or she can feel overwhelmed. So much is known that extracting the important from the irrelevant is difficult. The competent professional adopts or is taught a hierarchy of decision making to assist him or her in navigating through the confusion of too much information.

In addition, the learner begins to have a sense of responsibility for the outcome of a decision, and this emotional involvement is critical to the move to the competence stage. The dancer is now able to decide that dancing close to the judge of a dancing contest is the most important task and feels confident in doing so while dancing. Other components of the dance no longer require intense focus. The steps of the waltz are second nature, the synchronization with a usual dance partner is established, and the dancer rarely bumps into other couples on the dance floor. Thus, she or he is able to begin to plan and establish goal-directed behavior in the larger environment.

At this level, an occupational therapy practitioner working in a behavioral health setting has had experience with hundreds of clients and several dozen activities. Access to all of this information allows him or her to begin to construct a form of triage in activity selection. For example, a competent practitioner can interact with a client in a way that allows him or her to understand that the client's self-esteem is so damaged that an activity in

which a successful outcome is ensured is of primary importance. After that decision, an exploration of the type of activity in which the client might be motivated to engage might follow. In other words, it is a search for an activity that is meaningful to the client. The competent practitioner's task is then to adapt and grade the client's choice to ensure a positive outcome. The practitioner has an emotional stake related to both empathy for the client and a desire to make the right choice in activity with the client. Dreyfus and Dreyfus (1986) stated that many people do not develop beyond this level of skill because to do so would entail moving into intuitive levels of thought and action.

Stage 4: Proficient

At the proficient stage, the occupational therapy practitioner functions without a conscious reach for rules, situations, or hierarchies. *Intuition*, as described by Dreyfus and Dreyfus (1986), consists of a "holistic understanding" (p. 109) in which response to patterns occurs without having them deconstructed into component parts. It is knowing the right thing to do without thinking about why it is the right thing to do. It is akin to Csikszentmihalyi's (1990) description of the concept of *flow* as a seamless flow of activity. The proficient practitioner functions effortlessly. The proficient dancer is at one with his or her body, partner, the dance floor, and the entire experience in which they exist.

A proficient occupational therapy practitioner in behavioral health senses when a client is ready to tackle a more challenging task, tolerate an intervention about his or her behavior, or take an interpersonal risk. The practitioner does not break down the client's interactions or behavior into units but looks at the entire client moving through the environment. This level is difficult to explain to the novice student because it goes beyond the simple acquisition of thousands of hours of experience. It is a leap into the intuitive realm that many practitioners never make.

Stage 5: Expert

Dreyfus and Dreyfus (1986) stated, "When things are proceeding normally, experts don't solve problems and don't make decisions; they do what normally works" (p. 31). Being one with what one does is the essence of expertise. The move from proficiency to expertise mirrors that of the move from advanced beginner to competence. As the advanced beginner accrues more and more situations and rules, he or she groups them together to improve his or her decision-making skills. In the same manner, the proficient learner groups intuitive experiences into larger chunks so that thinking recedes and acting and living become one. As long as things unfold as usual, the expert will not make mistakes. The dancer on the floor will waltz in a way that all can recognize as expert, but to say why would be to break the experience into parts that would render it incomprehensible as a whole. If asked what makes her an expert, the waltzer may not be able to say because at this level, such a question is akin to asking her what makes her who she is.

An expert occupational therapy practitioner in behavioral health practice might be able to sense that a client is in acute distress even if the client is not manifesting symptoms. Many of my peers related experiences of becoming disquieted by the behavior of a client during a group. They could not tell me why, but they knew somehow that increased intervention or even intervention of a more restrictive nature might be necessary. They could not tell the client's psychiatrist why they requested an immediate consult, but in most instances, they were correct in their belief. They did not think but acted according to instincts they could not identify.

To explore the role of intuition in clinical reasoning, Chaffey, Unsworth, and Fossey (2010) conducted a qualitative study of occupational therapists who specialized in mental health. The authors based their work on the Cognitive Continuum Theory (CCT) of Hammond (1996), which had previously been used to study clinical reasoning in nursing. Their findings seem to validate Dreyfus and Dreyfus's (1986) description of the expert practitioner as a person who uses intuition to make clinical decisions. The work of this group continues currently (Chaffey, Unsworth, & Fossey, 2012) and is focusing on the contribution of emotional intelligence to intuition in clinical reasoning and reflective practice. The authors are also building on their use of the CCT in what appears to be an effort to create a new taxonomy. This work has the potential to add more dimensions to the body of knowledge in occupational therapy clinical reasoning and reflective practice.

The five stages from novice to expert, along with the concept of *reflective practice,* provide a structure for the discussion of the different types of reasoning occupational therapy practitioners use.

Types of Reasoning About Occupation and Related Activities

This section describes ways of looking at the complexities of clinical reasoning as they relate to occupational therapy. First, the *three-track mind,* or three tracks of reasoning—(1) procedural, (2) interactional, and (3) conditional—put forth by Fleming (1991) and expanded on by Mattingly and Fleming (1994) and Mattingly and Gillette (1991), are discussed. Their small qualitative study examined the reasoning of a small group of practitioners with a specialization in physical disabilities as they provided treatment. Second, three other tracks of reasoning are discussed: (1) pragmatic, (2) ethical, and (3) narrative. The subject of clinical reasoning is abstract, and readers are advised to relate the perspectives presented to their own thinking, reasoning, and decision-making processes.

Procedural Reasoning

When in Exercise 7.1 you engaged in thinking about the process of deciding to become an occupational therapy practitioner, you were engaging in *procedural reasoning,* the "dual search for problem definition and treatment selection" (Flemimg, 1991, p. 1008). The practitioner who thinks about the activities he or she might use with a client to improve the client's functional limitations is engaging in procedural reasoning. The evaluation process, focusing on the relationship between performance in daily life and the barriers to engagement and participation in daily activities, requires the ability to reason in a procedural way. The connection between this evaluation and the creation of an intervention plan is procedural as well.

Mattingly and Fleming (1994) distinguished between the procedural reasoning of an occupational therapy practitioner and that of a physician engaging in medical reasoning. The goal of medical reasoning is to postulate a diagnosis. Practitioners do not engage in diagnosis, but they work with the functional sequelae of diagnoses (A. C. Mosey, personal communication, 1986).

An experienced practitioner has a great deal of past information to which to refer to identify patterns and offer hypotheses about what might work with a client. Through a form of what I call *cognitive figure–ground,* which is reasoning to determine what is important and needs to be attended to and what to ignore, practitioners sort and sift through the information gathered while speaking with and observing a client. The practitioner pushes aside what he or she reasons to be irrelevant and extraneous to determine what is meaningful and worthy of attention. As Mattingly and Fleming (1994) stated, this type of thinking does not take place without the other two tracks operating in concert.

Interactional Reasoning

Interactional reasoning is all of the ways in which a practitioner decides how to communicate with and listen to a client. Relationships form the context within which an occupational therapy practitioner functions. During evaluation, the dialogue between practitioner and client is part of the intervention, and the way in which a practitioner interacts with a client can determine the efficacy of the entire course of intervention. An experienced practitioner develops what he or she would call an instinct for knowing how to speak with a client.

The most powerful and meaningful intervention is one that allows the client to determine what goals are important to him or her. Collaboration with a client is essential to this process. Beginning practitioners have to juggle so many new ideas, thoughts, frames of reference, and facts that the simple act of listening to the client's story can become lost. Yet, it is this very act that can lead the practitioner to a clear direction to take the client.

Knowing how to speak with a client allows the practitioner to provide encouragement and motivation in a positive manner. However, reasoning about the interaction is not to create a positive relationship. Often, the hardest concept for an occupational therapy student to grasp is that the job is rarely about being liked. A practitioner needs to be honest and say the things that will move a client to pursue his or her goals. For example, using interactional reasoning skills, the practitioner can judge the point at which he or she can push a client to

progress beyond the safety of moving only around the house or the limited interactions with a difficult spouse.

Interactional reasoning requires that a practitioner know himself or herself well. What a practitioner says has to match his or her personality and style, or he or she will not be taken as genuine. For example, both a sense of humor and a serious nature can be used to connect with a client. The question becomes "What do I need to communicate with this client, and how shall I express it so that it is coming from me?" In addition, the practitioner has to be able to observe the effect of his or her behavior on others and adapt or alter it when needed.

Conditional Reasoning

The holistic roots of the occupational therapy profession suggest the need for conditional reasoning because it provides the connection from meaning to action. *Conditional reasoning* is the ability to place thinking in an environmental context at the same time that thinking takes place in a context that is beyond the bonds of strict linear cognition. It is *phenomenological* (i.e., reality is what the client perceives), creative, and imaginative. It is the synthesis of all of the other forms of reasoning, some of them beyond what is known explicitly.

The phenomenology of the client is of paramount importance in conditional reasoning. The occupational therapy practitioner's task is to understand how the client makes meaning out of his or her life and its activities. The joy of working with clients comes from the moment when the narrative they are sharing rings with meaning for them and allows the practitioner a glimpse into their world, which is part of conditional reasoning. As with clinical reasoning, conditional reasoning is difficult to conceptualize; however, Case Example 7.1 may offer some insight into the notion of entering the client's world and connecting that world with action through conditional reasoning.

Mattingly and Fleming (1994) noted, "We think that conditional reasoning revolves around the ways that therapists think about which of the actions that the patient takes have potential for meaning-making" (p. 198). They believed that meaning making connects with activity in three ways: (1) intentionality, (2) habits, and (3) symbolic meaning. This connection is an integral one for

Case Example 7.1. Martha: Borderline Personality Disorder

Martha is a young woman with borderline personality disorder who refused to sit during her interview and became engrossed in telling me what it was like to be in her head: "It's like in the movies, when those whirling disks are chasing the star, and she just escapes one, when, just like that there's another and another, and she can't keep up. I feel like I'm being chased and captured."

Thanks to her eloquent metaphor, as her occupational therapist, I was able to ask her whether she wanted help learning how to control the whirling disks. For the first time during the occupational profile process, she sat down, made eye contact, and seemed to be listening to me. All at the same time, I watched her movements in space, I watched the room in which she sat, and I listened to her words. For a brief moment, I entered her world, and she was ready to begin to do the things she needed to do to decrease her disorganization and emotional pain.

practitioners. It is the framework for the jump from meaning to action.

Intentionality (i.e., when someone acts deliberately) implies choice. Consider the thinking involved in collaborating with a client about the choices he or she will make concerning purposeful activities and occupations. The occupational therapy practitioner's goal is to ensure that the client chooses activities that will allow him or her to move forward into his or her life, but the practitioner's ideas may not match those of the client.

For example, a weak grasp may preclude tooth brushing, but the client may want to be able to pick up a fork first. Furthermore, the practitioner may choose items or activities other than those chosen by the client, such as a pencil or pick-up sticks instead of a toothbrush or fork, because these items may have many useful applications and outcomes, an idea identified by Mattingly and Fleming (1994).

Most people's conception of occupational therapy practice is based on a linear progression of

activity. They may not be aware of the clinical reasoning in the form of conditional reasoning that is the impetus for the practitioner's choice of activities. What looks like playing pick-up sticks to a casual observer may mean independence in feeding to the practitioner and the client. The richness of the many layers of meaning for the client and the practitioner is often misperceived. When the practitioner explains to clients what he or she is doing and why, the practitioner lets clients into his or her phenomenology and provides them with the opportunity for greater understanding of the power of occupational therapy.

Habit is a word that has its origins in the very beginnings of occupational therapy. Habit training harkens back to the earliest days of the profession. Life is made up of a series of routines and rituals that simplify and secure meaning. Occupational therapy practitioners understand the importance of habits to people whose daily routines have been interrupted by disability. The meaning of a morning cup of coffee is far grander than the mechanics of the praxis that brings the coffee to the lips. Although the importance of praxis may not have been apparent when the person did not have to think about how his or her body moved in space, it is of the utmost importance when it prevents an activity from happening. On an even more ephemeral level, the *symbolic meaning* of activity is critical to the practitioner's clinical reasoning skills, because a person attributes significance or representative or figurative association with the activity.

Exercise 7.2. The Computer Expert

Read Case Example 7.2 and identify when the occupational therapy practitioner uses instances of procedural, interactive, and conditional reasoning.

Pragmatic Reasoning

Health care has undergone major changes since the inception of managed care, and these changes are taken into account by pragmatic reasoning (Schell & Cervero, 1993; Schell & Schell, 2008). Schell and Cervero (1993) identified pragmatism after they completed a literature review on the topic of clinical reasoning. *Pragmatic reasoning* considers the contextual issues affecting the patient now and

Case Example 7.2. Yeung: Depression

Working with **Yeung, age 14 years** with depression, made it clear to me that when a person thinks about his or her own thinking, it can result in unexpected outcomes. Yeung was brought to day treatment after an inpatient stay in the hospital for depression and a suicide attempt by hanging. When Yeung was 11 years old, his hand was caught in the washing machine at home, resulting in a complete amputation of his right (dominant) thumb. The thumb was replanted, but, although almost all such procedures in children are very successful (Sebastin & Chung, 2011), he never fully regained a good pincer grasp, and sensation was limited. In addition, Yeung seemed traumatized by all of the surgeries he had to endure after the replantation failure.

Yeung was of Chinese descent but had been born in the United States and spoke English as his primary and preferred language. His parents were bilingual but were not willing to participate in Yeung's treatment. In more than 20 years of employment, I have seen only 3 East Asian patients, despite a high concentration of ethnic Chinese living close to the hospital. I was unable to ascertain the reasons for the reluctance of Yeung's parents to participate, because they refused to respond to all attempts at contact.

At the time of our interview, Yeung was a student in middle school and was doing poorly because he had missed many days as a result of his depression. He has also previously lost many days while undergoing surgeries for his hand.

I reasoned that it would be important to find out what was important to Yeung before I decided on a plan of action. I noticed that he had some higher-level social skills that were evident when he entered my office, smiling and making eye contact with me. Perhaps these behaviors were automatic, but I would find that out as the interview progressed.

Yeung was very unhappy at school. He had become a victim of taunting and bullying, mostly because he tended to hide his thumb, which did not look very deformed to me. However, my years working with people with eating disorders had taught me just how distorted a self-image can become. It may have been possible that the sensory deficits were causing him to hide the digit from his peers. Children can be very cruel to anyone who seems different from them.

While we talked, I watched Yeung to see how he used the affected thumb and noticed that while he favored it, it did not look very abnormal to me. However, I know that subjective perception is key in defining the reality of a person. I decided not to pursue the behavior with the thumb, both at this point and during treatment, unless it was brought up by Yeung.

What emerged as we spoke was that Yeung appeared to be devastated by the loss of his ability to engage in his favorite video game, Halo 3.® When Yeung spoke about the game, he lit up but also started to slump in his chair and look down as he detailed his inability to play after the partial loss of sensation in his right thumb. The game had been updated to Halo 4 in 2012, but by then, Yeung was avoiding his Xbox® completely.

My reasoning after the interview followed this path: First, I believed that video gaming was an occupation for Yeung and that he had clearly identified it as meaningful. Second, video gaming was an occupation for Yeung in the sphere of play or leisure and social interaction. (Yeung used to play with friends in his neighborhood.) What I found puzzling was that despite the sensory limitations and weak pincer grasp, most children adapt well to hand difficulties and, without orthotics, can usually handle game controllers well. Why wasn't Yeung playing his favorite video game?

In Chapter 1, "Occupation, Activities, and Occupational Therapy," Hinojosa and Blount identified 6 reasons why occupational therapy practitioners use purposeful activities. Of those, I felt that the reason that dealt with directing attention to the accomplishment of an activity might be useful with Yeung. I deduced that he had stopped playing the video games because of his belief that he would not be able to work the game controller. Perhaps if we engaged in another activity that mimicked the hand movements necessary to work a game controller, I might be able to help Yeung transfer from my chosen activity to the video game device.

(Continued)

Case Example 7.2. Yeung: Depression *(Cont.)*

I wanted something that was realistic and meaningful but not related to computers and video gaming. I spoke with Yeung at length about his home life and the occupations in which he engaged. Although he spoke mostly of his Xbox games, he also said that he would like to build a computer of his own one day—a super computer with the power and graphics to handle all the online, graphics-rich video games.

Twenty years ago, I would have taken Yeung to our woodworking shop and have him use hand tools to demonstrate his ability to perform a video-gaming grasp, but now activities that have meaning are those that are related to the current social, economic, and cultural times. Thus, after meeting with Yeung, I went over to our Information Technology (IT) Department and spoke with the director. I asked whether they had any old computer parts that I could use for a patient who wanted to tinker. I left with armloads of chips and parts, along with a set of tools designed for working on computers. I applauded myself for thinking out of the box.

The next day, Yeung and I got to work. He seemed genuinely enthusiastic about the idea of working on the computer parts. I told him that the plan was to fix the parts according to diagrams the IT Department had given me. I went over the tools I had been given and showed him how to use them. I showed him the plans, and he was able to read and follow them without any problems. I was hoping that the occupational performance involved in the activity would distract him from defending his right hand and thumb. When Yeung reached for the tweezers, I was thrilled. He picked up a solder with tweezers in his left hand, but picked up the soldering gun with his right hand. He hummed as he engaged in the complex, bilateral purposeful activity of soldering pins in place on the computer board. He demonstrated advanced fine-motor skills.

I decided to say nothing about how this performance meant he could easily use the video game controller, because I felt it was too soon to push him. I knew that as our relationship grew, I would be able to suggest that he try to play Halo 3, or even Halo 4, once again.

In the 2 weeks that followed, Yeung demonstrated that he could handle even the most complicated computer-building skills. The IT director commented that he would gladly hire him, which I told Yeung, and he laughed. Our therapeutic relationship had progressed to the point where I felt I could push him to use the video game controller. I had borrowed an Xbox, loaded with the newest version of Halo, and when the time came, Yeung started to play with abandon, commenting on the game as he played, so that I would be made aware of all the nuances of his gaming. I felt a sense of mastery myself.

Many years later, Yeung had graduated from high school and was in school for computer repairs. We met on the street in the town near my hospital, and he approached me grinning. He told me about his success in computer work and told me that he had enjoyed our working together. He spoke of what was most meaningful in the encounter with me, and that was that I had allowed him to use a soldering iron when others believed him to be acutely suicidal. I had focused on the patient's occupational performance, and he had focused on the trust and relationship. I do not know what Yeung is doing today, but I learned a lot working with him.

in the future, the practitioner's personal context, and the practice environment's culture (Schell & Schell, 2008). It is similar to conditional reasoning in its recognition of the integration of environmental and personal factors, but it goes further to embrace the phenomenology of the practitioner, the input of the treatment team, and the political–economic factors of present-day health care (Schell & Schell, 2008).

Ethical Reasoning

Within the context of pragmatic reasoning is *ethical reasoning*, which deals with values relative to human conduct, with respect to the rightness or wrongness of certain actions, and the goodness or badness of the motives, means, and ends of such actions.

The mechanics of managed care and caps on reimbursement are often in conflict with both the needs of the client and the desire of the practitioner. How is reasoning affected when a therapist determines that a client requires 6 months of rehabilitation and the reimbursement is for only 10 visits? How does the therapist construct a context of improvement under these constraints? It is important for the therapist to advocate for the client, for example, when care of the client for 1 or 2 days will prevent or forestall a relapse or rehospitalization or when the client is being discharged before receiving the maximum benefits from the intervention if it is believed that he or she could benefit from additional treatment.

The opposite occurrence is just as common. The criteria for treatment at a partial hospital level of care are usually very specific. Often, a client no longer meets these criteria but has been certified for additional days of treatment. The right thing to do is discharge the client to a less structured level of care, which does not always happen.

The concept of ethics lies outside of the scope of this chapter, but it is another aspect of the complexity involved in clinical reasoning. The decisions practitioners make about what they do must be reasoned about in terms of whether they are the right things to do. Ethical reasoning is a part of this process.

Narrative Reasoning

> Whether I shall turn out to be the hero of my own life, or whether that station will be held by anybody else, these pages must show.
> —Charles Dickens, 1849/2000

Narrative reasoning uses a phenomenological process where the meaning of therapy is gained through stories (Mattingly, 1991). People are the heroes of their own lives, and the way they tell their stories has a lot to do with their perceptions of their own health and illness. Mattingly and Fleming (1994), Schell (2003a), and others have stressed the importance of the client's meaning making in clinical reasoning. Each client's story is unique and carries the seed of intervention. *Narrative* is the story a person tells of illness and wellness and how the practitioner

fashions a view of the client's future world. Often, a disparity exists between the client's vision and the reality of the course of treatment (Mattingly & Fleming, 1994; Schell, 2003a). For example, in the story of Yeung (Case Example 7.2), I envisioned him returning to his beloved video game. What occurred on the surface was what I had envisioned, but its meaning for Yeung was worlds apart from my view.

Listening for the meaning in the narrative requires the skills of an experienced clinician. Narrative reasoning exists on two levels: First is the life story of the client as it unfolds during evaluation and continues in treatment, and second is the narrative constructed by the practitioner as intervention is designed and implemented.

The key task for the occupational therapy practitioner who wishes to reason in a narrative form is to listen, listen, listen because the client's story emerges through his or her storytelling. A beginning occupational therapy student juggles so many impressions and ideas in his or her mind that the art of active listening can be lost. As experience makes it easier for the student to focus attention, he or she can truly concentrate on the client's story.

In my own work (Babiss, 2003), the story has become the main method for making decisions about ways of improving client outcomes. I let the client tell me how the next chapter of his or her story should proceed. Furthermore, this approach can be invaluable when a practitioner is troubled by some aspect of a client's treatment. In any case, it is always worth the time and effort to sit with a client and allow meaning to emerge. Often, the experience is intense when a client can see that you get it, and his or her world opens to you. In Case Example 7.3, narrative reasoning helped the practitioner enter her client's world to collaborate with him on the plot for his future, showing that it is crucial to know what the client's story is so that effective interventions can be made.

Again, the most crucial element in narrative reasoning is listening. Without hearing what the client with a disability is saying, a practitioner is unable to place his or her reasoning skills into that person's world. Peloquin (1993) addressed some of the viewpoints that interfere with the ability to establish a full understanding of the client in his or her narrative.

For example, when practitioners think of a client in terms of only his or her disability (e.g., "the right hemi"), they are engaging in *reductionistic think-*

Case Example 7.3. Chris: Interrupted History

Chris, age 19 years, is a handsome young man, who was a brilliant student with a few good friends, a loving mother, and an obsession with flying. In his first year of aviation school, he began to hear voices, which continued until he was forced to leave school and enter a psychiatric hospital. After an inpatient stay, the story he had written for himself—college graduate, pilot, husband, and father—was dashed. "I was going along fine, and then I was plucked out of life," he said with tears in his eyes. Chris's story highlights the temporal quality of narrative. He believed that his life was traveling a path whose trajectory was assured.

On hearing this narrative of an interrupted history, the practitioner reasoned that Chris's assertion that he had been "plucked" from life had some validity, but the practitioner believed that he had been removed only from the life he had envisioned. Together with Chris, the practitioner determined that the task ahead was to write a new story and allow the narrative to unfold in a different way.

In a review of a book of his short stories, the author William Trevor, as cited in Allen (1998), stated, "It's not as rose-tinted a world as most people would like it to be. But the people in my stories and novels are not ragingly desperate; they have . . . come to terms, and coming to terms in itself is quite an achievement" (p. 7). On the basis of that idea, Chris's main task would be to come to terms with what he could do now, and the practitioner's job would be to work with Chris to develop a different story in the context of real possibilities

The practitioner's narrative acknowledged the reality that Chris could not hope to fly again because of his psychiatric history. The practitioner's plan involved exploring with Chris the support activities involved in aviation. However, Chris's loss of narrative rendered cooperation difficult initially, but eventually he determined that he wanted to become involved in the construction of airplanes. This goal set the path that permitted the practitioner to work with Chris on constructing a daily life built around purposeful activities that would ensure that Chris's story would not face a major disruption.

For example, Chris worked out a daily schedule, independently figuring out that setting the alarm on his aviator's watch would remind him to take his medications, compliance with which was critical to maintaining his stability and function. Chris had a very supportive mother who was instrumental in providing a home environment in which Chris could remain independent but supported.

Together, Chris and the practitioner researched schools, and he chose one far from the hospital. He applied to the school, visited it with his mother, and was accepted. It was determined that he would remain at home until the next semester, 3 months away. During that time, Chris came to the hospital and practiced work and study skills. He wanted his story to be one of someone who could concentrate in school despite the voices, which still plagued him from time to time. He worked on the computer in the clinic and showed slight improvement with time.

In addition, Chris made friends with several other clients in treatment. His story of the roles that had been disrupted made it difficult for him to see himself as their peer. As time passed, however, he realized that he had more in common with them than he first had thought. The practitioner's story of Chris's life in the clinic before returning to school contained chapters on his connecting with other people, so she constructed group experiences and even the placement of chairs in the computer room to encourage spontaneous conversations.

The story ended for the practitioner when Chris and his mother moved to another state so that he could attend school. Chris's last letter told of his moderate success in school and that he had a few friends. He was still sad about the change in his circumstances, but it seemed that he had come to terms with his new story.

ing (i.e., oversimplifying a complex idea to fundamental components) or *monistic thinking* (i.e., perspective that things can be explained in terms of a single reality). This thinking leads to applying rote techniques and exercises (e.g., to increase strength or range of motion) that may not address the client's desires (e.g., to be able to stroke a pet). Thus, to engage in meaningful narrative reasoning, one has to take the time to hear the story.

Exercise 7.3. Clinical Reasoning and Activity Choice

Case Example 7.4 represents a unique instance of a person with both behavioral health and physiological concerns. Read through the case and think about the planning, performance, and reflection involved in working with this client.

The pragmatic realities of Gerard's case greatly hampered the realization of interventions that the treatment team reasoned to be meaningful. Gerard was discharged after 2 weeks because of insurance company constraints and a decrease in his acute psychiatric symptoms of anxiety and suicidal ideation. The treatment team, working in a behavioral health environment, reasoned that the most important task for Gerard was to accept the restrictions in his hand's range of motion so that he could make plans for avocational pursuits that accounted for his limitation in hand function. Without acceptance, Gerard would have no motivation to act in a goal-directed manner oriented toward the future.

A review of Gerard's history seemed to suggest that he was not deeply concerned with his lack of intimate social relationships and that attending a 12-step program (Alcoholics Anonymous) would not be a good choice for him. Gerard seemed motivated to interact only with family members and did not seem to value relationships outside of his family. Unfortunately, the treatment team did not get to enact many interventions with Gerard, beyond leaving him with the information about coming to terms with his hand injury.

New Directions in Clinical Reasoning

The new directions being taken by occupational therapy practitioners who address clinical reasoning hold great promise. In the recent past, in my opinion, work in the area of clinical reasoning in occupational therapy took a step toward a more reductionistic view of the phenomenon. Schell (2003a) began to look at clinical reasoning as a cognitive activity, which it is, and to suggest the use of mental models as a means of making practice more efficient. *Mental models* are a person's representation of the real world upon which he or she anticipates actions and consequences and prepares action.

Mental models were first suggested by the philosopher Craik (1967), who posited that people used a small-scale model of reality to be able to predict events and explain phenomena. Although Schell (2003a) acknowledged a drawback to fitting people into scripts and schemata, she was supportive of mental models.

I acknowledge that a thinking practitioner can do almost nothing to avoid categorizing and pattern recognition, but grave danger exists in adopting this habit as a means of making work more efficient. Johnson-Laird, Girotto, and Legrenzi (1998) warned against the hazards of reasoning using mental models. People who create mental models make very little explicit, because they focus on the implicit information in their models. This use of mental models creates an environment in which the possibility of considering alternatives that lie outside the mental model is diminished. Johnson-Laird et al. (1998) provided an example of a grievous error of this nature that occurred during the nuclear crisis at Three Mile Island. The rise in temperature in the plant was ascribed to a leak. The staff did not entertain other possibilities, which would have revealed that a valve was stuck in an open position. Their actions were guided by a faulty mental model, and the result was a major accident. Practitioners with less experience may welcome the ease of mental models, but the difficulty of changing one's models can make them too strong to reject.

The art of practice is born of treating each client as if he or she were a completely new experience because he or she is a new experience. If I start out working on pattern recognition and mental models, I may remain within this framework and never grow into a seasoned professional who has the ability to look outside of the cubbyholes I have created. A "typical hemi" is never just that. Schell and Schell (2008) rejected mental models and embraced the importance of the clinician's ability to search for evidence-based interventions as a major part of reasoning behavior.

Case Example 7.4. Gerard: Behavioral Health Hospitalization

Gerard, age 55 years, is a single man referred to the day program after an inpatient stay on the psychiatric department of a major hospital. This behavioral health hospitalization was his first.

The information collected during the occupational profile revealed a man of many facets. Gerard is medium height, slender, and graceful in his movements, all of which make his story more remarkable.

Gerard was a Vietnam War veteran, with the rank of captain. He watched as several of his men died in a helicopter that took off while he remained behind on orders from a superior. He commented that he has always felt guilty about this incident. After a 4-year tour, he returned home to find that his peers had gone to school, married, and moved on. He joined the city fire department, where he worked for 20 years in some of the most dangerous neighborhoods in the city. On retirement, he sold the condominium where he lived alone and moved into an apartment in the house of his sister and brother-in-law.

Gerard never married, which he attributed to his use of alcohol throughout most of his life. At the time of his admission to the day program, he had not had a drink for several months. He stated, "Alcohol is the thing that destroyed anything good in my life." Gerard identified as an asset his desire to spend time with his family and as a weakness a fear of close relationships with people other than his family.

In retirement, Gerard taught himself to use a computer and started to work in construction with his brother-in-law. This vocation contributed to his current difficulties. While working on his sister's house, he fell from the roof, fracturing his spine and crushing his right radius. Gerard's back healed, but he required surgery for his forearm, which has several internal stabiliza-tion devices in it. Gerard laughed ruefully as he said, "I set off the alarms at the airport now."

Although Gerard went to therapy after the surgery, he remained unable to use his hand for carpentry or to use the computer keyboard. Besides computers, he identified golf and carpentry as avocational pursuits, all of which have been greatly hampered by the lack of range of motion. Frustrated with the difficulties with his hand, Gerard contemplated suicide, which necessitated the inpatient hospitalization.

As he began to realize that he would not regain full use of his right hand, Gerard began to experience what he described as anxiety attacks. He then remembered that in his last few years at the fire department, he had become panicked and gone to speak with the fire department psychiatrist a few times. This was, however, Gerard's first inpatient and subsequent day hospital encounter.

It was clear that the therapist needed more information about the prognosis for Gerard's hand. She conducted a phone consultation with the occupational therapist who had treated Gerard. She reported that Gerard's internal fixation status would limit his wrist extension to 40° forever, but she believed that he could adequately accommodate for this with respect to the computer. Carpentry work, however, would be limited, unless he was able to change handedness for the use of tools.

Note. Before reading the rest of the case, answer the following questions: What is the priority need for intervention with Gerard? Why did you make this choice? Suspend pragmatic and ethical concerns and make activity choices to provide intervention in the priority area. Reason about the importance of social components for Gerard in planning choice of occupations.

Knowing More Than We Can Say

Thinking about the way you think, the act of *metacognition,* is a laborious task. When asked to think about the way in which you decided to pursue a career in occupational therapy, you could probably discern a linear path that you followed in making the decision. Identifying the intangible factors that affected your decision is not so straightforward an activity. Time spent examining the way in which your mind handles information and experiences can result in a substantial improvement in your ability to reason about activities.

A structured portal into your thinking about thinking is the examination of your style of learning new information. Learning-style models abound, and a student or practitioner who is interested in exploring how he or she learns what he or she knows is advised to choose a taxonomy that feels suited to his or her needs. Gardner (1983) and Kolb (1984) offered learning-style models based on types of intelligence and on experiential learning, respectively.

Gardner (1983) asserted that intelligence is not one discrete measurement but that it includes seven dimensions: (1) logical–mathematical, (2) linguistic, (3) musical, (4) spatial, (5) bodily–kinesthetic, (6) interpersonal, and (7) intrapersonal. For example, over time, I have come to know that my strongest areas of intelligence are linguistic and spatial. Therefore, when learning new material or working with new clients, I read and observe as much as I can. It is the reason I am drawn to qualitative, narrative information gathering. Kolb's (1984) work on experiential learning is similar to that of Schön (1983) because it is based on doing and reflection. He reasoned that people learn through doing and thinking about what they have done. For further information on learning styles, refer to Schell and Schell (2008).

A practitioner who wants to expand his or her ability to know without knowing and improve his or her prowess in the intuitive leaps that characterize a seasoned clinician is advised to practice some form of self-awareness technique. Meditation, yoga, and journal writing are all satisfactory means of expanding one's inner life through occupation. The more awareness you have of the ways in which you make sense of the world, the better your ability to understand how this view affects your reasoning.

Four-Quadrant Model of Facilitated Learning

Greber, Ziviani, and Rodger (2007a, 2007b) have presented a model of learning that uses teaching–learning approaches. They contended that this approach, the *Four-Quadrant Model of Facilitated Learning,* can enhance clinical reasoning and help organize choice of intervention with clients.

The theoretical framework of the model is Bandura's (1977) Social Learning Theory, which serves as the foundation of some acquisitional frames of reference (Mosey, 1986). The four quadrants, as a schematic (Greber et al., 2007a), contain several continua, ranging from learning that is initiated by the facilitator to learning that is initiated by the learner, from direct teaching methods to indirect teaching methods, and from teachers moving from leading learners to fading from them. This framework outlines a gradation of ability much like that from novice to experienced practitioner, but it clearly incorporates methods of learning that are based on social learning.

Greber et al. (2007a) explored several learning strategies to create the four strategy clusters that make up the quadrants. Thus, they contended that the model provides scaffolding for making clinical decisions about interventions with clients and that it enables practitioners to make accurate intervention choices. A practitioner can begin working with a client in direct teaching methods, demonstrating how things are done and giving concrete instructions and move all the way to the fourth quadrant in which the client is engaging in problem solving and questioning his or her own progress. The usefulness of this organization as it is applied to the teaching of occupations remains to be determined.

Case Studies: Clinical Reasoning in Action

I conclude this chapter with two examples of treatment interactions contributed by two occupational therapists. I asked each therapist to think and reason about the choices they had made. Case Example 7.5 provides a glimpse into the activity reasoning of a competent practitioner and Case Example 7.6, of an experienced practitioner. These two cases are very different. What they have in common is the therapists' desire to enter the client's world so that they could collaborate in the creation of a meaningful environment for the client. Each therapist used different forms of clinical reasoning to achieve his or her objectives. As you read, think about how you might have reasoned about each situation.

Summary

In this chapter, I explored the many facets of reasoning about activity. My goal was to increase awareness of the nature and importance of how you

Case Example 7.5. Jane: Cerebral Palsy

The following describes an assessment, treatment plan, and intervention conducted by Ann Winter, an occupational therapist who had worked many years as a certified occupational therapy assistant. Much of what she wrote included her reasoning, and I also asked her to think and write about the decisions she made in collaborating with this client. What follows is both an account of a creative competent practitioner and a metacognitive exploration of clinical reasoning. Winter's reflections about her choices, made after the treatment, are presented in italics.

Jane, age 17 years, was adopted from Korea. She was diagnosed with left hemiplegic cerebral palsy at age 8 months and acquired Prader–Willi syndrome when she was 3 years old in addition to an inoperable tumor on her hypothalamus. She has many of the symptoms and signs of congenital Prader–Willi syndrome, including low muscle tone; short stature; cognitive disabilities; problem behaviors; and a flaw in the function of the hypothalamus, resulting in chronic feelings of hunger.

Jane's biological brother, also adopted by the same American parents, displays no cognitive or physical disabilities. The ethnic disparity in the family is reported to have had no effect on Jane's social or school experiences. Jane's father has a drug and alcohol dependency and has emotionally abused Jane's mother for the past 15 years. Consequently, Jane's mother has assumed the majority of the responsibilities associated with Jane's care since infancy and currently has an order of protection against her husband. He has been out of the house for the past 6 months. There is no history of physical abuse to either child.

Jane's room is on the ground floor of a home that has been environmentally adapted to suit her needs in terms of bathroom requirements and front-door accessibility. She requires moderate assistance to rise from a sitting position; ambulate; and perform bed transfers, oral hygiene, dressing, showering, and toileting. She navigates independently in a motorized wheelchair when outside of her home. Her bedroom is adjacent to the den, which houses a television, computer, and stereo system, all of which Jane is able to operate.

Jane attends a Board of Cooperative Educational Services high school and participates in its 6-week summer session. She has been taking part in a prevocational program at her school during which she assembles parts for test tubes a full day once a week and receives a weekly paycheck. She spends the other days working on academics. Jane reads at a third-grade level, and she can perform single-digit addition and subtraction problems. She is unable to speak and must use an augmentative communication device to converse. She states that she enjoys communicating over the Internet and that she loves "looking things up." Jane's intelligence quotient was measured on a standardized intelligence test as 77. She continues to receive physical therapy at school, but much to her mother's opposition; occupational therapy services were discontinued 3 years ago because her therapist believed that Jane had reached a plateau in terms of skill acquisition.

Jane displays enthusiasm for school, and as long as her routine is not interrupted, she moves willingly through her day. Any change in routine, however, such as a different bus driver, brings on an emotional meltdown in the form of a temper tantrum, according to Jane's mother. In fact, on a few occasions, a change in bus driver resulted in Jane's mother having to miss a day of work.

Jane has two close female friends she has known since kindergarten, and whenever possible, their mothers take them to the mall. According to her mother, Jane has not demonstrated an interest in or curiosity about boys. The mother's extended family visits whenever possible. Jane receives home health care 3 hours a day, 4 days a week, and 8 hours on Saturday to help alleviate the strain on her mother. Jane's father does not visit nor does he contribute financially to the family.

Jane presents as a grossly overweight adolescent girl of short stature. At the onset of the evaluations, she did not appear timid or fearful in the presence of the evaluating therapist and did, in

(Continued)

Case Example 7.5. Jane: Cerebral Palsy *(Cont.)*

fact, seem to be excited by the attention. Although Jane is nonverbal, she demonstrated exuberance by smiling broadly and waving her arms up and down. Jane's left arm is much weaker than her left leg and only moves slightly in momentum with her body during her excitement. She is able to use her left arm as an assisting extremity for stabilization of objects in various tasks, such as eating or writing.

During the interview, Jane was cooperative for approximately 15 minutes, oriented to the reason for the interview, and adept in the use of her communication device. She used her right index finger to operate her communication device and computer. Because Jane cooperated for only a brief period, her mother had to complete various portions of the interview with Jane's approval. Jane made frequent nonverbal sounds, which her mother understood to mean that she wanted food. According to her mother, Jane requests food all day long, and as soon as she comes home from school, she either listens to music, logs on to the Internet, or watches television, while repeatedly making requests for food. Jane's mother told the therapist that Jane has an ongoing obsession with the stories she has watched on the Lifetime network. She speaks incessantly to her teachers about the melodramas, claiming that specific actors are actually involved in her life.

Evaluation

Jane was observed eating a lunch of scrambled eggs, using a gross grasp of her fork. Although she continually requests food and is morbidly obese, she is reportedly an extremely finicky eater and will eat only particular food items, such as eggs and pizza, without demonstrating satiety. After the evaluation, Jane was seated on the floor in front of the television in the den with moderate physical assistance from her mother. She was clad in a T-shirt and underpants, which her mother stated is her usual attire for home. Jane is unable to toilet herself independently, and this state of undress is a convenience strategy. Jane ambulates in a waddling, unsteady gait and exhibits classic Prader–Willi traits of obesity,

hypotonia, and dried saliva at the corners of her mouth. She wears bilateral ankle–foot orthotics to enhance ambulation stability while at school and outside. Jane requires only contact guarding when wearing the orthotics. At home, she requires minimal-to-moderate assistance for all transfers and ambulation and does not wear the orthotics.

The occupational therapist evaluated Jane at home because she had finished the school year and had not yet begun the summer program. The two assessments used in this evaluation were the Canadian Occupational Performance Measure (COPM; Law et al., 1998) and the Comprehensive Occupational Therapy Evaluation Scale (COTE; Brayman, Kirby, Misenheimer, & Short, 1976).

I chose COPM for this client because it is a client-centered interview, one in which the therapist elicits information that the client identifies as pertinent. This particular adolescent has not had many opportunities in her life to be heard in her own voice. She has had few opportunities to make her own choices; because of her physical, communicative, and mental limitations, she rarely gets a chance to express her desired occupations, dreams, and desires as an adolescent girl. At her age, many girls have already started to choose elective classes in school, get a driver's license, research potential colleges, and think about what to do on a Friday or Saturday night. This assessment enabled Jane to call the shots in terms of desired roles and satisfaction with the roles in which she currently engages in the home, school, and community. Although her mother was available to add information on issues that Jane was not interested in answering, such as household management, Jane clearly had much to say about her desired occupations. I did not want to oblige Jane to answer structured questions that limited her thought process or imagination.

I selected COTE for Jane because, given the time allotment, it allowed me to observe Jane and look for specific behaviors that would be pertinent to her occupational performance in interaction with people and objects in the environment and in daily life tasks. COTE is relatively easy to administer, and Jane's behaviors were observed throughout the

(Continued)

Case Example 7.5. Jane: Cerebral Palsy *(Cont.)*

entire process of interview, lunchtime, watching television, ambulating from kitchen to den, and operating her communication device. Therefore, COTE seemed to be an appropriate complement to COPM because it required no additional effort on Jane's behalf with regard to the overall assessment, and it still afforded me very pertinent data regarding Jane's appearance and behaviors such as activity level, interpersonal behaviors, and task behaviors.

COPM includes three sections: (1) Self-Care, (2) Productivity, and (3) Leisure. The client or caregiver prioritizes the occupations that the client needs or wants to perform within the client's typical daily routine. The respondent then rates the importance of each activity on a scale ranging from 1 to 10. Jane was able to participate in the interview by means of her communication device, and her mother continued when Jane decided that she was finished.

As noted before, I chose COPM because Jane has had limited opportunity to express her wishes for direction of treatment and self-selected priorities. Jane initially appeared to enjoy the fact that the interview was directed toward her and that she had the power to answer without judgment or censure.

The problems identified as Jane's priorities offer valuable insight. Jane would like to spend more time on prevocational skills; improve her ability to cope with changes in routines; expand her range of socialization; participate in more school activities, such as cheerleading, chorus, and acting; and increase her scope of hobbies beyond that of television and computer. Jane indicates that she would like to be an actress and that although she is in chorus and cheerleading at school, she does not get as many chances to participate in these activities as she would like. In addition, she has prevocational training only 1 day a week. As indicated on the scoring section of COPM, Jane believes that she does a good job at her prevocational activity but is not satisfied with the work.

I postulated that an increase in purposeful activities that Jane finds interesting, satisfying, and meaningful would lead to enhanced socialization opportunities, coping strategies, and variation in recreational hobbies because motivation is a key

element in the treatment of people with Prader–Willi syndrome. Thus, in pursuing activities that Jane finds interesting, valuable, and enjoyable and melding them into the repertoire of her desired occupations (as outlined in COPM), I hypothesized that she would be more likely to participate actively in those occupations and with a greater degree of satisfaction.

COTE is a behavioral rating scale used as an observation tool to identify behaviors relevant to a client's occupational performance in interaction with objects in the environment and daily life tasks. COTE consists of a single-sided sheet of paper that incorporates 26 behaviors divided into three areas: (1) General Behavior, (2) Interpersonal Behavior, and (3) Task Behavior. The occupational therapy practitioner applies a rating scale ranging from 0 to 5 to the client's level of functioning for each component of behavior (Brayman & Kunz, 2000).

I used COTE throughout the interview process, during which time Jane ate lunch, watched television, operated her communication device, and ambulated from the kitchen to the den. This tool was extremely helpful in evaluating Jane because it documented valuable information about her behaviors while imposing no further demands on her attention. Evaluating observed strengths and weaknesses makes treatment planning easier.

Jane's major identified areas of difficulty are independence, attention-getting behaviors, concentration, cooperation, decision making, coordination, and frustration tolerance. These behaviors correspond to the deficits indicated on COPM and, in particular, the problems that she experiences in coping with changes. Challenges presented to Jane in the form of a new task, alteration in a task, or unfamiliar peers and personnel may elicit an extremely negative response. It is therefore easier for those around her to play it safe rather than risk evoking a tantrum reaction from Jane.

Jane might benefit from treatment using interventions based on the Model of Human Occupation (MOHO; Kielhofner, 1995). According to MOHO, a person is perceived as an open and dynamic system in which the organization of

(Continued)

Case Example 7.5. Jane: Cerebral Palsy *(Cont.)*

cognitive processes, musculoskeletal integrity, and nervous system influences his or her ability to successfully explore the environment. MOHO suggests a human system that is not only in a constant state of organized process but also encompasses three subsystems: (1) the volition subsystem, which refers to a person's ability to anticipate, choose, experience, and interpret his or her own occupational behavior; (2) the habituation subsystem, which occurs when the human system acquires automatic and familiar performances as a result of recurrent patterns of occupational behavior; and (3) the mind–brain–body performance subsystem, which incorporates the biomechanical components of the person's physical and mental features.

The reason I chose MOHO as a frame of reference for Jane's treatment was that it focuses on interests, attraction, and preference for certain occupations and aspects of performance. The primary method for arousing motivation in adolescents with Prader–Willi syndrome is to focus on their interests. Another component of MOHO, values, will generally follow suit after interest has been established within the adolescent's personal convictions and sense of obligation toward an occupation that he or she finds pleasant or interesting. MOHO also incorporates occupational choice, and one of the key aspects of choosing MOHO was to allow Jane to give voice to what she finds meaningful and valuable in her life. Knowing Jane's personality traits and those of other people with Prader–Willi, I believed that motivation for occupation (Kielhofner, 1995) was the only way to elicit Jane's incentive to engage in desired occupations.

Clinical Reasoning About Activity and Use of Evidence-Based Support

By completing COPM, Jane was given an opportunity to prioritize her interpretation of the volitional structure of her life's routines. Providing a rationale for motivation is a key element in the treatment of people with Prader–Willi syndrome. Weber (1993) found that "based on past experiences, a combination of social reinforcement and token economy incentives work well to control and change behaviors" (p. 6).

In exploring occupations that she might find valuable, enjoyable, and interesting, I projected that Jane's sense of self-efficacy would improve. Moreover, the adolescent with Prader–Willi syndrome is most comfortable with routine and repetitiveness in daily occupations. To meld the performances that Jane chooses into a habituation process, the collaborative team involved in her progress will provide opportunity for increasing emotional adaptability by very slowly making changes in routine. (Ho & Dimitropoulos, 2010). Jane has many physical issues that must be considered when planning treatment, and her performance is greatly affected by the impairments associated with her dually diagnosed conditions. "Occupation requires us to use our bodies to traverse the geography and act upon the objects of a physical world" (Kielhofner, 1995, p. 116). Jane's mind–brain–body subsystem has affected her actions in an inefficient manner as a result of low tone, neurological deficits, and decreased cardiopulmonary energy. With the introduction of activity choices that address her volitional needs, I anticipated that she would move along the continuum from the current state of parent-asserted helplessness, observed incompetence, and inefficacy toward occupational exploration. It is likely that she will gain a sense of competence and eventual mastery over chosen occupations.

Jane demonstrates a zeal for occupations that she enjoys and for independent thought processes pertaining to attractions and interests that trigger personal convictions. According to COPM, Jane has the ability to attribute meaning to certain occupations in which she would like to be engaged. The COTE Scale revealed an adolescent girl who has a generally appropriate orientation to her situation and surroundings and the desire for increased socialization along with a highly animated and appealing affect.

After examination of the results of COPM and COTE, the primary areas in which Jane exhibits deficits are socialization, play or leisure exploration, and vocational exploration. These skill areas were clearly prioritized in the initial COPM assessment, and the deficits observed in interpersonal behaviors and task behaviors on COTE further support the concentration of intervention in

(Continued)

Case Example 7.5. Jane: Cerebral Palsy *(Cont.)*

these areas. Jane exhibited a lack of independent actions and self-assertion and a plethora of attention-getting behaviors (e.g., making noise and waving her arms) during the evaluation. Her task behavior demonstrated poor concentration, poor coordination, and inadequate decision-making abilities. She lost interest in the interview and had no coping mechanisms to implement when frustration emerged. Jane could benefit from activities that provide an opportunity to develop a sense of efficacy and control in achieving desired behavior outcomes (Kielhofner, 1995).

Socialization was deemed a priority to be addressed within the treatment plan, and vocational exploration was the next concern. The most likely scenario for Jane's future is to reside in a group home and work in a sheltered workshop. Jane is presently dissatisfied with the work that has been chosen for her; thus, this activity does not facilitate a sense of personal causation, values, and interest. A disconnection exists between the reality of her current and projected life management. Play and leisure exploration are Jane's concern and her mother's. It would benefit Jane both physically and socially to broaden her range of hobbies to include fewer sedentary interests. Adolescents with Prader–Willi syndrome can benefit from activities involving muscular strength, endurance, cardiovascular endurance, and coordination (Weber, 1993). Her current lack of incentive to actively explore her environment reflects a dysphoric attitude toward physical activity.

Treatment Planning

To facilitate improved socialization skills for Jane, the occupational therapist identified performance components that must be focused on, including increased problem-solving skills, attention span, interests in activities that Jane enjoys and that may be shared with others, social conduct, interpersonal skills, self-expression, coping skills and self-control for improved frustration tolerance, and assumption of roles for societal demands. Jane's strength, endurance, and gross motor coordination need to be addressed to enhance participation in many social activities.

When planning treatment of vocational performance, the occupational therapist must take into account many areas of concern, including deficits in fine and gross motor coordination, endurance, strength, attention span, problem solving, initiation of activity, role assumption of worker, interest in task, social conduct, interpersonal skills, self-expression, coping skills for transitioning to new tasks, time management, and the self-control to modulate behavior in response to new demands. Jane's present play and leisure activities require very little physical exertion. She identified interests in acting and cheerleading. She will have to work on improving strength and endurance, gross motor coordination, postural control, attention span, initiation of activity, and problem solving. She also needs to assume the role of an active participant; assess her values in determining that an activity is worth her effort; share her interest in the chosen activity; and improve social conduct, interpersonal skills, self-expression, coping skills, and self-control.

After identifying the areas requiring attention, the therapist identified two short-term and one long-term goal for Jane. The first short-term goal was with moderate verbal assistance, Jane will within 2 weeks identify two alternative strategies that she may implement when presented with a group task that she either is not interested in or does not want to complete. This goal was to help Jane enhance her problem-solving skills within a social context. The second short-term goal was with moderate assistance, Jane will within 1 week compile a list of at least 5 activities that she is interested in attempting and that require more than one person to perform. This goal was to help Jane increase self-expression pertaining to a social setting. The long-term goal was Jane will within 4 months demonstrate an improved ability to interact with peers in an appropriate contextual and cultural manner by participating in a group task consisting of at least 3 other group members. She will have close supervision for 20 minutes and require fewer than 3 verbal prompts to stay on task. This goal was to help Jane promote her role as a social participant.

The therapist decided to use a game called Guess What I Am Doing? to encourage players

(Continued)

Case Example 7.5. Jane: Cerebral Palsy (Cont.)

to guess what activity another player was miming. This activity is a form of charades, but it takes the game a few steps further into occupational reality. A minimum of 2 participants is needed. The game involves the following 7 steps:

1. The occupational therapy practitioner prints on index cards different tasks and activities that occur in everyday life. For example, a card could specify brushing one's teeth, washing dishes, or making a bed.
2. Each participant gets a card when it is his or her turn, and he or she must act out the task on the card.
3. The other participants write down what they think the actor is doing.
4. The actor then tells the group what he or she has performed.
5. The participants are then encouraged to applaud the actor.
6. After the performance, with the practitioner's assistance, the group discusses whether any components of the task have been omitted in the performance. For example, if the task is brushing teeth, perhaps the actor forgot to replace the toothpaste cap or rinse off the toothbrush.
7. It is then the next person's turn to give a performance.

I selected this activity for Jane because as indicated on COPM, she desires to participate as an actress in plays and make more friends. This activity gives Jane an opportunity to act and exhibit self-expression while integrating socialization skills into the group process. The game also gives Jane a chance to be part of the audience; therefore, she may practice waiting her turn, attending to task, and implementing problem-solving strategies if necessary during the course of the activity.

Guess What I Am Doing? has a great deal of importance related to Jane's projected future in a group home. Although I anticipated that she would enjoy the experience of role-playing within the socialization of a small group, the tasks that are to be enacted mimic activities that are a part of Jane's

daily routines. Furthermore, many of the tasks on the index cards can be modified to correspond to COPM's self-care and productivity sections. To become a successful member of a group home, it is in Jane's best interest to practice situations and tasks that may be expected of her. In this manner, she will help establish a sociocultural fit that will apply to current and future relationships and environments.

Intervention

The second visit with Jane took place in the late afternoon on a day on which she did not attend the summer program. Jane's mother invited Jane's two close girlfriends over, who knew ahead of time that they would be playing the Guess What I Am Doing? game. The activity encouraged participation and engagement because the girls appeared motivated to act out the situations and were eager to respond with their deductions. They giggled at each other's portrayals and could identify the tasks. The tasks were purposely very simple, such as brushing hair or washing face, to reduce possible frustration. The game addressed the priorities and goals because Jane was observed to wait her turn, interact appropriately, express herself, and clearly maintain attention for a full 10 minutes before she required redirection to the activity. She began to ask for food, and her mother told her that she would have to wait.

I would have preferred to field test the activity within the setting of Jane's summer program where there would have been more adolescent participants. The benefit to testing the game in Jane's home was that there was a high comfort level. Nonetheless, the school would have been a better environment in which to observe the efficacy of the game's components and how they relate to Jane's goals. The discussion component of the game (Step 6) is one that would be reserved for a group with a relatively high attention span and frustration tolerance. It was apparent that each participant wanted to take her turn as soon as the previous actor's task was identified. They did not have the tolerance or interest in discussing whether any aspects of the represented task were omitted in the performance.

Case Example 7.6. Mr. Lamb: Home Health

This case example was provided by Donald Auriemma, MSEd, OTR/L, BCN, who is an assistant professor of occupational therapy at York College of the City University of New York. He was pleased to write this case example because of his belief that the skill of reasoning about activities connects directly to the elegance of practice.

Mr. Lamb, at age 78 years, was referred for occupational therapy services through a certified home health agency. I began this journey with a review of the documentation package. A broadly written referral requested both evaluation and treatment of challenges to activities of daily living. Frequency of treatment was set at 2–3 times per week for 9 weeks. Mr. Lamb had arrived home after an inpatient stay for an exacerbation of congestive heart failure (CHF). His hospital stay was just one of several in the past few years for heart failure. An exacerbation of CHF was his primary condition; severe osteoarthritis was the secondary condition. Cardiac precautions were clearly indicated. Mr. Lamb's medication list was extensive. A preliminary picture was drawn of a person facing the challenges that the later stages of his diseases posed. I made an appointment for an initial evaluation.

As I approached his front door, I made my way up his 4-step stoop, and the absence of handrails stood out. In response to my knock, he called out for me just to walk in. A frail-appearing, well-spoken man welcomed me. The sight of this unkempt person sitting on a stained and tattered couch struck me. A musty smell and strong body odor permeated the room. Signs of years of neglect marked the first floor of his home. Mr. Lamb immediately offered an apology for not being able to walk over to open the door. A combination of limited range of motion and multiple sclerosis affecting both lower extremities along with compromised cardiovascular endurance had left him unable to ambulate.

Who was this man sitting in front of me, and how did his life situation lead to this unsettling picture? Mr. Lamb, an effective historian, provided a vivid history. As a child, he immigrated to the United States from South America. Raised by his grandmother, he lived a childhood marked by extreme poverty and a strong religious tradition. As a young adult with limited education, he learned a trade and worked as a machinist, an occupation he loved. It afforded him the ability to live out the dream of purchasing a home and raising a family. His 2 grown children live out of state. Proudly, he explained how in his middle years, he converted his oversized garage into a machine shop. There, for more than 20 years, he was able to support his family. Advancing CHF and osteoarthritis slowly robbed him of the ability to continue his business, maintain his home, move about, and ultimately perform much of his self-care.

He had been married for more than 40 years. His wife needed to work long hours in a hair salon she was trying to sell. Somberly, he described how he spent both day and night on his living room couch. For approximately the past 3 years, his wife had provided him with breakfast, lunch, a clean urinal, and a bedpan. He would stay alone until she returned from work. Recreation was watching television and an occasional visit from a friend or neighbor. His elderly wife usually returned home visibly exhausted. Because he was reluctant to burden his wife further with the assistance he needed, several days would go by before he had a bath or changed his clothes. A dust-covered standard walker stood in the corner of his room. It was the only piece of therapeutic equipment Mr. Lamb had.

Evaluation

During this visit, I completed the initial evaluation. The information I obtained helped me to understand better Mr. Lamb's challenges and assets. His roles as a husband, provider, friend, and neighbor were no longer satisfying. His ability to spend time in his machine shop as a leisure pursuit was gone. Participation in home maintenance, cleaning, and shopping was no longer possible. Rolling and sitting up in bed was possible, but ambulating was not. Physical assistance to transfer was required. If someone brought him food, he could feed himself. He could manage to

(Continued)

Case Example 7.6. Mr. Lamb: Home Health (Cont.)

dress his upper body, but he required assistance with his pants, shoes, and socks. Bathing was limited to sponging with assistance. He would toilet himself with the use of a bedpan and urinal. Deterioration in key performance components appeared to have greatly contributed to these performance area declines. Substantial limitations in range of motion were present in all extremities and trunk, more so in his lower extremities. General strength was fair-plus to good-minus. His endurance was very limited, with an estimated muscle endurance test level of 2.0–2.5. The high value he placed on self-reliance, ability to cope with demanding situations, interest in learning, strong interpersonal skills, and liberal health insurance were some of the outstanding assets.

Reasoning and Treatment Planning

I believed that a client-centered approach and early successes would lay the foundation for allowing Mr. Lamb to believe change was possible. This approach could motivate optimal participation and create an effective therapeutic relationship, thus maximizing his functional potential. Collaboration with Mr. Lamb revealed that functional mobility was his number one priority. My thoughts focused on adaptations, equipment, and instructed skills. Mobility options needed to match his physical capabilities and not place a dangerous demand on his compromised cardiac function. Sliding transfers and manual wheelchair use were chosen. Both could use the greater strength of and range in his upper extremities and allow for a rest period at any point when the physiological demand became too challenging.

Intervention

Mr. Lamb's couch no longer confined him. He achieved independence with a hospital bed, drop-arm commode, and manual wheelchair. He now slept on an electric hospital bed set up in his living room. Sleeping became more restful, and Mr. Lamb found it easier to breathe in a semi-reclined position. Using all four extremities, he could move about in a manual wheelchair, in a slow and effort-filled manner. Access to his living room, dining room, and kitchen was regained. Within 2 weeks, his world had expanded from his couch to the entire first floor of his home.

Mr. Lamb's next priority was to reduce the burden on his wife by gaining a greater capacity to perform his own self-care. A focus was placed partially on what compensatory treatments would best help meet his desires. Through training with the use of a dressing stick, sock aid, reacher, long-handled shoehorn, and buttonhook, he regained the ability to dress himself. Long-handled devices provided access to the distal parts of his body that limited joint range prevented him from reaching. Commode use replaced the need to use a urinal and bedpan. Wheelchair access to the kitchen sink afforded Mr. Lamb a consistent opportunity to sponge bathe and groom regularly. Now able to reach his refrigerator, Mr. Lamb could choose from a variety of prepared or simple-to-prepare foods. A reacher provided access to lightweight objects placed in closets.

During this same period, Mr. Lamb engaged in an exercise program designed to remediate endurance, range of motion, and muscle strength. Because of his frail health, frequent, brief, and mild bouts of exercise were thought to be the most beneficial and least risky. Therefore, the remediation program was split between being provided as a portion of the 3-times-a-week visits and a home exercise program that was performed on nontreatment days. I believed that even small gains in these components of performance would positively contribute to Mr. Lamb's regaining both the quantity and the quality of his functional abilities, and they did. These gains contributed to Mr. Lamb achieving independence in more physically demanding modified stand–pivot transfers. Manual wheelchair propulsion was performed with greater ease. Self-care activities were performed with a reduction in the number of rest periods required. Once again, Mr. Lamb was strong enough to open and close his heavy front door. Successes gained in the 6 weeks of the program continued to motivate Mr. Lamb.

(Continued)

Case Example 7.6. Mr. Lamb: Home Health (Cont.)

Mr. Lamb was encouraged to broaden his thinking. A 3-week window for occupational therapy was left. Cognizant of the limited remaining time and projected discharge date, his interest shifted to regaining access to his community. I judged his limited endurance and the 4 steps to enter his home to be his greatest challenges. The acquisition of a power wheelchair and a ramp constructed by a neighbor met these challenges. Power wheelchair use afforded Mr. Lamb access to his beloved machine shop. Traveling 4 blocks to the local shopping area became possible. Moving through his community allowed him to engage again with friends and neighbors with whom he had lost touch. His power wheelchair served him well for neighborhood travel. A solution for traveling longer distances was desired. Returning to driving seemed impossible. Car-related costs and the physical demands of placing a wheelchair into a car were beyond his economic and physical capabilities. Cab service costs could not fit within his limited budget. A referral to a city-based transportation service was pursued. This low-cost service broadened access beyond Mr. Lamb's immediate community. For the price of public transportation, he could travel throughout the city.

Termination of occupational therapy services occurred, as planned, in the 9th week of sessions. Contact with Mr. Lamb was maintained informally after his discharge through an occasional visit or crossing paths while I traveled through his neighborhood providing services to others. Despite the continuation of the destructive course of the CHF and osteoarthritis and several more hospitalizations, greater participation filled his remaining years. For years, it made my day brighter seeing him talking to neighbors in front of his home or traveling about his neighborhood.

reason about what you do with clients. The enormity of the responsibility for decisions made in collaboration is mitigated by a conscious attention to the task of clinical reasoning. One day, a student or client may ask why you did or said something as you go through your day as a practitioner. If you can answer the question, you will be on the way to becoming an expert practitioner who can balance self-awareness with an awareness of the client's needs within the realities of the environment. It seems a worthwhile goal to strive for the ability to reason with awareness.

Acknowledgments

I acknowledge the invaluable contribution of Ann Winter and Donald Auriemma, occupational therapists who willingly examined their practice and gave of their words and time.

References

Accreditation Council for Occupational Therapy Education. (2012). 2011 Accreditation Council for Occupational Therapy Education (ACOTE®) standards. *American Journal of Occupational Therapy, 66*(Suppl.), S6–S74. http://dx.doi.org/10.5014/ajot.2012.66S6

Agency for Healthcare Research and Quality. (2013). *About TeamSTEPPS*. Retrieved from http://teamstepps.ahrq.gov/about-2cl_3.htm

Allen, B. (1998, September 6). Fatal attraction [Review of the book *Death in summer* by W. Trevor]. *New York Times Book Review*, p. 7.

Babiss, F. (2003). *An ethnographic study of mental health treatment and outcomes: Doing what works.* New York: Haworth.

Bandura, A. (1977). *Social learning theory.* Englewood Cliffs, NJ: Prentice Hall.

Brayman, S. J., Kirby, T. F., Misenheimer, A. M., & Short, M. J. (1976). Comprehensive Occupational Therapy Evaluation Scale. *American Journal of Occupational Therapy, 30,* 94–100.

Brayman, S., & Kunz, K. (2000). The Comprehensive Occupational Therapy Evaluation Scale. In B. J. Hemphill (Ed.), *The evaluation process in psychiatric occupational therapy* (3rd ed., p. 270). Thorofare, NJ: Slack.

Chaffey, L., Unsworth, C. A., & Fossey, E. (2010). A grounded theory of intuition among occupational therapists in mental health practice. *British Journal of Occupational Therapy, 73,* 300–308. http://dx.doi.org/10.4276/030802210X12759925544308

Chaffey, L., Unsworth, C. A., & Fossey, E. (2012). Relationship between intuition and emotional intelligence in occupational therapists in mental health practice. *American Journal of Occupational Therapy, 66,* 88–96. http://dx.doi.org/10.5014/ajot.2012.001693

Clark, F. (2012). Beyond high definition: Attitude and evidence bringing OT in HD–3D. *American Journal of Occupational Therapy, 66,* 644–651. http://dx.doi.org/10.5014/ajot.2012.666002

Cohn, E. S. (1991). Clinical reasoning: Explicating complexity. *American Journal of Occupational Therapy, 45,* 969–971. http://dx.doi.org/10.5014/ajot.45.11.969

Coster, W. J. (2008). Curricular approaches to professional reasoning for evidence-based practice. In B. A. B. Schell & J. W. Schell (Eds.), *Clinical and professional reasoning in occupational therapy* (pp. 311–334). Baltimore: Lippincott Williams & Wilkins.

Craik, K. (1967). *The nature of explanation.* Cambridge, England: Cambridge University Press.

Csikszentmihalyi, M. (1990). *Flow: The psychology of optimal experience.* New York: HarperCollins.

Dickens, C. (2000). *David Copperfield.* New York: Modern Library Classics. (Original work published 1849)

Dreyfus, H., & Dreyfus, S. (1986). *Mind over machine: The power of human intuition and expertise in the era of the computer.* New York: Free Press.

Duncombe, L. (2008, December). *Nurturing professional and personal growth through reflective inquiry: A gift to fieldwork students and yourself.* Paper presented at a meeting of the Metropolitan Occupational Therapy Council, New York.

Fleming, M. H. (1991). The therapist with the three-track mind. *American Journal of Occupational Therapy, 45,* 1007–1014. http://dx.doi.org/10.5014/ajot.45.11.1007

Gardner, H. (1983). *Frames of mind: The theory of multiple intelligences.* New York: Basic.

Greber, C., Ziviani, J., & Rodger, S. (2007a). The four-quadrant model of facilitated learning (Part 1): Using teaching–learning approaches in occupational therapy. *Australian Occupational Therapy Journal, 54*(Suppl. 1), S31–S39. http://dx.doi.org/10.1111/j.1440-1630.2006.00558.x

Greber, C., Ziviani, J., & Rodger, S. (2007b). The four-quadrant model of facilitated learning (Part 2): Strategies and applications. *Australian Occupational Therapy Journal, 54*(Suppl. 1), S40–S48. http://dx.doi.org/10.1111/j.1440-1630.2006.00558.x

Hammond, K. R. (1996). *Human judgment and social policy irreducible uncertainty, inevitable error, unavoidable injustice.* London: Oxford University Press.

Ho, A. Y., & Dimitropoulos, A. (2010). Clinical management of behavioral characteristics of Prader–Willi syndrome. *Neuropsychiatric Disease and Treatment, 6,* 107–118. http://dx.doi.org/10.2147/NDT.S5560

Johnson-Laird, P. N., Girotto, V., & Legrenzi, P. (1998). Mental models: A gentle guide for outsiders. *Sistemi Intelligenti, 9*(68), 33.

The Joint Commission. (2013). *Top performers on joint commission key quality measures.* Retrieved from http://www.jointcommission.org/about/JointCommissionFaqs.aspx?CategoryId=52#11

Kielhofner, G. (1995). *A model of human occupation* (2nd ed.). Baltimore: Williams & Wilkins.

Kolb, D. A. (1984). *Experiential learning.* Englewood Cliffs, NJ: Prentice Hall.

Law, M., Baptiste, S., Carswell, A., McColl, M. A., Polatajko, H., & Pollock, N. (1998). *Canadian Occupational Performance Measure* (3rd ed.). Ottawa, Canada: CAOT.

Mattingly, C. (1991). What is clinical reasoning? *American Journal of Occupational Therapy, 45,* 979–986. http://dx.doi:10.5014/ajot.45.11.979

Mattingly, C., & Fleming, M. H. (1994). *Clinical reasoning: Forms of inquiry in a therapeutic practice.* Philadelphia: F. A. Davis.

Mattingly, C., & Gillette, N. (1991). Anthropology, occupational therapy, and action research. *American Journal of Occupational Therapy, 45,* 972–978. http://dx.doi.org/10.5014/ajot.45.11.972

Mosey, A. C. (1985). A monistic or a pluralistic approach to professional identity? [Eleanor Clarke Slagle Lecture]. *American Journal of Occupational Therapy, 39,* 504–509. http://dx.doi.org/10.5014/ajot.39.8.504

Mosey, A. C. (1986). *Occupational therapy: Configuration of a profession.* New York: Raven.

Peloquin, S. M. (1993). The patient–therapist relationship: Beliefs that shape care. *American Journal of Occupational Therapy, 47,* 935–942. http://dx.doi.org/10.5014/ajot.47.10.935

Polanyi, M. (1962). *Personal knowledge: Towards a post-critical philosophy.* Chicago: University of Chicago Press.

Rogers, J. C. (1983). Clinical reasoning: The ethics, science, and art [Eleanor Clarke Slagle Lecture]. *American Jour-*

nal of Occupational Therapy, 37, 601–616. http://dx.doi.org/10.5014/ajot.37.9.601

Schell, B. A. B. (2003a). Clinical reasoning and occupation-based practice: Changing habits. OT Practice, 8, CE-1–CE-8.

Schell, B. A. B. (2003b). Clinical reasoning: The basis of practice. In E. B. Crepeau, E. Cohn, & B. Schell (Eds.), Willard and Spackman's occupational therapy (10th ed., pp. 131–139). Philadelphia: Lippincott Williams & Wilkins.

Schell, B. A., & Cervero, R. M. (1993). Clinical reasoning in occupational therapy: An integrative review. American Journal of Occupational Therapy, 47, 605–610. http://dx.doi.org/10.5014/ajot.47.7.605

Schell, B. A. B., & Schell, J. W. (Eds.). (2008). Clinical and professional reasoning in occupational therapy. Baltimore: Lippincott Williams & Wilkins.

Schön, D. (1983). The reflective practitioner: How professionals think in action. New York: Basic.

Sebastin, S., & Chung, K. C. (2011). A systematic review of the outcomes of replantation of distal digital amputation. Plastic and Reconstructive Surgery, 128, 723–737. http://dx.doi.org/10.1097PRS.0b013e318221dc83

Weber, R. C. (1993). Physical education for children with Prader–Willi syndrome. Palaestra, 9(3), Article 11. Retrieved from http://www.thefreelibrary.com/Physical+education+for+children+with+Prader-Willi+syndrome.-a013254215

CHAPTER 8.

APPLICATION OF ACTIVITIES TO ENHANCE OCCUPATIONAL PERFORMANCE

Nancy Robert Dooley, PhD, OTR

Highlights

✧ Use of occupations, purposeful activities, and activities
✧ Activity as a means
✧ Purposeful activity as a means
✧ Occupation as a means
✧ Occupation as an end
✧ Power of occupation's related activities
✧ Addressing occupational needs at the organization level
✧ Addressing occupational needs at the population level.

Key Terms

✧ Activities
✧ Activity as a means
✧ Activity synthesis
✧ Co-occupation
✧ Culture
✧ Enabling activities
✧ Forensic settings
✧ Just-right match
✧ Occupational performance
✧ Occupational profile
✧ Occupation as an end
✧ Occupation as a means

✧ Occupations
✧ Occupation's related activities
✧ Preparatory methods
✧ Pragmatic reasoning
✧ Purposeful activities
✧ Purposeful activity as a means
✧ Sensory diet
✧ Sensory integration
✧ Simulated activities
✧ Subcomponent skills
✧ Theoretical reasoning

This chapter discusses the many ways that occupational therapy practitioners use occupations and activities to enhance occupational performance, specifically emphasizing the practitioner's use of occupations, purposeful activities, and activities centered on the client's needs and therapeutic goals. Practitioners select the appropriate therapeutic medium based on sound reasoning and reflection. This chapter presents a brief introduction to theoretical reasoning and its importance to developing and implementing effective interventions, how to select therapeutic activities that are meaningful to the client as well as relevant to his or her life and preferred occupations, and the influence of activity choice on the therapeutic relationship.

Next, some of the challenges and pragmatic and cultural considerations that occupational therapy practitioners must deal with to provide appropriate, effective intervention are presented, followed by four perspectives on providing occupational therapy: (1) activity as a means, (2) purposeful activity as a means, (3) occupation as a means, and (4) occupation as an end. The chapter ends with a discussion of the therapeutic power of activities and the use of occupational therapy at the organizational and population levels.

Use of Occupations, Purposeful Activities, and Activities

Every day, occupational therapy practitioners choose the best occupation, purposeful activity, or activity to meet the therapeutic goals of their clients. For students and beginning practitioners, making this choice can be anxiety provoking and overwhelming. It is difficult for new practitioners to take into consideration theoretical reasoning while simultaneously addressing clients' occupational needs as well as relevant elements of the environment and culture.

Whether practitioners intervene or consult in health care, education, or community settings, their clients have occupational performance problems. These problems can be the result of deficits in their brains and other parts of their bodies in endless combinations. Clients come from extremely diverse backgrounds and environments that may be different from the practitioner's.

In addition, clients and families expect practitioners to be experts at providing therapy in a client-centered manner that respects the client's particular wishes, needs, and interests. Payers and employers expect practitioners to fill specified numbers of therapy minutes, often with limited resources or planning time. Practitioners are under ever-increasing pressure to assist clients in achieving occupational performance goals quickly and efficiently. Choosing therapeutic activities is crucial to a successful outcome for the occupational therapy process, namely that the client be able to engage or reengage in desired roles and occupations.

Occupational therapy practitioners believe in the value of activity as an effective tool for facilitating change and growth. Consequently, practitioners use activities to enhance people's ability to engage in the occupations that they need and choose to do. Depending on client needs, practitioners provide interventions using *occupations* (i.e., activities that are personally meaningful to the person who voluntarily engages in them out of personal choice or sociocultural necessity), *purposeful activities* (i.e., when a person engages in activities out of personal choice and values those activities), or *activities* (i.e., a wide range of actions that a person takes to accomplish or perform something) to enhance clients' occupational performance. *Occupational performance* is "the ability to perceive, desire, recall, plan and carry out roles, routines, tasks and subtasks for the purpose of self-maintenance, productivity, leisure and rest in response to demands of the internal and/or external environment" (Chapparo & Ranka, 1997, p. 60).

Occupational therapists with the assistance of occupational therapy assistants begin intervention by first assessing the client's situation to decide which interventions might be most effective to meet the client's unique needs. After completing a comprehensive evaluation, the therapist in collaboration with the assistant develops an appropriate intervention plan to enhance occupational performance.

Intervention may involve the use of a specific occupation, purposeful activity, or activity as the therapeutic medium. In other words, the practitioner may use an occupation valued by the client, a purposeful activity selected by the therapist but motivating to the client, or an activity for its own characteristics to meet therapeutic goals. The client engages in the occupation, purposeful activity, or

---

Exercise 8.1. Observing a Therapy Session

Observe a therapy session with an experienced occupational therapy practitioner. As the session begins, the practitioner may ask the client a few questions, perhaps there is a momentary pause, and the practitioner then suggests an activity. Why do you think the practitioner selected this activity? How does it relate to the client's occupational performance? As you watch the therapy session evolve, you might observe a brief interaction in which the activity plan is modified using the client's input. The practitioner then launches into a newly synthesized activity that meets the client's needs, helps move him or her toward one or more goals, and is often fun or engaging. Briefly describe how the use of activity supported the development of the client's occupational performance and his or her future ability to engage in an occupation.

Cohn (1991) suggested that experienced practitioners must explicate, or uncover, their reasoning processes to assist students or newer practitioners in developing their professional skills. Refer to Fleming's introduction to practitioners' clinical reasoning processes for further details. In addition, it is important for novice practitioners to understand *activity synthesis,* which is changing or modifying a specific activity so that person can engage in it successfully, and how it is used by expert practitioners.

When an occupational therapy practitioner is planning occupations, purposeful activities, and activities for an occupational therapy session, five important variables must be considered: (1)

Exercise 8.2. Reasoning Process

Step 1: With a small study group, watch a video of an occupational therapy session. Stop the video at various points and discuss what you think the occupational therapy practitioner may have been thinking at that moment. Think of each of these points as places where the practitioner had several options. With your small group, discuss what else the practitioner could have done at that moment. Take a few of your group's suggestions and talk about how the therapy session would have been different if these options had been taken. Do you think these choices would have been beneficial?

Step 2: Discuss with your group what would be helpful as you learn to make occupation, purposeful activity, or activity choices based on a client's needs. Identify a list of questions that you would ask the practitioner about what he or she did. Discuss possible answers to these questions. The focus here is on activity synthesis. Although activity synthesis uses information gained from an activity analysis, the process of closely examining an activity to distinguish its component parts requires clinical reasoning to guide the reconstruction or reconfiguration of the activity.

Occupational therapy education programs often use activity analysis to teach entry-level students about choosing occupations, purposeful activities, and activities for therapeutic use. Are these assignments helpful? What else could be used? Does activity analysis adequately address how to reconstruct activities for therapeutic means?

---

activity to acquire skills, complete tasks, fulfill life roles, and assume or resume participation in meaningful occupations.

Occupational therapy practitioners use a wide range of occupations, purposeful activities, and activities when providing intervention. Learning to choose and use them effectively is not easy. Experienced practitioners collaborate with clients and their significant others to combine and modify ideas in endless variations to meet the demands of each distinct situation. Experienced practitioners learn this expertise through clinical experience, observation of other practitioners, and ongoing reflection about the interventions they provide (Schell, 2014; Schell & Schell, 2008).

In contrast, most occupational therapy students spend hours creating intervention plans in which they decide what activity choices or occupation to present to a client. They often come to class after a Level 1 fieldwork session and say that practitioners "just come up with something to do." In fact, it is so difficult to see the thinking processes of occupational therapy practitioners that when Fleming (1991)—who was one of the first researchers to study the reasoning process in occupational therapy—initially investigated clinical reasoning, she wondered whether their thinking processes were "inconsistent or scattered" (p. 1007)

theoretical reasoning, (2) client needs and desires, (3) influence of activity choices on the therapeutic relationship, (4) pragmatic considerations, and (5) cultural considerations.

Theoretical Reasoning

As described in Chapter 1, "Occupation, Activities, and Occupational Therapy," an occupational therapy practitioner chooses activities based on theoretical rationales, or *theoretical reasoning* (i.e., hypothetical thinking), whether it takes the form of a frame of reference, model, or paradigm. The practitioner is not just keeping a client busy or guessing at what might be helpful. Within the occupational therapy team, the occupational therapist is responsible for choosing a frame of reference. The occupational therapy assistant should have a working knowledge of the frame of reference to implement related activities accordingly.

In choosing a frame of reference, one of the first questions a therapist asks is whether the person appears capable of remediating the client factors or performance skills that are preventing engagement in desired occupations. If that is not the case, a frame of reference that takes a compensatory approach may be appropriate. Considerations such as diagnosis, prognosis, and available intervention time and resources come into play in this decision.

The Well Elderly study conducted by Clark and colleagues (1997) at the University of Southern California is one example of the value of basing therapeutic activities and occupations on a defined theoretically based perspective. In this study, 361 community-dwelling, low-income older adults benefited substantially more from occupational therapy than from social activities provided and supervised by nonprofessional staff.

For readers who are new to occupational therapy, it is important to provide some context for this research study. The Well Elderly study caused a stir in the occupational therapy community for several reasons. The results were published in *JAMA,* putting evidence regarding the power of occupational therapy in front of an audience of physicians, powerful gatekeepers in the health care system. Additionally, the study was, at the time, the largest grant-funded clinical trial of occupational therapy and the first time that occupational therapy was being tested for use with relatively healthy older adults. Participants in the study tended to have chronic conditions, but they were not acutely ill or referred to occupational therapy in a traditional way.

Results indicated that skilled occupational therapy provided within a theoretical framework, Lifestyle Redesign, was effective at producing changes in participants. The members of the experimental occupational therapy group made improvements in physical and mental health and occupational functioning that were sustained over time and cost-effective (Clark et al., 2001; Hay et al., 2002). Another important finding was that the control group in which generic activities were provided demonstrated no statistically significant differences from the control group that did nothing (Clark et al., 1997). The authors obtained similar results in a follow-up study that offered the program to a more diverse population (Clark et al., 2011). The value of activity engagement from an occupational therapy perspective is so much more than keeping busy.

Client Needs and Desires

Although a theoretically based intervention is important, client needs and desires are the center of the occupational therapy process. The challenge for occupational therapy practitioners is to continually select therapeutic activities that are meaningful to the client and relevant to his or her life, experiences, hopes, and dreams, resulting in therapy that is tailored to the person through activity choices and the client's preferred occupations.

When a practitioner has limited or no planning time, it is easy to slip into a rut of providing the same activities to similar clients on a caseload, whether the clients like or find meaning in them or not. Practitioners must collaborate with the client, caregivers, or both in choosing activities for use in practice settings (Figure 8.1). This collaboration requires the occupational therapy practitioner to give the client the opportunity to express him- or herself.

At times, occupational therapy practitioners will say they are too busy or stressed to create new treatment activities for every client, so they fall back on a small repertoire of exercises and enabling or simulated activities. The idea that "one size fits all" does not work well in occupational therapy. In my

Figure 8.1. After collaborating with her client, the practitioner found that a valued activity was preparing food, which also provided opportunities for family interactions.

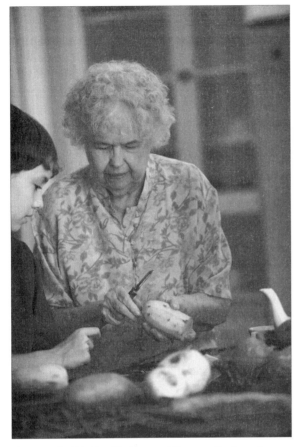

Source. Public Health Image Library, Centers for Disease Control and Prevention. Photo by Cade Martin and provided by Dawn Arlotta.

experience teaching occupational therapy assistants to become occupational therapists, I often hear complaints that occupational therapists in some settings write the same goals with seemingly little regard for patient needs. Individualizing goals may help occupational therapists and occupational therapy assistants in the activity selection process.

Take my friend, Anne, an occupational therapist who recently died from amyotrophic lateral sclerosis (ALS). In the space of a few months, Anne had to give up her practice as a key team member on an acute geropsychiatry inpatient unit. When a fall caused a fractured hip, she became an occupational therapy client. She was having trouble with upper-extremity coordination and weakness. The usual occupational therapy inter-

vention plan would call for activities of daily living (ADL) retraining to achieve some improvement in ADL functioning. But Anne had been trying that for several months at home and found activities such as bathing and dressing herself exhausting. She preferred to focus her limited energy on ways to help engage in more satisfying activities such as doing crossword puzzles, sharing jokes via email, or helping to create videos for occupational therapy students. Engaging in occupations she found meaningful gave Anne much more satisfaction at the end of her life.

Occupational therapists can avoid creating impersonal or generic goals (which may lead to impersonal or generic activities) by attending to the client's *occupational profile*. Obtaining an occupational profile is a key element of the occupational therapy evaluation process. The information contained in an occupational profile is invaluable for helping to choose activities. Therapists want to know who the person is and why he or she is seeking services. What circumstances have caused a change in his or her ability to engage in daily occupations? What are the person's priorities, and what is his or her occupational history? All of these factors give the occupational therapist a baseline for establishing context for each client.

As described in Chapter 7, "Clinical Reasoning and Reflective Practice," a client-centered interview such as the Canadian Occupational Performance Measure (COPM; Law et al., 1990) may be used to determine a client's priorities, values, and interests. For new therapists and students, the Occupational Self-Assessment Version 2.2 (OSA; Baron, Kielhofner, Iyenger, Goldhammer, & Wolenski, 2006) can be easier to use than the COPM because it consists of specific questions related to each subsystem of the Model of Human Occupation (Kielhofner, 2008). Like the COPM, the OSA has clients rate the degree to which something is a problem and the importance the client places on that problem. The OSA is useful for many groups of people, including adults living in a shelter for homeless families (Helfrich & Chan, 2013), adults with serious and persistent mental illness in a day program (Curral et al., 2012), and older adults in community settings (Nakamura-Thomas & Kyougoku, 2013). More attention to the occupational profile would have helped in Case Example 8.1.

Case Example 8.1. Robert: Activities for Thumb Opposition

Robert, age 64 years and an otherwise healthy, right-handed man, had reconstruction surgery of the right carpometacarpal joint to ease pain and regain mobility lost as a result of osteoarthritis at the base of his thumb. The occupational therapist's goal, based on a biomechanical frame of reference, was for Robert to achieve full thumb opposition to all fingertips. He had most trouble opposing to the fifth digit. Robert's therapist asked him to complete simulated activities, such as using a pegboard or nuts-and-bolts board, at the outpatient clinic.

At home, he wanted to resume activities that he valued such as cooking, gardening, caring for his dog, helping with household chores, and playing cribbage in a weekly league. He also had to go back to work soon, where he would need to handle money, complete paperwork, and use a computer smoothly and efficiently.

Robert came away from this experience with a limited view of occupational therapy. He felt that the occupational therapist only focused on restoring mobility in his thumb and that the activities were boring and irrelevant. The therapist did not help him get back to what he needed and wanted to do in his everyday life. Unfortunately, Robert's experience may not be atypical. In my experience, simply educating the client about why some therapy sessions consist of less meaningful activities goes a long way.

Note that Robert's therapy sessions consisted of contrived activities, not occupations or purposeful activities. Students often describe their disappointment at seeing occupational therapy sessions that "look like physical therapy." When asked to explain what they have seen, students often describe clients engaging in rote exercises or activities that lack personal meaning. When occupational therapy practitioners use activities without connecting them to everyday life and what the client needs and wants to do, they may be doing a disservice to their profession. However, in this case, Robert's hand motion and strength improved and he was able to resume his usual occupations. Robert's case is discussed further later in the chapter.

Influence of Activity Choices on the Therapeutic Relationship

Occupational therapy practitioners' activity choices affect the therapeutic relationships they are trying to build with clients. For example, asking a child to do activities he or she does not like or does not find fun often results in refusal, tears, or limited attention, whereas doing activities he or she likes results in the child being engaged (Figure 8.2). Adults are more likely to initially go along with activities they do not value or understand, but they may later complain that their occupational therapy session was stupid, childish, or boring. Adolescents, however, will often express the same complaints loudly and immediately. When this situation occurs, occupational therapy practitioners have to work extra hard to provide meaningful activities to rebuild any therapeutic rapport that they may have established up to that point.

In addition, if a client experiences an occupational therapy intervention as boring, stupid, or just puzzling, the practitioner involved is doing a disservice to the profession. Practitioners have been trying to explain our services and our unique contributions to society since 1917. We all must do our part in this effort, and our first audience is our clients.

Pragmatic Considerations

Although occupational therapy practitioners strive to use occupations as a means to achieve maximal

Figure 8.2. A child actively engaged in an activity that he finds interesting.

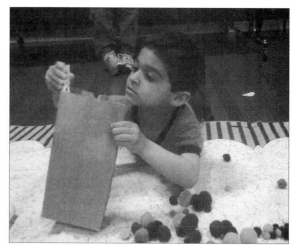

Source. N. R. Dooley. Used with permission.

participation in daily life, pragmatic considerations do not always make this type of intervention possible. Schell defines *pragmatic reasoning* as reasoning about the contextual issues affecting clients now and in the future, the practitioner's personal context, and the practice environment's culture and describes it as another variable affecting the activity synthesis and activity choice process (Schell & Schell, 2008).

For example, occupational therapy practitioners specializing in hand therapy must often follow strict protocols set by surgeons. Practitioners working in public schools must make their goals and interventions relate to the students' ability to access their education (Bazyk & Case-Smith, 2010).

In addition, pragmatic considerations such as limitations in space, time, or materials may constrain practitioners' choices. For example, if an occupational therapy assistant is unable to see a skilled nursing facility resident during morning bathing and grooming, she may ask the client to stand for an activity that has similar task demands to combing hair or brushing teeth at the sink. Or, if the client's roommate is sleeping, making her room unavailable for a session addressing lower body dressing and use of adaptive equipment, the session may take place in a public room. Because the session would not be appropriate in a public area, the practitioner might use a contrived activity with a long-handled reacher, such as having the client pick up various items off the floor and bring them to her lap. Engaging in activities requires interaction with other people, the physical and social environment, and the context that is within and surrounds a person (American Occupational Therapy Association [AOTA], 2014).

The intervention environment can serve as a pragmatic limiter in contemporary occupational therapy practice. Certain spaces and places provide opportunities for many different activities, whereas others are more restrictive. For example, occupational therapy practitioners working in *forensic settings,* which are service delivery sites that work with and include clients who are at risk for offending or who have a history of offending, are familiar with the long list of materials their clients are not allowed to have and learn to work around this limitation.

Many occupational therapy practitioners work in cramped, crowded, or changing work spaces. For example, a practitioner working in an urban school department shares a therapy space, which is a former storage closet, with a physical therapist and a speech–language pathologist; therefore, the practitioner must consider the presence of other people when planning activities. Although the practitioner may prefer *sensory integration* (i.e., a person's ability to use sensory input from within the body and from external stimuli) as a theoretical framework, she must account for available space when making decisions about what can and cannot be done with students. No swinging or riding scooter boards will happen in that converted closet.

Exercise 8.3. Influence of a Restrictive Environment

An occupational therapy assistant is working in a rehabilitation hospital with Damon, who has cognitive and physical impairments after a traumatic brain injury caused by a motorcycle accident. The assistant and Damon's occupational therapist have collaborated to develop an intervention plan based on a cognitive frame of reference. Damon has progressed through several purposeful activities related to shopping and money management. The occupational therapy assistant would like to challenge Damon with the unpredictable distractions and physically close quarters of a real urban convenience store because he will be returning to that environment in about a week. However, facility policies related to payment and liability prohibit patients from leaving the hospital grounds. Describe at least 5 ways for the occupational therapy staff to further challenge Damon without violating this policy. Compare your thoughts with your classmates' answers.

You are likely to find that this learning exercise prompts a wide variety of ideas and possibilities. Indeed, your professional colleagues are great resources for imaginative activity ideas. Everyone's brain works a little differently, and everyone has different life experiences to call on. In Damon's case, the setting that seemed restrictive may still provide opportunities for occupation-based interventions. For instance, does the hospital have a cafeteria or a gift shop?

Cultural Considerations

Consideration of the client's culture adds another dynamic to the process of planning for and synthesizing activities to use in occupational therapy.

Note that culture is much more than ethnicity. Culture encompasses all the learning about doing that people pass down to new members of a group of people. Richardson (2001) provides a comprehensive definition of *culture* that is useful for occupational therapy practitioners:

> Culture is the material form assumed by humanity's social activity. If it is what we produce, this production has specific aims. In particular, culture is shaped by the form of whatever we create in the course of our social lives to serve or respond to the purposes of social communication: the way we build our houses, the way we eat our food, the way we establish work patterns, practice religion or create art are all elements of culture. Almost all human activity serves culture in one way or another and results in the production of cultural evidence. This, not the fact of culture itself, is what really distinguishes us as a species. But it is not the activity itself; it is the way we carry it out that imprints social forms with characteristic cultural patterns that may be said to constitute the essential element that defines the human being and provides the evidence—as provisional as it may be—that we exist as a species apart. (p. 10)

A funny example happened one night when I was at my children's elementary school. I was attending a program for parents when I learned about the rules of an activity in that setting. While walking down the hallway, I ran my fingers along the painted brick wall. My daughter told me I should not do that; it was not allowed. At first, I did not know what she was talking about. She said, "You can't touch the walls in the hallway, and you have to walk on the middle squares," meaning of the tile floor. Still puzzled, I finally figured out that teachers or the principal had made a rule to prevent students from touching the walls as they walked from place to place. To my daughter, about age 6, this rule, specific to the culture of her school, was well ingrained in her as a member of that culture. That evening, I entered a new culture and did not know the rules. Likewise, cultural missteps can happen to occupational therapy practitioners entering new

schools, skilled nursing facilities, or homes. Occupations and activities chosen for their therapeutic value must fit the culture of the person and the setting.

An occupational therapy assistant working in a skilled nursing facility recently told me about her client whose usual mode of dress was to wear a sari. Some occupational therapy practitioners may have insisted that the client don Western clothing because that is all the practitioner knows how to do. Instead, this practitioner learned about donning Indian attire from her client and from a staff member. Soon, the client was completing her own upper- and lower-body dressing with adaptations the practitioner and client made together to accommodate physical limitations after surgery. A bonus for the practitioner was that she felt enriched by her new knowledge of Indian culture. The same learning may be needed when addressing meal preparation, religious participation, or any number of other areas.

Working in Jamaica, I learned the importance of playing dominos in that culture. As a child, I played dominos as just another game. Although Americans from other ethnic backgrounds certainly did, I did not know adults who played dominos. I learned that, for the men I met, the dominos would be held in one hand rather than standing them up to face the player as I had done as a child. Also, playing dominoes was an occupation that men routinely engaged in at the end of the work day. Adapting ways to hold the dominos for a player with limited use of one hand would allow him to feel a lot more normal, like a member of the group (Figure 8.3).

A new approach to activities can also serve as an intentional means of change within an organization's culture. In Case Example 8.2, the occupational therapy practitioner brings the culture of occupational therapy, including doing activities with people and facilitating their engagement in occupations, to a setting that is nontraditional for occupational therapy and had previously been dominated by staff doing activities for residents.

Although many occupational therapy interventions are provided in hospitals or centers, Cecilia's focus with Erika was to work on real-life activities within her actual community environment. It is often easy to pick out practitioners working in nontraditional roles by their propensity to do things

Figure 8.3. Bingo, like dominoes, can be an important social activity.

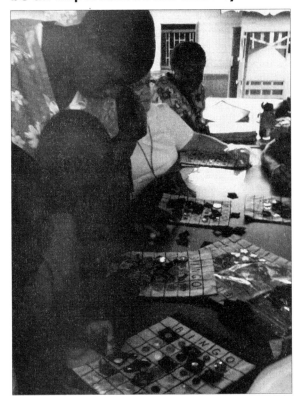

Source. N. R. Dooley. Used with permission.

with clients instead of for clients, as Erika's case illustrates.

The following sections discuss the use of activity, purposeful activity, and occupation as the means as well as occupation as the end that occupational therapy practitioners use to help clients achieve participation in their desired occupations.

Activity as a Means

Activity as a means occurs when the practitioner selects an activity on the basis of its characteristics to achieve therapeutic goals. As described earlier, activities involve various actions that a person takes to accomplish or perform something. *Simulated,* or *enabling, activities* (i.e., activities that imitate real activities) provide opportunities for the client to practice motor, cognitive, or psychosocial skills.

Simulated activities were popular in the 1980s when occupational therapy practitioners were trying to make the profession more objective and measurable so that it would fit more easily into the

---

Case Example 8.2. Erika: Anxiety Taking the Bus

Erika, age 33 years, is a mother of 3 children and lives in a family shelter for people with disabilities who is diagnosed with social anxiety disorder. She can live there for up to 8 weeks while looking for permanent housing. The shelter director has told her that she qualifies for a public transportation pass to save money when she rides the bus. However, after a few days, the director cannot understand why Erika has not obtained the bus pass.

Cecilia, an occupational therapy assistant and case manager at the shelter, meets with Erika and learns that a major barrier is Erika's anxiety about taking the bus into the city to get the pass. Erika comes from a rural area and has forced herself over the past several months to take local buses after she lost her car.

Although Cecilia could quickly get the pass for Erika, she knows by doing so, she will miss an opportunity to help Erika gain new skills and increase her self-confidence as well as confidence in using public transportation. Cecilia helps Erika break up the activity of getting a bus pass into manageable tasks. Together, they plan and time the route, make transfers, and ride a bus to obtain the bus pass. Cecilia gradually withdraws her support until Erika can go anywhere by bus by herself.

Afterward, Erika said it was not as bad as she thought it would be. However, she admitted she did not know whether she would ever have done it without Cecilia's help.

---

dominant medical model. At that time, it became popular to use cones, blocks, puzzles, and other therapeutic activities to try to develop *subcomponent skills,* which are the parts of the whole that contribute to the whole skill when combined. On the basis of learning theories, simulated activities frequently involved practice and repetition. The value of this practice is supported by various practitioners who have reported that clients need repetition to incorporate new skills or performance patterns into their daily lives (Ma & Trombly, 2002; Mosey, 1986).

Preparatory methods are preliminary techniques that are used to prepare a client for a specific treatment and are appropriate and effective occupational therapy interventions (AOTA, 2012). For example, a client with hemiplegia may need scapular mobilization before she can use her affected arm to dress or put dishes in an overhead cabinet. A child with attention problems or learning disabilities may participate more efficiently in class after receiving joint compressions or other sensory stimulation as part of a *sensory diet,* which is a personalized activity plan that addresses a person's sensory needs so that he or she can stay focused and organized throughout the day. Ultrasound and splinting are effective techniques for people recovering from hand injuries or surgeries.

However, preparatory methods generally do not stand alone as occupational therapy for billing purposes or for the integrity of the profession. Whenever an occupational therapy practitioner provides a preparatory modality or activity, it is critical that the client and his or her caregivers understand the relationship between participation in the activity and the long-term therapeutic goals. In Case Example 8.3, a practitioner uses an activity as the means to therapeutic ends and considers several pragmatic factors during the activity-planning process.

In the case of Mrs. Harris, a colleague videotaped an occupational therapy session that I supervised with the occupational therapy assistant. At the time, I thought the simulated activity was appropriate and met the client's needs. Later, however, while showing the video to students, I thought using the real occupation would have made a better therapy session. In reality, the pragmatic limitations made the contrived activity the best choice at the time. In addition, Mrs. Harris knew why she was doing the activity and was able to problem solve with the occupational therapy assistant to make her transition to the real occupation smoother. Now, I think of that session as appropriate for the time and place as well as client needs.

Purposeful Activity as a Means

Purposeful activity as a means occurs when the client selects an activity that has a meaningful outcome to achieve therapeutic goals. Although some occupational therapy practitioners who work in a rehabilitation setting use exercise and repetition, a substantial body of evidence is accumulating that

---

Exercise 8.4. Adaptation in Everyday Activities

Create some purposeful activities for Robert in Case Example 8.1 to replace enabling or simulated tasks during the therapy session. Because you are seeing Robert in an outpatient clinic for 30 minutes at a time, most of his hand use will happen in the course of his daily activities at home rather than in the brief intervention with you. Recommend some occupations that Robert can complete as he goes about his day so that he can continue to gain pain-free opposition of the thumb to each finger. You may need to suggest adaptations to his usual movements so that the desired motions are included.

---

shows that participation in real activities in context is most effective in building motor and cognitive skills (Latham, 2008).

In Exercise 8.4, you created purposeful activities for Robert that he considers both meaningful, enjoyable, and relevant. The purposeful activity also meets the client's needs (Figure 8.4). By recommending ways for Robert to incorporate therapeutic hand movements into his everyday routines, you suggested occupation-based interventions that will help stretch the benefits of occupational ther-

Figure 8.4. An alternative purposeful activity for a younger person would be preparing a pumpkin for Halloween. This activity is an occupation-based intervention that extends the benefits of occupational therapy beyond the therapy session.

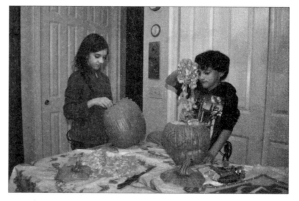

Source. N. R. Dooley. Used with permission.

Case Example 8.3. Mrs. Harris: An Activity That Suits Client Needs and Considers Pragmatic Limitations

Mrs. Harris, age 83 years and a skilled nursing facility resident, was recovering from a long period of bed rest after cardiac surgery and complications, including respiratory failure. She also had substantial range-of-motion limitations resulting from arthritis in many joints and a severe hearing loss. When she was finally able to stand with a walker for short periods of time, her goal was to return home with family. She would be alone for several hours a day and wanted to be able to pour herself a drink or fix a quick snack.

Working together, the occupational therapist and the occupational therapy assistant decided that having Mrs. Harris practice activities at a kitchen counter would meet her needs to pour a drink and fix a snack. However, the only kitchen counter available in the facility was in a resident dining room that was often occupied by residents, staff, and guests. The noise level would make it very difficult to communicate with Mrs. Harris, and there would be no privacy. In addition, the practitioners concluded that having Mrs. Harris pour a drink would introduce too

much variability for her movement and balance abilities at the time.

Therefore, using a rehabilitative frame of reference, the practitioners devised an activity to simulate working at a kitchen counter. The practitioners decided to use a card table in Mrs. Harris's room with the bedside water pitcher, two water glasses, two plates, and materials needed to prepare a peanut butter sandwich. All the materials were placed on the locked bedside table, which was adjusted to counter level. During the treatment session, Mrs. Harris moved the pitcher filled with water and place it on the table. Next, she moved the glasses to the table. Standing at the bedside table, she prepared a peanut butter sandwich and cut it in half, placing a half sandwich on each plate. She then delivered each plate to the table. Sitting down, she poured the water.

This activity provided Mrs. Harris the opportunity to practice moving items with one hand while maintaining her balance with the other hand on her walker.

---

apy well beyond Robert's 30-minute visits. More importantly, using real occupations in the intervention plan will help him to see occupational therapy's importance and role in helping him return to his valued life roles.

Case Example 8.4 describes how an occupational therapist used a purposeful activity to help a young adult reestablish a productive place in society. Purposeful activities require a complex interplay of physical, cognitive, perceptual, and psychosocial skills and have the potential to produce change in a person. By choosing tasks in the areas of social participation and leisure, Karen used a real occupation to help Gerry gain the physical and emotional skills needed to engage in some of the roles he had lost.

The best way to effect change and restore meaning in life is to listen carefully to clients and tailor interventions to each person's life and contexts. Even when clients cannot communicate verbally, they can usually express their activity preferences. Clients will

select participation in specific activities they enjoy when they are given choices or opportunities.

For instance, in Case Example 8.5, our team of occupational therapists gave a group of nonverbal adults with disabilities the opportunity to participate in music and movement sessions. Even though we expected weeks or months to pass before anyone would participate, 2 or 3 clients immediately expressed their activity preference by attending the first session, and they continue to attend the sessions. (*Note:* Therapy Missions is a nonprofit organization that aims to provide occupational and physical therapy to underserved populations around the world; see www.therapymissions.org.)

Occupation as a Means

Occupational therapy practitioners use *occupation as a means* when the therapeutic medium is the

Case Example 8.4. Gerry: Using Purposeful Activity Within the Context of Occupation

Karen met Gerry when she was a young occupational therapist working at a long-term care facility where he resided. **Gerry was 22** when a diving accident left him with a spinal cord injury and quadriplegia. His parents' home was not physically accessible, and he had many assistance needs. He had been living in the facility for about 6 months when Karen began her long campaign to reengage Gerry in life. At first, she stopped by his room only to talk because Gerry would not come out of his room or attend any activities. Eventually, Gerry agreed to go to the break room with Karen while she had some coffee. They talked about common interests and began to establish rapport. Gerry would not have a beverage because he was embarrassed about needing an adapted cup as a result of his limited hand grasp.

Eventually, Karen got Gerry to try playing table tennis. With the paddle strapped to Gerry's hand, they played brief games on half of the table. His strength and endurance improved as they played for many weeks. When Gerry began beating Karen at every table tennis game, he had to find more worthy opponents. Gerry began to see himself as a capable person again when he participated in the popular and age-appropriate game. This participation was the start of Gerry's engagement in a series of new activities that helped him to live a more satisfying life. He eventually got a job working as the facility's telephone operator.

Case Example 8.5. Therapy Missions in Jamaica

When leading a **Therapy Missions** group working in Jamaica, I was part of a team of occupational therapists educating caregivers at a residential facility for adults with various disabilities affecting their physical, cognitive, and sensory systems. We were using the Person–Environment–Occupation Model (Law et al., 1996) and had success with simple musical instruments and songs with movement that were familiar to the Jamaican residents and caregivers.

We had planned a smaller group for the most impaired residents, believing they needed a quieter space and fewer people. This subgroup consisted of adults who were nonverbal. They had been institutionalized in less humane facilities for most of their lives and demonstrated behaviors associated with that situation. Caregivers reported that these residents "never did anything." We had seen them spend a lot of time lying on the ground, self-stimulating, or pacing.

We discussed with the staff and leadership that it might take weeks or even months for people to become engaged in group activities. As an initial activity, we had decided to offer a modified bingo game (Figure 8.5). We were very pleasantly surprised when 2 or 3 of these residents joined in the music and movement group the next morning. One man even came to sit about 2 feet from me. As of this writing, 3 months since this activity program began, staff reports that some residents are now feeding themselves and sitting with other members of the community. They continue to participate daily in the movement and music group. Others continue to play bingo.

client's actual occupation. Occupational therapy practitioners have embraced the use of real-life and community-based occupations, which is considered by many to be consistent with the fundamental assumptions of occupational therapy. Moreover, such occupations and their related activities support the use of contextually relevant pursuits that facilitate a client's use of physical, cognitive, perceptual, and psychosocial skills to interact with his or her environment. In Case Example 8.6, the practitioner devises an activity that promotes social and cognitive skills in a teenager with autism.

People perform better under normal, contextually relevant circumstances. As Julian's example illustrates, school-based occupational therapy provides opportunities to help a client participate in real-life roles. Everything takes place in the client's actual environment, and occupational therapy

Figure 8.5. While playing Bingo, players interact and socialize in a culturally appropriate manner.

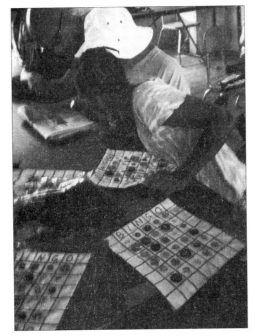

Source. N. R. Dooley. Used with permission.

practitioners schedule therapy sessions so that they coincide with client's daily routines. At an early morning therapy session, a practitioner would address bathing and dressing routines. In the afternoon or early evening, cooking a meal would be relevant. Observing a student at school recess gives the practitioner real information about the child's physical and social adaptation on the playground. Working in these environments is different from working in an outpatient clinic, where a client may be scheduled anytime throughout the day. These clinical settings are often plain and sterile, and there may be specified protocols to follow.

Listening to clients and their caregivers helps occupational therapy practitioners create solutions that enable clients to engage in their own recovery process. When a practitioner actively listens to a client and his or her caregivers, he or she can discover the client's occupations and use them as the therapeutic medium, such as in Case Example 8.7.

Our society expects young adults to be productive. Besides lacking the proprioceptive input that Jack needed, the existing groups at the day program did not provide him with a feeling of satisfaction, productivity, or self-worth. When he began

Case Example 8.6. Julian: Real-Life Engagement

Julian, age 16 years and diagnosed with autism works with his registered occupational therapist, Cyndi, who specializes in working with children with severe developmental disorders. Cyndi wanted to use an occupation that would allow Julian to practice communication skills, organization, following directions, and completing multistep tasks.

Julian enjoys interacting with staff and helping them arrange events. The teachers and therapy staff at Julian's school order a take-out lunch every Friday. Julian's job is to knock on each classroom door; make eye contact with the teacher; and ask, "Are you ordering lunch today?" Cyndi has created an order sheet that Julian follows. He crosses off the staff member's name if he or she is not ordering. Otherwise, the staff member writes in the order and gives Julian the money. Julian repeats this process for each classroom. Before Julian could carry out his assignment in the context of the real school hallways and classrooms, Cyndi coached him through various activities in the occupational therapy room. She then accompanied him on the job and gradually withdrew her support.

to work for the center, was paid, and had people depend on him, however, Jack could see himself as a whole person.

Occupation-based intervention requires practitioners to use occupations from the person's life as a part of the intervention. Therefore, the practitioner must attend to cues from the client about occupations the client does or would like to do. Practitioners do not always have to generate novel activities for clients. Often, the client and his or her family have an existing set of occupations or activities that will work well to facilitate desired changes.

In addition, the client may find it easier to engage in familiar and routine tasks that are part of other occupations than new tasks or unfamiliar activities. Moreover, recipients of occupational therapy services often have difficulty following through

Case Example 8.7. Jack: Developing Skills

Jack, age 28 years and diagnosed with autism, attends an adult day program where most of the other clients have mental illness or acquired brain injuries. Jack's occupational therapy program focuses on skill development. A Level II occupational therapy assistant student at the center noticed that Jack had a hard time concentrating in many group activities such as crafts and games. When he was overstimulated or having trouble engaging in an activity, Jack sought almost constant reassurance from group leaders and began to make odd noises that got louder and louder. He had a history of occasionally being physically aggressive when he was frustrated. The student noticed that Jack was always eager to push people in wheelchairs and do other tasks that involved movement or resistance. Jack often asked the staff for jobs to complete and said that he liked to help.

On the basis of this observation of Jack's interest, the student met with the occupational therapist. Together, they decided to use occupations consistent with Jack's strengths and interests as the therapeutic medium. They selected activities that provided strong sensorimotor input, requiring Jack to do heavy work. Some selected occupations were carrying groceries, moving boxes, helping with holiday decorations, pushing the lunch cart, and carrying plates. Jack's success at these occupations led to part-time employment in a maintenance position at the adult day program.

with home exercise programs; one way to overcome this problem is to use familiar everyday tasks or occupations instead.

When practitioners work in skilled nursing facilities, a common complaint takes the form of "I can't get Mrs. Smith to do anything." Karen, an occupational therapy assistant with 33 years of experience, sees this problem as a personal challenge to take on these clients. She does not have any magic tricks but uses some simple ideas to get residents moving again. The first is talking and listening. What does this person value? Who are the important people in his or her life? What can be learned by observing the person and his or her room, personal items, or photographs? If someone just wants to talk, Karen will use the conversation as an opening to begin to create rapport and wait for a natural activity to present itself. The resident may discuss a valued occupation or role; for example, Mrs. Smith might say that she misses her grandchildren. Karen will then use that information to synthesize an activity that supports the desired role and incorporates a therapeutic goal (Figure 8.6). In the case of Mrs. Smith, her limited standing balance and upper-extremity strength could be addressed while baking cookies for her grandchildren's visit (i.e., occupation as a means).

Figure 8.6. Mrs. Smith's limited standing balance and upper-extremity strength could be addressed while baking cookies for her grandchildren's visit.

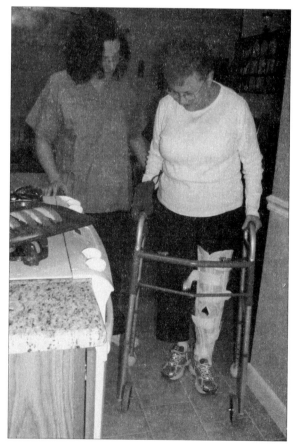

Source. N. R. Dooley. Used with permission.

Exercise 8.5. Home Activity Program for Shoulder Injury

After Tom's shoulder injury and rotator cuff repair, his occupational therapist focused on his gaining another 30° of shoulder flexion and returning to normal strength. Tom, however, cared about moving normally when he took off his suit jacket at work or when he wrote on a whiteboard during presentations and meetings. He was concerned about his ability to perform normal daily activities and relieve his family of hiring expensive help for yard work or snow removal. He also really wanted to go along when one of his sailing friends needed a crewmember. Initially, his occupational therapist used a biomechanical approach and prescribed several exercises to help him gain range of motion and then strength in his dominant shoulder.

Tom is a working adult with responsibilities in child rearing and other instrumental activities of daily living. Think about all the possible occupations that could be used or adapted so that he works on shoulder range of motion or strength. Name at least 15 ways for him to incorporate your suggestions into his daily routine so that a home exercise program just happens and is not an added chore in already busy days. How would you upgrade or downgrade these occupations or activities to meet his therapeutic needs?

As a means of engagement, it is often easier to persuade people to help others than it is to convince them to do something for themselves. For example, Karen might say, "I know you don't feel like exercising today, but I need help with all these plants." Mrs. Smith could work on her standing balance and upper-extremity strength by watering the plants in the occupational therapy clinic. As Mrs. Smith's tolerance for standing activities improves, the activity could be expanded to include trimming dead leaves, transplanting plants, or weeding outdoors at a raised flowerbed (purposeful activities as a means).

Karen often tells students that she does not mind when a skilled nursing facility resident says, "I have to go to the bathroom." Students tend to wonder why she wants to facilitate an activity that may be difficult, smelly, or dirty. What Karen knows is that she has the chance to help the resident engage in a purposeful activity of his or her choice while Karen observes the

Exercise 8.6. Responding to a Client's Activity Cues

Think about an older adult who has been admitted to a skilled nursing facility for short-term rehabilitation. She is debilitated after a hip replacement and pneumonia. What occupations are suggested by these client statements?
- "I'm thirsty."
- "I'm cold."
- "It's too hot in here."
- "I look terrible."

What occupational performance skills could be observed by enabling the client to participate in the occupations you described for each statement?

resident's abilities and difficulties with various underlying skills. Because the resident requests the activity and it takes place in his or her current living environment, it not just an activity but a true occupation.

Marsha is a registered occupational therapist working in an urban school system. She has a large caseload of elementary school children and relatively few resources. The school system requires occupational therapy practitioners to intervene with children in the classroom whenever possible. One of Marsha's favorite places to work with her elementary school students is the art classroom. In collaboration with the art teacher, Marsha can ensure that children with special needs participate in the same projects and activities as the other children by suggesting activity adaptations. The art teacher can also use these activity adaptations to enhance participation for children who do not qualify for occupational therapy services. In addition, one scheduling problem, working around special classes such as music and art, was eliminated.

Occupation as an End

Occupation as an end is the practitioner's use of a purposeful, meaningful activity that, when completed, will provide the client with the capacity to perform an occupation. As discussed in Chapter 1, "Occupations, Activities, and Occupational Therapy," most daily activities are mundane. Likewise, most occupations are routine. However, occupational therapy practitioners may need to adapt clients' occupations or related activities to address their therapeutic goals.

Exercise 8.7. School-Based Activities

Divide into small groups. Compete with classmates to see which group can identify the greatest number of activities that would help facilitate handwriting in an elementary school student. In your groups, consider the various reasons why a child might have a problem with handwriting. Then create a list of activities for addressing difficulties with handwriting when it is not caused by difficulty with fine motor coordination. Compare the activity lists.

For example, clients with orthopedic conditions, traumatic conditions, or burns commonly have to execute specific actions in therapy. Rather than asking the client to participate in rote exercises that focus on the problem areas, the practitioner can creatively adapt one of the client's own occupations to ensure it includes the required actions. Listening to the client, caregiver, or both is still essential when adapting or modifying an occupation and its related activities.

Case Example 8.8 and Case Example 8.9 illustrate the use and adaptation of people's existing occupations to work toward therapeutic goals and allow them to engage in their desired occupations and roles. These scenarios also demonstrate how occupational therapy intervention for the *co-occupation* (i.e., when 2 or more people share participation in an occupation physicality, emotionality, and intentionality) of caregiving may benefit clients and family members.

In early intervention programs, occupational therapy practitioners use everyday tasks in their natural settings to help children from birth to age 3 years engage in their appropriate occupations of play, self-care, and social participation. Parenting can be stressful, but meeting the needs of a child with medical problems or developmental disabilities can be truly overwhelming. Practitioners in early intervention use a family-centered approach to help parents and caregivers maximize their children's abilities and minimize disruptions in daily routines (see Case Example 8.10). Parents and caregivers may need to learn how to hold a child, position a child, and engage a child in play.

At the other end of the life span, adults with dementia or other degenerative diseases also require care from others. Case Example 8.11 describes a

Case Example 8.8. Patricia: Maintaining Involvement in a Valued Occupation

Patricia, age 65 years, is a newly retired financial planner who has osteoarthritis and is troubled by pain and stiffness in her hands and knees. Patricia's most cherished role is being a caregiver for her only granddaughter. It is difficult for her to manipulate the sticky tape on disposable diapers, and a squirming and crying baby make the situation more taxing. A lot of the baby clothes her son and daughter-in-law sent over had multiple snaps in the inseams of pants and pajamas.

Working with her occupational therapist, who decided to use an ecological theoretical perspective (Dunn, Brown, & McGuigan, 1994; Dunn, Brown, & Youngstrom, 2003), Patricia found that diapers with Velcro tabs were easier to handle and more adjustable. The therapist also suggested finding baby clothes with fewer snaps. Patricia was thrilled to follow that recommendation because it reinforced her valued and longstanding leisure occupation of thrift store shopping. Patricia loves to buy the baby gently used clothes that she knows she will be able to use.

home-based occupational therapy consultation in a memory disorders clinic.

Anyone who has had a new baby or a frail elder in his or her home knows that sleep is an easily disrupted part of daily life that is extremely important. Lack of restful sleep makes other activities more difficult and contributes to a lower quality of life. Case Example 8.12 illustrates how an occupational therapist helped restore sleep to the life of a family caregiver.

Power of Occupation's Related Activities

The power of an *occupation's related activities,* that is, using therapeutic activities that are associated with an occupation, enhances the applicable and efficacy of the intervention. Activities are therapeu-

Case Example 8.9. Ian's Mom: Stress With a Premature Child

Ian was born at 28 weeks' gestational age and was being seen by an occupational therapist in a neonatal intensive care unit. Although this situation is always stressful, Ian's mother was having additional difficulty with her son's premature birth because she had previously had another son who died in the neonatal intensive care unit after living only 1 day. She also reported that she felt guilty and wondered what she had done to precipitate another premature birth.

When the medical team agreed that Ian should try bottle-feeding, the occupational therapist sat with the mother and baby to evaluate and facilitate the process. The occupational therapist showed her how to hold Ian to maximize his breathing and swallowing. When his suck was weak, the therapist showed her how to use her fingers to support Ian's oral musculature and control his chin. In a few days, the therapist encouraged Ian's mother to show another relative the special techniques for feeding him. These positive experiences helped Ian maximize his nutrition and increased his mother's sense of self-efficacy in caring for him.

Case Example 8.10. Kara: Early Intervention Services

At 30 months of age, Kara was receiving early intervention occupational therapy services to help bring her fine motor, visual–perceptual, and self-care skills to an age-appropriate level. Kara had a new baby brother and was having trouble coping with the new demands on her parents' attention. The occupational therapist saw that Kara liked playing with a baby doll, emulating what her mother and father did. The therapist suggested they provide real diapers, clothes, and a doll stroller so Kara could take care of her doll. They were able to address all of Kara's problem areas with creative play that the toddler loved. Kara's engagement with caring for the doll helped to give her mother a break so that she could feed the baby or put him down for a nap. As Kara's fine motor and perceptual skills improved, the therapist talked to her mother about the next steps, for example, introducing doll clothes with snaps or buttons.

tic when an occupational therapy practitioner uses them as directed by theoretical guidelines for intervention and as they relate to the client's current or future occupations. A practitioner skillfully uses activities as directed by theoretically based guidelines to ensure that the client's therapeutic goals are achieved. The activities, although selected to relate to a person's occupations, must be expertly applied so that the client accomplishes his or her goals. At times, the goal is the ability to perform an occupation. At other times, the goal is to participate in the occupation with adaptation or modification. Unfortunately, sometimes the therapeutic goal is to replace the occupation with one the client is able to perform. In all cases, therapy is directed by sound theoretical principles and a concern for the person's current and future occupations.

Occupational therapy practitioners' use of activities in the real world involves creating the *just-right match* (i.e., when the treatment and how it is delivered address the client's need to facilitate positive change) among the client, the frame of reference that guides intervention, the context, the activity, and the service delivery model. The ultimate goal of an occupational therapy intervention is for the client to engage in occupations, and as stated throughout this book, one specific and valuable tool is purposeful activity.

An occupational therapy practitioner selects purposeful activities consistent with the theoretical base of the frame of reference. A practitioner selects an activity because of its therapeutic value. The activity has two distinct sets of goals. First are the client's goals. These client-centered goals are influenced by the client's abilities, needs, desires, motivations, and limitations. Second are the therapeutic goals set by the practitioner, which are influenced by the service delivery model and where it is applied, the resources available to support the intervention, and the practitioner's knowledge and skills (Schell & Schell, 2008).

As illustrated in this chapter, activities at an appropriate level of challenge that fit the needs and desires of the client and his or her family and work well within their life roles and contexts can

Case Example 8.11. Mr. and Mrs. Sweeney: A Husband With Alzheimer's Disease

Mr. Sweeney, age 67 years, who has mild-to-moderate Alzheimer's disease, lives with his wife in their own home. He is retired from his job as a journalist and editor. His wife has already cared for his mother, who had Alzheimer's disease and died several years earlier.

Mrs. Sweeney was cheerful and patient with her husband but also recognized his decline and dreaded going down the road that she had traveled with her mother-in-law.

Paying the bills had always been one of Mr. Sweeney's jobs, and he got upset when he saw his wife doing it. Mrs. Sweeney was frustrated because she knew he would make mistakes in bill-paying tasks and might get angry when he could not recall the next step in the activity.

The consulting therapist used cognitive and contextual evaluation and activity analysis to suggest ways to structure the activity and break down the tasks so that Mr. Sweeney could still participate. Mrs. Sweeney maintained control of the finances to prevent errors, and Mr. Sweeney signed the checks and applied stamps and return address stickers to the envelopes. They felt satisfied that they could do an occupation together, and the stress level around this household chore greatly decreased.

Exercise 8.8. Developing Fine Motor Coordination

Think about all the possible everyday activities that could be used or adapted to help a 3-year-old boy develop fine motor coordination. They could be part of self-care, play, or any other area of occupation. Name at least 20. How would you upgrade or downgrade these activities? What suggestions could you make to his caregivers to help incorporate your suggestions into the family's daily routine?

At one time in occupational therapy history, arts and crafts activities were a primary treatment modality. Engagement in these activities reinforces hand skill development, builds the ability to concentrate and follow written directions, and fosters values for creativity and effective use of leisure time. Arts and crafts projects can build self-esteem at any age through the completion of a project, either to keep or to give as a gift. Even so, over time and with an increasing emphasis on working within the medical model, occupational therapy practitioners abandoned or deemphasized the use of arts and crafts as a primary treatment modality.

In some situations, occupational therapy practitioners do not have to provide new activities for their clients. They may facilitate someone's engagement in client-identified occupations through adaptations or contextual changes, as shown in Case Example 8.15 and Case Example 8.16.

Addressing Occupational Needs at the Organization Level

Thus far, the examples in this chapter have dealt with occupational therapy for individuals or groups. Occupational therapy services may also be provided at the organization level, such as businesses (AOTA, 2010). A common application of occupational therapy expertise in this arena is in suggesting activity or workstation adaptations when carpal tunnel syndrome or other repetitive strain injuries are prevalent as a result of computer use (Case Example 8.17).

Similar routines could be incorporated into the work days of hair stylists, dentists, and dental hygienists, who spend long hours in repetitive hand use, often with awkward wrist positions or stooped

be powerful in building a sense of competence. When occupational therapy practitioners, clients, and families can harness that power, the full range of motor, cognitive, emotional, and social benefits of activity engagement is realized. It is hoped that a heightened level of participation and sense of competence carry far beyond the walls of an occupational therapy clinic or intervention setting, as seen in the next two case examples. Case Example 8.13 demonstrates how the use of a related activity resulted in Sean achieving the balance and motor skills needed to ambulate while playing. In Case Example 8.14 an arts and crafts project leads to a client's new occupation.

Case Example 8.12. Mrs. D'Ambra: A Husband With Moderate Dementia

Mrs. D'Ambra, age 71 years, was caring for her husband, who had moderate dementia. She felt relatively satisfied with their daily routine, in which Mr. D'Ambra went to an adult day program 3 days a week so that she could run errands and have a few hours to herself. Mrs. D'Ambra thought her husband was relatively content, but she felt worn out. He would take a short nap most afternoons, but she felt that she could never nap herself and leave him unsupervised.

They lived in an apartment on the first floor off a long hallway. The problem came at night when Mr. D'Ambra tended to get out of bed and wander into the hallway. Once in the hallway, he could not recognize his own door because they all looked the same. In addition, all the apartment doors would be locked, and the only door that would open was the fire door at the end of the hallway, leading him out to the cold night, close to the road, in his pajamas. Mr. D'Ambra had been discovered by chance outside one night, and his wife was terrified that he could die or be seriously injured if it happened again.

She told the occupational therapist who made a home visit that she did not sleep well because she knew from experience that she might not wake up if her husband got up at night. Mrs. D'Ambra had begun to push the kitchen table against the apartment door and pile the chairs on and around it. If he tried to get out the door, she would hear him moving the furniture and get up.

The occupational therapist discussed her concern that blocking the door, although it seemed to help keep Mr. D'Ambra inside the apartment, was dangerous in other ways. The neurologist had previously suggested a door alarm, but Mrs. D'Ambra felt it was too expensive. The occupational therapist suggested attaching a string of large bells to the door so that Mrs. D'Ambra would hear the door opening. Mrs. D'Ambra was not sure that this would work, but then she remembered that her daughter had used a baby monitor for her children. Mrs. D'Ambra liked her own solution best, because she could keep the monitor right on her bedside table and control the volume herself. A follow-up call a month later revealed that the monitor was working well, Mrs. D'Ambra was sleeping better, and she felt more effective as a caregiver.

---

shoulder postures. In addition, a real break should be provided between appointments or tasks. These breaks, although short, could be used to perform neck, shoulder, and arm circles that help counteract the static postures that contribute to repetitive strain injuries. If these exercises are to be successfully incorporated into the day's routine, all members of a work unit need to follow them. Signs around the workplace, computer screen savers, and other cues could be used to make hand-saving techniques just as normal as hand-washing behaviors in health care, childcare, and food preparation settings.

Addressing Occupational Needs at the Population Level

Occupational therapy interventions for populations are meant to help an entire group of people rather than individuals (AOTA, 2010). For example, occupational therapy faculty and students at the New England Institute of Technology have developed a summer day camp program for children living in a nearby family shelter. The camp provides safe and developmentally appropriate play and social participation opportunities for these homeless children. Innumerable unserved or underserved populations could benefit from occupational therapy services in some form. Case Example 8.18 describes the organization's provision of such services in Mexico. Therapy Missions was formed by several therapists after they made their initial visit to Mexico.

Closer to home, many children and adults with disabilities lack sports and leisure participation opportunities. Occupational therapy practitioners or students can consult with sports programs or facilities to maximize participation for all. Case Example 8.19 describes the benefits of sports participation for a child with disabilities.

Case Example 8.13. Sean: A Premature Child

Sean was born at 28 weeks' gestational age weighing 2 pounds, 10 ounces. He required a ventilator for several days and supplemental oxygen for about 8 weeks. He was later diagnosed with bronchopulmonary dysplasia and plagiocephaly for which he wore a cranial remolding orthosis (helmet).

Sean did very well at home and only needed occupational therapy from the early intervention team. With early intervention, his upper-extremity muscle tone gradually normalized, and he was more capable of transitioning to developmentally appropriate positions using typical movement patterns.

Sean was always attracted to a wooden rocking horse that belonged to his older sister. When he was about 15 months old, he would crawl over to the rocking horse and pull himself to stand. He relied on his parents to put him on the horse and safely support him while he rode it. However, he did not like to wait for help; he was intrinsically motivated to get on that horse and stay on it. His occupational therapy practitioner developed a home intervention program where Sean's parents could play with him imaginary games while supporting him on his rocking horse. He built his strength, balance, coordination, and other skills while his mother and father gradually downgraded the level of support they provided. Improvement in his sitting and standing balance and his ability to ambulate was observed. When

Figure 8.7. Cowboy Sean on his rocking horse.

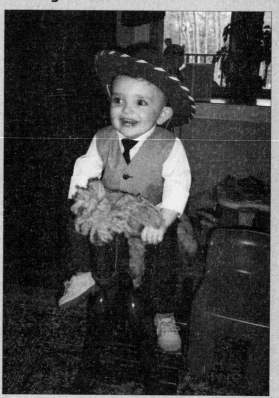

Source. N. R. Dooley. Used with permission.

he mastered the activity of riding the rocking horse, Sean had to show his skill to everyone who came to the house (Figure 8.7).

To say that adolescents or young adults have a lot to adjust to after a spinal cord injury is an understatement. One very important change that occurs after such an injury is the limited access they have to social and recreational activities. Community organizations exist around the country that help people with spinal cord injuries adjust to their new lives. Organizations such as Empower Spinal Cord Injury in Boston, and Adapted Sports in Crested Butte, CO, provide much-needed services to teens and adults with paraplegia and quadriplegia. Some of the possibilities for wheelchair sports were shown to the general public in the documentary film *Murder-*

ball (Shapiro, Mandel, & Rubin, 2005), which showcased athletes playing wheelchair rugby at an international level. Although no occupational therapy practitioners are depicted in the movie, many opportunities for professional or volunteer involvement with these and other sports exist.

Summary

All activities have the potential to be important and meaningful therapeutic modalities when used by occupational therapy practitioners. Using theoretically based guidelines for intervention,

Case Example 8.14. Alice: Learning a New Activity and Developing an Occupation

Alice, age 65 years, has a history of strokes and many other medical problems. She attends an adult day program and receives help with several daily activities. She uses a wheelchair but transfers independently and lives in her own home with support from aides.

Alice was one of the first people at the adult day program to get involved in making blankets for recent immigrants who lacked warm clothes and household goods. The occupational therapy assistant students and I taught Alice and several others to make "no-sew" fleece blankets and adapted the tasks as needed so people with many different functional abilities and impairments could participate. Alice became an advocate for the project, recruiting her many friends at the center to help. It was very important to her to feel useful, and she often discussed her gratitude for the help she has received from others.

The blanket donation project was only a beginning for Alice. After completing the project, she asked for help getting to the fabric store so she could make blankets for her home health aides. She altered the shape and size to make herself a cape to wear in cold weather when she rides in the van in her wheelchair. She explained how coats were never very practical considering her size and physical limitations. The cape keeps her hands and whole body warm. After being away from the center for several weeks, I returned one morning to hear Alice calling me and wheeling right over. It was a rainy day, and she had to show me her latest creation—a new cape with water-repellent fabric on one side and fleece on the other.

Case Example 8.15. Marcus: A "Sit Down" Comic

Marcus, age 26 years, has an acquired brain injury. At an adult day program for people with such injuries, Marcus, who uses a power wheelchair, is the comedian of the group and says he wants to be on stage. He appeared at an open mic night at a local comedy club and got some laughs. Now, his goal was to win the cash prize offered at the club once a month.

Working with an occupational therapy practitioner, Marcus used a computer to write down and fine-tune his jokes. While watching Marcus practice his act, the practitioner determined that he could remember the beginning, but his attention skills were not perfect, and he began to ramble toward the end. He and the practitioner collaboratively determined that he could tape a cue card to his pants and refer to it to keep on track while on stage. Marcus invited everyone to the next open mic night, and he has won several cash prizes since then.

Staff at the day program knew that Marcus made some female program members uncomfortable when he told sexually inappropriate jokes during leisure or cooking groups. With prompting, Marcus recognized that he needed to learn the proper time and place for his jokes. The occupational therapist developed a cuing system that was agreed on by Marcus and the staff so that he could receive the limit setting that he sometimes needed, without embarrassment.

practitioners promote change using occupations, purposeful activities, and activities, in the context of real life. Purpose in doing the activity must be inherent for activity participation. Practitioners skillfully use occupations and activities to facilitate a client's participation in his or her daily life. The variety of interventions is limited only by their imagination.

Case Example 8.16. Walter: Developing Socially Appropriate Behavior

Walter, age 53 years and diagnosed with bipolar disorder, was an active participant in a psychosocial clubhouse. He was very sociable and funny, but his participation in social activities was limited by his need to leave 3 mornings a week to go to renal dialysis.

Having gained some insight into his tendency to ramble in conversation, Walter admitted that he did not always know when he needed to "reel it in." He wanted to make the most of his time at the center and did not like it when other members interrupted him so that someone else could talk. As a consulting occupational therapist, I suggested that when we were in group activities together, I would do a hand motion to simulate reeling in a fish. Walter thought that was a great idea because it appealed to his sense of humor and pride. After trying the agreed-on cue, we decided that the first cue would simply be the reeling-in gesture. If Walter did not notice that, the group leader would speak his name, then make the hand signal. It worked like a charm.

Case Example 8.17. Preventing Repetitive Strain Injuries in the Workplace

In a workplace in which people use computers all day, an occupational therapist may recommend changing the height of monitors, the ergonomic demands or position of the keyboards, or the amount of time spent at computer terminals. Desks and chairs can be changed or adjusted to provide adequate ergonomic seating support. Occupational therapists can teach workers to schedule regular rest and stretch breaks. For example, workers can use timers that go off at specific intervals and cue workers to stand up and do stretches derived from yoga poses. These or other fun activities encourage changes in posture and gross mobility rather than concentrated use of the hands. Evidence-based practice has shown yoga to be an effective, nonmedical intervention for carpal tunnel syndrome (Garfinkel et al., 1998; Huisstede et al., 2010). Additionally, an occupational therapist could recommend that the management team bring in a yoga instructor to conduct classes on a weekly basis or reimburse employees for the cost of yoga classes.

Case Example 8.18. Therapy Missions in Mexico

In 2007, **Carol Doehler, Dahlia Castillo,** and other occupational therapists offered their services to the Fundación Integra (hereafter called Integra) in Juárez, Mexico. Integra is a community-based agency established by the families of people with disabilities. In Mexico, children with disabilities other than blindness are not allowed to go to school. Many such children thus do not leave their homes. Furthermore, rehabilitation for adults with physical disabilities is very limited. Some may be given a wheelchair, but few buildings or public services are wheelchair accessible.

Parents and other family members bring people to Integra, where they learn and carry out therapeutic exercises and participate in horseback riding or water activities. Integra has intermittent services from a physiatrist, but it has no professional rehabilitation therapists.

Using a developmental approach, the American occupational therapists quickly noticed that many of the children who visited Integra had no outlets for play. One of the first interventions for this population was to teach parents and other caregivers how to help the children access toys and play in developmentally sound and therapeutic ways. Various toys and positioning devices were purchased or created so that the children could try to play. By helping the parents think about play as a normal and beneficial occupation for their children, the therapists empowered parents to expand therapeutic activities into their home lives and to strengthen their community by sharing ideas with each other.

Although Integra has functioned as a home base for the visiting therapists, the entire population of people with disabilities in Juárez is being served by the education of families and other caregivers.

Case Example 8.19. Matt: A Child With Cerebral Palsy

Matt, an 11-year-old boy with cerebral palsy with left hemiparesis, began receiving occupational and physical therapy as an infant and has since been diagnosed with attention-deficit/hyperactivity and sensory processing disorders. Matt's parents tried to get him involved with various activities and sports with little success due to Matt's poor motor control of the left side of his body.

Matt's occupational therapist suggested that they send him to a martial art class and said she would work with him on mastering the motor skills needed for the class. Matt has been participating in karate classes 3 times a week since age 4 years. His differences were never seen as a barrier to his participation in all the class activities, just as challenges to overcome. A few activities were initially adapted for Matt's participation, but now he independently engages in classes, tournaments, and social events at the martial arts academy.

Matt has been discharged from all therapies and at 11 has just earned his black belt. He is adept at cartwheels, flips, and other acrobatics—not bad for a boy whose doctors thought might never walk.

References

American Occupational Therapy Association. (2010). Standards of practice for occupational therapy. *American Journal of Occupational Therapy, 64*(Suppl.), S106–S111. http://dx.doi.org/10.5014/ajot.2010.64S106

American Occupational Therapy Association. (2012). Physical agent modalities. *American Journal of Occupational Therapy, 66*, S78–S80. http://dx.doi.org/10.5014/ajot.2012.66S78

American Occupational Therapy Association. (2014). Occupational therapy framework: Domain and process (3rd ed.). *American Journal of Occupational Therapy, 68*(Suppl. 1), S1–S48. http://dx.doi.org/10.5014/ajot.2014.682006

Baron, K., Kielhofner, G., Iyenger, A., Goldhammer, V., & Wolenski, J. (2006). *A user's manual for the Occupational Self Assessment (OSA) (version 2.2).* Chicago: Model of Human Occupational Clearinghouse, Department of Occupational Therapy, University of Illinois.

Bazyk, S., & Case-Smith, J. (2010). School-based occupational therapy. In J. Case-Smith & J. C. O'Brien (Eds.), *Occupational therapy for children* (6th ed., pp. 713–743). Maryland Heights, MO: Mosby/Elsevier.

Chapparo, C., & Ranka, J. (1997). The occupational performance model (Australia): A description of constructs and structure. In C. Chapparo & J. Ranka (Eds.), *Occupational performance model (Australia). Monograph 1* (p. 60). Sydney: Occupational Performance Network. Retrieved from http://203.17.62.122/opma/index.php/au/home/definitions

Clark, F., Azen, S. P., Carlson, M., Mandel, D., LaBree, L., Hay, J.,... Lipson, L. (2001). Embedding health-promoting changes into the daily lives of independent-living older adults: Long-term follow-up of occupational therapy intervention. *Journals of Gerontology, Series B: Psychological Sciences, 56*, 60–63. http://dx.doi.org/10.1093/geronb/56.1.P60

Clark, F., Azen, S. P., Zemke, R., Jackson, J., Carlson, M., Mandel, D.,... Lipson, L. (1997). Occupational therapy for independent-living older adults. A randomized controlled trial. *JAMA, 278*, 1321–1326. http://dx.doi.org/10.1001/jama.1997.03550160041036

Clark, F., Jackson, J., Carlson, M., Chou, C.-P., Cherry, B. J., Jordan-Marsh, M.,... Azen, S. P. (2011). Effectiveness of a lifestyle intervention in promoting the well-being of independently living older people: Results of the Well Elderly 2 Randomised Controlled Trial. *Journal of Epidemiology and Community Health, 66*, 782–790. http://dx.doi.org/10.1136/jech.2009.099754

Cohn, E. S. (1991). Clinical reasoning: Explicating complexity. *American Journal of Occupational Therapy, 45*, 969–971. http://dx.doi.org/10.5014/ajot.45.11.969

Curral, M. R., Maia, D., Lopes, R., Fonseca, S., Ferreira, P., Rodrigues, S., ... & Roma Torres, A. (2012). Multidisciplinary assessment of patients in day hospital (DH) of psychiatry department at the Hospitalar Center of São João. *European Psychiatry, 27*, 1.

Dunn, W., Brown, C., & McGuigan, A. (1994). The ecology of human performance: A framework for considering the effect of context. *American Journal of Occupational Therapy, 48*, 595–607. http://dx.doi.org/10.5014/ajot.48.7.595

Dunn, W., Brown, C., & Youngstrom, M. J. (2003). Ecological model of occupation. In P. Kramer, J. Hinojosa, & C. B. Royeen (Eds.), *Perspectives in human occupation: Participation in life* (pp. 222–263). Philadelphia: Lippincott Williams & Wilkins.

Fleming, M. H. (1991). The therapist with the three-track mind. *American Journal of Occupational Therapy, 45*, 1007–1014. http://dx.doi.org/10.5014/ajot.45.11.1007

Garfinkel, M. S., Singhal, A., Katz, W. A., Allan, D. A., Reshetar, R., & Schumacher, H. R., Jr. (1998). Yoga-based intervention for carpal tunnel syndrome: A randomized trial. *JAMA, 280,* 1601–1603. http://dx.doi.org/10.1001/jama.280.18.1601

Hay, J., LaBree, L., Luo, R., Clark, F., Carlson, M., Mandel, D.,... Azen, S. P. (2002). Cost-effectiveness of preventive occupational therapy for independent-living older adults. *Journal of the American Geriatrics Society, 50,* 1381–1388. http://dx.doi.org/10.1046/j.1532-5415.2002.50359.x

Helfrich, C. A., & Chan, D. V. (2013). Changes in self-identified priorities, competencies, and values of recently homeless adults with psychiatric disabilities. *American Journal of Psychiatric Rehabilitation,* 16(1), 22–49.

Huisstede, B. M., Hoogvliet, P., Randsdorp, M. S., Glerum, S., van Middelkoop, M., & Koes, B. W. (2010). Carpal tunnel syndrome. Part I: Effectiveness of nonsurgical treatments—A systematic review. *Archives of Physical Medicine and Rehabilitation, 91,* 981–1004. http://dx.doi.org/10.1016/j.apmr.2010.03.022

Kielhofner, G. (2008). *Model of Human Occupation: Theory and application* (4th ed.). Philadelphia: Lippincott Williams & Wilkins.

Latham, C. A. T. (2008). Occupation: Philosophy and concepts. In M. V. Radomski & C. A. T. Latham (Eds.), *Occupational therapy for physical dysfunction* (6th ed., pp. 340–357). Philadelphia: Lippincott Williams & Wilkins.

Law, M., Baptiste, S., McColl, M., Opzoomer, A., Polatajko, H., & Pollock, N. (1990). The Canadian Occupational Performance Measure: An outcome measure for occupational therapy. *Canadian Journal of Occupational Therapy, 57,* 82–87. http://dx.doi.org/10.1177/000841749005700207

Law, M., Cooper, B., Strong, S., Stewart, D., Rigby, P., & Letts, L. (1996). The Person–Environment–Occupation Model: A transactive approach to occupational performance. *Canadian Journal of Occupational Therapy, 63,* 9–23. http://dx.doi.org/10.1177/000841749606300103

Ma, H. I., & Trombly, C. A. (2002). A synthesis of the effects of occupational therapy for persons with stroke, Part II: Remediation of impairments. *American Journal of Occupational Therapy, 56,* 260–274. http://dx.doi.org/10.5014/ajot.56.3.260

Mosey, A. C. (1986). *Psychological components of occupational therapy.* New York: Raven.

Nakamura-Thomas, H., & Kyougoku, M. (2013). Application of occupational self assessment in community settings for older people. *Physical and Occupational Therapy in Geriatrics, 31*(2), 103–114.

Richardson, M. (2001). *The experience of culture.* Thousand Oaks, CA: Sage.

Schell, B. A. B. (2014). Professional reasoning in practice. In B. A. B. Schell, G. Gillen, & M. E. Scaffa (Eds.), *Willard and Spackman's occupational therapy* (12th ed., pp. 384–397). Philadelphia: Wolters Kluwer Health/Lippincott Williams & Wilkins.

Schell, B. A. B., & Schell, J. W. (2008). *Clinical and professional reasoning in occupational therapy.* Philadelphia: Lippincott Williams & Wilkins.

Shapiro, D. A. (Director/Producer), Mandel, J. (Producer), & Rubin, H. A. (Director). (2005). *Murderball* [Motion picture]. Los Angeles: THINKFilm.

CHAPTER 9.

FACILITATING OCCUPATIONAL PERFORMANCE

Margaret Kaplan, PhD, OTR

Highlights

✧ Facilitating occupational performance
✧ Using activities to elicit greater effort, repetition, or duration than traditional exercise
✧ Using activities to provide graded challenges
✧ Using activities to develop effective strategies for performance skills.

Key Terms

✧ Client factors
✧ Cognitive–behavioral strategies
✧ Cognitive Orientation to Daily Occupational Performance
✧ Cognitive strategies
✧ Compensatory approaches
✧ Dynamic Interactional Model
✧ Electromyographic activity
✧ Goal objects and tools
✧ Graded challenges
✧ Habituate

✧ Instrumental activities of daily living
✧ Interpersonal strategies
✧ Just-right challenge
✧ Metacognition
✧ Motor strategies
✧ Occupation-as-means
✧ Passive range of motion
✧ Performance skills
✧ Regulatory conditions
✧ Sensory strategies
✧ Strategies

The end goals of all occupational therapy are improved occupational performance, engagement, and participation in society. To improve occupational performance, occupational therapists determine which areas of occupation are meaningful to a client and which have become difficult for him or her to perform. Interventions include the development of compensatory strategies, selection and modification of available assistive devices, design and fabrication of unique assistive devices, modification of the context, and focused practice of relevant tasks.

This chapter begins by describing the use of occupation and related activities as means (Case-Smith, 2010; Trombly Latham, 2008), in which occupational therapy practitioners design activities to provide structured challenges to reduce specific impairments in client factors and improve specific performance skills. Three ways to use occupations and their related activities to improve a client's internal factors (e.g., promote interest, challenge performance level, and develop effective cognitive or motor strategies) are identified. Each approach is discussed separately beginning with the use of activities to facilitate a client's increased effort, repetition, and length of participation in a therapeutic activity. Examples include physical activity for adults and play behaviors for children.

The next section describes how to use activities to provide a graded challenge to clients. It discusses various regulatory conditions that an occupational therapy practitioner can use to engage the client in the activity, including goal objects and tools, rules, supporting structures, environmental context, and the practitioner.

The final section presents how to use activities to promote development of effective strategies for performance skills. The strategies described are motor, cognitive, interpersonal, and sensory. In each section, the focus is on the use of occupations and their related activities as effective therapeutic mediums that address the unique needs of each person.

Facilitating Occupational Performance

Occupational therapy practitioners facilitate improvement of occupational performance through balanced interventions that maximize the client's potential to improve *client factors,* which are "specific capaci-

ties, characteristics, or beliefs that reside within the person and that influence performance in occupations" (American Occupational Therapy Association [AOTA], 2014, p. S7), and *performance skills,* which are "goal-directed actions that are observable as small units of engagement in daily life occupations" (AOTA, 2014, p. S7; i.e., factors internal to the client). They also seek to minimize activity limitation through *compensatory approaches,* which are interventions that modify the environment or teach the client adapted procedures to substitute for loss of function (i.e., factors external to the client). Occupational therapy practitioners balance these internally and externally directed interventions to promote performance of occupations that will enhance participation in family and community settings (Figure 9.1).

Improvements in internal factors are critical to the occupational therapy process because they enable clients to perform an infinite number of tasks in a variety of situations. Such improvements empower them to create and discover unanticipated occupations and roles. Practitioners who work with children often use play activities as a means to facilitate and encourage the development of more mature performance skills (internal factors). A careful balance is planned to present a client with the *just-right challenge*—one that is neither so far above the client's present abilities that it is frustrating nor so far below that new learning does not occur.

Occupation-as-means refers to intervention in which the occupational therapy practitioner selects therapeutic activities based on a client's occupational interests and needs. That is, the occupation itself is the means of therapy. Practitioners use a client's occupation by selecting related activities in the therapeutic process in three major ways to promote improvements in a client's internal factors.

1. Practitioners present an activity to promote the interest level that enables a client to exert more effort, complete more repetitions of a desired behavior, or sustain performance for a longer duration.
2. Practitioners manipulate a selected activity and environmental conditions to present graded challenges to specific skills.
3. Practitioners select activities that will provide problems that challenge a client to develop effective cognitive or motor strategies that he or she can generalize to a variety of future situations.

Figure 9.1. Activity-based intervention in occupational therapy is a balance between internally and externally directed interventions to improve performance in areas of occupation and, ultimately, participation in valued roles.

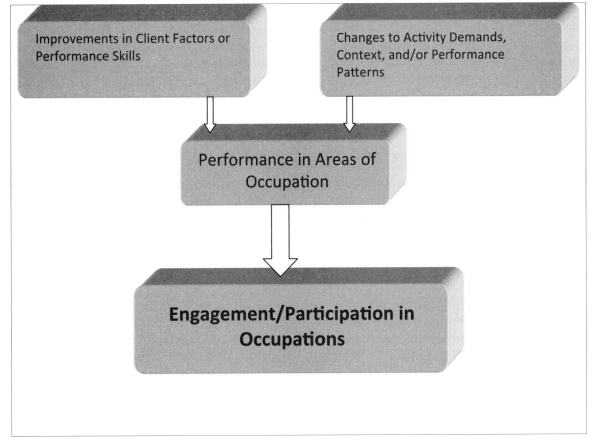

Source. M. Kaplan. Used with permission.

Although categories overlap, it is critical that occupational therapy practitioners understand the types of occupation-as-means and their related activities. Further, practitioners need to understand when each type of occupation-as-means may be most appropriate and which concepts are relevant to apply when using activities in each of these three ways.

Critical interventions exist to enable clients to improve their performance in selected activities. If underlying impairments remain unchanged, however, these improvements are not likely to be generalized and make their way into the performance of other occupations. When a practitioner determines that a client demonstrates the potential to improve underlying factors or performance skills, the client deserves the opportunity to work toward such restoration of foundational motor, cognitive, or interactive capacities.

Using Activities to Elicit Greater Effort, Repetition, or Duration Than Traditional Exercise

Rather than giving a client an exercise, practitioners can use an activity that increases the client's motivation to encourage greater effort, increase repetition, and extend endurance. Historically, the earliest use of activities in occupational therapy may have been as a medium to facilitate improvement in underlying client factors and performance skills (Taylor, 1929). Research findings (Bloch, Smith, & Nelson, 1989; Kircher, 1984; Steinbeck, 1986) have indicated that healthy adults exert greater cardiovascular and muscular effort, as evidenced by faster heart rate and increased *electromyographic activity* (i.e., measurement of electrical activity

Exercise 9.1. Personal Goals

Think about the goals you would set for yourself or a loved one, if faced with limitations in activity performance. Suppose your friend cannot perform *instrumental activities of daily living* (i.e., daily life activities that require more complex interactions than routine activities of daily living) because his organizational and problem-solving skills have been affected by a traumatic brain injury. If he exhibits the potential to improve these underlying cognitive skills, would an occupational therapy program consisting only of specific task practice be sufficient?

What if your younger sister demonstrates impairments in hand coordination that limit her ability to learn handwriting skills? You would want occupational therapy to offer her the opportunity to improve her underlying limitations in addition to specific handwriting practice or use of adapted writing utensils.

Suppose your grandfather has survived a stroke with intact cognition. He demonstrates some movement throughout his paretic left arm but cannot use the arm for task performance. Would you be satisfied with an occupational therapy program that is limited to teaching one-handed self-care techniques?

produced by skeletal muscles) in selected muscles, when performing activities that they perceive to be fun (e.g., jumping rope) compared with exercises with similar motor components (e.g., jumping in place). Using activities as interventions is relevant when treatment goals are to improve cardiopulmonary and specific muscle endurance.

Performance of interesting or personally meaningful activity also promotes greater repetition and prolonged duration of physical output than performance of routine exercise programs (DeKuiper, Nelson, & White, 1993; Hsieh, Nelson, Smith, & Peterson, 1996; Lang, Nelson, & Bush, 1992; Miller & Nelson, 1987; Nelson et al., 1996; Riccio, Nelson, & Bush, 1990; Steinbeck, 1986; Yoder, Nelson, & Smith, 1989). This fact is well understood in current popular culture, as evidenced by the use of dance routines and embedded games during aerobic exercise and muscle-toning sessions at community fitness centers. When muscle endurance or joint flexibility is a treatment goal, it is

advantageous for the client to produce more repetitions over a longer duration of actions that demand optimal levels of muscle output or soft tissue elongation (Downey & Darling, 1994). When seeking to decrease distal limb edema, repetitive isotonic contractions of muscles in the targeted body segment are a recognized complement to medical and positioning interventions (Artzberger & White, 2011; Cooper, 2008).

For example, to improve range for overhead reach and stretch painful muscles, one client found that putting dishes away on high shelves provided repetitive reaching during a task that was necessary and important to her. She also found that a Pilates exercise routine enabled her to engage in the exercises recommended by the practitioner more regularly and for longer periods than did a standard exercise regimen (Earley & Shannon, 2006).

Research findings have provided evidence that people with disabilities exhibit greater range of motion (i.e., perform closer to their maximum potential) when engaged in interesting activities than when performing under conventional exercise conditions. In one study, van der Weel, van der Meer, and Lee (1991) encouraged children with cerebral palsy who exhibited right hemiparesis to perform actively the forearm movements of pronation and supination. While performing in the experimental condition, the children were instructed to use a drumstick to bang on drums that were positioned to require full forearm range of motion. During the control condition, the same children were instructed to move the drumstick back and forth as far as they could in the frontal plane. Range of movement was substantially greater during drum banging than during the abstract exercise condition.

Sietsema, Nelson, Mulder, Mervau-Scheidel, and White (1993) produced similar findings in their study of forward reach in adults with hemiparesis caused by traumatic brain injury. Neurodevelopmental treatment strategies were used to prepare study participants for forward reach from the sitting position. In the exercise condition, participants reached out their hands as far as they could in a rote manner. In the activity condition, they reached forward to control Simon,® a popular computer-controlled game that challenges players to repeat its sequences of flashing lights and sounds by pressing colored panels. Data collected through computerized motion analysis revealed that participants displayed much greater mobility when engaged in the activity than when they attempted to reach forward in an exercise context.

Other researchers have found greatly improved motor performance in adults after a stroke when using postural control strategies and reaching and manipulating objects when the objects are the actual objects they use during a task versus practicing movements that are similar to those used in a task (Chen, Lin, Chen, & Wu, 2008; Lin, Wu, Chen, Chern, & Hong, 2007), as in Case Example 9.1.

In pediatric intervention, the use of playful, inviting sensory integration equipment serves, in

Case Example 9.1. Jack: Stroke

Jack is a 75-year-old man who sustained a stroke with resulting left-side hemiparesis and is now receiving occupational therapy in an inpatient rehabilitation unit. Goals were to increase standing balance, sustained visual attention to both right and left fields, and fine motor coordination, especially during bilateral tasks. Jack was able to stand for less than 5 minutes during manipulation tasks; then he needed to stop and sit down to rest. He needed frequent verbal cues to attend to the left visual field.

The occupational therapist learned from Jack that he liked to fish and had made his own fishing poles in the past. Jack thought that he could sand and refinish poles and might be able to fish next spring. The occupational therapist positioned the fishing pole at a standing-height table extending across both the right and the left sides of the table. Jack was able to stand and work on the fishing pole for 20 to 25 minutes without asking for a rest break, and he maintained visual attention to both sides of the visual field to sand the pole and apply varnish. Jack continued work on the pole, resanding and applying more varnish, and was able to maintain his standing balance for 20 to 30 minutes at a time. He required much less cuing to search both sides of the visual field for the pieces and supplies he needed.

part, to pique children's interest in and sustain their performance of activities that provide vestibular, tactile, or proprioceptive stimuli that they might otherwise avoid. The introduction of imaginative play may engage the child still further, thus encouraging longer duration of involvement and expenditure of greater effort during treatment sessions. Increased practice of gross motor developmental actions within the context of a nontherapy, gamelike group event resulted in greater improvements in skill acquisition in young children with Down syndrome than for those who received only physical therapy (Fiss & Effgen, 2008). For children with burns, a therapy program consisting of child-chosen games using clay, playdough, and puzzles produced a statistically significant decrease in pain perception and an increase in functional hand use compared with children who received rote exercise (Omar, Hegazy, & Mokashi, 2012).

What makes an activity engaging enough that it will entice a person to continue a performance while repetitively performing a prescribed exercise or practicing a new skill? The answer depends on each person. A person's interest in specific activities is influenced by a complex array of factors, including his or her cultural background, age, prior experiences, and current abilities. In addition to these factors, developmental level must be taken into account when providing choices of activities to children. Usually, the practitioner engages the child by making the purpose of the activity clear, for example, "Let's build a garage for your car," "Let's make a valentine's card for Mom," and "Stay on the boat [bolster], here come some waves, don't fall in the water." Depending on the developmental level, the introduction of pretend play and social play can provide an additional level of interest and motivation that increases the effort or duration of the activity engagement (Humphry, 2002; Humphry & Wakeford, 2006). As children get older, the judicious use of small groups can be extremely effective in modeling behavior and motivating children to participate with peers.

In their attempt to create activities that will entice clients to perform repetitive practice of specific movements or skills, occupational therapy practitioners may be tempted to present tasks that are so contrived that they hold little meaning for their clients (Fisher, 1998). If an occupational therapy activity does little to engage the client, no advantage exists in choosing such an activity over exercise as an intervention.

The occupational therapy practitioner must learn as much as possible about each client's previous skills, interests, and activity background. This information, combined with knowledge of the person's current strengths and limitations, is critical to setting feasible treatment goals. Parents and family members can be invaluable in providing insight into what engages a child who appears to have little interest in his or her environment. A favorite object from the home or classroom can be used to develop an activity (e.g., "Let's put your doll to sleep" or "Can you help your teddy bear to draw a picture?"). Although this background information may also be helpful when selecting therapeutic activities, activities that engage the client do not necessarily need to be related to a client's prior repertoire of activity interests. "It does not matter whether one originally wanted to do the activity, whether one expected to enjoy it, or not. Even a frustrating job may suddenly become exciting if one hits upon the right balance" (Csikszentmihalyi & Csikszentmihalyi, 1988, p. 32).

For many adults, an enabling activity need not have been a favorite prior pastime. In fact, sometimes a well-meaning practitioner is disappointed to learn that selecting a favorite task as a therapeutic intervention frustrates clients rather than brings them pleasure. The client who worked as an electrician may become disheartened to see that simple wiring tasks are now excessively challenging. The avid puzzle solver may be dismayed to be practicing crossword puzzles designed for children. The match between an activity's intrinsic interest level and the person's understanding of why the practice is important is key in determining how successful an activity will be in eliciting pleasure during sustained performance. As in all other aspects of occupational therapy, active involvement in the total therapeutic process enhances a client's motivation to participate (Figure 9.2).

Occupational therapy practitioners must consider a few critical words of caution when using activities to elicit repetitive performance of prescribed movement sequences. First, repetitive movements must be performed only from a position of optimal alignment. The practitioner must avoid activities that are ergonomically unsound while providing appropriate therapeutic positioning and handling

Figure 9.2. Client engaged in sanding and finishing a fishing pole using repetitive reach, grasp, and manipulation activities while increasing standing balance and tolerance.

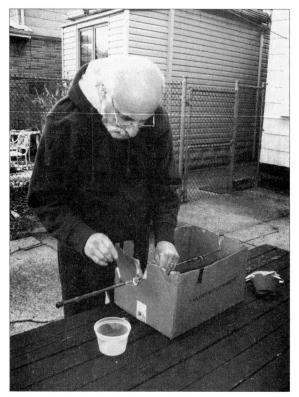

Source. M. Kaplan. Used with permission.

to enhance the client's performance and comfort. Second, therapeutic activities should not be introduced unless the client demonstrates adequate prerequisite factors and skills.

For example, introducing a task that requires repetitive active reaching has no therapeutic value unless the client exhibits the necessary joint play and muscle distensibility that will allow adequate *passive range of motion* (i.e., the moving of a joint without exertion by the client that usually occurs when a therapist manually moves the client's body part) at all the joints of the shoulder complex. Third, practitioners need to remember that repetition must occur naturally within the activity performance. For example, setting up a checkerboard affords the opportunity for repetitive practice of reach, grasp, and release. The activity component, however, is maintained only if the initial placement of game pieces is followed by an actual game of checkers (with a family member, a volunteer, or another client). To foster even more repetition, a practitioner may be tempted to ask a client to remove the checkers from the board and set them up again. Although this contrivance may be effective once or twice, it quickly reduces what may have begun as an interesting activity to a rote exercise that is unlikely to maintain the client's interest over time.

Using Activities to Provide Graded Challenges

Repetition alone will not promote improvement in all client factors and performance skills. When client goals are to enhance muscle strength, range of motion, balance, coordination, manipulation, social skills, or other skills that have the capacity to improve on a continuum, practice sessions must use activities that provide incremental increases in appropriate demands, that is, *graded challenges.* The key to effectively using activities to provide graded challenges is the occupational therapy practitioner's identification of a specific, relevant continuum on which gradations are introduced.

For example, if the client's goal is to improve active hip and pelvic mobility when sitting, placement of activity objects in relation to the client will represent a relevant continuum. Because the weight or size of activity objects will essentially be irrelevant to the specific performance of active hip motion, these factors will not be manipulated when making incremental changes to the activity demands.

Gentile's (1972, 1987) concept of *regulatory conditions* refers to those environmental features that directly influence a person's choice of strategies for performing a selected task. When designing activities to present graded challenges, practitioners determine which features in the environment and the selected task are regulatory to the skills they seek to challenge (Sabari, 1991). A variety of regulatory conditions (goal objects and tools, rules, supporting structures, the practitioner, and environmental context) can be manipulated to influence the performance requirements for engaging in therapeutic tasks (Figure 9.3).

Goal Objects and Tools

Goal objects and tools are items that a person must act on or manipulate within the course of task performance. These objects and tools can be adapted according to size, shape, weight, and texture (AOTA, 1993; Trombly Latham, 2008). In addition, their position in relation to the person will greatly influence which movements and balance adjustments will be required for task performance. Goal objects may also vary between being static, such as a jar of paint placed next to an easel, and being in motion, such as a ball during a game of catch or the action figures in a computer game. When goal objects are moving, their trajectories may be either predictable or unpredictable. Each variation places different demands on the person's requirements to use perceptual–motor skills and timing.

Rules

Rules guide performance of hobbies, crafts, games, and sports. Creative adaptations to rules can tailor an activity to allow for grading along dimensions as varied as turn taking, cognitive complexity,

Figure 9.3. Regulatory conditions that can be graded to alter an activity's performance requirements.

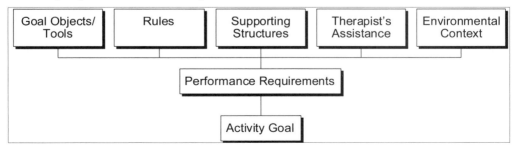

Source. M. Kaplan. Used with permission.

social interaction, use of imagination, and specific motor skills.

Supporting Structures

Supporting structures can be graded to provide incremental challenges to balance and dynamic motor performance. Whether a supporting structure is a chair, a bolster, a floor surface on which the client stands, or a piece of suspended play equipment, the occupational therapy practitioner can create variations in shape, weight, texture, base of support, and degree of external support. In addition, supporting structures can be graded along a continuum, beginning with stationary support to increasingly unstable or dynamic surfaces.

The Practitioner

The occupational therapy practitioner may also be viewed as a regulatory condition that influences the client's performance requirements. Practitioners can vary the ways in which they provide instructions and feedback and the ways in which they provide physical handling to support or assist a client in task performance. Such assistance is graded down incrementally to provide clients with opportunities to develop increasing ability in the skill on which their intervention is focused (Figure 9.4).

Figure 9.4. Child practicing a strategy of balancing objects with "bigger" on the bottom.

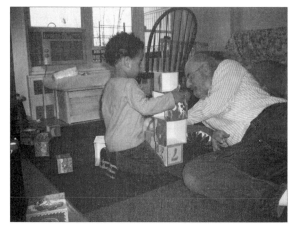

Source. M. Kaplan. Used with permission.

Environmental Context

The environmental context introduces a variety of additional regulatory conditions. Competitive noises or visual distractions place higher demands on attentional skills and can be graded through adaptations to the setting in which therapeutic intervention is provided. Physical obstacles, even when they are not central to the actual activity, can be used to pose graded cognitive, perceptual, and motor challenges. Several client factors and corresponding regulatory features are appropriate to adjust when the intervention is designed to present relevant, graded challenges (Table 9.1).

Case Example 9.2 provides a clinical example of how one occupational therapist uses activity grading within a group setting to assist clients in achieving specific goals related to trusting others and developing a repertoire of wellness behaviors.

Precautions for Graded Challenges

Precautions similar to those described when using activities to promote repetitive, sustained performance also hold true when occupational therapy practitioners present activities as a series of graded challenges. The practitioner must ensure that in any activity requiring movement, the client is performing from a position of optimal body alignment. Particularly when grading is achieved by altering a support surface or by introducing objects that have been strategically placed in increasingly more challenging locations, the practitioner must pay close attention to the client's general body posture and to maintaining appropriate alignment of specific body segments. If the practitioner does not, what he or she planned as a therapeutic intervention may promote inefficient and potentially harmful motor strategies.

Before selecting a treatment sequence for graded activity performance, the occupational therapy practitioner must determine whether the client demonstrates the potential to benefit from this type of intervention. Simply providing increasingly difficult challenges does not always result in functional improvements. The practitioner must collaborate with other team members to determine what combination of medical, orthotic, physical, and educational measures should precede or accompany graded activity performance.

Occupational therapy practitioners should strive to avoid two common mistakes when using activity

Table 9.1. Regulatory Features of Tasks That Correspond With Grading to Challenge Specific Client Factors or Skills

Factor	Intervention Strategies
Figure–ground perception	• Complexity of the visual background, similarity between the visual background and the key foreground object (provided in real-life hide-and-seek games or paper-and-pencil puzzles)
Active ROM: Shoulder flexion	• Height of object placement
Active ROM: Finger flexion	• Size of handles to grasp
Strength of specific muscles	• Placement of objects in relation to gravity (from gravity eliminated to lightweight objects to be moved against gravity) • Increased weight (resistance) against gravity • Length of lever arm (from short resistance arm to progressively longer resistance arm)
Praxis	• Complexity of a novel motor task
Fine motor coordination and dexterity	• Size and shape of tool (from gross to fine grasp) • Size, texture, and shape of objects to be manipulated • Increased demands on speed of performance • Increased demands on manipulation of objects
Standing balance	• Size and stability of base of support (from larger, most stable base to smaller, less stable base) • Amount of weight shift required in all planes of motion (achieved through placement of goal objects in relation to the person)
Attention span	• Increased time necessary to complete a task
Social interaction	• The interactive nature of tasks, which may progress from parallel task performance alongside another person, to activities requiring dyadic interaction, to activities requiring increasing amounts of sharing views and feelings with one or more persons

Note. ROM = range of motion.

grading as a therapeutic intervention. First, activity grading becomes counterproductive when the client perceives it as an unfair "tease." In this situation, a well-meaning but overzealous practitioner constantly upgrades the challenge of therapeutic tasks so that the client never achieves the satisfaction of performing activities more easily.

For example, after struggling to achieve improved reach in the context of making a macramé rug, the client deserves an opportunity to work with the materials positioned within reasonable distance. The practitioner, however, in an attempt to continually challenge the client's improving abilities, constantly repositions the wall-mounted rug so that it is always just out of comfortable reach. Blanche (2008) has warned practitioners who use toys as lures to motivate young children to reach or ambulate that the practice becomes misguided if, in an attempt to upgrade the child's efforts, the practitioner constantly moves the toy farther and farther away as the child approaches.

A second problem occurs when a client is participating in an occupational therapy program designed to promote improvements in multiple areas. For example, a child may be working to improve cognitive and gross mobility skills. It would be a mistake to grade treatment activities so that cognitive and gross mobility challenges are simultaneously increased. Rather, the practitioner should account for the likelihood that increased demands in one skill domain might have a negative effect on the child's demonstrated skills in other domains. Consider how you might function if you were challenged to your ultimate limits in trying to perform a triple-axel ice skating jump. Would that be the best moment for you to grapple with a difficult mathematics problem?

Similarly, a woman who demonstrates dual problems with balance and fine hand coordination may recently have achieved the ability to sit unsupported in a standard chair. When confronted with a challenging task in which she must manipulate objects with both hands, however, her ability to function at her highest level in maintaining sitting balance may be temporarily diminished.

In another example, a young woman who has survived a traumatic brain injury may demonstrate

Case Example 9.2. Cynthia: Activity Grading

Cynthia is coordinating a relaxation group for 6 members who attend an outpatient community mental health day program. All clients are considered to have serious mental illness. This group is part of a larger wellness program in which participants are learning to manage their psychiatric symptoms and develop healthier lifestyles. Group members exhibit difficulty committing themselves to new styles of behavior and to exposing their vulnerabilities to others. Cynthia will grade the group's activities along a continuum of increasing trust within a group framework and use the clients' strengths and interests in maintaining good health to motivate interest.

At the first session, the group members are required to take off their coats (hanging them on wall hooks that are clearly visible in the same room) and sit in a circle on wooden chairs. Initial activities include practicing deep-breathing strategies and performing active stretching of neck muscles. At subsequent sessions, clients also remove their shoes to practice foot and ankle stretches and then

progress to facial exercises with eyeglasses removed. Cynthia encourages group members to appreciate the humor in their facial expressions of frowning, grinning, and pouting to enhance their level of trust and comfort in doing awkward and unfamiliar movements.

Gradually, larger body movements are added to the group repertoire. Eventually, Cynthia demonstrates relaxation activities performed supine on a floor mat and encourages group members to try these in private at home as well. Cynthia is alert to the discomfort that her clients might feel, especially when a new activity is added. She is mindful that it takes time to learn to relax and extends the time for each relaxation technique in response to the group's behaviors.

An ultimate goal of this grading process is for clients to reach a level of comfort at which they are able to sufficiently trust the group to engage in a full repertoire of relaxation exercises considered to be popular and healthful in society at large and to use these techniques to relieve stress or symptoms in their daily lives.

problems related to socially appropriate behavior and cognitive processing and motor control. When the treatment emphasis is on upgrading demands for social interaction, the intellectual and motor challenges of a group activity must be kept as simple as possible. The skillful practitioner knows how to alter a task's regulatory conditions so that when grading up on one domain, demands to other domains are kept at manageable levels. In many cases, the practitioner will structure the activity so that competing demands are temporarily graded down.

Using Activities to Develop Effective Strategies for Performance Skills

Participation in activities is an essential method of assisting the client with developing strategies that will result in improved occupation performance skills. For many people, the essential occupational therapy goal is to develop performance

skills through a process of learning. Teaching and learning as part of occupational therapy intervention are necessary for clients of all ages whose goals are to improve postural control, motor control, cognitive abilities, interpersonal skills, and coping mechanisms. Neither activity repetition nor activity grading may be a sufficient intervention when the therapeutic goal is to assist clients in learning and generalizing effective strategies for their performance of daily tasks.

Strategies are organized plans or sets of rules that guide action in a variety of situations (Sabari, 2011). Everyone has developed a variety of strategies that serve as foundational guidelines for effective participation in daily activities. Many of these strategies have been so well learned that they seem to be automatic. Without them, however, the challenges of performing occupations would be overwhelming.

Children learn strategies by experimenting with movement and manipulation of objects and by using verbal and nonverbal communication to perform actions and obtain desired results. Most children learn effective strategies over time with practice and support from adults. Children with motor and cognitive impairments often have difficulty in learning new strategies and may need specific help to consider and try new ways of doing things.

Motor Strategies

Motor strategies include the vast repertoire of kinematic and kinetic linkages that underlie performance of skilled, efficient movement. For example, when reaching forward to turn on the computer, the strategy of anteriorly tilting the pelvis ensures sufficient mobility of the trunk and scapula. The strategy of abducting and upwardly rotating the scapula enhances the smooth mobility of the arm's trajectory (Neumann, 2002). Specific hand-shaping (Jeannerod, 1990) and visual guidance (Shumway-Cook & Woollacott, 2007; Wing & Frazer, 1983) strategies enable the index finger to reach the start button with minimal effort.

Other motor strategies include those automatic plans of action that enable people to maintain their balance throughout infinite varieties of environmental support and challenges to their centers of mass. In addition, people routinely implement strategies that will ensure their "postural readiness" (Zhang, Abreu, Gonzales, Huddleston, & Ottenbacher, 2002) to perform desired tasks. Think about the task of turning on the computer. What strategies do you use for establishing a base of support and alignment of body segments that ultimately make it easier and more efficient to accomplish this goal?

Cognitive Strategies

Cognitive strategies include the multiple and varied tactics people use to facilitate processing, storage, retrieval, and manipulation of information. What cognitive strategies have you found to be useful in negotiating the academic demands of being a college or graduate student? Sitting close to a lecturer and jotting down questions to ask after class may be effective strategies that enable one to process information in a large, noninteractive class setting. Regularly reorganizing and rewording class notes aid in storing course information. Categorizing and drawing one's own visual models may

be helpful in storing, retrieving, and manipulating information.

Cognitive strategies influence people's performance of all activities, whether simple or complex. Grocery shopping can be achieved more efficiently if one uses the strategies of taking a kitchen inventory, generating a shopping list, organizing the list according to the supermarket layout, and assembling appropriate discount coupons. When basic self-care tasks are challenging to people because of brain injury or developmental disabilities, selection and use of appropriate cognitive strategies make it possible to achieve independence and autonomy.

Interpersonal Strategies

Interpersonal strategies assist people in their social interactions with other people. During childhood and adolescent development, and every time people join a new group, people learn the normative practices of social engagement in a given context. Interpersonal strategies are required for forming and maintaining friendships, for expressing one's opinions in various situations, for enlisting assistance from strangers or family members, and for conducting routine transactions within one's community.

Many people requiring occupational therapy intervention can benefit from the opportunity to develop more effective interpersonal strategies. For example, children with autism are taught social skills strategies using explicit teaching and practice. In addition, they can more successfully maintain those skills when also taught self-monitoring strategies (Loftin, Odom, & Lantz, 2008).

Sensory Strategies

Sensory strategies include the methods people use to modulate their awareness of the myriad sensory stimuli and input in their surroundings. At times, a person may need to *habituate,* or screen out, for example, the light touch of his or her shirt sleeve on the skin or the birds chirping outside the classroom window. At other times, it is important to attend carefully to certain sensory aspects of the environment such as the teacher giving out instructions for homework or the status of the walk–don't walk light at the corner.

If people have difficulty in processing and regulating sensory input, an occupational therapy practitioner can help them find the type and pattern of sensory input that allows them to pay attention to necessary stimuli and screen out those that may be distracting. A practitioner can practice methods of regulating arousal by using deep touch pressure and proprioceptive input to calm and focus a client or by using some movement activities to alert the client. In addition, the Alert Program has been developed to help children recognize their arousal states and teach self-regulatory sensory strategies (Williams & Shellenberger, 1996). This program uses cognitive and sensory strategies to improve a child's ability to match level of alertness to the demands of the situation or task.

Using Activities in Developing Strategies in Occupational Therapy Practice

When using activities to develop strategies in occupational therapy practice, the occupational therapy practitioner should view the strategies as frameworks rather than as recipes. Strategies provide the client with foundational skills that are meant to be adapted to the ever-changing demands of the occupations in which he or she engages and the infinite variations of multiple environments. In addition, some strategies may have a negative effect on a person's future success or well-being. Therefore, the practitioner must guide clients toward developing strategies that are likely to have long-term positive implications.

People develop strategies through a process of encountering problems, implementing solutions, and monitoring the effects of the solutions. In child development, an experienced adult might guide his or her child through problem-solving activities and structure learning environment by selecting, focusing, and organizing incoming stimuli (Toglia, 2011). For example, both practice and assistance in developing neuromotor strategies for postural control are important to a child's ability to develop reach and grasp (Duff & Charles, 2004). When children have difficulty with postural control, they tend to move less; explore the environment less; and therefore have less practice with postural control, reaching, and manipulation.

In therapy, practitioners set up the environment and use feedback to facilitate the child's search for a solution to what he or she wants to do (Kaplan,

2010). Children with neuromotor problems often have particular difficulty in developing anticipatory postural control and require encouragement to practice developing strategies in multiple contexts (Valvano, 2004). The importance of practicing postural control strategies as part of goal-directed tasks requiring movement has been documented in children with cerebral palsy (Palisano, Snider, & Orlin, 2004; Westcott & Burtner, 2004).

Children with Asperger's syndrome (Gillberg, 2003), developmental coordination disorder, and learning disabilities (Taylor, Fayed, & Mandich, 2007) have been described as having difficulty in modifying ineffective strategies during motor tasks and handwriting. *Cognitive–behavioral strategies* are an intervention approach that focuses on using the client's intellectual reasoning to develop skills and abilities. They can be used to help children state the goal of the action explicitly, make a plan, and evaluate their own performance. The child is taught to evaluate the result, think of a different method, or modify his or her technique during the next attempt (Sangster, Beninger, Polatajko, & Mandich, 2005).

Strategy development continues throughout people's lives. New jobs, new relationships, and new hobbies present people with new sets of problems to be solved. Changes in their physical status, concomitant with normal aging, disease, or disability, create the need for altered strategies when performing familiar tasks.

Sometimes people are able to get advice or instruction to guide them in the formation of new strategies. For example, one's success in tennis will be enhanced if one learns, early on, some basic rules about postural set, kinematic linkages, and offensive and defensive tactics. Facility at the computer keyboard will be promoted if one practices touch-typing techniques. Ergonomic strategies for the positioning of workstation materials will have a positive impact on one's long-term visual and musculoskeletal health. A coworker's advice about how to interact with a particular administrator will guide one in developing effective on-the-job strategies.

Vygotsky (1978) believed that children learn through social interactions. Parents and others intuitively understand and provide the just-right challenge (Case-Smith, 2010) for their child and encourage a new skill by providing enough support for the child to try it. The adult withdraws the support or grades down the level of support as the child no longer needs it. For example, Gina's parents see that she can stand by the furniture and take steps sideways. She is starting to let go with one hand and turn to look around the room. They encourage her to let go with both hands and take a step toward them. At first, they stay barely one step away with arms outstretched to catch her. As she gains confidence in taking one step without support, they move further and further away. If Gina was not ready to take a step on her own, this activity would not be a just-right challenge. If her parents asked her to take 10 steps rather than 1 on the first attempt, the challenge would be far beyond her capabilities.

How does an occupational therapy practitioner use activities to assist clients in developing useful strategies? He or she structures tasks in a safe environment that provides clients with opportunities to try different solutions to actual problems. In addition, the practitioner selects activities in accordance with each client's goals. For example, for Trina, a preschool child with balance dysfunction, the problem was to figure out how to stay upright while pushing a doll carriage. Instead of providing solutions, the practitioner offered Trina suggestions through physical handling and artful structuring of the play situation (Pierce, 1997). Specifically, the practitioner would stabilize Trina at her hips and have objects (e.g., blanket, bottle, toys) at her waist level for Trina to pick up and place in the doll carriage.

In another example, for Scott, a young adult with schizophrenia, a set of problems was presented to help him successfully work as a salesperson in the hospital-run thrift shop. Problems included the challenge of interacting appropriately with customers and maintaining interest in work when business was slow. The practitioner assisted Scott in reflecting on the efficacy of the solutions he chose and helped him determine strategies that might guide his future performance in this job and other work experiences. The ultimate goal in this type of activity intervention is for the client to develop strategies that can be generalized to a wide variety of occupations and environments.

Self-awareness and self-monitoring skills are critical prerequisites to a person's ability to generate and apply appropriate strategies. *Metacognition*

(Katz & Hartman-Maier, 1998) is the knowledge and regulation of personal cognitive processes and capacities. It includes an awareness of personal strengths and limitations and the ability to evaluate task difficulty, plan ahead, choose appropriate strategies, and shift strategies in response to environmental cues. The Alert Program (Williams & Shellenberger, 1996) has been successfully used to help children with emotional and sensory processing disturbances recognize their own need for self-regulation and generate effective cognitive and sensory strategies that help them match their own alertness to the demands of the situation or task (Barnes, Vogel, Beck, Schoenfeld, & Owen, 2008).

Toglia's (2011) *Dynamic Interactional Model* for people with cognitive impairments caused by brain injury emphasizes the importance of metacognition. In this treatment approach, occupational therapy intervention begins by helping clients develop insight about personal strengths and deficits through a program that challenges them to estimate task difficulty, predict outcomes, and evaluate personal performance. The practitioner then has the client perform tasks that have been synthesized to present specific challenges and that guide the client in selecting appropriate strategies for meeting these challenges. Self-review of one's performance and guided planning for tackling the challenges of future tasks are key factors in the therapeutic process.

The *Cognitive Orientation to Daily Occupational Performance* is a strategy-based skill acquisition approach. This approach is based on the cognitive–behavioral work of Meichenbaum (1977) and Feuerstein, Haywood, Rand, Hoffman, and Jensen (1986) and has been studied with children with developmental coordination disorder. The three objectives are (1) skill acquisition, (2) cognitive strategy development, and (3) generalization and transfer. The child sets the goals with help from the practitioner, using the Canadian Occupational Performance Measure (Law et al., 2005). The practitioner engages in ongoing performance analysis to ensure that the child's motivation is maintained; he or she understands the task requirements; and there is a balance of child ability, task demands, and environmental conditions to support occupational performance. The child is taught to use a line of self-talk that includes questions such as, "What do I want to do?" "How am I going to do it?" and

Case Example 9.3. Joey: Developing Alternative Strategies

Joey is a 6-year-old boy who has been referred to occupational therapy because his excessive activity level, impulsiveness, and motor incoordination are affecting his ability to function successfully in his first-grade classroom. The occupational therapist has determined that Joey has difficulty identifying environmental cues that are important to successful activity outcomes. Therefore, one occupational therapy goal is to help him develop strategies to improve his ability to match his motor acts to the requirements of the task.

Because Joey demonstrates great interest in throwing balls and bean bags, the occupational therapist presents a problem. She informs Joey that the clown (a cardboard cutout with a hole for the mouth) has not eaten today and is very hungry. A bucket of "chocolate-flavored" beanbags that are the clown's favorite food is placed at a distance from the clown that the therapist judges to be challenging but still close enough for Joey to be able to throw the food through the clown's mouth. The therapist asks Joey, "What shall we do?" By asking Joey to tell her what he intends to do before he does it, the therapist ensures that he focuses on the relevant characteristics of distance, size, and position of the clown's mouth and the size and weight of the beanbags. His interest level in the activity will help him learn to screen out extraneous environmental stimuli.

After Joey throws the food, he must tell the occupational therapist what happened. To help him learn to assess his own performance, the therapist gives such feedback as "You threw the food too hard" or "Look at the mouth when you throw." The therapist can also help Joey learn to modify his strategies as needed by encouraging him to try another way or asking him, "What can you do differently?"

The occupational therapist creates a safe environment with a playful atmosphere in which Joey can feel comfortable experimenting and making mistakes. In this way, Joey will learn to engage in the following strategies:

- Focus on characteristics that are relevant to the task,
- Assess his behavior and actions about outcome and performance, and
- Implement changes in his behavior and actions on the basis of the assessment.

The occupational therapist has also collaborated with Joey's teacher to develop ways of encouraging Joey to use these strategies during classroom activities.

"How well did my plan work?" This approach has been used to address motor problems (Taylor et al., 2007) and handwriting problems (Banks, Rodger, & Polatajko, 2008; see also Case Example 9.3).

The use of activities to stimulate strategy development requires extensive knowledge and creativity. Whether the intervention is directed toward developing motor, cognitive, interpersonal, or sensory strategies, the practitioner must be an expert about that area of function. A thorough knowledge base, skill in analyzing performance, and the ability to anticipate how environmental and task demands are likely to affect function are required for effective intervention.

A key component is that activity challenges must be presented in a safe environment that allows for mistakes, self-reflection, and dynamic interaction with the occupational therapy practitioner. Although providing this type of activity intervention in a naturalistic environment has value, the practitioner must consider that public spaces may be embarrassing places for clients to be developing basic strategies.

For example, a supermarket or public library may not be an appropriate place to try new motor or cognitive strategies. Rather, the practitioner can simulate challenges in the client's home or in the therapy setting, where it may be emotionally and physically safer to begin the process of strategy development. Once the client has sufficiently mastered the necessary strategies, it is then advisable to provide opportunities to practice in real-world environments (Figure 9.5).

Figure 9.5. Child learning the strategy of keeping one's "eye on the ball" and counting 1, 2, 3 to the ball toss.

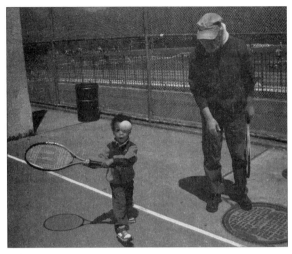

Source. M. Kaplan. Used with permission.

Summary

The use of activities as interventions to improve client factors or develop performance skills is an important component of occupational therapy intervention. On the basis of a client's goals, the practitioner determines whether the activity program will be structured to elicit repetition or longer duration of a desired behavior, present graded challenges to specific skills, or provide problems that challenge the client to develop appropriate strategies.

Regardless of the treatment setting, client background, or type of activity intervention, several criteria must be met. First, the client must be ready to participate in the selected activity. Prerequisite skills for performance must be assessed and interventions instituted to reduce physical, cognitive, or emotional factors that might hinder performance. Such constraints to performance can render an activity intervention useless or even harmful to a client.

Second, the activity must be synthesized for each person. This synthesis is necessary to ensure that the activity will be useful in developing skills that are specifically relevant to that person and will meet the third criterion, which is that the activity must provide some level of inherent interest to the person. In addition, the client must understand the dual purpose of the activity. Many clients are con-

fused by the occupational therapy process. When an occupational therapy intervention is designed to promote improvements in underlying client factors or performance skills, clients need to be able to differentiate the underlying therapeutic purposes from the activity itself.

Finally, occupational therapy intervention to improve client factors or performance skills is never isolated from the projected impact on a client's ability to perform meaningful tasks. The ultimate goal is always to facilitate performance of occupations and roles that are meaningful to the person in the context of his or her life.

Acknowledgments

I acknowledge Suzanne White, MA, OTR, for providing the case example about Cynthia.

References

American Occupational Therapy Association. (1993). Position paper: Purposeful activity. *American Journal of Occupational Therapy, 47,* 1081–1082. http://dx.doi.org/10.5014/ajot.47.12.1081

American Occupational Therapy Association. (2014). Occupational therapy framework: Domain and process (3rd ed.). *American Journal of Occupational Therapy, 68*(Suppl. 1), S1–S48. http://dx.doi.org/10.5014/ajot.2014.682006

Artzberger, S. M., & White, J. (2011). Edema control. In G. Gillen (Ed.), *Stroke rehabilitation: A function-based approach* (3rd ed., pp. 307–325). St. Louis: Elsevier/Mosby.

Banks, R., Rodger, S., & Polatajko, H. J. (2008). Mastering handwriting: How children with developmental coordination disorder succeed with CO-OP. *OTJR: Occupation, Participation and Health, 28,* 100–109. http://dx.doi.org/10.3928/15394492-20080601-01

Barnes, K. J., Vogel, K. A., Beck, A. J., Schoenfeld, H. B., & Owen, S. V. (2008). Self-regulation strategies of children with emotional disturbance. *Physical and Occupational Therapy in Pediatrics, 28,* 369–387. http://dx.doi.org/10.1080/01942630802307127

Blanche, E. I. (2008). Play in children with cerebral palsy. In L. D. Parham & L. S. Fazio (Eds.), *Play in occupational therapy for children* (2nd ed., pp. 375–393). St. Louis: Mosby.

Bloch, M. W., Smith, D. A., & Nelson, D. L. (1989). Heart rate, activity, duration, and affect in added-purpose versus single-purpose jumping activities. *American Journal of Occupational Therapy, 43,* 25–30. http://dx.doi.org/10.5014/ajot.43.1.25

Case-Smith, J. (2010). Development of childhood occupations. In J. Case-Smith & J. C. O'Brien (Eds.), *Occupational therapy for children* (6th ed., pp. 56–83). Maryland Heights, MO: Mosby/Elsevier.

Chen, H. C., Lin, K. C., Chen, C. L., & Wu, C. Y. (2008). The beneficial effects of a functional task target on reaching and postural balance in patients with right cerebral vascular accidents. *Motor Control, 12,* 122–135.

Cooper, C. (2008). Hand impairments. In M. V. Radomski & C. A. Trombly Latham (Eds.), *Occupational therapy for physical dysfunction* (6th ed., pp. 1132–1170). Baltimore: Lippincott Williams & Wilkins.

Csikszentmihalyi, M., & Csikszentmihalyi, I. S. (Eds.). (1988). *Optimal experience: Psychological studies of flow in consciousness.* New York: Cambridge University Press.

DeKuiper, W. P., Nelson, D. L., & White, B. E. (1993). Materials-based occupation versus rote exercise: A replication and extension. *OTJR: Occupation, Participation and Health, 13,* 183–197.

Downey, J., & Darling, R. (Eds.). (1994). *Physiological basis of rehabilitation medicine* (2nd ed.). Boston: Butterworth-Heinemann.

Duff, S. V., & Charles, J. (2004). Enhancing prehension in infants and children: Fostering neuromotor strategies. *Physical and Occupational Therapy in Pediatrics, 24,* 129–172. http://dx.doi.org/10.1300/J006v24n01_06

Earley, D., & Shannon, M. (2006). The use of occupation-based treatment with a person who has shoulder adhesive capsulitis: A case report. *American Journal of Occupational Therapy, 60,* 397–403. http://dx.doi.org/10.5014/ajot.60.4.397

Feuerstein, R., Haywood, H. C., Rand, Y., Hoffman, M. B., & Jensen, M. R. (1986). *Learning Potential assessment device manual.* Jerusalem: Hadassah-Wizo-Canada Research Institute.

Fisher, A. G. (1998). Uniting practice and theory in an occupational framework [1998 Eleanor Clarke Slagle Lecture]. *American Journal of Occupational Therapy, 52,* 509–521. http://dx.doi.org/10.5014/ajot.52.7.509

Fiss, A. C., & Effgen, S. K. (2008). Effect of increased practice using sensorimotor groups on gross motor skill acquisition for children with Down syndrome. *Pediatric Physical Therapy, 20,* 112–113.

Gentile, A. M. (1972). A working model of skill acquisition with application to teaching. *Quest, 17,* 3–23. http://dx.doi.org/10.1080/00336297.1972.10519717

Gentile, A. M. (1987). Skill acquisition: Action, movement, and neuromotor processes. In J. H. Carr, R. B. Shepherd, J. Gordon, A. M. Gentile, & J. N. Held (Eds.), *Movement science: Foundations for physical therapy in rehabilitation* (pp. 111–187). Rockville, MD: Aspen.

Gillberg, C. (2003). Deficits in attention, motor control, and perception: A brief review. *Archives of Disease in Childhood, 88,* 904–910. http://dx.doi.org/10.1136/adc.88.10.904

Hsieh, C. L., Nelson, D. L., Smith, D. A., & Peterson, C. Q. (1996). A comparison of performance in added-purpose occupations and rote exercise for dynamic standing balance in persons with hemiplegia. *American Journal of Occupational Therapy, 50,* 10–16. http://dx.doi.org/10.5014/ajot.50.1.10

Humphry, R. (2002). Young children's occupations: Explicating the dynamics of developmental processes. *American Journal of Occupational Therapy, 56,* 171–179. http://dx.doi.org/10.5014/ajot.56.2.171

Humphry, R., & Wakeford, L. (2006). An occupation-centered discussion of development and implications for practice. *American Journal of Occupational Therapy, 60,* 258–267. http://dx.doi.org/10.5014/ajot.60.3.258

Jeannerod, M. (1990). *The neural and behavioral organization of goal-directed movements.* Oxford, England: Clarendon.

Kaplan, M. (2010). A frame of reference for motor skill acquisition. In P. Kramer & J. Hinojosa (Eds.), *Frames of reference for pediatric occupational therapy* (pp. 390–424). Baltimore: Lippincott Williams & Wilkins.

Katz, N., & Hartman-Maier, A. (1998). Metacognition: The relationships of awareness and executive functions to occupational performance. In N. Katz (Ed.), *Cognition and occupation in rehabilitation: Cognitive models for intervention in occupational therapy* (pp. 323–342). Bethesda, MD: American Occupational Therapy Association.

Kircher, M. A. (1984). Motivation as a factor of perceived exertion in purposeful versus nonpurposeful activity. *American Journal of Occupational Therapy, 38,* 165–170. http://dx.doi.org/10.5014/ajot.38.3.165

Lang, E. M., Nelson, D. L., & Bush, M. A. (1992). Comparison of performance in materials-based occupation, imagery-based occupation, and rote exercise in nursing home residents. *American Journal of Occupational Therapy, 46,* 607–611. http://dx.doi.org/10.5014/ajot.46.7.607

Law, M., Baptiste, S., Carswell, A., McColl, M. A., Polatajko, H., & Pollock, N. (2005). *The Canadian Occupational Performance Measure* (4th ed.). Ottawa: CAOT Publications.

Lin, K. C., Wu, C. Y., Chen, C. L., Chern, J. S., & Hong, W. H. (2007). Effects of object use on reaching and postural balance: A comparison of patients with unilateral stroke and healthy controls. *American Journal of Physical Medicine and Rehabilitation, 86,* 791–799. http://dx.doi.org/10.1097/PHM.0b013e318151fb81

Loftin, R. L., Odom, S. L., & Lantz, J. F. (2008). Social interaction and repetitive motor behaviors. *Journal of Autism and Developmental Disorders, 38,* 1124–1135. http://dx.doi.org/10.1007/s10803-007-0499-5

Meichenbaum, D. (1977). *Cognitive–behavioral modification: An integrative approach.* New York: Plenum Press.

Miller, L., & Nelson, D. L. (1987). Dual-purpose activity versus single-purpose activity in terms of duration of task, exertion level, and affect. *Occupational Therapy in Mental Health, 7,* 55–67. http://dx.doi.org/10.1300/J004v07n01_04

Nelson, D. L., Konosky, K., Fleharty, K., Webb, R., Newer, K., Hazboun, V. P., . . . Licht, B. C. (1996). The effects of an occupationally embedded exercise on bilaterally assisted supination in persons with hemiplegia. *American Journal of Occupational Therapy, 50,* 639–646. http://dx.doi.org/10.5014/ajot.50.8.639

Neumann, D. A. (2002). *Kinesiology of the musculoskeletal system: Foundations for physical rehabilitation.* St. Louis: Mosby.

Omar, M. T., Hegazy, F. A., & Mokashi, S. P. (2012). Influences of purposeful activity versus rote exercise on improving pain and hand function in pediatric burn. *Burns, 38,* 261–268. http://dx.doi.org/10.1016/j.burns.2011.08.004

Palisano, R. J., Snider, L. M., & Orlin, M. N. (2004). Recent advances in physical and occupational therapy for children with cerebral palsy. *Seminars in Pediatric Neurology, 11,* 66–77. http://dx.doi.org/10.1016/j.spen.2004.01.010

Pierce, D. (1997). The power of object play for infants and toddlers at risk for developmental delays. In L. D. Parham & L. S. Fazio (Eds.), *Play in occupational therapy for children* (pp. 86–111). St. Louis: Mosby.

Riccio, C. M., Nelson, D. L., & Bush, M. A. (1990). Adding purpose to the repetitive exercise of elderly women through imagery. *American Journal of Occupational Therapy, 44,* 714–719. http://dx.doi.org/10.5014/ajot.44.8.714

Sabari, J. S. (1991). Motor learning concepts applied to activity-based intervention with adults with hemiplegia. *American Journal of Occupational Therapy, 45,* 523–530. http://dx.doi.org/10.5014/ajot.45.6.523

Sabari, J. (2011). Activity-based intervention in stroke rehabilitation. In G. Gillen (Ed.), *Stroke rehabilitation: A function-based approach* (3rd ed., pp. 100–116). St. Louis: Elsevier/Mosby.

Sangster, C. A., Beninger, C., Polatajko, H. J., & Mandich, A. (2005). Cognitive strategy generation in children with developmental coordination disorder. *Canadian Journal of Occupational Therapy, 72,* 67–77. http://dx.doi.org/10.1177/000841740507200201

Shumway-Cook, A., & Woollacott, M. (2007). *Motor control: Translating research into clinical practice* (3rd ed.). Baltimore: Lippincott Williams & Wilkins.

Sietsema, J. M., Nelson, D. L., Mulder, R. M., Mervau-Scheidel, D., & White, B. E. (1993). The use of a game to promote arm reach in persons with traumatic brain injury. *American Journal of Occupational Therapy, 47,* 19–24. http://dx.doi.org/10.5014/ajot.47.1.19

Steinbeck, T. M. (1986). Purposeful activity and performance. *American Journal of Occupational Therapy, 40,* 529–534. http://dx.doi.org/10.5014/ajot.40.8.529

Taylor, M. (1929). Occupational therapy in industrial inquiries. *Occupational Therapy and Rehabilitation, 8,* 335–338.

Taylor, S., Fayed, N., & Mandich, A. (2007). CO-OP intervention for young children with developmental coordination disorder. *OTJR: Occupation, Participation and Health, 27,* 124–130.

Toglia, J. P. (2011). The dynamic interactional model of cognitive rehabilitation. In N. Katz (Ed.), *Cognition, occupation, and occupation across the life span: Neuroscience, neurorehabilitation, and models of intervention in occupational therapy* (3rd ed., pp. 29–72). Bethesda, MD: AOTA Press.

Trombly Latham, C. (2008). Occupation: Philosophy and concepts. In M. V. Radomski & C. Trombly Latham (Eds.), *Occupational therapy for physical dysfunction* (6th ed., pp. 339–357). Baltimore: Lippincott Williams & Wilkins.

Valvano, J. (2004). Activity-focused motor interventions for children with neurological conditions. *Physical and Occupational Therapy in Pediatrics, 24,* 79–107. http://dx.doi.org/10.1300/J006v24n01_04

van der Weel, F. R., van der Meer, A. L. H., & Lee, D. N. (1991). Effect of task on movement control in cerebral palsy: Implications for assessment and therapy. *Developmental Medicine and Child Neurology, 33,* 419–426. http://dx.doi.org/10.1111/j.1469-8749.1991.tb14902.x

Vygotsky, L. S. (1978). *Mind in society: The development of higher psychological processes.* Cambridge, MA: Harvard University Press.

Westcott, S. L., & Burtner, P. A. (2004). Postural control in children: Implications for pediatric practice. *Physical and Occupational Therapy in Pediatrics, 24,* 5–55. http://dx.doi.org/10.1300/J006v24n01_02

Williams, M., & Shellenberger, S. (1996). *How does your engine run? A leader's guide to the Alert Program for Self-Regulation.* Albuquerque: Therapy Works.

Wing, A. M., & Frazer, C. (1983). The contribution of the thumb to reaching movements. *Quarterly Journal of Experimental Psychology: Human Experimental Psychology, 35*(A), 297–309. http://dx.doi.org/10.1080/14640748308402135

Yoder, R. M., Nelson, D. L., & Smith, D. A. (1989). Added-purpose versus rote exercise in female nursing home residents. *American Journal of Occupational Therapy, 43,* 581–586. http://dx.doi.org/10.5014/ajot.43.9.581

Zhang, L., Abreu, B. C., Gonzales, V., Huddleston, N., & Ottenbacher, K. J., (2002). The effect of predictable and unpredictable motor tasks on postural control after traumatic brain injury. *Neurorehabilitation, 17*(3), 225–230.

CHAPTER 10.

GROUP PROCESS, OCCUPATION, AND ACTIVITY

Jeff Tomlinson, MSW, OT, FAOTA, and Suzanne White, MA, OTR/L

Highlights

- ✧ Group formation
- ✧ Defining groups in occupational therapy
- ✧ Therapeutic activity groups
- ✧ Group development
- ✧ Group norms
- ✧ Practitioner's role in groups
- ✧ Group membership
- ✧ Member roles
- ✧ Levels of group interaction
- ✧ Group process
- ✧ Group decision making
- ✧ Group problem solving
- ✧ Therapeutic factors
- ✧ Occupational therapy task groups
- ✧ Common group problems.

Key Terms

- ✧ Active listening
- ✧ Affection stage
- ✧ Altruism
- ✧ Associative groups
- ✧ Basic cooperative groups
- ✧ Behavioral roles
- ✧ Catharsis
- ✧ Closed groups
- ✧ Control stage
- ✧ Developmental groups

- ✧ Effectance
- ✧ Empathy
- ✧ Existential factors
- ✧ Experiential learning
- ✧ Formal groups
- ✧ Group
- ✧ Group building and maintenance roles
- ✧ Group cohesion
- ✧ Group development
- ✧ Group thinking

❖ Heterogeneous group composition
❖ Homogeneous group composition
❖ Imitative behavior
❖ Inclusion stage
❖ Individual roles
❖ Informal groups
❖ Interpersonal learning
❖ Interpretation
❖ Naturally occurring groups
❖ Mature groups
❖ Moral treatment movement
❖ Nominal group technique
❖ Norms
❖ Open groups
❖ Parallel groups
❖ Parallel process
❖ Process commentary
❖ Supportive cooperative group
❖ Therapeutic activity groups
❖ Third ear
❖ Task roles
❖ Transferential dynamics
❖ Universality

Figure 10.1. Naturally occurring groups form around children's play.

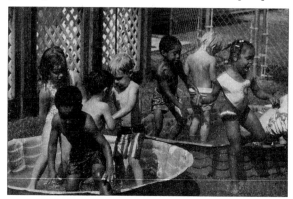

Source. Public Health Image Library, Centers for Disease Control and Prevention. Photo by Jim Gathany.

This chapter discusses the dynamics of therapeutic activity groups. Activity group process is defined, and the key concepts in designing occupation-based therapy groups are covered. These concepts include group development, norms, group membership and roles, levels of group interaction, group decision making, and common group dynamics problems. In addition, strategies are presented on how to become a leader of an occupational therapy group by using self-reflection to learn to both participate in and observe group dynamics.

Also discussed are the therapeutic and curative factors of groups that make the group a meaningful growth-producing experience using activities as therapeutic modalities and how to address common group dynamics problems. Although these concepts are often discussed in relation to verbal group therapies, this chapter explores how they are applied in the context of activity and social participation.

Group Formation

Activities are the building blocks of occupation, and because people are social animals, they naturally form groups to complete activities associated with an occupation. Therefore, the purpose of any group is for people to engage in activities together.

Naturally occurring groups (i.e., groups formed for a particular purpose unique to their environmental context and that function accordingly, such as families or elementary school classes; Figure 10.1) can be *informal* or *formal*. Informal groups often occur spontaneously in settings such as playgrounds, schools, workplaces, religious centers, and health clubs and on the Internet.

Examples of more structured, or formal, groups are families, classrooms, school sports teams, special interest clubs (e.g., chess or gardening), scouting organizations, volunteer community task forces, political action groups, and workplace teams and committees. Many social venues, such as parties, concerts, plays, tours, movies, religious organizations, and sporting events, are examples of large formal groups. These types of groups are often planned by large organizations, well in advance, for the purpose of fundraising or as profit-making business ventures (Figure 10.2).

An increasing number of groups, formal and informal, are Web-based, such as online learning sites, blogs and forums, shopping sites, e-mail groups, and social and personal networks. These virtual groups may not require the face-to-face aspect crucial to some definitions of a *group*. All of these group activities may fall under occupations of social participation, leisure, or work, among others, depending on the design, purpose, and context of the group.

Common to all groups are necessary communication, social, and emotional regulation skills (Ameri-

Figure 10.2. Sometimes groups from to support a cause. After completing a walk for the National Alliance on Mental Illness, group members celebrate their accomplishment with a group photograph.

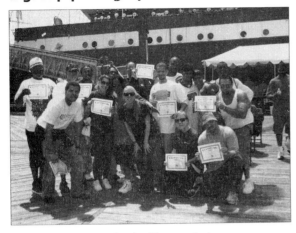

Source. S. White. Used with permission.

can Occupational Therapy Association [AOTA], 2014). In addition, environment, performance context, and cultural considerations are critical to both naturally occurring groups and *therapeutic activity groups,* defined and discussed later. Furthermore, not all groups are formed to produce positive outcomes. Although not a focus of this chapter, "negative" groups such as violent antisocial gangs and organized crime organizations also exist.

Defining Groups in Occupational Therapy

Several useful definitions of *group* are found in the occupational therapy literature. A *group* is "a gathering of three or more people joined together for a joint face-to-face purpose for a continuous period of time" (Donohue & Greer, 2004, p. 226). According to Barbara Posthuma (2002), a *group* is a sum of its parts: a collective of individual persons participating together. Gail Fidler (1969) stated that a *group* is a therapeutic intervention.

Occupational therapy practitioners function as members of many groups in the workplace. Practitioners are often part of a large organization, for example, a school system, hospital, home care agency, or university. They are also part of a smaller group in their occupational therapy department,

and often they are one member of an interdisciplinary team composed of people from several professions. Membership on a committee or task force may be an additional type of group participation in which practitioners engage at work. However, occupational therapy's primary interest in groups, and the engagement in occupations within groups, is their value as an intervention that affects the group members. Thus, knowledge of how to plan and deliver group occupations is critical for all occupational therapy practitioners.

Therapeutic Activity Groups

Therapeutic activity groups are usually planned groups that are held in a particular setting or treatment environment context, designed for a therapeutic purpose with a specific, selected population of participants. An occupational therapy practitioner designs these groups around members' interests, common needs and problem areas, or treatment goals.

Haiman (1989) recommended that in the planning of groups, occupational therapy practitioners consider the demographics of the population being served, the average length of treatment in the group's setting, and other services already available to group members. In addition, practitioners should acknowledge the regulatory and financial constraints of the setting. In some settings, funds are available to purchase supplies to augment the group's purposes; in other settings, the group is mainly verbal, because such funds may not be available.

Haiman provided a four-step process for the clinical decision making that leads to developing a group protocol:

1. Consider the practice model, or frame of reference, that will provide guidance for how to conceptualize what problems the group will address and how.
2. Identify what specific information is necessary to know about the potential members of the group.
3. Conduct a program assessment to identify the setting's existing services so that the new group can provide services not currently offered in the setting.
4. Prepare or design an appropriate protocol for the group.

Occupational therapy practitioners typically name their groups after the primary activity that will be used therapeutically or the performance skills that will be enhanced during the group treatment sessions. Some common examples of occupational therapy groups are exercise, cooking, and dressing groups in rehabilitation centers. Schools often have gross motor skills and sensory motor skills groups. Community day treatment programs frequently use budgeting, wellness, and stress management groups. Some settings include assessment or evaluation groups and treatment groups. Participation in an activity group is most often voluntary but may sometimes be required as part of an intervention plan or program.

Typically, one or two practitioners, who are the designated group leaders, lead occupational therapy groups. Groups consist of 5 to 10 group members. In the occupational therapy literature, 8 is considered the optimal size for therapy groups (Fidler, 1969), but smaller or larger groups may be designed for specific purposes in various treatment settings. Practitioners might also limit the group size to suit the purpose of the activity, such as a community outing. In this case, the group might be smaller to allow closer supervision. Case Example 10.1 depicts the work of an occupational therapy practitioner with groups in a typical day.

One challenge facing occupational therapy practitioners is that they must design therapy groups that meet the needs, concerns, and intervention goals of both the individual members and the entire group. In addition, according to Donohue and Greer (2004), when providing therapeutic activities, practitioners must attend to five major components:

1. The activity
2. Occupational therapy practitioner's use of self as a leader
3. Group members as participants
4. Group process or interactions
5. Group culture and physical context.

The Activity

In occupational therapy groups, the focus is often primarily on the activity (as opposed to the self, which is the primary focus in psychotherapy and social support groups). This focus on activity stimulates interest and often leads to continued sustained

> ### Case Example 10.1. Yohanan: Mental Health Day Program
>
> **Yohanan is an occupational therapist** in a mental health day program treating adults with chronic mental illness. The clients in the day program have myriad deficits, including in social skills and activities of daily living performance. Yohanan leads 2–3 groups each day that address these deficits, including social skills, cooking skills, problem-solving skills, instrumental activities of daily living skills, exercise, cognitive skills, and a men's mutual support group. Each group takes advantage of group interaction around purposeful activities.

engagement in a meaningful activity (Figure 10.3). Engagement in an activity allows clients to focus on the tasks and to work toward the achievement of successful end results.

Group activities are designed by an occupational therapy practitioner to incorporate individual treatment goals, such as performance skills, including returning to work, computer use, and cooking, while working on performance areas of cognitive, sensory modulation, and communication skills. Group activities also provide a forum for the obser-

Figure 10.3. Group members join together to finish a craft project. Completion requires cooperation and sharing of responsibilities.

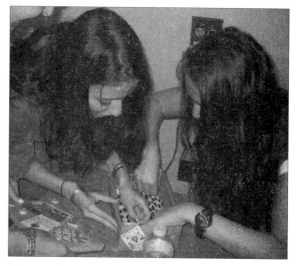

Source. S. White. Used with permission.

vation of a person's behavior in the here and now of the group.

Exercise 10.1. Naturally Occurring Group History

In a group of 3 or 4 students, briefly describe some of the naturally occurring groups in which you participated during early childhood, childhood, adolescence, and young adulthood. Note similarities and differences, including the environmental or cultural context of the groups. Alternatively, interview another student, a neighbor, a friend, or a relative about his or her participation in groups while growing up.

Practitioner's Use of Self as a Leader

When leading a group, the practitioner is the group's planner, convener, and facilitator. Beginning each group with introductions and a clear statement of the group's purpose and goals maximizes its therapeutic potential by encouraging participation in a safe secure environment. The group leader functions as a technical expert and role model for appropriate participation in all group discussions and activities.

Group Process

Group process feedback, although often focused on the activity of the group and participation within the group, also provides the occupational therapy practitioner and other group members with critical opportunities to provide feedback to individual group members. Feedback to individual members and to the group as a whole is usually concrete, task focused, and behavior based, but it may also be about the process observed within the group. Group process feedback is discussed in greater detail later in the chapter.

Group Culture and Physical Context

As groups are formed, they develop their own unique goals and norms. These norms, often facilitated by the practitioner, encourage participants' appropriate interactions and involvement in the activity. The practitioner supports the group by ensuring that group members have adequate meeting space and the materials or supplies needed to engage in the activity.

Exercise 10.2. Relationship of Activity Groups to Areas of Occupation and Performance Skills

For the groups you recalled in Exercise 10.1, delineate the group activities in which you participated, and classify them by the areas of occupation under which they fall. Where possible, also state the performance skills involved in the activities performed in these groups. Prepare to share this information in a group discussion.

Group Development

Many social scientists have studied groups and identified stages in the development of group interaction. This information has been summarized in occupational therapy texts (Cole, 2012; Howe & Schwartzberg, 2001; Posthuma, 2002). Three pioneers in analyzing and articulating phases of *group development* are Bruce Tuckman (1965), Roy Lacoursiere (1980), and William Schutz (1958).

Tuckman (1965) named the stages of group development *forming, storming, norming,* and *performing.* Lacoursiere (1980) labeled these stages *orientation, dissatisfaction, resolution, production,* and *termination.* The stages described by Tuckman and Lacoursiere were given convenient, self-explanatory descriptive names. Each theorist identified an initial formative phase. In the second stage of group development, each articulated a period of turbulence and disagreement, followed by smoother periods during which most of the group's work is accomplished. Schutz (1958) described the stages as *inclusion, control,* and *affection.* During the *inclusion stage,* group members are concerned with acceptance and belonging in the group as it forms. During the *control stage,* group members focus on issues regarding leadership and authority. During the final *affection stage,* group members are primarily concerned with the emotional attachments between members.

Schutz's (1958) theory of group development is innovative because he identified these stages as a cycle that recurs during the life of the group (Posthuma, 2002). At times of stress or crisis in the group, a reversion to one of the earlier group phases (often that of turbulence or control) frequently occurs. Because of these cycles, the group stages can be viewed as moving through phases that recur. In therapy groups that have many members with impaired social skills, it is possible that the turbulent second stage and the camaraderie of the production or affection stages develops slowly or cannot fully develop.

Most authors (e.g., Johnson & Johnson, 2013; Kaplan, 1988) who study group development have now also incorporated Lacoursiere's (1980) idea of a final termination, or adjourning, stage, in which the group moves toward a sense of closure. The termination phase occurs as the group completes its work (e.g., planning a special project), when the allotted number of sessions for the group ends (e.g., the end of a semester or school year), or whenever group leaders or group members change.

Occupational therapy practitioners can organize activities to support and resolve each of the stages. For example, during the forming stage, a practitioner designs activities to build familiarity or rapport among the members. The practitioner can prepare questions related to theme group goals for the members, such as, "What is something you can do that you are proud of?" for a work exploration group. Next, the practitioner divides the group into pairs and gives them questions to discuss and answer with each other. Afterward, the group comes back together and the pairs give summaries of what they learned about the partner. These types of activities allow the group to begin the forming phase of getting to know each other and feeling a sense of belonging to the group as a whole.

The relationship between a group leader and group members evolves with each developmental stage of the group. Early in the group's development, members often demonstrate greater levels of dependence on the leader. At later stages, group members may be very independent. Group members at some point will usually challenge the leadership role, most frequently during the phase of discord in the group's development. Group leader-

---

Exercise 10.3. Identifying Group Stages

Reflect on and briefly describe one team experience or group project in which you have participated. How did the initial forming phase feel? Was there a phase of discord? Did the group achieve a sense of unity and affection as you worked on tasks together? Was there a clear termination phase? Compare your notes with a partner, in a class discussion, or with a supervisor.

---

ship challenges are discussed later in the chapter, along with the practitioner's role in groups, group roles, and common group problems.

Group Norms

In any group involving occupation, rules guide behavior and actions within, and at times outside, the group. These rules of behavior are called *norms*. The institution that the group works within may, in part, hand down the norms of the groups. The group's leaders or the group members generate other norms. In the initial sessions, group norms need to be established. The norms of the greatest importance relate to the safety and dignity of the group members and to the maintenance of the group's cohesion and functioning.

Group norms have a strong influence on shaping group members' behavior (Figure 10.4). One method of ensuring that group norms are established is to explicitly state them. Asking group members to discuss their values helps to clarify and build agreement to accept and follow the norms. Writing and displaying the norms on a bulletin board in the group room helps the group refer back to them if a member questions a norm or a norm needs reinforcement. Important explicit norms usually include respect, confidentiality within the group, active participation, mistakes are okay, and have fun. The need for individual members to be accepted by the group and maintain their membership in the group strengthens the force of norms on shaping behavior and conformity within the group. When membership in the group is very attractive, the group's norms will hold greater influence over the members, as demonstrated in Case Example 10.2.

In occupational therapy groups, certain values are implicit norms. These values include engaging in activities, interdependence, and a client-centered approach to therapeutic relations. The group setting provides an invaluable opportunity for refining members' perceptions of independence. Through collaborative relations with others in groups, the members have the opportunity to realize the existential reality of interdependence, that is, the reality that in human society, people are never completely independent but rather rely on each other for the satisfaction of many of their needs. Therefore, one of the core values of occupational therapy groups is not independence but,

Figure 10.4. Groups have their own norms supporting active participation, acceptance of differences, and having fun.

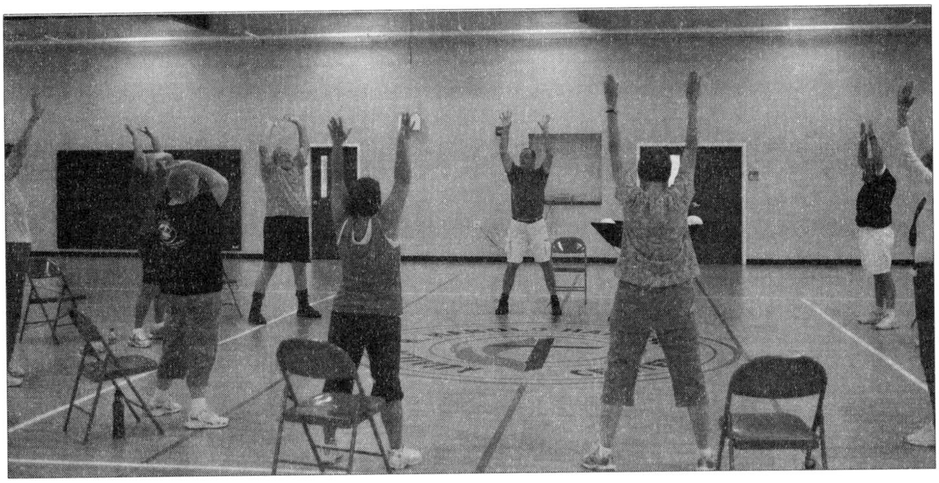

Source. Public Health Image Library, Centers for Disease Control and Prevention. Photo by Amanda Mills.

Case Example 10.2. Christopher: Conduct Disorder

Christopher is a 14-year-old high school freshman with conduct disorder. Christopher is struggling with destructive and attention-seeking impulses that have made it very difficult for him to attend school and participate in classroom activities.

Christopher has been invited to join an after-school group that is coordinated by an occupational therapy assistant. The group uses skateboarding; interactive party video games; and popular music such as house, hip-hop, and reggae to facilitate social interaction among the members. Christopher is immediately very attracted to both the activities and the other members, and he finds himself looking forward to the after-school group. Initially, he dominates materials and attention. Other group members, through both verbal feedback and modeling, give Christopher a clear message about the group's norms regarding respect as demonstrated by sharing and taking turns. Although Christopher struggles to control his impulses, he finds the group very important to him and works harder to follow the group's norms concerning these behaviors.

---

more accurately, successful and balanced interdependence. For group members who may be adjusting to diminished abilities or radically changed life circumstances, this reframing of values is critical.

Practitioner's Role in Groups

Fidler (1969) stated that the overall role of the group leader, in this case the occupational therapy practitioner, is not that of a treatment giver but rather that of an agent in maximizing the group's therapeutic learning potential. The group leader's responsibilities may include the selection of group members, the provision of adequate meeting space and materials, the initial establishment of the goals and norms for the group, and the responsibility to function as a technical expert and a role model for appropriate participation in the group.

Some effective techniques that may be used by the leader to model appropriate group behaviors are self-disclosure ("I wonder if anyone else felt . . ."), self-reflection ("I felt . . . when . . ." "I thought . . ." or "What do you think of Joe's idea?"), and empa-thy (Cole, 2012; Posthuma, 2002). The practitioner's role is to be an effective helper in the group, which Davis (2011) described as facilitating and assisting rather than controlling, using active listening, and using empathy. *Active listening* involves restatement of the problem, a statement of reflection on it, and also a statement clarifying it. *Empathy* is described as listening to others with the *third ear* (Reik, 1948), which is attuned to the feelings of others and the meaning of the feelings for others, so that the leader can describe what it is like to be in the situation of another group member.

A leader and all group members can facilitate development of maturity in groups by attending to and modeling desired member behaviors during group sessions. This modeling of behavior often involves being an active participant rather than a silent observer, giving objective and constructive positive or negative feedback to others, and being receptive to feedback oneself (Cole, 2012; Figure 10.5).

Being an active participant requires the occupational therapy practitioner to exercise good clinical judgment about his or her level of participation. The practitioner needs to be competent in the activity while noticing each member's verbal and nonverbal reaction to the activity and the group. The practi-

Exercise 10.4. Group Leadership

Select 2 or 3 groups you have been a part of, and reflect on the relationship between the group leader and group members. Did this relationship involve the group leader's facilitating and assisting the group members? If not, reflect on the differences in your groups. If you have been a leader in a group, reflect on how you would have incorporated a more facilitating style. Share your thoughts in classroom discussion or with your supervisor.

tioner's participation allows the group members to learn vicariously through him or her. However, the practitioner should not overwhelm the group with skills too sophisticated for the members to copy or get so involved in the activity that he or she forgets to notice the group's reaction.

In groups that use activities, interactions develop around the activities. These interactions occur in behaviors, feelings, and group roles. The three distinct types of roles, each of which may be modeled

Figure 10.5. A group of older adults participate in an activity using a large, multicolored tarpaulin. While engaged in the activity, some participants are more active than others, and each encourages other members to participate.

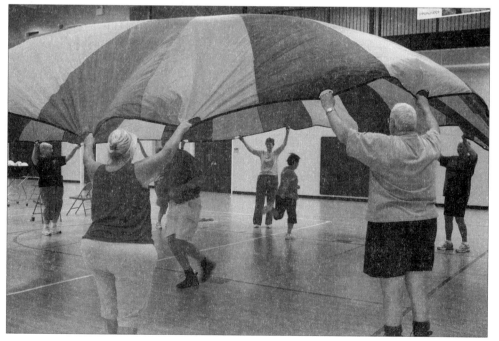

Source. Public Health Image Library, Centers for Disease Control and Prevention. Photo by Amanda Mills.

Figure 10.6. A group often forms around a common purpose. Here, members who do not know each other sit at a table to discuss and plan a project.

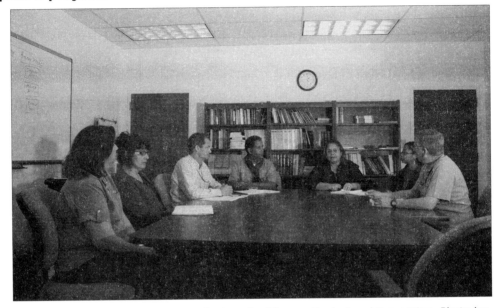

Source. Public Health Image Library, Centers for Disease Control and Prevention. Photo by Amanda Mills.

by the group leader, are discussed in detail later in the chapter (Cole, 2012; Posthuma, 2002).

Group Membership

One of the immediate considerations in planning a group is its membership. In a naturally occurring group, the members select each other. This formation is either through an attraction between the members (i.e., a social desire to spend time together), a perception that the group will help them in some manner, or an attraction to the group's activity. In the latter scenario, members come together out of a shared interest in the activity itself, and most often, group members are drawn together without knowing each other before their participation in the group (Figure 10.6).

Groups may have either formal or informal membership. Many therapy groups are formal in membership: The occupational therapy practitioner or other staff selects the clients, the group recognizes the practitioner or other staff member as the leader, and their participation in the group is formally recognized. In groups with formal membership, norms and expectations about attendance are usually formalized as well. In groups that have

informal membership, such as a cancer survivors' support group, the practitioner allows members to attend or not attend group sessions, as they desire.

In groups that have formal membership, the group may be either closed or open to new members (Case Example 10.3). *Open groups* allow new members to join throughout the group's life span. *Closed groups,* however, begin with a set membership and do not allow any new members to join. A group that is designed so that members acquire new information or skills in a sequential, or developmental, manner, such as an introductory pottery class, may choose a closed format because new members would be entering in the middle of a process and might not fully benefit from the group.

In formal groups, therapists must take into consideration many factors in the selection of the group members, including

- Client's therapy needs and individual goals,
- Whether the client's needs are better served in a group or in individual sessions, and
- The client's ability to participate in groups.

In some settings, the occupational therapist may begin the treatment planning process by collecting data on the service needs of the population in the

Case Example 10.3. Flo: Groups

Flo, an occupational therapy practitioner, leads both a social skills training group and a psychoeducational group, in which she is currently teaching budgeting skills, at a mental health day program. The social skills training group encourages members to bring to each group examples of difficult interpersonal situations that they have encountered since the last group meeting. The group then selects a different social situation, and each member works at mastering communications that are more effective. The format of the group is consistent from week to week; however, the specific content of the group varies and often has little relationship to the prior week's group session.

In the psychoeducational group, Flo is teaching budgeting skills that build developmentally on the content learned from the previous session. In the first group session, the members learned how to keep records of money they spent. In the second session, the members learned how to separate these expenditures into different categories. In the third session, the members learned how to collect the different expenditure categories into fixed monthly expenses and variable expenses.

Any client who asked to join the budgeting skills group at the third session would be at a great disadvantage because he or she would not have learned the content of the previous group sessions. However, the psychoeducational social skills group could function as an open group, admitting new members at any time.

setting and then conducting a needs assessment. The therapist then matches the service needs of the clients with the existing therapy programming and ultimately identifies unmet areas of intervention, which could lead to the planning of new treatment programming, including groups. During this process of identifying unmet treatment needs, the occupational therapist most likely will have identified a potential group of members based on the needs assessment.

One aspect of group membership that occupational therapists need to consider is homogeneous versus heterogeneous group composition. *Homogeneous group composition* means that certain relevant qualities of the group members are the same or very similar (e.g., a particular condition). *Heterogeneous group composition* means that certain identified qualities of the group members are substantially different. The relevant qualities or client factors to consider for homogeneity in groups may include age, gender, education, level of experience in an occupation, common treatment problems and goals, medical condition, or level of functioning.

Both types of group composition have advantages and disadvantages. In a more homogeneous group, members may be better able to identify with each other and develop group cohesion quickly, so that group tasks are more readily accomplished. Heterogeneous groups, however, provide a variety of experiences, knowledge, and unique contributions that a practitioner can use to stimulate the group and may provide a richer problem-solving base when difficulties in task performance or other conflicts arise.

Another important consideration for the occupational therapy practitioner is what the number of clients should be to provide the most appropriate group experience. For many occupational therapy groups, 6–8 members is considered optimal. In psychoeducational groups, in which more of a classroomlike process exists, the group may be much larger and still work successfully. The practitioner should take into consideration how much assistance the members may need during tasks and the nature of the activity to engage an adequate number of members in relation to the number of group leaders.

Member Roles

In groups, members will assume different *behavioral roles,* or patterns of behavior, as a result of their character and individual needs or of the group's dynamic pressures and demands. This process of assuming a certain role or roles in a group usually occurs without the members' awareness. Benne and Sheats (1948) set forth a long list of the roles that frequently occur in groups. More recently, three main types of roles have been identified—(1) task roles, (2) group building and maintenance roles, and (3) individual roles (Cole, 2012; Posthuma, 2002).

Task roles relate to facilitating completion of the group's tasks:

- *Initiator–contributor.* Helps provide initiative in the group, suggests new ideas, and contributes frequently
- *Information seeker.* Often asks for information from others in the group
- *Information giver.* Frequently provides information to the group
- *Opinion seeker.* Often solicits opinions from other group members
- *Opinion giver.* Frequently expresses his or her own opinions and beliefs
- *Elaborator.* Often further explains a point made by another member of the group
- *Coordinator.* Organizes information, plans, and events for the group
- *Orienter.* Summarizes to help keep the group organized and points out when the group strays from its original focus
- *Evaluator–critic.* Provides judgmental feedback to the group or its members
- *Energizer.* Provides encouragement or a boost to help the group move forward with tasks
- *Procedural technician.* Provides detailed information about how to get tasks done and may give out task supplies
- *Recorder.* Keeps notes or records of events in the group, either in writing or by memory.

Group building and maintenance roles focus on the functioning of the group process:

- *Encourager.* Provides verbal encouragement and support to group members
- *Harmonizer.* Tries to smooth over conflicts in groups and maintain peace
- *Compromiser.* Gives up a position or power to help resolve group conflict
- *Gatekeeper–expediter.* Facilitates communication between members
- *Standard setter.* Communicates standards for performance in the group
- *Observer–commentator.* Makes comments on observations of events in the group
- *Follower.* More passive than the other members and goes along with group decisions.

Individual roles focus on the individual members and their own issues and needs; these roles frequently disrupt or impede progress with the group:

- *Aggressor.* Forceful and outspoken in the group, often to the detriment of others or to the group
- *Blocker.* Frequently raises negative objections, opposition, or obstacles to group movement or group efforts
- *Recognition seeker.* Frequently acts in ways that draw attention to himself or herself
- *Self-confessor.* Uses the group to get personal issues off his or her chest
- *Playboy or playgirl.* Stays on the periphery of the group; offers little to the group, as if above or different from the rest of the group; and often jokes off topic
- *Dominator.* Often tries to control the events or members in the group
- *Arguer.* Frequently takes an opposing viewpoint for the purpose of disagreement to continue group discussion; may plead special interests or causes.

Roles are not mutually exclusive. Members may take on multiple roles within the group, either simultaneously or on an alternating basis. One group member may be both an information giver and an information seeker (task roles), a harmonizer (group building and maintenance role), and occasionally a self-confessor (individual role).

Communication within the group may be enhanced or disrupted by the roles individual group members take on during the group's activity performance. In the following sections, we expand on group interaction and communication.

Levels of Group Interaction

Occupational therapy practitioners consider interaction skills in relation to activity groups in occupational therapy. Donohue (2003, 2005, 2006, 2013; Donohue, Hanif, & Wu Berns, 2011) expanded the original work of Mosey (1970) and Parten (1932) to describe five levels of *developmental groups* that Mosey proposed assist a person in developing group interaction skills in a sequential manner. These group levels can also be used as a framework by which the relative maturity of a group's interaction may be gauged (Mosey, 1970). Thus, developmental groups can serve as a structure for creating, organizing, and understanding the social interaction skills in other types of activity groups as well. The five group levels are (1) parallel, (2) associative, (3) basic cooperative, (4) supportive cooperative, and (5) mature; they are listed in order from the simplest level to the highest level of interaction among group members. In this framework, the role of the leader and interactions with the leader are considered.

In *parallel groups,* minimal conversation and minimal sharing of activities occur, so the occupational therapy practitioner encourages and reinforces appropriate behaviors and social interactions. An example of this type of group is a wellness chair yoga group. *Associative groups* have brief shared interaction and cooperation among members; therefore, the practitioner sets up, encourages, and reinforces social interaction and sharing of tasks. An example of this type of group is a leisure exploration, playing a game of tag. In *basic cooperative groups,* members are beginning to engage in joint decision making and interact with others with more social awareness, so the practitioner encourages group problem solving. An example of this type of group is a leisure activity, playing Jenga group (a game in which each person takes a turn from removing a block from a tower of blocks and places it on the top).

Supportive cooperative group members share ideas and feelings and are able to fulfill one another's interaction needs; however, the activity becomes secondary to these group members, so the practitioner is an advisor and coparticipant in the group. An example of this type of group is a women's group. In *mature groups,* members take on a variety of roles, and a balance exists between the activity and member satisfaction. Therefore, the practitioner functions simply as a group member and provides mutual reinforcement of appropriate behavior within the group. An example of this type of group is a community government group.

Using this framework in occupational therapy groups, group members' interaction abilities and limitations are matched with the leader's design for purposeful activities. Usually, groups do not operate on one level of developmental interaction within the session. When two levels are in operation, the occupational therapy practitioner can encourage the subgroup operating at the lower developmental level to model the behavior of peers operating at a higher level. The practitioner can reinforce the higher level peer functional participa-

tion skills by pointing out their positive results or asking them to help the lower functioning member. These bilevel groups then offer a spectrum of levels of participation.

In addition to providing the basis for a session, the levels can be used to organize weekly programming, especially on a short-term unit with rapid turnover. For example, Monday's schedule has mainly parallel focus groups. As the week goes by, stages of higher-level groups are part of the program design. By Friday, a practitioner can design a mature group such as a weekend planning group, knowing the members have the interaction skills needed to follow through on independent purposeful activities, such as a Saturday night movie and pizza party.

Exercise 10.5. Developmental Groups and Levels of Communication

From your own experience of participating in groups, find examples of each of Donohue's (2003, 2005, 2006, Donohue et al., 2011) developmental group types. Identify the levels of communication most often used in each group type. Compare your findings in a group discussion.

Group Process

The structure, task behaviors, and process of the group are three intertwining aspects of an activity group (Posthuma, 2002). Occupational therapy practitioners must be aware of many phenomena that exist in any group that interacts around a task. The first and most obvious element of this interaction is the content of the communication—the objective or factual record of what is stated between members of the group. The second set of phenomena that requires attention is the process of group communications—how events unfold in the group and what unspoken meaning these events may have.

Process Content

Process considerations include questions such as "Who made the statement?" "To whom was the statement made?" "What was the timing of the communication?" "What was the tone of the communication?" and "What could be a manifest reason for the communication?"

Therapists who are process-oriented are concerned not primarily with the verbal content of a patient's utterance, but with the "how" and the "why" of that utterance, especially insofar as the how and the why illuminate aspects of the patient's relationship to other people. Thus, therapists focus on the meta-communication aspects of the message and wonder why, from the relationship aspect, a patient makes a statement at a certain time in a certain manner to a certain person. (Yalom, 1995, p. 131)

The occupational therapy practitioner's interest in the group process includes an understanding of the dynamics of the group, how it evolves and responds, and its structure. Beyond the communication process between group members, the practitioner is concerned with the effect of the activity demands on the process of the group. In other words, How do the activity demands of the group's occupation affect communication? Does the activity facilitate or even require communication? How much communication? What style of communication? How frequent? Does the task require collaboration? Do the group's activity demands require communication and collaboration only at the beginning of the activity or during several steps of the activity?

In addition to imposing communication demands on the members, the inherent qualities of some activities will also elicit different member behaviors, such as quiet individual parallel performance, serious outcome-driven team collaboration, or loose and boisterous play.

Process Commentary

The literature on group process is focused mostly on psychotherapy groups and groups in which verbal interaction is the primary or sole group activity. In psychotherapy groups, a technique called *process commentary* is a central therapeutic intervention that involves the giving of immediate feedback to the group on its current group process. The group leader uses process commentary to help group members develop better insight and understanding of manifest behaviors. Initially, the group leader introduces the technique of process commentary to the group by stopping the current group activity and making comments about what seems to be occurring. Even-

tually, clients may contribute to this effort to gain insight by offering their own comments on what seems to be happening in the group.

Process commentary is not a natural social behavior in most groups. In ordinary social groups, members do not normally make comments on the group's process and underlying events. Occupational therapy practitioners involved in facilitating natural activity groups in more natural contexts may find process commentary inappropriate to the group type or group setting. In many occupational therapy groups, however, process commentary is a critical and fundamental therapeutic technique.

Yalom (1995) gives process commentary a primacy in interpersonal psychotherapy groups:

Process is not just one of many possible procedural orientations; on the contrary, it is indispensable and a common denominator to all effective interactional groups. . . . A process focus is the one truly unique feature of the experiential group . . . where else is it permissible, in fact encouraged, to comment, in depth, on the here-and-now behavior, on the nature of the immediately current relationship between people? (p. 137)

When does the occupational therapy practitioner use process commentary? In many types of groups engaged in occupations, the practitioner judiciously uses process commentary as an intervention strategy. The therapist may determine that the activity demands, communications, and relationships that evolve around the activity are therapeutic in themselves.

In some group scenarios, the members of the group may not have the capacity to use or benefit from such an insight-oriented metacognitive task as process commentary. Process illumination may raise group members' anxiety levels, initially cause some confusion, or be met with some resistance from group members. With some populations who respond to stress poorly or in a nonadaptive manner, this type of intervention may not be indicated.

In addition, during the early stages of group formation and development, members may not be ready for the task of receiving and considering process comments. As the group becomes comfortable with process commentary and experiences, members may eventually welcome this exercise and benefit from this intervention, and the members may even occasionally initiate their own process.

In some instances, the occupational therapy practitioner may conclude that the group members can benefit from process commentary. When group members have the cognitive ability to reflect on the events within the group and the psychological ability to tolerate some anxiety created by the reflection on members' actions, the members may develop further understanding or insight. Process commentary should not be the primary tool of occupational therapy groups, but rather one of many potential tools the practitioner might use to maximize the members' learning from an activity. Taylor (2008), in discussing the therapeutic intentional relationship in occupational therapy, recommended that practitioners balance the group's "activity focus" with an "interpersonal focus." Indeed, the activity itself may be the focus of the process commentary. What kind of reaction has the activity stimulated in the group members? What have they learned in the process of doing the activity with others in the group?

Occupational therapy practitioners may use process comments at any point during group activities. When the practitioner introduces process comments during the activity, the activity is usually stopped. The comment may be made during the activity when a problem has arisen or when an important event has occurred in group relations and communications. Conversely, the practitioner may find that the activity is proceeding smoothly and that stopping the group to make comments would be disruptive. In this case, the practitioner may decide to wait until the end of the session to comment. The practitioner must then leave adequate time at the end for group members to respond to and discuss his or her comments.

Interpretation

Another intervention that an occupational therapy practitioner may use in groups is interpretation. *Interpretation* is the group leader's offering of an understanding or insight that he or she has reached during the group activity or the interactions around the activity. The practitioner usually presents interpretations to group members as a hypothesis in the form of a question or statement.

For example, "It seemed to me that some people in the group were a little frustrated with the shortage of materials needed to complete the job." Inter-

pretations offered in this form encourage members to reflect on the statement made by the practitioner and allows those unprepared for the content of the interpretation to reject the hypothesis at that time. For the practitioner, the rejection of an interpretation may either mean that the practitioner was wrong in his or her conclusion or that group members may not have reached the same awareness or acceptance of the information in the content of the interpretation. Again, as with process commentary, the use of interpretation as a therapeutic intervention in activity groups must be preceded by a careful evaluation of the group members' cognitive and psychological capacity to respond effectively to the technique.

Group Decision Making

Any group that is involved in occupations will have to make decisions, including what occupation to select. Other decisions regarding occupation may include time, place, materials, procedures, division of labor, roles, and the projected outcome. The occupational therapy practitioner may have to make early formative group decisions. For example, he or she may make decisions about a therapy group's purpose and membership criteria even before group members are identified.

The process by which the group makes decisions can itself be an important therapeutic modality. Who will assume leadership roles in the occupation? How will group members be involved in decisions? Providing group members with an opportunity to resolve these decisions, whether individually or as a group, can offer an excellent opportunity for personal growth. Johnson and Johnson (2013) listed seven methods for group decision making:

1. Decision by authority without discussion
2. Decision by authority after discussion
3. Identification of an expert member who leads the group decision
4. Identification of an average of the members' opinions
5. Decision by a minority of the group
6. Democratic decision—a majority of the group by vote
7. Consensus.

Another form of decision making, similar to the democratic decision, is the supermajority (two-thirds) vote. This approach helps to empower the subgroups that tend to be in the minority in many of the group's decisions and requires the group to discuss a matter and negotiate long enough to build a larger subgroup of support for a position.

It is well understood that member involvement in group decisions improves interest and motivation to actively participate in the group activity. It also helps members to feel that they are part of the group, enhancing their sense of affiliation and thereby improving group cohesion. In addition, involving group members in the decision-making process improves the amount and quality of information included in the final decision; each member brings a unique combination of knowledge and experience to the group. Groups that are more heterogeneous in background and experience have the advantage of a broader knowledge base for group decision making. The collective knowledge of the group, and the diversity of that knowledge, is one of the group's main assets and should be used when making group decisions.

Throughout the course of a group, the group leader must make careful decisions concerning when it is appropriate for group problems and decisions to be delegated to the group. Although the democratic process of voting to make group decisions may seem to make the most logical sense, scholars of democratic government have talked at length about the tyranny of the majority—the concern that members of a group who find themselves in the minority on repeated votes or on key issues may feel estranged or disenfranchised from the group. Whenever a group uses votes to reach group decisions, the group leader should be actively concerned about the impact that the voting process will have on group cohesion and membership. In fact, the group leader may find that even when the group uses voting for some decisions, other decisions central to individual rights and membership must be made by consensus, as demonstrated in Case Example 10.4.

Group decision making by consensus is often considered the gold standard, because all members have, by definition, reached agreement on a decision, and the estrangement of group members is therefore avoided. However, decision making by consensus is often a very lengthy, deliberative process that requires extensive collaboration and compromise, and even conflict resolution, between and among members or subgroups. When a group decision has to be reached in a timely manner, a consensus pro-

---

Case Example 10.4. Carla: Group Decision Making

Carla, an occupational therapist leading a group in a day program for elderly people, found that the members often disagreed on many matters they had to decide. Many of these decisions seemed rather simple and could have been easily made by herself, for example, what activities the group would engage in at the next session. Presenting each decision to the group, however, provided the members with an opportunity to discuss the matter and develop stronger relationships within the group, as well as feel more ownership for the group's activities.

Then a subgroup of women in the group expressed the idea that the group was involved more in female gender–related activities and felt that the minority subgroup of male members might be more comfortable with forming a separate group to pursue activities that were more related to their gender. One more vocal female member suggested that this issue be put to a vote. Carla suggested that this was a very important issue and should be discussed further and decided by full consensus because any of the individual male members might feel a strong affiliation with the group and choose not to leave. In addition, Carla recognized that there might be some underlying gender relationship issues that should be explored and discussed further.

---

cess may not be feasible. Many decisions may not practically be reached by consensus, particularly in larger groups. On more serious or controversial issues, true consensus decision making in which all members in a group agree may be rare.

A group's effectiveness in decision making is, of course, dependent on the quality of the group's overall functioning. Very large groups might find that consistent involvement of all members in all decisions is too cumbersome and difficult. In these instances, delegating certain decisions and responsibilities to a committee or subgroup may be a more appropriate use of time and resources. Groups that are experiencing repeated or extreme conflict around an issue at hand, or around other issues, will usually have difficulty with the decision-making process. At such a time, the occupational therapy practitioner must make a thorough assessment of the nature of the conflict and the group's process and development. Any thoughts about changing the group's method for making decisions must be given careful consideration. Another important aspect of group decision making is the client factors supplied by the members. For example, the capacity for clients to participate cognitively in decisions varies. Groups that have members with cognitive impairments may depend on many decisions made at an authority level by the group leader.

Group Problem Solving

For a group to creatively solve a problem, the steps taken must be followed within a very cooperative group context. The group should be supportive and not overly pressured. If group members feel threatened or not supported, they will be less likely to take risks with creative suggestions. Diverse viewpoints and suggestions must be encouraged. Controversy and debate must be allowed, supported, and tolerated. Finally, the group must be allotted appropriate time to reflect on the diverse ideas developed in the group.

Group engagement in decision making is an excellent opportunity for teaching and modeling effective problem solving because it parallels individual problem solving. The occupational therapy practitioner can lead the group through the five steps of problem solving:

1. Clearly identifying the problem and its implications
2. Brainstorming potential actions or solutions
3. Assessing different possible solutions
4. Selecting the solution
5. Implementing the solution and reassessing.

A stated norm for the group that allows for further interaction is when any member has the right to veto a project if they hate it. This norm allows for a more positive attitude toward less-valued projects (i.e., the client knows that he or she will not be forced to follow through with a project just because the group discusses it) and provides an escape if the project is abhorrent to the client (e.g., a client with anorexia who does not want to engage in food preparation). Consensus can be more easily reached by eliminating the "hated" project, the unanimous consensus for one project, and a popularity vote among several projects.

Nominal (i.e., in name only) *group technique* is a structured variation of a large-group discussion to reach consensus. The technique considers the natural tendency to follow *group thinking,* which is a group norm that militates against critical thinking. It prevents domination of the discussion by a single person, encourages all group members to participate, and results in a set of prioritized solutions or recommendations that represent the group's preferences. By having the group members write their answers first, natural bias is diminished. It allows for a greater diversity of concerns to be raised and for the group to get a broader view of the issues and allow for all the members' opinions to be stated. The following is the four-step process to conduct nominal group technique (Centers for Disease Control and Prevention, 2006):

1. *Generating ideas.* The leader presents the question or problem to the group in written form and reads the question to the group. The leader directs everyone to write ideas in brief phrases or statements and to work silently and independently. Each person silently generates ideas and writes them down.
2. *Recording ideas.* Group members engage in a round-robin feedback session to concisely record each idea (without debate at this point). The leader writes an idea from a group member on a flip chart that is visible to the entire group and proceeds to ask for another idea from the next group member, and so on. There is no need to repeat ideas; however, if group members believe that an idea provides a different emphasis or variation, they can include it. The process continues until all members' ideas have been documented.
3. *Discussing ideas.* Each recorded idea is discussed to determine clarity and importance. For each idea, the leader asks, "Are there any questions or comments group members would like to make about the item?" This step provides an opportunity for members to express their understanding of the logic and the relative importance of the item. The creator of the idea need not feel obliged to clarify or explain the item; any member of the group can play that role.

4. *Voting on ideas.* Each member of the group votes privately to prioritize the ideas. The votes are tallied to identify the ideas that are rated highest by the group as a whole. The leader establishes what criteria are used to prioritize the ideas. To start, each group member selects the most important items from the group list and writes one idea on each index card. Next, each member ranks the five ideas selected, with the most important receiving a rank of 5, and the least important receiving a rank of 1.

After members rank their responses in order of priority, the leader creates a tally sheet on the flip chart with numbers down the left-hand side of the chart, which correspond to the ideas from the round-robin. The leader collects all the cards from the participants and asks one group member to read the idea number and number of points allocated to each one, while the leader records and then adds the scores on the tally sheet. The ideas that are the most highly rated by the group are the most favored group actions or ideas in response to the question posed by the leader.

Therapeutic Factors

A variety of processes inherent to working in a group foster learning, growth, and development for individual group members. Yalom (1995) described 11 of these therapeutic factors that make group membership and group treatment so potentially powerful, efficient, and dynamic:

1. Instillation of hope
2. Universality
3. Imparting information
4. Altruism
5. Corrective recapitulation of the primary family group
6. Development of socializing techniques
7. Imitative behavior
8. Interpersonal learning
9. Group cohesiveness
10. Catharsis
11. Existential factors.

In addition to Yalom's list, we have added two more therapeutic factors that are specific to groups that use an occupation or a specific activity:

12. Effectance (Schwartzberg, Howe, & Barnes, 2008; White, 1959, 1971)
13. Experiential learning (Schwartzberg et al., 2008).

Instillation of Hope

Groups provide mutual support and assistance that inspire hope in their members. Members often find hope in observing other group members with similar problems who have made progress. Yalom (1995) recommended that group leaders capitalize on this dynamic by pointing out members' progress or achievements. Member performance during an activity in the group is an excellent opportunity to demonstrate actual progress and surreptitiously instill the hope in other group members that they may achieve the same progress.

Universality

Universality is consensual validation, which can be very comforting to group members and may foster feelings of connection. Many people come to groups feeling isolated and different from others because of an illness, disability, or unique set of life problems. Even though a person may have some knowledge of stories and demographics of others in similar situations, the group experience delivers this information in a more intimate and personal format. When group members can directly hear, or more importantly, see, other group members with similar problems struggle with an activity, they may realize they are not alone in this experience. They may also see that others with similar problems are progressing.

Imparting Information

The group is a natural context for imparting information by both group leaders and group members. Group leaders, including occupational therapy practitioners, are a great source of information. They may have added experience or educational resources to which the members have not yet had access. However, one potential pitfall arises when the group leader is identified as an expert. In groups in which people are struggling with disability and dependency on others, the group expert may encourage or prolong that dependency role, which may in turn stunt the group's development. In addition, the establishment of the group leader as an expert risks creating an informational orthodoxy that prevents the introduction of alternative views or suggestions.

Group members should thus be acknowledged as invaluable sources of information. In the early stages of group development, when the members first assume that the occupational therapy practitioner or group leader will simply deliver the information and resources necessary for the group, group members may not recognize that they themselves may hold most of the information and resources needed to accomplish the group's tasks. The group may slowly begin to realize its own potential, a process that may need to be facilitated by the group leader.

This process begins with the group leader's genuinely acknowledging each group member's unique value and imparting this information to the group. In addition, the group leader can take a Socratic approach to facilitate information sharing and establish that as a collective, the group has extensive knowledge. Using this method, the group leader asks group members carefully formed questions that allow the group to reveal its knowledge.

This approach goes against an assumption often manifest in group members that the occupational therapy practitioner or group leader is the expert and that they are in attendance to learn from the leader. The group members indeed begin to realize that they can learn from each other. This realization of group efficacy promotes group development toward more advanced levels of functioning and encourages group therapeutic factors. The realization that group members can learn from each other may also dispel assumptions that practitioners and members have about disability and knowledge.

Altruism

Group endeavors in occupations and specific activities provide repeated opportunities for members to assist each other and experience *altruism* (i.e., helping others with no regard to personal benefit). During this process, members may experience giving and receiving firsthand. The very act of helping others can be cathartic and often motivates the giver toward further development of interpersonal relationship skills.

Corrective Recapitulation of the Primary Family Group

Therapists believe that some group experiences can be seen by the members as a recreation of one's own family of orientation. The family is the first social group to which a person belongs. The person's experiences in this group, both positive and negative, shape cognitive and emotional schemas and thus influence his or her perceptions, understanding, and responses in all subsequent social groups.

Although occupational therapy groups are not usually intensive interpersonal experiences designed to foster *transferential dynamics* (which are redirections of feelings and ideas from childhood toward another object or therapist), an activity group provides opportunities for some members to re-experience the patterns of behavior and interpersonal interactions they had in previous relationships. A skilled occupational therapy practitioner recognizes these transferences as opportunities for group members to develop awareness of and reflect on these patterns, gain insight into the meanings within these patterns, and work eventually to correct maladaptive responses or develop more adaptive responses.

Development of Socializing Techniques

The group, especially when engaged in an occupation or a specific activity, provides a rich laboratory for members to develop interpersonal skills, that is, improve social skills. For members who are extremely anxious in social situations, involvement in the occupation or activity offers an opportunity to divert the focus away from the face-to-face eye contact and social demands of reciprocal verbal exchange. The task focus provides a natural reason for interpersonal interaction, and verbal responses can take place within the context and experience of the task (Figure 10.7).

Imitative Behavior

The activity group provides a natural context for members to practice *imitative behavior,* that is, mimicking the actions of others, by observing both communication and performance skills of other group members. It offers repeated opportunities for members to practice new behaviors and enhance

Figure 10.7. During a fun activity, group members respond to each other while focusing on their own actions.

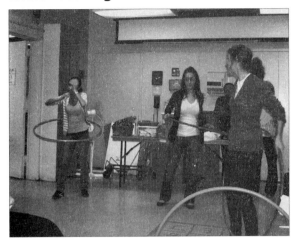

Source. K. Buckley. Used with permission.

their social perceptions, thereby shaping and increasing each member's repertoire of behaviors.

Interpersonal Learning

Social groups provide opportunities for members to learn about themselves through interactions with others, or *interpersonal learning*. Activity groups add another dimension to interpersonal learning through the shared experience of performing an activity. Through collaboration and interdependence while working on an activity, activity group members can learn much more about group productivity and their relations with others (in the group) compared with members of a social group.

Group Cohesion

Although group cohesion is a therapeutic factor, it is also a critical aspect during the forming or orientation stage of group development and essential to group function during later stages of conflict. *Group cohesion* is the extent to which members feel connected to each other and feel a bond with the group as a whole. Cohesion reflects the quality of the individual member's relationship with the group. Group cohesiveness is an essential underpinning for sustaining membership when problems or conflicts arise and a critical foundation for the effective operation of many other therapeutic factors.

Catharsis

The group can provide stimuli for *catharsis* (i.e., working through feelings) for its members. Such stimuli may include the recapitulation of previous relationships, which leads to the expression of deeply held feelings about previous life events and current events within the group.

Existential Factors

When Yalom (1995) added *existential factors,* he suggested that the group provides opportunities for its members to identify core life issues that have more meaning and relevance than day-to-day trivialities. Thus, members learn that they are ultimately responsible for how they live out their lives.

Effectance

Effectance is the idea that people are naturally drawn toward activity. Therefore, the availability of the opportunity to participate in activity is in itself strongly self-motivating (Schwartzberg et al., 2008; White, 1959, 1971).

Experiential Learning

Effective learning often takes place through actual "doing" rather than through reading about or attending a lecture about an activity. In groups in which members participate in occupations and specific activities, the group provides not only opportunities for learning social skills but also a forum for learning about occupation through interaction with the activity. These activities provide members with safe, supported opportunities to explore occupation, interact with the materials and particular qualities of activities, and realize their own interests and the other individual client factors that affect performance (Schwartzberg et al., 2008).

When a group member engages in an occupation as part of a group, he or she is participating voluntarily in accomplishing something that he or she finds meaningful and that is socioculturally relevant. Participation is personally fulfilling and is grounded in place, social group, and cultural meaning (Pierce, 2001).

Therapeutic Factors Summary

Groups engaged in occupation may include any of the therapeutic factors, although those involving more intensive psychodynamic processes, such as recapitulation of the family or catharsis, are less likely to be operative in occupation-focused groups. The immense potential power of group treatment is largely the result of therapeutic factors, whether in a psychodynamic group or a task group.

Occupational Therapy Task Groups

The history of the focus on occupational therapy task groups can be traced back to its roots in the *moral treatment movement* of the 1830s, when groups of people worked together on particular activities that were important to maintaining their community. By the mid-20th century, occupational therapy recognized the importance of socialization and group process in task groups. Group cohesiveness is now believed to be needed for effective treatment using activities in groups (Howe & Schwartzberg, 2001).

Fidler (1969) posited that occupational therapy task groups consist of "active involvement in doing." Her seminal article described the relationship among feelings, thoughts, actions, and group task performance creating excellent learning opportunities. For example, task groups can be structured to allow sharing of responsibilities and accomplishments, behavioral trial and error, problem solving, and feedback on actions within the group.

Task groups can also be structured for gradation of engagement in concrete social interactions; new learning; engagement with nonhuman objects and the environment; and sheltered opportunities for reality testing of behaviors, actions, feelings, and perceptions of both self and others (Fidler, 1969). Group members become aware of their limitations and abilities and develop their functional capacities through concrete, reality-based task achievement.

Cole (2012) outlined a seven-step format for organizing the structure of an occupational therapy task group (Exhibit 10.1). This format allows the leader and the clients to have the full benefit of the therapeutic group process. Because occupational therapy uses everyday activities as the source of therapy, clients often only see the con-crete aspect of the group activity (e.g., the steps taken to make an origami crane). Clients usually do not see the more abstract opportunity to measure behavioral change, such as the depressed person's ability to concentrate better, or to create symptom relief as a result of attention being diverted from a problem and directed toward active engagement in a task.

Cole's format begins with the occupational therapy practitioner briefly introducing himself or herself and the group members, and stating the therapeutic goal of the session task. The activity, which is the main part of the session, is then introduced. Here, the practitioner uses his or her knowledge of task analysis and synthesis, environmental adaptation, and therapeutic use of self, among other factors, in designing this task portion of the session to maximize the therapeutic value.

During processing, clients share their own work and experience with each other. They are then given the opportunity to reflect on how effectively they work together and the value of doing tasks with or in the presence of others. They are asked to reflect on any feelings that the activity may have evoked in them. Did those feelings support or interfere with the client's functioning or the overall functioning of the group?

The ultimate goal of the task group is to generalize the session to everyday life and increase function outside the treatment setting. This goal is accomplished by summarizing the session with a mental review in which everyone thinks back to what has happened and summing up how the session met the goal. The review encourages home-

---

Exercise 10.6. Formulating an Occupational Therapy Group Protocol

Design an occupational therapy task group. Succinctly state the name of the group, incorporating occupational therapy into the title; describe the population for which the group is designed; describe group membership; state the group's purpose; list group goals (2 short-term goals matched with 2 long-term goals); briefly list the group activity procedures (for an activity to be performed in 1 group session); specify requirements for space, supplies, equipment, and cost; and list any references or sources needed for the creation of the group.

Exhibit 10.1. Cole's 7-Step Format for Group Leadership

Total group session time is 1 hour.

1. Introduction
20%
- Introduce yourself and members.
- Briefly outline the session and set the mood.
- Warm-up (optional): Short, attention getting, relaxes participants and prepares them for more in-depth group activity.
- Review homework or commitment.
- Introduce the activity, task, and goals for the session.

2. Activity (consider the following when planning the activity)
50%
- Complex process in cooperation.
- Knowledge of each member.
- Diagnosis.
- Strengths and limitations both physical and mental.
- Long- and short-term goals.
- Activity analysis and synthesis.
- Understanding of group dynamics.
- Therapeutic use of self.
- Adaptation of the activity, environment, or self.

3. Sharing
- End products are shared with the group.

4. Processing
- Allow members to share own work and experience.
- Acknowledge members' contributions.
- Reflect on how effectively the members work together.
- What skills are needed to increase function of the group in the future?
- How do members feel about the session?
- Do those feelings support or interfere with the group function?
- Discuss nonverbal aspects observed.
30%
- Any group curative factor?

5. Generalizing
- To everyday life and to increase function outside the treatment setting.

6. Application
- How does what has been learned apply to his or her life?

7. Summary (may be done by group member)
- Mental review of the group to the activity.
- Sum up the "meta issues" or general principles (resemble the original goals).
- Include and allow for the unexpected or unplanned events.
- Prepare for next week by asking for next step in personal goal (homework or commitment).
- End on time.

---

work to be carried out by the group members and use of the lessons learned in this session going forward. Case Example 10.5 describes a task group.

Common Group Problems

Groups provide many therapeutic intervention opportunities for the group leader. Leading groups, however, also presents the occupational therapy practitioner with a unique set of problems. This section provides an overview of some common problems characteristic of and inherent in groups, such as issues with group formation, conflict, decision making, dependency, apathy, and parallel process.

Problems With Group Formation

Many problems can occur with group formation. Such issues can affect group functioning and successful participation in occupations. How are members recruited? The enrollment of inappropriate members can severely affect early group development and functioning and may contribute to serious conflict within the group. Clearly articulating the criteria for group membership, both inclusionary and exclusionary, is critical to prevent such situations. In addition, when enrolling a person in a group, it is essential that the group's purpose and general goals be clearly shared with the potential member. Clients often enter groups because of an interest in being with the group leader

> ## Case Example 10.5. Ruth: Participating in Groups
>
> **Ruth is newly retired** and lives alone, and she keeps very busy with a variety of activities. Her clowning class is her favorite activity. This group meets every other week and shares ideas on costumes, tricks, and antics that are involved in clowning. She finds that participating in these activities with others is very beneficial for her. The clowning class allows Ruth a liberating permission to be playful and spontaneous and have fun. In addition, the group provides her with an opportunity to socialize and form new friendships in her postwork retiree life.

or a particular group member. Members may also be strongly attracted to the group's activity without understanding its therapeutic purpose.

Closely related to the issue of member recruitment is the frequent challenge of activity selection in a heterogeneous group. When a group is formed of members who have a wide variety of individual interests and skills, selecting commonly shared occupations may be difficult. After careful discussion and exploration of different occupations, some groups may conclude that membership must be re-formed around the occupations in which the members can better share participation.

Finally, early in group formation, norms and rules regarding attendance and punctuality must be articulated clearly. Inconsistent attendance sends an unspoken message that the group is not valued and erodes group formation and the development of cohesion. Late arrivals and frequent departures from the group can be very distracting to group members. Although group leaders may negotiate attendance and punctuality rules in some groups, once the rules are set, they should be consistently enforced.

Problems in Group Process

Conflict and decision making

Problems in the group process (e.g., conflict) are often inevitable. As previously discussed, group theorists suggest that conflict is one of the normal stages of group development. Conflict in a group is a natural interpersonal event that provides a therapeutic opportunity for the individual members involved, and for the group as a whole, to learn from the immediate moment and to develop further through successful conflict resolution. Appropriate management of conflict begins before the conflict arises, with successful development of roles, relationships, norms, and cohesion in the group. These elements help prepare the group to weather conflict and maintain a commitment to participation in the group. Rules regarding mutual respect among the members and limits on destructive language and behavior are essential in successful conflict resolution.

Once conflict has occurred, the group leader may have to actively reinforce the rules, especially when conflicts resurface. The group leader should respond positively by suggesting that conflict is natural and offering a constructive opportunity for group development. The group leader should then assist the group in a structured negotiation of the conflict, using the same steps set forth for group decision making. This problem-solving approach includes clear identification of the conflict, recognition of opposing viewpoints, brainstorming for possible solutions, and group selection of a resolution to the conflict.

Dependency

Dependency can also be a difficulty and is a dynamic common to all groups. Dependency can be seen as a developmental phase of the group. As discussed previously with regard to the occupational therapy practitioner's role in the group, the first stage of the group members' development in relation to the group leader is dependence (Posthuma, 2002). The group members feel and enact a dependence on the group leader. Members interact little with the other group members and look only to the leader for direction and answers.

In groups made up of people with disabilities, this stage of group development may be prolonged. The group leader should recognize that this stage is natural but should foster growth toward more functional interdependence. Group members' strengths and abilities should always be considered in the selection of group activities. These assets should be repeatedly recognized and celebrated by the group. The leader should at times redirect questions and requests back to the group members. These techniques will foster experiences within the group in which the members begin to recognize the individual and collective skills that they bring to the group (Posthuma, 2002).

Apathy

Some groups may experience apathy or amotivation. When apathy or amotivation arises, the leader should evaluate whether it is caused by the illness that group members are struggling with, such as depression, negative symptoms of schizophrenia, or residual deficits of brain injury. Apathy or amotivation may also arise from issues such as frustration with an activity in the group, selection of an activity that is not attractive to the group, or anticipation of failing by the group members. Apathy may also arise out of interpersonal conflicts within the group followed by failures at attempts to resolve these conflicts. Groups in which the members experience repeated futility in problem solving have a high potential for apathy. Apathy in the group requires careful assessment by the group leader, along with the selection of strategies that are unique to that situation. For example, changes in the group's activity, with a concomitant infusion of greater energy through the activity, may be helpful in reducing group apathy.

Parallel process

Parallel process, is when group leaders or members interact in a setting other than the activity group. The events and process in one setting can spill over to the other setting. Group leaders, including occupational therapy practitioners, can be affected both positively and negatively by the organizations for which they work. When group leaders experience certain strong dynamics within an organization, it is not unusual for them to carry that experience into their work and even into the activity group. For example, in an organization in which the group leader experiences a hostile work environment and lack of support by a supervisor or coworkers, it would not be unusual for the group leader to come to the group feeling that he or she is not safe or in reasonable control of events. That feeling may be unconsciously transmitted to the group members in a variety of ways.

Parallel process can also occur among group members. Issues that have arisen elsewhere in the treatment milieu or in previous groups may easily spill over into the activity group. Careful evaluation and recognition of these problems are essential. When the group leader brings organizational problems into the group, he or she must recognize it and work to prevent it from occurring again. When the leader recognizes that members are bringing issues into the group from other settings, it should also be confronted. Whenever possible, group members should be encouraged to maintain the boundaries of the group and prevent outside matters from infringing on its tasks. In occupational therapy groups, this encouragement can be especially important for clients who need to develop the ability to focus on an activity and complete it despite the existence of current problems or stressors.

Summary

Therapeutic activity groups present multidimensional opportunities for individual members' interpersonal development and growth during engagement in occupation. Many levels of interpersonal communication, a variety of roles, multiple therapeutic factors, and opportunities for group leadership and decision making are some of the critical areas of learning that are experienced during the complex process of treatment in a therapeutic activity group. Group treatment using occupation can be one of the most efficient and dynamic means of achieving individual goals in many treatment settings.

References

American Occupational Therapy Association. (2014). Occupational therapy framework: Domain and process (3rd ed.). *American Journal of Occupational Therapy, 68*(Suppl. 1), S1–S48. http://dx.doi.org/10.5014/ajot.2014.682006

Benne, K. D., & Sheats, P. (1948). Functional roles of group members. *Journal of Social Issues, 4,* 41–49.

Centers for Disease Control and Prevention. (2006). *Evaluation Briefs: Gaining consensus among stakeholders through the nominal group technique.* Retrieved from http://www.cdc.gov/healthyyouth/evaluation/index.htm

Cole, M. B. (2012). *Group dynamics in occupational therapy: The theoretical basis and practice application of group intervention* (4th ed.). Thorofare, NJ: Slack.

Davis, C. M. (2011). *Patient practitioner interaction: An experiential manual for developing the art of health care* (5th ed.). Thorofare, NJ: Slack.

Donohue, M. V. (2003). Group profile studies with children: Validity and reliability in children's groups. *Occupational Therapy in Mental Health, 19,* 1–23. http://dx.doi.org/10.1300/J004v19n01_01

Donohue, M. V. (2005). Social Profile: Assessment of validity and reliability in children's groups. *Canadian Journal of Occupational Therapy, 72,* 164–175. http://dx.doi.org/10.1177/000841740507200304

Donohue, M. V. (2006). Interrater reliability of the Social Profile: Assessment of community and psychiatric group participation. *Australian Occupational Therapy Journal, 54,* 49–58. http://dx.doi.org/10.1111/j.1440-1630.2006.00622.x

Donohue, M. V. (2013). *Social Profile: Assessment of social participation in children, adolescents, and adults.* Bethesda, MD: AOTA Press.

Donohue, M., & Greer, E. (2004). Designing group activities to meet individual and group goals. In J. Hinojosa & M. Blount (Eds.), *The texture of life: Purposeful activities in occupational therapy* (2nd ed., pp. 226–261). Bethesda, MD: AOTA Press.

Donohue, M. V., Hanif, H., & Wu Berns, L. (2011). An exploratory study of social participation in occupational therapy groups. *Mental Health Special Interest Section Quarterly, 34,* 1–3.

Fidler, G. S. (1969). The task-oriented group as a context for treatment. *American Journal of Occupational Therapy, 23,* 43–48.

Haiman, S. (1989). Selecting group protocols: Recipe or reasoning. *Occupational Therapy in Mental Health, 9*(4), 1–14. http://dx.doi.org/10.1300/J004v09n04_01

Howe, M. C., & Schwartzberg, S. L. (2001). *A functional approach to group work in occupational therapy* (3rd ed.). Philadelphia: Lippincott.

Johnson, D. W., & Johnson, F. P. (2013). *Joining together: Group theory and group skills* (11th ed.). Upper Saddle River, NJ: Pearson Education.

Kaplan, K. L. (1988) *Directive group therapy: Innovative mental health treatment.* Thorofare, NJ: Slack.

Lacoursiere, R. (1980). *The life cycle of groups.* New York: Human Sciences Press.

Mosey, A. C. (1970). The concept and use of developmental groups. *American Journal of Occupational Therapy, 24,* 272–275.

Parten, M. (1932). Social participation among preschool children. *Journal of Abnormal and Social Psychology, 28,* 136–147. http://dx.doi.org/10.1037/h0074524

Pierce, D. (2001). Untangling occupation and activity. *American Journal of Occupational Therapy, 55,* 138–146. http://dx.doi.org/10.5014/ajot.55.2.138

Posthuma, B. H. (2002). *Small groups in counseling and therapy* (4th ed.). Boston: Allyn & Bacon.

Reik, T. (1948). *Listening with the third ear: The inner experience of a psychoanalyst.* New York: Grove Press.

Schutz, W. (1958). The interpersonal underworld. *Harvard Business Review, 36,* 123–135.

Schwartzberg, S. L., Howe, M. C., & Barnes, M. A. (2008). *Groups: Applying the functional group model.* Philadelphia: F. A. Davis.

Taylor, R. R. (2008). *The intentional relationship: Occupational therapy and the use of self.* Philadelphia: F. A. Davis.

Tuckman, B. W. (1965). Developmental sequence in small groups. *Psychological Bulletin, 63,* 384–399. http://dx.doi.org/10.1037/h0022100

White, R. W. (1959). Motivation reconsidered: The concept of competence. *Psychological Review, 66,* 297–333. http://dx.doi.org/10.1037/h0040934

White, R. W. (1971). The urge towards competence. *American Journal of Occupational Therapy, 25,* 271–280.

Yalom, I. D. (1995). *Theory and practice of group psychotherapy* (4th ed.). New York: Basic Books.

CHAPTER 11.

REDESIGNING LIFESTYLES: USING ACTIVITIES TO MEET OCCUPATIONAL NEEDS

Lisa E. Cyzner, PhD, OTR

Highlights

✦ Understanding disability
✦ World Health Organization models
✦ Exploration and integration of perspectives
✦ Occupational Therapy Reflective Staircase: Framework to help people construct and reconstruct their lifestyles
✦ Using the Staircase in clinical practice: The process.

Key Terms

✦ Activity reasoning process
✦ Bereavement
✦ Bottom-up approach
✦ Co-occupations
✦ Cultural production
✦ Dichotomous identity
✦ Disability
✦ Educative environment
✦ Environmental factors
✦ Figure
✦ Figure–ground

✦ Functional limitations
✦ Ground
✦ Medical model of disability
✦ Narrative
✦ Occupation
✦ Occupational Therapy Reflective Staircase framework
✦ Producing culture
✦ Sensory defensiveness
✦ Social model of disability
✦ Top-down approach

Four life perspectives—physical, psychological, philosophical, and sociological—should be integrated into occupational therapy evaluation, intervention, and projected outcomes when addressing the multifaceted needs of people with disabilities. This chapter concentrates on the psychological, philosophical, and sociological perspectives. Integral to planning and provision of activities that can lead to rebuilding or reformulation of a client's occupations is that occupational therapy practitioners must embrace these perspectives and understand the constructs that are the foundation for each. Equally important is recognizing that the process of integrating these perspectives must be individualized for each client.

This chapter begins by discussing the *International Classification of Impairments, Disabilities and Handicaps* (*ICIDH*), first published by the World Health Organization (WHO) in 1980 and later published as the *International Classification of Functioning, Disability and Health* (*ICF;* WHO, 2001). Within this document is a continuum that was designed to cultivate a more uniform terminology for health professionals. The application of the *ICIDH* with respect to the occupational therapy profession and information about *ICF* are examined. The *ICF* includes concepts of impairment and disability similar to the *ICIDH;* however, it also includes how these concepts can be paired and grouped with concepts related to functioning. Information is then provided regarding the *International Classification of Diseases, Tenth Revision* (*ICD–10;* WHO, 1990), with further discussion on the complementary nature of the *ICD–10* and *ICF.*

The *ICF* can provide information about a person's ability to function with his or her health conditions as delineated by the *ICD–10,* which can be applied to occupational therapy, including information related to activities and participation with respect to function. The *ICF* also emphasizes contextual factors such as environmental and personal considerations similar to the exploration of context in the occupational therapy literature and its direct use in daily practice.

Many of these aforementioned components of the *ICF* and others are reflective of the domain of concern of the occupational therapy profession and the history of the profession in developing a common language, first with *Uniform Terminology* (American

Occupational Therapy Association [AOTA], 1979, 1989, 1994), followed by the *Occupational Therapy Practice Framework: Domain and Process* (the *Framework;* AOTA, 2002, 2008, 2014). These documents have further supported the goal of the profession to not only incorporate terminology from the *ICF* but also to have a platform from which to provide the greater community of health professionals with a better understanding of the occupational therapy profession, its domain of concern, and the populations with whom occupational therapy practitioners work in a multitude of settings.

Over the past several years, the occupational therapy profession has witnessed a reemphasis on and return to its roots of occupation. Occupational therapy practitioners must consider how a client's occupations are affected not only by underlying performance components but also by the person's disability and how his or her life has been affected. By using a top-down approach during the evaluation process, a therapist first should ascertain a person's ability to perform certain life roles and the meaning attached to these roles. This evaluation, in turn, helps determine activities to be integrated as part of the intervention process, again setting the foundation for helping the person return to engagement in meaningful occupations.

After discussing this foundational information, the chapter then explores in depth the psychological, philosophical, and sociological perspectives as they relate to people with disabilities and the occupational therapy process that evolves. The first presented is the psychological perspective. Parkes and Weiss (1983) presented a continuum of the grieving process that people with disabilities experience. This grieving process involves a person letting go of one set of assumptions and adopting another set when coming to terms with a loss, such as when acquiring a disability. Each person's movement along this continuum toward emotional acceptance and adoption of a new identity will be different, and some may never reach these levels. Thus, occupational therapy practitioners must have a deep understanding of the client's emotional exploration of loss. In addition, the choice of activities for intervention must be meaningful and relate to where clients are in their grieving process, that is, the activity must match a client's interests and emotional state.

The second perspective presented is the philosophical perspective. The philosophical concept of *figure–ground* is described and is related back to the psychological continuum, because the assumptions people make when they carry out their daily activities are part of their *ground,* or what they do not plan or think about but is part of their automaticity or habits.

The third perspective is the sociological perspective. Disability is described as a culture, because people often define much of what they do through their own culture or what society has deemed acceptable.

The information discussed so far can be applied to occupational therapy practice through the *Occupational Therapy Reflective Staircase framework,* which helps people construct and reconstruct their lifestyles using activities. This framework's process is similar to engaging in the clinical reasoning process when planning activities for people with disabilities to help them construct or reconstruct their lifestyles. Finally, a worksheet is provided for occupational therapy practitioners to use in daily practice (see Appendix 11.A).

Understanding Disability

It is important to understand that the totality of the impact of serious physical impairment on conscious thought, as well as its firm implantation in the unconscious mind, gives disability a far stronger purchase on a person's sense of who and what he or she is than do any social roles—even key ones such as age, occupation, and ethnicity. Thoughts about one's sense of self can be manipulated, neutralized, and suspended. Therefore, a person may be able to adjust his or her self-perception to develop self-identity as a person with a disability (Murphy, 1990).

In his book *The Body Silent,* Robert Murphy (1990), a retired professor from the Department of Anthropology at Columbia University, described his experiences living with a chronic illness as the most challenging journey of his life. Invoking this metaphor of a journey, he took readers with him as he related how every aspect of his life was affected after learning he had a spinal cord tumor that eventually caused quadriplegia. If life is the journey, the body is the vessel through which we experience life. The body is our physical, psychological, philosophical, and sociological connection to the world through which we strive to create meaningful lives.

Occupational therapy practitioners working with people who have disabilities must use a multifaceted approach in incorporating the physical, psychological, sociological, and philosophical perspectives into evaluation and intervention using purposeful activities to support engagement in occupations. By helping people engage in activities, practitioners operate within the domain of our profession.

In a sense, we can embrace Murphy's (1990) anthropological perspective as a way to individualize our approach. The journey is different for each person: For some, it begins at birth; for others, it begins after a traumatic event. The families, friends, and significant others of people with disabilities are part of this journey as well, often engaging in *co-occupations* (i.e., 2 or more people sharing participation in an occupation), such as caregiving, with their loved one.

For many, the journey is a lifelong process of living with a chronic illness. Regardless of the timing or process of this journey, practitioners must recognize how essential occupations, and the activities that compose them, are to a person's identity and sense of competence and meaning in his or her daily life (AOTA, 2014).

World Health Organization Models

In an effort to provide a framework for health professionals who provide services for people with disabilities, WHO (1980) published the *ICIDH.* Complete with definitions and information regarding the consequences of disease, the *ICIDH* presented a continuum—an illness trajectory—through which health professionals could communicate by using more uniform terminology than had been used in the past (Knussen & Cunningham, 1988; Rogers & Holm, 1994; Wood, 1980; Figure 11.1).

Impairment, disability, and handicap are all considered to be consequences of disease. Rogers and Holm (1994) cautioned that in the *ICIDH* these concepts are defined only in terms of dysfunction; aspects of remediation or compensation are not discussed. However, the *ICIDH* definitions are useful in laying the groundwork for exploring the physical, psychological, and sociological perspectives affected by disability. Moreover, Coster and Haley (1992)

Figure 11.1. *ICF* continuum.

Disease $\Rightarrow$ Impairment $\Rightarrow$ Disability $\Rightarrow$ Handicap

Source. L. Cyzner. Used with permission.

Note. ICF = International Classification of Functioning, Disability and Health (World Health Organization, 2011).

noted that although the *ICIDH*'s continuum is hierarchical in that each of the four components represents "increasingly complex, integrated activities" (p. 13), health professionals should not necessarily view it as linear.

Coster and Haley (1992) explained that even though a person presents with problems indicative of a certain component or level of the *ICIDH* model, one cannot presume that person also has problems indicative of another component along the continuum. They provided the example of a child with a below-elbow amputation resulting from trauma (an impairment) who can perform with his prosthesis all activities of daily living (ADLs) independently. Thus, although this child has an impairment, he would not be considered disabled because he is able to independently perform all of his ADLs. Therefore, occupational therapy practitioners have to think and question themselves about what a person is and is not able to do. They also need to take into account what a person chooses to do and what level of assistance may or may not be needed.

Another model of disablement proposed by Nagi (1965, 1991) links impairment with disability through functional limitations. *Functional limitations* encompass a person's ability to perform tasks and to carry out those obligations that are part of his or her roles or daily activities.

WHO published the *ICIDH* in 1980 for trial purposes. After multiple revisions based on field testing and international consultation, WHO approved the latest version—the *ICF*—for use on May 22, 2001. In this version, the one continuum, which includes the concepts of impairment, disability, and handicap, was replaced with a two-level, or two-part, system: Part 1 is functioning and disability, and Part 2 is contextual factors. Each part has several components. Within this classification and further breakdown

of the components, the concepts of impairment and disability are still used; however, they are paired and grouped with other concepts related to functioning so that the presentation and relationship of all of these concepts are no longer linear as the original continuum suggested (Figure 11.2).

The 10th revision of the *ICF*, the *ICD–10*, also developed by WHO, is used to classify health conditions such as diseases, disorders, and injuries. The *ICD–10* and the *ICF* are therefore complementary because *ICF* can provide information on a person's ability to function with his or her health conditions. Because of this, the *ICF* is now viewed more as a component of health classification rather than of consequences of disease. According to WHO (2001), it is considered a multipurpose classification and conceptual framework that can be used in a variety of contexts related to health care, including management of health care systems; prevention and health promotion programs; and research related to such entities as health care evaluations, health care policy, and applied research to meet the changing needs of society.

Table 11.1 (WHO, 2001, p. 14) provides an overview of the *ICF*, outlining its overall organization and structure. The *ICF* provides information related to human functioning and to restrictions of human functioning that can be used by a variety of disciplines. Part 1, functioning and disability, has two components: (1) body functions and structures and (2) activities and participation. Applying directly to occupational therapy, the information related to activities and participation encompasses a range of domains covering many aspects of functioning, including looking at functioning from both the individual's and society's perspective.

Therefore, the components of Part 1 can be used to indicate a problem, impairment, activity limita-

Figure 11.2. Interactions between the components of *ICF*.

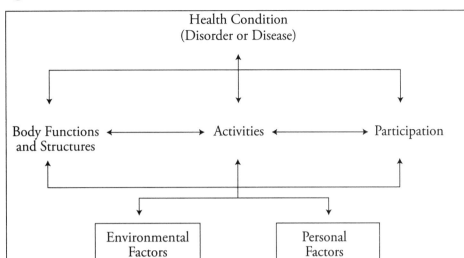

Source. From *International Classification of Functioning, Disability and Health* by the World Health Organization, 2001, p. 26. Geneva: Author. Used with permission.

Note. ICF = International Classification of Functioning, Disability and Health (World Health Organization, 2001).

Table 11.1. Overview of *ICF*

	Part 1: Functioning and Disability		**Part 2: Contextual Factors**	
Components	Body Functions and Structures	Activities and Participation	Environmental Factors	Personal Factors
Domains	Body Functions Body Structures	Life Areas (Tasks, Actions)	External Influences on Functioning and Disability	Internal Influences on Functioning and Disability
Constructs	Change in Body Functions (Physiological) Change in Body Structures (Anatomical)	Capacity Executing Tasks in a Standard Environment Performance Executing Tasks in the Current Environment	Facilitating or Hindering Impact of Features of the Physical, Social, and Attitudinal World	Impact of Attributes of the Person
Positive Aspect	Functional and Structural Integrity Functioning	Activities Participation	Facilitators	Not Applicable
Negative Aspect	Impairment Disability	Activity Limitation Participation Restriction	Barriers/ Hindrances	Not Applicable

Source. From *International Classification of Functioning, Disability and Health* by the World Health Organization, 2001, p. 14. Geneva: Author.

Note. ICF = International Classification of Functioning, Disability and Health (World Health Organization, 2001).

tion, or participation restriction, which can all be summarized under the umbrella concept of disability. These components can also be used to indicate aspects of health that are not related to a problem or impairment, which can be summarized under the concept of functioning (WHO, 2001). As mentioned previously, it is important that practitioners continue to ask themselves what a person both can and cannot do. In addition, it is vital to include and evaluate contextual factors and how these also affect a person's performance of ADLs. The information gained from this questioning is integral to evaluation, intervention planning, and intervention provision.

Part 2 of the *ICF,* contextual factors, includes environmental factors and personal factors. A person's level of functioning and disability is considered an interaction between health conditions, such as disease, illness, or injury, and contextual factors, such as how the environment affects functioning and disability. In the occupational therapy literature, the Ecology of Human Performance Framework (Dunn, Brown, & Youngstrom, 2003) similar to what WHO (2001) described, gives equal value to four constructs that are essential for intervention: (1) person, (2) context, (3) task, and (4) performance.

This framework emphasizes the role of context because, according to its developers, context is often neglected by occupational therapy practitioners and by other programs and professions (Dunn, Brown, & McGuigan, 1994; Dunn et al., 2003). Tham and Kielhofner (2003) agreed and noted that, specifically regarding research related to disability, occupational therapy as a profession lacks empirical documentation of how social context influences occupational performance for people with disabilities.

According to WHO (2001), *environmental factors* are factors from a person's immediate and surrounding environments that affect all the components of functioning and disability. Although personal factors are included and would be considered here, they are not classified in the *ICF* because, as WHO (2001) explained, they contain too much variance related to social and cultural differences. Yet, information related to both social and cultural factors is vital to practitioners because these factors can greatly affect how they work with people and their families and what practitioners' and families' expectations are relative to intervention. Social and cultural factors can also affect a person and his or her family's view of functioning and disability, which has a direct influence on intervention choices, activities integrated into the intervention itself, modifications to the person's environment, or all of these.

As described previously, *ICF* sections and components particularly related to activities and participation and contextual factors have direct application to occupational therapy practice. It is recommended that readers consult the short version of the *ICF* (WHO, 2001) for further detail on all of its components, multiple usages of the classification, and other applications to practice.

To expand on the relationship between the *ICF* and occupational therapy practice, Donald J. Lollar (2003) described the following in his Foreword to *Perspectives in Human Occupation: Participation in Life:*

> Two major tenets of the new system are that the environment and contextual factors play a crucial role in human function generally and in disability specifically. Second, the outcomes for all people are framed as societal participation. These two components of the new *ICF* have been the essence of occupation and occupational therapy since their inception: (a) participation and (b) society. This framework allows occupation and occupational therapy to take a leadership role as the field of health and disability moves beyond body function to embrace the assessment of classification of health status. The coding system will allow both positive and negative elements of the environment to be included for research, policy development, and program implementation. Evaluation of activity limitations can now be balanced between domains of individuals and their environment. New assessment tools and procedures will grow from this model and occupational therapists will be at the forefront. (pp. vii–viii)

As noted, many of the *ICF*'s components appear similar to those areas of human experience in which occupational therapy practitioners have expertise. They reflect elements of the domain of concern (Mosey, 1996) and the *Framework* (AOTA, 2014). The *Framework* includes language to aid practitioners in explaining occupation to their community, particularly how occupation relates to the provision of occupational therapy intervention. Furthermore, it was designed to help the profession to profess its role in "promoting the health and participation of persons, groups, and populations through engagement in occupation" (AOTA, 2014, p. S2).

The *Framework* was also designed to be more universal, that is, it incorporated terminology from the *ICF* so that other health professionals could understand it and in turn understand more about the profession of occupational therapy, its domain of concern, the client populations with whom practitioners work, and the various settings in which practitioners work on a daily basis. The *Framework* includes revisions necessary to update language and concepts that are part of both current and emerging practice of occupational therapy (AOTA, 1994, 2002, 2008; Hinojosa, Kramer, Royeen, & Luebben, 2003; Luebben, 2003; Youngstrom, 2002).

Thus, considering all of these documents, occupational therapy as a profession has witnessed the reemphasis on (and essentially a return to) its roots of occupation. In addition to taking into account physiological and participatory concerns, practitioners must also consider the larger activity performance areas—occupations—as they are affected by a disability, and not just their underlying performance components (Baptiste, 2003; Clark et al., 1997; Coster, 1998; Jackson, Carlson, Mandel, Zemke, & Clark, 1998; Padilla, 2003; Wood, 1998).

Whether the performance of an activity is related to such occupations as work, play, leisure, social participation, or ADLs, some members of the occupational therapy profession have advocated that practitioners look at these areas first—along with considering context—rather than initially evaluating, and subsequently basing treatment on, problems related to the underlying components affecting the performance. This approach is known as a *top-down approach* to evaluation rather than a *bottom-up approach*, which focuses on the underlying components (Coster, 1998; Ideishi, 2003; Kramer & Hinojosa, 2010; Latham, 2008; Trombly, 1993, 1995).

When using a top-down approach with a client, the occupational therapist initially tries to determine a person's ability to perform certain roles and the meaning attached to those roles. The therapist ascertains this information to determine what activities the person may want to address in occupational therapy sessions. The roles and related activities in which a person engaged before becoming disabled or before coming to occupational therapy (as a result of a recent event or more chronic disability) become the focus of evaluation. If the occupational therapist determines that a difference exists among past, present, and future role performances, then treatment should be implemented. The occupational therapist explores with the client the role performances and occupations the client wants to do and investigates why he or she is unable to do them. This exploration aids in helping the client understand the need for treatment and what the focus of treatment will be (Hinojosa, Kramer, & Crist, 2014; Latham, 2008; Trombly, 1993, 1995).

The occupational therapist can organize his or her practice through the implementation of one of three approaches: (1) top-down, (2) bottom-up, or (3) contextual (Ideishi, 2003; Weinstock-Zlotnick & Hinojosa, 2004). Regardless of the approach chosen, all practitioners share a common concern for occupation and have the goal of helping people engage in meaningful occupations.

Ideishi (2003) noted,

> the challenge for the occupational therapist is to transform and articulate our theoretical concepts into daily practice. If we can articulate what we do and why we do it, our clients, our communities, our colleagues in other disciplines, and the institutions that pay for our services will understand the unique contribution that occupational therapy provides society. (p. 294)

Because the *ICF* is a global taxonomy, it challenges the profession of occupational therapy to clarify definitions related to occupation and activities. Occupation is considered to be the core of our profession because it is made up of the daily tasks and purposeful activities, whether mundane or of great importance, that are meaningful to people and are a part of who they are (AOTA, 2012; Hinojosa et al., 2003). Throughout the history of the profession, occupation has been used as both a means during intervention processes and an end, which is the goal of interventions—that clients can return to old occupations or choose new directions regarding their choices and participation in daily life tasks. Several people at the forefront of clarifying definitions used in occupational therapy have contributed valuable discussion, with many suggesting that the concept of *occupation* be defined as a process and activity, or as one component (Hinojosa & Blount, 2008; Hinojosa et al., 2003; Latham, 2008).

Whatever a practitioner's view, the highest goal of occupational therapy intervention is to help a person participate in meaningful occupations, resulting in participation in life (Ideishi, 2003). Yet, little documentation of efficacy regarding occupation, the practice of occupation, and the relationship of occupation to disability exists (Padilla, 2003). Furthermore, WHO (2001) professed through the *ICF* that the medical model of disability be integrated with the social model of disability. WHO (2001) defined the *medical model of disability* as

> a problem of the person, directly caused by disease, trauma or other health condition, which requires medical care provided in the form of individual treatment by professionals. Management of the disability is aimed at cure or the individual's adjustment and behaviour change. Medical care is viewed as the main issue, and at the political level the principal response is that of modifying or reforming health policy. (p. 18)

It defined the *social model of disability* as

> a socially created problem, and basically as a matter of the full integration of individuals into society. Disability is not an attribute of an individual, but rather a complex collection of conditions, many of which are created by the social environment. Hence the management of the problem requires social action, and it is the collective responsibility of society at large to make the environmental modifications necessary for the full participation of people with disabilities in all areas of social life. (p. 18)

If occupational therapy as a profession embraces this integration of models, which also appears to be at the core of its philosophical underpinnings, and wants to align itself with the leaders who affect health policy, management, and outcomes, then it must be clear in its definitions and able to explain its models of intervention to society at large. Practition-

ers need to be able to demonstrate how occupational therapy's emphasis on occupation and social justice (the support of social policies, actions, and laws that permit people to participate in occupations that are personally meaningful and purposeful) reflects larger, universally accepted models such as WHO's. The occupational therapy profession's view of health reflects that of the WHO models. WHO stated that a person's health can be affected by the inability to carry out activities and participate in life situations related to environmental barriers and by problems that occur with body structures and body functions (AOTA, 2014; WHO, 2001).

Exploration and Integration of Perspectives

For occupational therapy practitioners working with people with disabilities, the four perspectives—physical, psychological, philosophical, and sociological—must be brought together and merged, because they are inextricably linked within the whole person. In the following sections, the foundational construct of these perspectives are individually discussed. This chapter focuses on psychological, philosophical, and sociological perspectives, as the physical perspective is extensively discussed in other chapters of this text. Occupational therapy practitioners understand physical impairment and disability but must integrate this understanding with other perspectives. The practitioner integrates these perspectives to address the unique needs of each individual. Each perspective offers insight into the ways of looking at the problems of living with a disability and the way in which a person with disabilities represents his or her life and its challenges.

A Psychological Continuum: The Disability Process

Much of the psychological literature describing people's reactions to disability and the processes they undergo, including the tasks of grieving continuum (Parkes & Weiss, 1983), can be found in the areas of bereavement and loss as well as stress and coping (Bennett, Gibbons, & Mackenzie-Smith, 2010; Carroll, 1961; Clegg, 1988; Knussen & Cunningham, 1988; Lazarus & Folkman, 1991; Parkes, 1998). Clegg (1988) defined *bereavement* as a state that follows an actual or perceived loss, including changes in

Figure 11.3. The tasks of grieving by Parkes and Weiss (1983).

Intellectual recognition and explanation of loss	$\Rightarrow$	Emotional acceptance	$\Rightarrow$	Adoption of a new identity

Source. L. Cyzner. Used with permission.

all dimensions of a person's life—physical, psychological, and behavioral—as a result of this loss. People may display their reactions to this actual or perceived loss through social, cognitive, physical, and emotional behaviors. Thus, again, one is reminded of the integration of the models of disability both from the individual and the societal perspectives.

Parkes and Weiss's (1983) tasks of grieving continuum was specifically developed from research related to bereavement (Figure 11.3), with some research related to the bereavement process of study participants who had acquired disabilities. According to Clegg (1988), people tend to live each day on a set of assumptions; these assumptions can be disrupted when one faces a loss (also see the "Philosophical Underpinnings: Self, Skills, and Ideas" section that follows). She further explained that Parkes and Weiss (1983) viewed the grieving process as part of a person's letting go of one set of assumptions and adopting another set when coming to terms with a loss as occurs with a disability. Parkes and Weiss (1983) believed that a person must go through this grieving process before truly accepting the loss. They stated that a person facing a recent loss must first try to make sense of what has happened to begin to answer the omnipresent question "Why?"

People then move along the continuum toward emotional acceptance when they begin to feel less of a need to avoid reminders of the loss, which may evoke other painful feelings and emotional responses, including denial. Some people with a disability who receive occupational therapy will never fully come to emotional acceptance. The same may be true for parents of a child born with a disability; one who acquires a disability; or one with a disability that develops over time, such as a learning disability or autism spectrum disorder. For many of these people, the process may be slow. Each person's experience and ways of dealing with loss are unique, and

practitioners must be vigilant about and sensitive to their place along this continuum.

At the end of the continuum, Parkes and Weiss (1983) described the adoption of a new *dichotomous identity,* that is, "maintaining one identity while acting in another" (p. 159). In addition, a person's identity reflects a personal set of assumptions or ideas that affect his or her choices and activity selections. This emphasis on choice in engaging in meaningful activity is central to the profession of occupational therapy. Whether activities are used in evaluation or in treatment to remediate or compensate for a disability, the activities chosen must be meaningful to the person. Once again, occupational therapy practitioners are reminded that as they help a person with disabilities reenter society and rebuild a life, occupation is the process and activities are the means. The choice of activities for treatment as part of helping a person reconstruct a lifestyle after a disability is specific to the person (AOTA, 1993), meaning the activities must match the person's interests.

Philosophical Underpinnings: Self, Ideas, and Skills

The philosophical underpinnings of a person's actions include his or her sense of self and skills. The concept of *figure–ground,* which originated in philosophy and means differentiating between foreground and background ideas, forms, and objects, has a direct application to understanding how a disability affects a person's physical and psychological well-being and how a person learns to cope with the loss (Bateson, 1972, 1979; Idhe, 1991; Popper, 1985, 1992). Similar to the ideas presented by Parkes and Weiss (1983), the assumptions on which people operate and carry out their daily activities are part of their *ground,* that is, what they do not consciously think about throughout the course of the day. The

Figure 11.4. We tend to live by a certain set of assumptions and attach our ideas and skills.

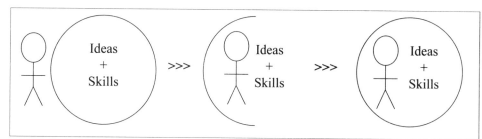

Source. L. Cyzner. Used with permission.

ground is background knowledge; it is what people often take for granted. Even habits can become part of a person's background knowledge.

It is not until a person experiences an event that brings about change—or "rupture"—that he or she sees the figure (Idhe, 1991; G. Moglia, personal communication, April 22, 1998). In other words, the *figure* (i.e., the object, idea, or illustration that is important or conspicuous against the background) must be brought out of the background for a person to realize all that he or she does automatically. Thus, when a person becomes disabled—and can no longer perform activities as before—the disability becomes part of the figure. A person may realize what he or she had taken for granted in the past. Trying to go back to the ground is often a difficult journey.

Related both to the concept of figure–ground and to the idea that a person tends to live by a certain set of assumptions is that a person also tends to adhere to the belief that his or her ideas and skills—and many daily activities—define who he or she is (Figure 11.4). Essentially, a person embodies ideas. If a person relinquishes an idea or a skill—especially if he or she loses a skill and can no longer perform an activity in the accustomed way—then a piece of who he or she is dies (Idhe, 1991; G. Moglia, personal communication, April 22, 1998; Popper, 1985, 1992).

Although it is very hard to do, a person can only begin to critique the ideas and skills needed to engage in activities when he or she is able to view those same ideas and skills outside of himself or herself. It is a difficult process because a person must accept that some of his or her ideas are fallible and that often mistakes must be made to learn about himself or herself. It is only then, however, that a person can improve on his or her ideas and skills (Popper, 1985, 1992).

This process appears analogous to a person's accepting that he or she may not be able to perform an activity the way he or she used to or learning that he or she can still perform the same activity but that modifications may have to be made for it to be carried out independently. A person may need assistance to continue to participate in an activity that was part of his or her daily occupation before the disability. Furthermore, if the symptoms of people living with chronic illness progress, then the level to which they may be able to perform certain activities will change. As the conditions change, so may the need for modifications or assistance.

The occupational therapy literature contains many examples of this theme of embodiment of ideas and skills; a few are presented here. In her 1993 Eleanor Clark Slagle lecture "Occupation Embedded in a Real Life: Interweaving Occupational Science and Occupational Therapy," Florence Clark (1993) presented the story of Professor Penny Richardson of the University of Southern California. She poignantly told of the process that Professor Richardson went through to rediscover herself, to realize how she had defined herself before surviving the traumatic event of an aneurysm, and what she would have to do to discover a new self. Clark described how, by using *narrative* (telling stories), she was able to help Richardson through the process of recovery and "how rehabilitation can be experienced by the survivor as a rite of passage in which a person is moved to disability status and then abandoned" (p. 1067). Professor Richardson made Clark aware "that occupations were important because they marked the new you versus the old you" (p. 1072). These statements not only echo the information presented in the tasks of grieving as described by Parkes and Weiss (1983) but also the notion that a person's ideas and skills—his or her occupations and the activities that constitute them—define who he or she is.

Similarly to Clark (1993), Price-Lackey and Cashman (1996) presented information gained from life history interviews to describe how Jenny Cashman (the second author of the work and a graduate student in library science and archeology) experienced and adapted to a traumatic brain injury. They presented Jenny's use of daily activities that had meaning to her and a narrative construction to help her in her recovery process to regain a sense of identity. As Robert Murphy (1990) described, Jenny also viewed her recovery process as a challenging journey. The following is an excerpt from Jenny's postscript regarding her head injury experience, which was included in the article:

> The process of healing and redefinition has also been a profound experience, providing new depth and richness to my life. The fact that my life has changed is no longer a source of grief to me, but something I embrace. I am writing again—not in the way I wrote before, but in a new way, and that feels like a gift. . . . I am at this point, working on a book about my experience and my journey. It is somehow fitting that I celebrated my 5-year anniversary of my accident on an archeological dig in Egypt. The joy this gave me makes it clear that I have found my new path, so I have committed to working on the excavation for at least the next five campaigns. Then I'll see what happens next. Life is, after all, an eternal process of being and becoming. (p. 312)

Both Price-Lackey and Cashman (1996) suggested the following to practitioners:

- It is important for practitioners to understand what daily activities their clients engaged in before their illness or disability. This information is important because descriptions of patterns of activities (i.e., occupations) may inform practitioners about their client's self-identities, which is integral to the recovery process.
- Goal setting should be a collaborative effort between the practitioner and the client.
- In intervention, occupational therapy practitioners should take into account both the doing

aspects of occupations and the narrative meaning the client expresses regarding his or her daily occupations. By doing so, practitioners can truly begin to value the personal meaning that daily, purposeful activities bring to their clients' lives.

Occupational therapy practitioners do not have to look only to the literature to find examples of the embodiment of ideas and how people attach their ideas to themselves as a way of forming and re-forming their identities. They can see examples in their everyday practice and in themselves. However, until a practitioner understands this concept within himself or herself, it is very difficult to recognize the impact of attaching one's ideas to oneself in helping others.

Related to this idea, it is important that occupational therapy practitioners determine what type of learner their client may be or what type of learning style may affect his or her intervention and recovery process. Practitioners must also understand that a person's learning style may evolve as intervention progresses. Thus, it is essential to create an environment in which a person feels comfortable learning and can learn through trial and error, creating his or her own knowledge as he or she begins to construct or reconstruct a lifestyle required by living with a disability.

Perkinson (1984, 1993) described what he called an *educative environment,* which may be valuable to practitioners as they help others learn new skills or relearn old ones in new ways. Although Perkinson mainly seemed to be describing the environment created by a teacher for his or her students, his ideas seem applicable to practitioners determining what type of intervention environment to set up for their clients, whether children or adults. Perkinson (1993) suggested that when making decisions about the environment needed to help people learn, practitioners create

- An environment in which people will feel free to "disclose their present knowledge" (p. 34);
- An environment that provides critical feedback regarding people's present knowledge (which can come from a variety of sources); and
- A supportive environment, so that people can accept criticism about their present knowledge and begin to eliminate errors.

Occupational therapy practitioners must question whether their client truly understands what he or she has been asked to do. They must ask themselves, "Because my client can perform a certain action while engaging in an activity (chosen by the client), does he or she really understand why I have asked him or her to perform this activity in a certain way?" In other words, can practitioners assume that if they set up behavioral objective A, they will get outcome B (Perkinson, 1993)? Practitioners must be sure that the client understands why he or she is performing a certain activity and for what purpose. The person can then begin generalizing the knowledge learned from the experience of performing this activity during treatment to other activities he or she wants to do in daily life. Again, an activity match must exist among the activity itself, the underlying reasons for performing it, and the person.

Exercise 11.1. Modifying Activities

Imagine experiencing a temporary loss of ability such as a painful shoulder that limits your ability to reach, drive, and don a coat, for example. List ways to modify these activities while you are healing.

Sociological Perspective and Personal Transformation

A person's sociological perspective, particularly his or her culture, can be transformational for his or her integration into society. Disability can, in many ways, be described as a culture (Balcazar, Suarez-Balcazar, Taylor-Ritzler, & Keys, 2010; Campbell & Oliver, 1996). All of us can probably think of at least one activity they do that has been defined by their culture—and perhaps by society—or even an activity in which they may actually resist engaging because their culture has deemed it unacceptable. Reflecting on the disability movement in Britain and disability movements in general, Campbell and Oliver (1996) described these movements as redefining "the problem of disability as the product of a disabling society rather than individual limitations or loss, despite the fact that the rest of society continues to see disabled people as chance victims of a tragic fate" (p. 105).

For a person with a disability, redefining himself or herself may include a sociological process that involves realizing that a portion of his or her personal issues surrounding disability may, in fact, be political

(Campbell & Oliver, 1996). These types of issues give rise to social movements. This change process within a person with disabilities has two components: (1) The person becomes aware of the changes in himself or herself and (2) is cognizant of how these changes affect society. Campbell and Oliver (1996) described this duality as transforming both a personal and a social consciousness, "promoting self-understanding as a platform for change" (p. 145).

Certainly, this idea has influenced American society with the passage of the Americans With Disabilities Act of 1990 and the Individuals With Disabilities Education Act Amendments of 1997 (Bailey & Schwartzberg, 2003; Bazyk & Case-Smith, 2010; Metzler, 1997, 1998). Much of the lobbying for passage of these laws came from advocacy groups, often consisting of people with disabilities and their families. Active participation in advocacy groups and other organizations often becomes a highly valued activity for people with disabilities.

In deciding how to describe this change process to others in their book, Campbell and Oliver (1996) mentioned that they resisted separating information and issues surrounding disability, including social theory, political history, action research, individual biography, and personal experience. Each of these areas related to disability influences the other, which is reflected in what appears to be yet another continuum regarding disability, looking at changes occurring on both a personal and a social level. Thus, it appears that two smaller continua that are more limited in scope are representative of the sociological perspective of disability and the change process associated with it. Here, I concentrate on a personal transformation continuum that eventually also affects the social transformation process (Figure 11.5).

For personal transformation to occur, Campbell and Oliver (1996) suggested that first, a person may deny the existence of a problem. His or her initial response may be to assimilate with the rest of society and view having a disability as part of his or her identity. Campbell and Oliver (1996) suggested that a person must then be grateful and reasonable. The person with a disability must somehow learn to balance accepting and being grateful to people who want to help them and simultaneously being reasonable and more conscious of what to accept and even tolerate from society, including, for example, knowing when to report discriminatory acts.

Figure 11.5. Personal transformation continuum.

Denial ⇒ Be Grateful and Reasonable ⇒ Bearing Witness ⇒

Understanding Ourselves ⇒ Fighting Back

Source. L. Cyzner. Adapted from ideas presented by Campbell and Oliver (1996).

The next stage of the personal transformation process is that of bearing witness. This stage begins to bridge from the personal transformation to the social transformation, which is the act of sharing experiences with others, especially those who have encountered similar problems, including problems related to social issues. Practitioners can see how sharing this information may become vital for those with whom they work, helping each client to establish resources and reestablish connections with the world. Usually, a person can learn the most from others with similar disabilities, such as information about what type of wheelchair lift to install in a van or what grocery store is the most easily accessible and accommodating to a person with disabilities.

Next along this continuum is that a person with a disability must learn to understand himself or herself and to differentiate between personal problems and problems caused by a disabling society. A person can arrive at the final stage, fighting back, especially against societal stereotypes, by rejecting what he or she believes is the dominant disabling culture, getting involved in *cultural production* (e.g., the arts) as a way to express what has happened in his or her life, and getting involved in political organizations to increase empowerment (Campbell & Oliver, 1996). *Producing culture* is thinking about one's values and collective norms and rules and how they influence actions and facilitate participation in social and cultural relations. Speaking from their personal experience, Camp-

bell and Oliver (1996) described, like many others, a difficult journey.

Parallels Among Perspectives

When reflecting on the four life perspectives that affect the activity performance of a person with disabilities, one can see the parallels among them. They overlap in the change processes that take place in the person, and these processes often occur simultaneously. Because changes occur within the person and the environment, *disability* can be viewed sociologically as a "gap between a person's capabilities and the demands of the environment" (Committee on a National Agenda for the Prevention of Disabilities, 1991, p. 1). Thus, to help a person construct or reconstruct a lifestyle and ultimately occupations using activities, occupational therapy practitioners must take into account information from all four of these perspectives. This information can be gained in many ways, most often through clinical interviews with the person, his or her family, significant others, and other caregivers.

The overriding theme for the *activity reasoning process* (i.e., thinking about an activity to form a logical conclusion or judgment regarding its usefulness as a therapeutic intervention) goes back to the question presented earlier in the chapter: What is the person able and not able to do with respect to his or her activity performance? These overlapping perspectives are represented in Figure 11.6. Practitioners also consider, but are not limited to, a person's resources; background knowledge; the client factors of values, beliefs, and spirituality; level of assistance needed; the person's own understanding of what he or she feels able to do; and the person's level of motivation. As always, each person's experiences, feelings, and life situation will be unique.

Exercise 11.2. Cultural Significance

Think of an example of an activity you engage in only because of its cultural importance. When did you start engaging in this activity? Could it become important to you for other reasons? What are they?

Figure 11.6. Integration of the continua from the four life perspectives.

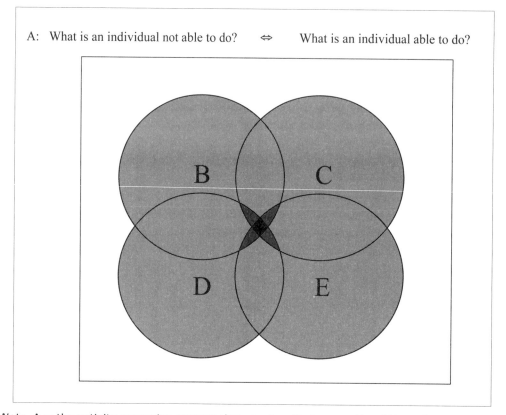

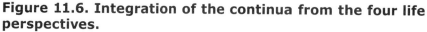

Note. A = the activity reasoning process that requires that occupational therapists continually ask the question, What is the individual able to do, and what is an individual not able to do regarding his or her activity performance? B = the physical; C = the psychological; D = the philosophical; E = the sociological perspectives.

Source. L. Cyzner. Used with permission.

Occupational Therapy Reflective Staircase: Framework to Help People Construct and Reconstruct Their Lifestyles

The Occupational Therapy Reflective Staircase framework was developed to help people construct and reconstruct their lifestyles. Philosopher Karl Popper believed that in order to learn, people have to criticize their ideas and look for errors. People often learn best through the process of trial and error. It is very difficult, however, for people to criticize their own ideas or to make other guesses about ways in which to solve problems when they are used to addressing problems in a certain manner.

Popper (1985, 1992) thus described one way in which people can learn more (and gain knowledge) about how to address their problems, accepting the idea that they may never find a true solution. Pop-per explained that once a person has identified a problem, he or she should make guesses about how to address it and criticize each of these guesses. By discovering solutions to problems, people advance knowledge. G. Moglia (personal communication, June 1, 1998) then used the metaphor of a staircase to explain Popper's ideas and formulated a process that can be used in occupational therapy.

Using the Staircase in Clinical Practice: The Process

The process for the Occupational Therapy Reflective Staircase framework involves six steps:

1. Identifying the problem,
2. Making a guess to address the problem,
3. Performing an activity to address the problem,

Figure 11.7. Occupational therapy reflective staircase.

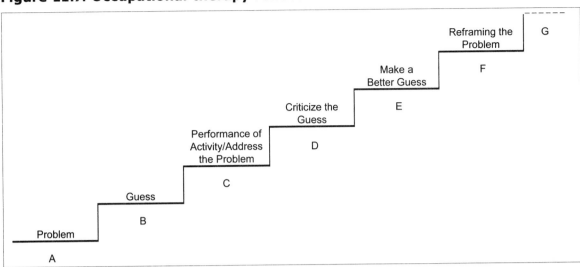

Note. Adapted and integrated for practice from the ideas of Moglia (personal communication, 1997, 1998), Popper (1985, 1992), and Schön (1983).

4. Criticizing the guess,
5. Making a better guess, and
6. Reframing the problem if necessary (Figure 11.7).

This process is continual and evolves at each step of the reflective staircase. The staircase has no finite end; it is only a process by which to reach better guesses (G. Moglia, personal communication, September 10, 1997; Popper, 1985, 1992). Therefore, as people ascend the staircase and are able to see their mistakes, they identify new or deeper problems and make better guesses.

Identifying the Problem

As part of the evaluation process, occupational therapists can ask several questions regarding a client's current and past level of activity performance. Therapists seek to determine through both interview and observation of activity performance what the client is able and unable to do. More specifically, they seek to determine what the client (or caregiver) identifies as a problem related to activity performance that is interfering with the client's ability to function as independently as possible (based on the activity chosen).

A related question is, What purpose does the activity serve? For example, is the activity part of a person's daily routine, is it a leisure activity, or is it an activity that aids the caregiver in assisting

the person? Answering this question assists occupational therapy practitioners in differentiating between activities and occupations, that is, trying to uncover what makes the activity personally meaningful to the person, which drives engagement in the activity itself (AOTA, 2002, 2008, 2014). In addition, practitioners must consider the underlying problems, performance skills and patterns, and contextual factors, remembering that occupations are grounded in place, social group, and cultural meaning (Hinojosa & Blount, 2014; Pierce, 2001). The focus will be different for each person, and the occupation that the activity relates to may be different as well. For example, for one person, reading a book may be a pleasure; for another, it may be considered part of his or her work or education. It is important to have a clear description and understanding of the problem before proceeding with the rest of the process.

Consider Case Example 11.1 and Case Example 11.2. (*Sensory defensiveness* is a defensive reaction to sensations that most people would not consider noxious; Wilbarger & Wilbarger, 1991, 1997.) Embedded within them are problems the practitioner may choose to address as part of helping clients construct or reconstruct their lifestyles using activities. More than likely, the practitioner would need more information to develop a complete intervention plan. As mentioned earlier, to provide a truly client-centered process, the practitioner should include how these activities relate

Case Example 11.1. Mr. Johnson: Paraplegia

Mr. Johnson, age 28 years, recently acquired paraplegia after a motor vehicle accident. Before his accident, he was a manager of a local business supply store. He has been referred by his physiatrist for inpatient occupational therapy now that he has stabilized; it has been determined that it is safe for him to participate in a rehabilitation program.

During an interview, Mr. Johnson tells you that he lives alone and plans on returning to his apartment upon discharge. His nearest relatives are 400 miles away. On weekends, close friends and family have been visiting him in the hospital. His initial requests during your occupational therapy evaluation are that he wants to be able to dress and bathe himself. At this time, he is completely reliant on others to carry out these daily living tasks for him. Moreover, later in the interview, Mr. Johnson mentions having been a member of a men's sports league before his accident and that he has enjoyed competitive sports since childhood.

Case Example 11.2. Karen: Sensory Defensiveness

Karen, age 5 years, attends public school in a regular education classroom. On initial evaluation, you determine that she is sensory defensive. She was initially referred to you, the school occupational therapist, by her prekindergarten teacher. Her teacher reports that Karen refuses to participate in most of the daily activities in which the children engage, such as arts and crafts and snack preparation, and she becomes upset (e.g., crying, running around the room while attempting to find a place to hide) when she sees that she might have to touch any type of messy materials such as glue or cookie dough. Also, she is fearful of playing on any moving playground equipment, resulting in her playing alone during recess. She has difficulty making friends. Her mother also tells you that Karen is unable to do many self-care activities independently, such as buttoning her shirt. You also notice that she uses a very weak grasp when drawing with crayons. Karen tells you that when she grows up, she wants to be an artist.

to a person's engagement in occupations that are purposeful and meaningful. These scenarios may, however, help stimulate readers' thinking in using the framework presented and in beginning to see the importance of the integration of the person with the context and environment and with his or her occupations (AOTA, 2014; Christiansen & Baum, 1997; Christiansen, Baum, & Bass-Haugen, 2005; Law, Baum, & Dunn, 2005).

After reading the case examples, ask yourself, What is one potential problem related to activity performance that could be addressed in occupational therapy? What occupations may be affected? What other information might you need? Then describe the problem in your own words (see Appendix 11.A for more guidance).

Making a Guess to Address the Problem

To begin making a guess about how to address the problem, the initial question one should ask at this point in the process is, What is constraining activity performance? Similar to using the top-down approach described earlier, after determining the

meaning attached to a person's activities and roles, the occupational therapist must explore with the person (or the caregiver, or both) the possible reasons why he or she is unable to carry out certain activities described as problems. This exploration helps form the focus of treatment (Latham, 2008; Trombly, 1993, 1995).

As described in Chapter 1, "Occupation, Activities, and Occupational Therapy," occupational therapy practitioners must remember that their clients may not actively think about the importance of the activities they engage in on a daily basis until they are not able to do them anymore. This perception may very well indicate a potential problem in and of itself. For practice, readers should think about this problem when reviewing the case example describing Mr. Johnson.

Several guesses or strategies may be used to address the problem related to activity performance. For example, the practitioner may choose to modify the activity, provide adaptive equipment, modify the environment, or provide physical assistance to help a person perform an activity that he or she has identified as part of his or her lifestyle. Client factors, including but not limited to values and beliefs and body functions, must be continuously taken into account as part of this client-centered process (AOTA, 2014). This entire thought process is similar to the description earlier in this chapter of how the *ICD–10* and *ICF* can be complementary as the practitioner considers a person's functioning given his or her described health conditions. Note, however, that observation is fundamental because the occupational therapist can never make the assumption that the expected problems for a given condition or disability will be the actual problems the client presents with during the evaluation process.

Exercise 11.3. Guessing

Considering the two case examples presented, think about what some of your possible guesses may be to address the problems you have described. Remember that one guess is not necessarily the only correct guess; several ways to address the problem may exist.

Also, when comparing the two scenarios, other issues may affect your thinking. For example, Mr. Johnson appears concerned with reconstructing certain activities that were part of his lifestyle before his accident. This issue will have a direct impact on his occupational performance. Karen, however, may possibly never have constructed certain lifestyle activities or engaged in certain occupations because of her sensory defensiveness.

For example, because she has avoided touching many objects, the musculature in her hands may not have fully developed, which would affect her fine motor performance and choice of fine motor activities and thus directly affect her play or education. You must also consider the necessity of co-occupation and these clients' interrelationship with their caregivers. In addition, societal expectations should be taken into account. For example, as a society, we seem to expect that a child will socialize with peers on the playground at school. However, Karen is playing alone out of possible fear or anxiety related to accessing the playground equipment based on her sensory needs and probable related social–emotional needs as well. Playing on the playground with peers is within her sociocultural context, yet she does not participate in active, meaningful engagement. Occupational therapists must be careful not to use sociocultural expectations to dictate treatment but to help guide their guesses as part of the evaluation process.

For example, Mr. Johnson may present with substantial physical needs that need to be addressed. After further interview and exploration, the problem may be how his acquired disability is affecting him from an emotional standpoint. Or, it may be how he now perceives himself fitting in or no longer fitting into the social contexts that appear to have been important in his daily life, such as participating in a variety of sports-related events and leagues since childhood (Slater & Meade, 2004). For Karen, her emotional reactivity appears to be as much of a potential problem or barrier to her functioning in school as her physical or sensory-based needs. These outward behaviors may be influencing her socially and her overall occupational performance as a student at school.

Performing an Activity to Address the Problem

Practitioners must observe people performing the activity to determine whether their guess regarding the problem was appropriate. Thus, the practitioner can reflect on the performance to move to the next step of criticizing the guess. In the case of Mr. Johnson, the practitioner may be able to observe him in the clinic. For Karen, it may be more helpful to observe her in her natural context at school.

Criticizing the Guess

Criticizing the guess is crucial to helping a person construct or reconstruct his or her lifestyle using activities because this point on the staircase is where the person may see the figure (as described earlier) of what he or she is still not able to do as a result of the disability. Furthermore, if errors were made during the performance of the activity, it is important to allow the person to see the error (Popper, 1992) and help him or her gain knowledge from the performance, thereby becoming involved in the process and in goal setting. Occupational therapy practitioners can also gain valuable knowledge by examining their guesses and attempting to figure out why they were or were not appropriate or why they did or did not work in addressing the identified problem.

Making a Better Guess

Making a better guess involves several issues. Perhaps the activity chosen to address a problem was

---

Exercise 11.4. Providing Feedback

Think about how you would provide feedback regarding errors or mistakes to both Mr. Johnson and Karen during their performance of activities.

For example, if Mr. Johnson attempted to use adaptive equipment during a dressing activity, using it in such a way that he expended too much energy, how would you make him aware of this problem? How could you use the activity as an element of change, helping him learn energy conservation techniques to incorporate into his lifestyle? If Karen continued to use a weak or incorrect grasp of her pencil or crayons, how would you make her aware of this problem? How could you place this problem in context for her so she sees the connection between working on her grasp and success in school? How could you help her understand the meaning behind what she is being asked to do? How could you address her emotional challenges, mainly her level of competence and self-esteem, that affect her occupational performance?

Furthermore, because she is sensitive to touch, would you physically cue her to place her fingers differently on the shaft of the pencil, or would you need to devise other cuing systems, such as modeling the grasp needed so that she can visually monitor the change needed for more successful activity performance? What feedback could you give to Mr. Johnson's and Karen's caregivers that may help them facilitate the process in the more natural context outside of the clinic, which may ultimately affect Mr. Johnson's and Karen's choices of occupations, confidence in their performance, and level of independence?

Providing feedback is an important part of the process of helping your clients redefine their identities or discover their identities for the first time, which can ultimately help lead to greater satisfaction because they have been involved in the process and goal setting.

---

appropriate (i.e., within the person's capabilities with or without modifications), but the conditions (e.g., the amount of time needed to perform the entire activity) or the context in which it was performed needed to be changed or modified. Maybe a different, related activity would better match the person's or caregiver's current needs. In the case of Mr. Johnson, other types of issues are evident.

For example, he has requested that the occupational therapist help him work on bathing and dressing in the hospital, yet at this point he is dependent on others to help him with these ADLs. If you chose to start with these activities based on Mr. Johnson's request, would you also need to consider first involving others in the process given his great need for assistance? Would you need to find out more about where he may transition to after his rehabilitation program (because working on bathing in the clinic may be very different from that at home)? For Karen, given her multiple needs, what context would be best to address her needs? Would she perform differently in the clinic setting compared with the school setting, where her level of anxiety may be more heightened and observable?

Only by making these better guesses—and thus seeking more in-depth information—can occupational therapy practitioners help clients move along the staircase so they can continue to construct or reconstruct their lifestyles—and ultimately their occupations—and help them in their personal search for meaning and sense of purpose.

Reframing the Problem

When making better guesses is not effective (because, for example, the original problem is not the one that needs to be addressed first to effect change, the original problem has changed, or deeper problems underlie the original problem), occupational therapy practitioners may have to reflect on all they have done and reframe the problem (Schön, 1983).

For instance, after initiating treatment, an occupational therapist begins to realize that a client's depression is affecting physical activity performance more than the therapist had detected on initial evaluation. Thus, the client may need to address the depression before continuing treatment or concurrently with treatment, possibly by seeking help from other professionals. If reframing the problem is necessary, practitioners must ask themselves the following questions:

- Did you take into account all of the possible activity demands?
- Is the person only physically unable to perform the activity (or elements of a larger activity), or are other life perspectives or issues affecting performance? For example, does the person have low levels of motivation and meaning, difficulty reaching emotional acceptance of the disability,

difficulty separating ideas from self to learn, or all of these challenges?

- What other performance patterns may need to be taken into account, for example, habits, routines, roles, and rituals? Have these patterns changed or evolved over time as a result of the disability; living with the disability; or engaging in the occupational therapy evaluation, intervention, and outcome process?
- Is the underlying problem in the environment or the objects used in the activity, not the person's physical or psychological capabilities?
- Can the person perform the first element of the activity but has trouble with the next element, making the activity more complex?

Summary

Occupational therapy practitioners must learn to consider the four life perspectives and how these perspectives can affect people with disabilities and the activity choices they make in their lives. The Occupational Therapy Reflective Staircase—incorporating the process from identifying the problem, making a guess, performing an activity, criticizing the guess, and making a better guess through reframing the problem—can help guide us as we learn to help people with disabilities construct or reconstruct their lifestyles using activities on the way to mastering the occupations they value. Popper's (1992) ideas about examining oneself and learning highlight this active change process:

> We can bestow a meaning upon our lives through our work, through our active conduct, through our whole way of life, and through the attitude we adopt toward our friends and our fellow men and toward the world. . . . In this way the quest for the meaning of life turns into an ethical question—the question "What tasks can I set myself in order to make my life meaningful?" (pp. 138–139)

References

American Occupational Therapy Association. (1979). *Occupational therapy output reporting system and uniform terminology for reporting occupational therapy services*. Rockville, MD: Author.

American Occupational Therapy Association. (1989). Uniform terminology for occupational therapy (2nd ed.). *American Journal of Occupational Therapy, 43,* 808–815. http://dx.doi.org/10.5014/ajot.43.12.808

American Occupational Therapy Association. (1993). Position paper: Purposeful activity. *American Journal of Occupational Therapy, 51,* 864–866.

American Occupational Therapy Association. (1994). Uniform terminology for occupational therapy (3rd ed.) *American Journal of Occupational Therapy, 48,* 1047–1054. http://dx.doi.org/10.5014/ajot.48.11.1047

American Occupational Therapy Association. (2002). Occupational therapy practice framework: Domain and process. *American Journal of Occupational Therapy, 56,* 609–639. http://dx.doi.org/10.5014/ajot.56.6.609

American Occupational Therapy Association. (2008). Occupational therapy practice framework: Domain and process (2nd ed.). *American Journal of Occupational Therapy, 62,* 625–683. http://dx.doi.org/10.5014/ajot.62.6.625

American Occupational Therapy Association. (2012). *Policy 1.12 Occupation as the common core of occupational therapy policy manual.* Bethesda, MD: Author.

American Occupational Therapy Association. (2014). Occupational therapy practice framework: Domain and process (3rd ed.). *American Journal of Occupational Therapy, 68*(Suppl. 1), S1–S48. http://dx.doi.org/10.5014/ajot.2014.682006

Americans With Disabilities Act of 1990, Pub. L. 101–336, 42 U.S.C. § 12101.

Bailey, D. M., & Schwartzberg, S. L. (2003). Section 504 and Americans With Disabilities Act. In D. M. Bailey & S. L. Schwartzberg (Eds.), *Ethical and legal dilemmas in occupational therapy* (2nd ed., pp. 34–57). Philadelphia: F. A. Davis.

Balcazar, F., Suarez-Balcazar, Y., Taylor-Ritzler, T., & Keys, C. (2010). *Race, culture and disability: Rehabilitation science and practice.* Sudbury, MA: Jones & Bartlett.

Baptiste, S. E. (2003). Client-centered practice: Implications for our professional approach, behaviors, and lexicon. In P. Kramer, J. Hinojosa, & C. B. Royeen (Eds.), *Perspectives in human occupation: Participation in life* (pp. 264–277). Philadelphia: Lippincott Williams & Wilkins.

Bateson, G. (1972). *Steps to an ecology of mind.* San Francisco: Chandler.

Bateson, G. (1979). *Mind and nature: A necessary unity.* New York: Dutton.

Bazyk, S., & Case-Smith, J. (2010). School-based occupational therapy. In J. Case-Smith & J. C. O'Brien (Eds.), *Occupational therapy for children* (6th ed., pp. 713–743). Maryland Heights, MO: Mosby/Elsevier.

Bennett, K. M., Gibbons, K., & Mackenzie-Smith, S. (2010). Loss and restoration in later life: An examination of dual process model of coping with bereavement. *Omega, 61,* 315–332.

Campbell, J., & Oliver, M. (1996). *Disability politics: Understanding our past, changing our future.* London: Routledge.

Carroll, T. J. (1961). *Blindness: What it is, what it does, and how to live with it.* Boston: Little, Brown.

Christiansen, C. H., & Baum, M. C. (Eds.). (1997). *Occupational therapy: Enabling function and well-being.* Thorofare, NJ: Slack.

Christiansen, C., Baum, M. C., & Bass-Haugen, J. (Eds.). (2005). *Occupational therapy: Performance, participation, and well-being* (3rd ed.). Thorofare, NJ: Slack.

Clark, F. (1993). Occupation embedded in a real life: Interweaving occupational science and occupational therapy [1993 Eleanor Clarke Slagle Lecture]. *American Journal of Occupational Therapy, 47,* 1067–1078. http://dx.doi.org/10.5014/ajot.47.12.1067

Clark, F., Azen, S. P., Zemke, R., Jackson, J., Carlson, M., Mandel, D.,...Lipson, L. (1997). Occupational therapy for independent-living older adults. A randomized controlled trial. *JAMA, 278,* 1321–1326. http://dx.doi.org/10.1001/jama.1997.03550160041036

Clegg, F. (1988). Bereavement. In S. Fisher & J. Reason (Eds.), *Handbook of life stress, cognition, and health* (pp. 61–78). Chichester, England: John Wiley.

Committee on a National Agenda for the Prevention of Disabilities. (1991). Executive summary. In A. M. Pope & A. R. Tarlov (Eds.), *Disability in America* (pp. 1–31). Washington, DC: National Academies Press.

Coster, W. (1998). Occupation-centered assessment of children. *American Journal of Occupational Therapy, 52,* 337–344. http://dx.doi.org/10.5014/ajot.52.5.337

Coster, W. J., & Haley, S. M. (1992). Conceptualization and measurement of disablement in infants and young children. *Infants and Young Children, 4,* 11–22. http://dx.doi.org/10.1097/00001163-199204000-00004

Dunn, W., Brown, C., & McGuigan, A. (1994). The ecology of human performance: A framework for considering the effect of context. *American Journal of Occupational Therapy, 48,* 595–607. http://dx.doi.org/10.5014/ajot.48.7.595

Dunn, W., Brown, C., & Youngstrom, M. J. (2003). Ecological model of occupation. In P. Kramer, J. Hinojosa, & C. B. Royeen (Eds.), *Perspectives in human occupation: Participation in life* (pp. 222–263). Philadelphia: Lippincott Williams & Wilkins.

Hinojosa, J., & Blount, M. L. (2008). Occupation, purposeful activities, and occupational therapy. In J. Hinojosa & M. L. Blount (Eds.), *The texture of life: Purposeful activities in occupational therapy* (3rd ed., pp. 1–28). Bethesda, MD: AOTA Press.

Hinojosa, J., & Blount, M. L. (2014). Occupation, activities, and occupational therapy. In J. Hinojosa & M. L. Blount (Eds.), *The texture of life: Purposeful activities in occupational therapy* (4th ed., pp. 1–16). Bethesda, MD: AOTA Press.

Hinojosa, J., Kramer, P., & Crist, P. (2014). Evaluation: Where do we begin? In J. Hinojosa, P. Kramer, & P. Crist (Eds.), *Evaluation: Obtaining and interpreting data* (4th ed., pp. 1–20). Bethesda, MD: AOTA Press.

Hinojosa, J., Kramer, P., Royeen, C. B., & Luebben, A. J. (2003). Core concept of occupation. In P. Kramer, J. Hinojosa, & C. B. Royeen (Eds.), *Perspectives in human occupation: Participation in life* (pp. 1–17). Philadelphia: Lippincott Williams & Wilkins.

Ideishi, R. I. (2003). Influence of occupation on assessment and treatment. In P. Kramer, J. Hinojosa, & C. B. Royeen (Eds.), *Perspectives in human occupation: Participation in life* (pp. 278–296). Philadelphia: Lippincott Williams & Wilkins.

Idhe, D. (1991). *Instrumental realism: The interface between philosophy of science and philosophy of technology.* Bloomington: Indiana University Press.

Individuals With Disabilities Education Act Amendments of 1997, Pub. L. 105–117, 20 U.S.C. § 1400 *et seq.*

Jackson, J., Carlson, M., Mandel, D., Zemke, R., & Clark, F. (1998). Occupation in lifestyle redesign: The Well Elderly Study occupational therapy program. *American Journal of Occupational Therapy, 52,* 326–336. http://dx.doi.org/10.5014/ajot.52.5.326

Knussen, C., & Cunningham, C. C. (1988). Stress, disability, and handicap. In S. Fisher & J. Reason (Eds.), *Handbook of life stress, cognition, and health* (pp. 335–350). Chichester, England: John Wiley.

Kramer, P., & Hinojosa, J. (2010). Philosophical and theoretical influences on evaluation. In J. Hinojosa, P. Kramer, & P. Crist (Eds.), *Occupational therapy evaluation: Obtaining and interpreting data* (3rd ed., pp. 21–40). Bethesda, MD: AOTA Press.

Latham, C. A. T. (2008). Occupation: Philosophy and concepts. In M. V. Radomski & C. A. T. Latham (Eds.), *Occupational therapy for physical dysfunction* (6th ed., pp. 340–357). Philadelphia: Lippincott Williams & Wilkins.

Law, M., Baum, M. C., & Dunn, W. (2005). *Measuring occupational performance: Supporting best practice in occupational therapy* (2nd ed.). Thorofare, NJ: Slack.

Lazarus, R. S., & Folkman, S. (1991). The concept of coping. In A. Monat & R. S. Lazarus (Eds.), *Stress and coping: An anthology* (3rd ed., pp. 189–206). New York: Columbia University Press.

Lollar, D. J. (2003). Foreword. In P. Kramer, J. Hinojosa, & C. B. Royeen (Eds.), *Perspectives in human occupation:*

Participation in life (pp. vii–viii). Philadelphia: Lippincott Williams & Wilkins.

Luebben, A. J. (2003). Ethical concerns: Human occupation. In P. Kramer, J. Hinojosa, & C. B. Royeen (Eds.), *Perspectives in human occupation: Participation in life* (pp. 297–311). Philadelphia: Lippincott Williams & Wilkins.

Metzler, C. (1997). A better idea. *OT Week, 11,* 14–15.

Metzler, C. (1998). Key issues in IDEA. *OT Week, 12,* 10.

Mosey, A. C. (1996). *Applied scientific inquiry in the health professions: An epistemological orientation* (2nd ed.). Bethesda, MD: American Occupational Therapy Association.

Murphy, R. F. (1990). *The body silent.* New York: W. W. Norton.

Nagi, S. Z. (1965). Some conceptual issues in disability and rehabilitation. In M. B. Sussman (Ed.), *Sociology and rehabilitation* (pp. 104–113). Washington, DC: American Sociological Association.

Nagi, S. Z. (1991). Disability concepts revisited: Implications for prevention. In A. M. Pope & A. R. Tarlov (Eds.), *Disability in America* (pp. 309–327). Washington, DC: National Academies Press.

Padilla, R. (2003). Clara: A phenomenology of disability. *American Journal of Occupational Therapy, 57,* 413–423. http://dx.doi.org/10.5014/ajot.57.4.413

Parkes, C. M. (1998). *Bereavement: Studies of grief in adult life.* Madison, CT: International Universities Press.

Parkes, C. M., & Weiss, R. S. (1983). The recovery process. In C. M. Parkes & R. S. Weiss (Eds.), *Recovery from bereavement* (pp. 155–168). New York: Basic Books.

Perkinson, H. J. (1984). *Learning from our mistakes: A reinterpretation of twentieth century educational theory.* Westport, CT: Greenwood.

Perkinson, H. J. (1993). *Teachers without goals, students without purposes.* New York: McGraw-Hill.

Pierce, D. (2001). Untangling occupation and activity. *American Journal of Occupational Therapy, 55,* 138–146. http://dx.doi.org/10.5014/ajot.55.2.138

Popper, K. R. (1985). *Popper selections* (D. Miller, Ed.). Princeton, NJ: Princeton University Press.

Popper, K. R. (1992). *In search of a better world: Lectures and essays from thirty years.* London: Routledge.

Price-Lackey, P., & Cashman, J. (1996). Jenny's story: Reinventing oneself through occupation and narrative configuration. *American Journal of Occupational Therapy, 50,* 306–314. http://dx.doi.org/10.5014/ajot.50.4.306

Rogers, J. C., & Holm, M. B. (1994). Accepting the challenge of outcome research: Examining the effectiveness of occupational therapy practice. *American Journal of Occupational Therapy, 48,* 871–876. http://dx.doi.org/10.5014/ajot.48.10.871

Schön, D. A. (1983). *The reflective practitioner: How professionals think in action.* New York: Basic.

Slater, D., & Meade, M. A. (2004). Participation in recreation and sports for persons with spinal cord injury: Review and recommendations. *NeuroRehabilitation, 19,* 121–129.

Tham, K., & Kielhofner, G. (2003). Impact of the social environment on occupational experience and performance among persons with unilateral neglect. *American Journal of Occupational Therapy, 57,* 403–412. http://dx.doi.org/10.5014/ajot.57.4.403

Trombly, C. A. (1993). Anticipating the future: Assessment of occupational function. *American Journal of Occupational Therapy, 47,* 253–257. http://dx.doi.org/10.5014/ajot.47.3.253

Trombly, C. A. (1995). Occupation: Purposefulness and meaningfulness as therapeutic mechanisms [1995 Eleanor Clarke Slagle Lecture]. *American Journal of Occupational Therapy, 49,* 960–972. http://dx.doi.org/10.5014/ajot.49.10.960

Weinstock-Zlotnick, G., & Hinojosa, J. (2004). Bottom-up or top-down evaluation: Is one better than the other? *American Journal of Occupational Therapy, 58,* 594–599. http://dx.doi.org/10.5014/ajot.58.5.594

Wilbarger, P., & Wilbarger, J. L. (1991). *Sensory defensiveness in children aged 2–12: An intervention guide for parents and other caretakers.* Santa Barbara, CA: Avanti Educational Programs.

Wilbarger, P., & Wilbarger, J. L. (1997). *Sensory defensiveness and related social/emotional and neurological problems (Course syllabus).* Oak Park Heights, MN: Professional Development Programs.

Wood, P. H. N. (1980). Appreciating the consequences of disease: The international classification of impairments, disabilities, and handicaps. *WHO Chronicle, 34,* 376–380.

Wood, W. (1998). It is jump time for occupational therapy. *American Journal of Occupational Therapy, 52,* 403–411. http://dx.doi.org/10.5014/ajot.52.6.403

World Health Organization. (1980). *International classification of impairments, disabilities, and handicaps.* Geneva: Author.

World Health Organization. (1990). *International classification of diseases* (10th rev.). Geneva: Author.

World Health Organization. (2001). *International classification of functioning, disability and health—Short version.* Geneva: Author.

Youngstrom, M. J. (2002). *Report of the chairperson of the commission on practice, III.C. to the representative assembly (RA Charge No. 2002M29).* Bethesda, MD: American Occupational Therapy Association.

Appendix 11.A. The Occupational Therapy Reflective Staircase Worksheet

Name: _____

Age: _____

Brief activity history: _____

Concerns, needs, wants, and priorities of the person that could guide evaluation, treatment, and possible outcomes related to activity performance: _____

Concerns, needs, wants, and priorities of the caregiver or significant other involved, which could guide evaluation, treatment, and possible outcomes related to activity performance: _____

Additional notes (e.g., you may want to include medical precautions, disposition plans, contexts in which activities are usually performed, other factors that may affect activity performance): _____

Identify the problem (related to activity chosen together with the person):_____

Make a guess:_____

Perform the activity to address the problem: _____

Criticize the guess: _____

Make a better guess:_____

Reframe the problem if needed: _____

CHAPTER 12.

INDEPENDENCE: SIMULATION OF LIFE ACTIVITIES TO OCCUPATIONS

Anita Perr, PhD, OT, ATP, FAOTA

Highlights

✧ Process to reintegrate clients into natural contexts
✧ Goal of occupational therapy intervention: Participation in real-life activities and occupations
✧ Independence and optimal participation
✧ Dependent or independent?
✧ Habilitation and rehabilitation: Transition process and simulation at each level of transition
✧ Simulation to improve occupational performance in areas other than occupational therapy
✧ Simulation in occupational therapy
✧ Advanced assistive technologies and simulation
✧ Real life.

Key Terms

✧ Avatars
✧ Brain–computer interface
✧ Computer simulation
✧ Contrived activities
✧ Dependence
✧ Exploratory play
✧ Habilitation
✧ Haptics
✧ High-fidelity simulation technology
✧ Independence
✧ Optimal participation
✧ Physical interactive simulation
✧ Real life

✧ Rehabilitation
✧ Role play
✧ Simulation
✧ Subskills
✧ Technology abandonment
✧ Transition process
✧ Virtual
✧ Virtual interactive gaming technology
✧ Virtual online worlds
✧ Virtual reality
✧ Virtual reality therapy
✧ Visual interactive simulation

This chapter discusses the importance of activities in the *habilitation* (i.e., learning and incorporating new skills into life) or *rehabilitation* (i.e., relearning skills previously known and part of life) process and in preparation for real-life occupation. Many textbooks concentrate only on occupational therapy and its use of activities in controlled environments, such as an occupational therapy clinic or lab or in a patient's room, but this chapter addresses the value of client-centered activities as part of the end goal of occupational therapy, namely, a client's return to real life.

Real life involves participation in activities or occupations outside the controlled therapeutic environment. It often requires that a client engage in activities that he or she commonly performed in specific contexts and settings before his or her illness or injury. Real life takes place in and around the home, in familiar and new places in the person's community, and in locations at great distances from home. Often, real life for a client with disabilities also requires that he or she engages in new occupations or performs activities in new ways.

This chapter begins with a discussion of simulated activities as a therapeutic modality to prepare a client for participation in occupations in the natural environment and describes the steps leading to performing occupations in real life. Next, the chapter discusses the goal of occupational therapy and presents a view that independence for a person is defined from the person's perspective rather than by his or her ability to perform a specific activity or task.

Finally, a summary of habilitation and rehabilitation discusses the nature of the transition process and simulations at each level of that process. Simulations used in areas other than occupational therapy are outlined before occupational therapy simulations (including smartphone and tablet applications, virtual reality, interventions that simulate real life, and simulations that ensure activities are purposeful) are discussed. The chapter concludes with a discussion of advanced assistive technologies and simulation.

Process to Reintegrate Clients Into Natural Contexts

Occupational therapy practitioners assume a critical role in the process of integrating a client into

his or her natural contexts. Using the therapeutic value of simulated activities, the practitioner works in collaboration with the client, caregivers, significant others, and other professionals to match the client's engagement in an activity with particular therapeutic goals. *Simulation* is the copied representation of the functioning by other means. A synonym for *simulated* is *virtual*.

The process by which a client reintegrates into his or her environment involves a series of transitions along a continuum of activities that includes five steps:

1. Performance of *contrived activities,* which are the clinical activities practitioners use in place of the actual end goal of the treatment session, in a clinical or controlled environment (e.g., stacking blocks)
2. Performance of simulated activities in a clinical environment (e.g., role playing a job interview with other clients)
3. Performance of simulated activities in a real environment (e.g., pretending to brush teeth at the bathroom sink)
4. Performance of real activities in a simulated environment (e.g., shaving at the sink in the occupational therapy clinic)
5. Performance of real activities in an actual environment (e.g., taking a bus to school or making a meal at home).

Figure 12.1 illustrates this process of a client's reintegration into his or her environment. Simulations are a central concept in these transitions.

Goal of Occupational Therapy Intervention: Participation in Real-Life Activities and Occupations

The overall goal of occupational therapy is for each client to participate in real-life activities and occupations that he or she needs or wants to participate in, in the environments where they usually take place, with or without other people. The United Nations (UN) Convention on the Rights of Persons With Disabilities is based, in part, on the principle of full and effective participation and inclusion in society (United Nations, 2006). Participation is central to the functioning described in the *International*

Figure 12.1. Client reintegration into his or her environment. Transitions along a continuum of activities move from contrived simulations to real-life occupations.

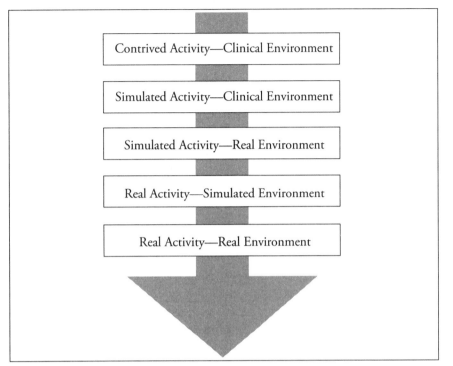

Contrived Activity—Clinical Environment

Simulated Activity—Clinical Environment

Simulated Activity—Real Environment

Real Activity—Simulated Environment

Real Activity—Real Environment

Source. A. Perr. Used with permission.

Classification of Functioning, Disability and Health (*ICF;* World Health Organization, 2001). The *ICF* model of functioning and disability describes the interactions among the person, the activities, and the contexts. The *ICF* acknowledges that biological and societal influences cannot be addressed separately but must both be addressed when discussing participation.

Through a collaborative process, the client (and possibly the client's caregivers) and occupational therapy practitioner identify and develop goals that meet the client's needs, address his or her specific environmental and personal factors, and are meaningful to the client.

Independence and Optimal Participation

Optimal participation means that the person participates in the activities he or she desires at the level he or she is able. Many people assume that real-life functioning means that a client can function independently. To accomplish this objective,

some occupational therapy practitioners focus on the client's developing the ability to complete tasks by himself or herself. This objective, however, is only relevant if it is acceptable to and appropriate for the client. The concept of independence is of major importance because many people associate independence with the ability to perform or complete specific tasks, activities, or occupations.

Occupational therapy practitioners define the concept of independence from the client's perspective. A client's independence is not based on his or her performance of various tasks; rather, *independence* is the ability to execute the task in a manner that is acceptable to the client. For many people, what is important is the ability to direct the type and style of assistance being received. Each person individually operationalizes the concept of independence for himself or herself— that is, the way one person defines *independence* may be different from another person's definition (American Occupational Therapy Association, 2002, 2014).

For example, a person may consider herself independent in managing her own meals if she can open containers, prepare cold foods, and cook hot foods. Another person might consider himself independent by eating in restaurants or having food delivered. The person in the first example might not consider this situation as independence because it does not include food preparation. The definition changes depending on the person's own interests, values, and priorities. What is important is the person's optimal participation. Optimal participation means that an occupational therapy practitioner considers the client's culture, support systems, and values when assessing a client's independent functioning.

The concept of independence becomes increasingly complex when activities are adapted or assistive devices are used. Society often views people with disabilities differently from people without disabilities, judging people with disabilities according to different standards. Many people view those with disabilities as limited in their participation if they use an adaptation or assistive device. For instance, a person who had a brain injury may use an assistive technology device to track appointments and keep lists of instructions for completing daily tasks. People without disabilities may judge this person to be limited or dependent. A person without a disability may use a similar device to track his or her schedule, yet others perceive this person as using technology to its fullest. Such double standards illustrate how society may judge people with disabilities (and perceive their level of independence) unfairly.

When independence is a goal, occupational therapy practitioners may modify environmental factors, use assistive technology, or integrate compensatory strategies to facilitate the client's participation in an activity. For instance, one goal for a person paralyzed after a cervical spinal cord injury may be to perform household maintenance activities independently. In this situation, independence requires the use of a wheelchair (i.e., assistive technology). From a practitioner's point of view, this client is independent in household maintenance when he or she performs the activities using the wheelchair. The use of a compensatory strategy or device, then, does not negate a person's independence; rather, such strategies or devices are simply the means to be independent.

Some clients may not be capable of or desire full independence. In this situation, the occupational therapist begins by evaluating the client to identify the steps in the process that are limited; the physical, sensory, cognitive, or psychosocial impairments that limit performance; and the obstacles to independence. In collaboration with the client, the occupational therapy practitioner develops realistic goals whether they are independence, partial performance, or the ability to instruct someone or something in his or her care. The practitioner may intervene by simplifying the activity to match the client's level of function, thus encouraging his or her participation. In addition, the practitioner may adapt the activity, manipulate the context, or teach the client to use assistive devices and compensatory techniques to facilitate task performance. The practitioner may also train the client to instruct others to help meet his or her needs.

The occupational therapist and client determine the client's potential for independence, and they select activities that lead to this goal. For example, a client may want to move from his bed to the toilet in the bathroom by walking, but the evaluation reveals poor sitting balance and coordination as well as an inability to stand with or without assistance. The evaluation also reveals good safety judgment and memory. Together, the occupational therapist and the client determine that a wheelchair will be necessary to move from the bed to the toilet in the bathroom. They expect that the client will be able to complete wheelchair transfers to and from his bed independently, perhaps using a sliding board (Figure 12.2). They decide that a reasonable short-term goal is performance of toilet transfers following setup with a sliding board and that a reasonable long-term goal is independent toileting, including transfers, lower-extremity garment management, and hygiene.

In therapy, the client performs activities to improve his sitting balance, including activities that he can perform at home with his family (i.e., contrived activities). In therapy, he practices transfers to and from various surfaces other than the toilet (i.e., simulated activities in the clinical environment). At home, he practices only toilet transfers with his attendant (i.e., simulated activities in the real environment), not lower-extremity garment management or hygiene after toileting. Later in therapy, he will practice transfers and lower-extremity garment management (i.e., real activities in a simulated environment). Eventually, he will

Figure 12.2. A young man with sitting balance and coordination problems works on integrating upper- and lower-body movements while practicing a sliding-board transfer with his outpatient occupational therapist.

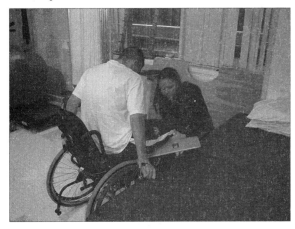

Source. A. Perr. Used with permission.

perform toileting at home (i.e., an occupation in the real environment).

Another example demonstrates a young man who has reached the end goal of therapy, which is to transfer from his wheelchair to his car in the parking lot of his apartment building (Figure 12.3). His use of the wheelchair, protective gloves, and a sliding board make him independent.

A client who does not wish to perform all aspects of his or her daily activities personally may still exert control over his or her routine by determining

Figure 12.3. A man transfers independently to his car.

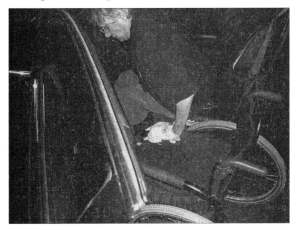

Source. A. Perr. Used with permission.

which activities to delegate to others. The occupational therapy intervention may include activities that help the client improve the clarity and manner in which he or she gives instructions to caregivers. For example, the occupational therapy practitioner and client may engage in role play to optimize client–caregiver interactions. These activities begin as simulations, such as role playing in a controlled environment, then transition into real life as the client directs the caregiver at home. The goal of many clients, however, is to become as independent as possible. Case Example 12.1 describes real-life activities that require assistance and the client's definition of independence.

Case Example 12.1 illustrates three crucial points. First, Daphne actively participates in some tasks and delegates others to her roommate. Second, Daphne's delegation does not diminish her sense of independence because she retains control over which tasks she delegates. Third, Daphne con-

Case Example 12.1. Daphne: Wheeled Mobility Evaluation

Daphne, age 28 years, has juvenile rheumatoid arthritis. During the rehabilitation process, Daphne participates in a seating and wheeled mobility evaluation and eventually receives a power wheelchair and seating system that enable her to negotiate smooth and uneven terrain both indoors and outside. She is able to transfer independently to and from her wheelchair.

Daphne has not been able to position her wheelchair for charging, connect her wheelchair to the battery charger in the evening, or unplug the charger and position the wheelchair for her transfer in the mornings. Daphne lives with a roommate who assists her with these activities. Daphne considers herself an independent person and hopes that she can devise a method to charge her wheelchair herself. For now, she is satisfied with her roommate assisting her, which allows her to spend her time on other tasks. Currently, this aspect of her real life is one in which she uses assistance. Her independence hinges on her ability to instruct her roommate in the appropriate care or assistance she requires.

tinues to strive for even greater independence for the future. Daphne is not independent in performing the task of wheelchair maintenance. Although she requires help in managing the maintenance of her wheelchair, she is independent in managing her routine in this area.

This case example illustrates independence for a person with a disability. Consider your own life. How do you define independence for yourself in relation to your family and your schoolwork? Think about whether you perform activities yourself or with others. Do you perform activities with help from others, or do you let other people perform the activities for you?

You may consider yourself independent because you have the freedom and the responsibility to make your own decisions, prioritize your activities, and accept the consequences of your decisions. In the same manner, a person with a disability may experience independence through personal performance, through the decision to delegate a time-consuming or difficult task, and by directing others to meet his or her needs. In addition, context can change your definition of independence.

Exercise 12.1. Life as a Student

Consider life as a student away from home. The context in which you perform activities has changed, and the human environment no longer includes your parents. Answer the following questions. How do you define your new level of independence? Does this independence differ from the independence you had living at home with your family? If so, in what ways? Consider your level of freedom. Who controls or directs your activities and your occupations? Consider the different ways in which people with disabilities may experience independence.

Dependent or Independent?

Independence may seem like a simple concept on the surface, yet the more one explores it, the more complex it becomes. In addition, understanding your own values concerning dependence and independence and being aware that they may be different than your client's is an important attribute to develop for occupational therapy practitioners.

Exercise 12.2. Independent Meal Preparation

1. Answer the following questions about you; be open-minded, and take the time to think carefully about your answers:
   • What is independent meal preparation?
   • Does independent meal preparation require cooking? Using a microwave oven? Using the stovetop or range? Following a recipe? Does preparation of a cold meal count?
   • Does independent meal preparation include getting packages from cabinets and the refrigerator and opening them, or is it still independent meal preparation if someone else cooks and puts together the meals and you merely put them on the table?
   • Does independent meal preparation require independently obtaining the food? Does it require shopping? Making a shopping list? Carrying food home?
   • Is it independent meal preparation if you order a meal from a restaurant or from a local delivery service? Does money management matter, or can a personal assistant pay for the meal? Can you run a tab that someone else pays and still be independent?
2. Select one of the following clients with a disability and answer the preceding questions for him or her: a woman who has had a stroke resulting in left hemiparesis, a young man diagnosed with depression, or a young woman with cerebral palsy resulting in spastic diplegia.

Are your answers from the exercise different for the client than for you? Why would a person with a disability be held to a different standard than the one we hold for ourselves? Planning for your client to order food or for the client to organize having someone else prepare meals is an appropriate activity. You have to know your client and his or her family members, support system, and needs, and then plan treatment accordingly.

Similar questions can be asked for every activity. Why is it acceptable for people without disabilities to hire a maid, but so important for clients with disabilities to be able to make a bed or iron a shirt? What is actually important depends on the client and his or her own situation. The occupational therapy practitioner should not force his or her values on a client. The role of the practitioner is to help a client meet his or her needs as he or she defines them, so if the ability to manage household help is what is important to the client, then that is what is important for the occupational therapy practitioner to consider.

Exercise 12.3. Independent Home Management

1. Answer the following questions about you:
   • What is independent home management?
   • Do you have to be able to mow a lawn?
   • What if you live in an apartment and have no lawn?
   • What if you hire someone to mow your lawn?
2. Select another client from Exercise 12.2, and answer the previous questions for him or her.

Are your answers different for this client compared with the client you selected in Exercise 12.2? The client's neighbor may have a lawn care service, or a teenager in the neighborhood may do the work. If this choice is acceptable for the neighbor, is it acceptable for your client? What if no one else in the neighborhood receives this service?

Habilitation and Rehabilitation: Transition Process and Simulation at Each Level of Transition

During the habilitation or rehabilitation process, a series of transitions occur. These transitions take place at each stage in which a person masters a new skill or gains the ability to instruct another in the assistance that is needed. Simulations are frequently used to make each transition easier (see Figure 12.1). The chronology of these transitions generally moves a person from *dependence* (difficulty in performing or inability to perform life skills) to the ability to perform desired occupations or instruct others in any assistance that is needed. Each step along the way involves a transition, and at the completion of each transition, the person is closer to independent participation. At each transition, the client actively participates in selecting and performing activities to promote the acquisition of occupational performance skills toward an agreed-upon goal.

Transition Process

Although people try to place events in a sensible order, the transition process during habilitation or rehabilitation often does not occur in an orderly and predetermined fashion. For example, some people start the process with total dependence and may require contrived activities in the clinic or other externally structured environments to master initial subskills. Contrived activities can be meaningful to the client if he or she understands their place in the overall treatment plan. The client should understand that these activities are temporary and transitional in nature and provide an opportunity for him or her to learn occupational performance skills that he or she will later integrate into the performance of occupations in his or her natural environment (Case Example 12.2).

Other people may start somewhere further along the continuum and focus on learning or relearning

---

Case Example 12.2. Dana: Severe Anxiety

Dana, age 44 years, experiences severe anxiety when he takes the elevator to his job on the 15th floor of a high-rise office building. Dana's goal is to take the elevator by himself without feeling anxious. Presently, however, he becomes physically ill when simply contemplating the idea. Because of his inability to use elevators, the occupational therapist has decided to initiate intervention by engaging Dana in simple, nonthreatening activities that involve the elevator.

Dana and his therapist discuss the activities, and with Dana's input, they make slight modifications. They decide on the following: Dana will watch the elevator doors open and close, watch people get on and off, push the button to summon the elevator, and quickly walk on and off the stationary elevator. During these activities, the therapist encourages Dana to discuss his level of comfort or discomfort, and the therapist in turn provides support and encouragement. Although contrived, these activities are meaningful to Dana and actively engage him.

skills in a simulated environment. Still others start at different points in different performance areas. For example, one client may be dependent in one area such as dressing and be further along the continuum in another area such as work activities and computer use. Here, the difference in performance level may be because the person has relatively intact fine motor coordination for computer use but impaired balance and gross motor performance, which he or she needs for dressing while sitting on the edge of the bed.

The transition process varies among clients. Moreover, discrepancies occur between the expectations and the actual progress made by each client. No one can say exactly how long a person will stay in any stage of the process or whether he or she will move forward and backward several times. Some people never make the journey all the way to being able to do all desired activities without assistance; they continue to require or choose to use assistance. Remember that the definitions of independence depend on the client's views.

Instead of following a neat, linear, and predictable timetable, the process of habilation or rehabilitation sometimes moves forward, sometimes backward, and sometimes in a spiraling pattern. The occupational therapy practitioner sets goals and expectations in conjunction with the client based on a wealth of information, including the practitioner's previous experiences, the client's current level of functioning, the context, and the practitioner's knowledge of body structures and functions. The practitioner adjusts treatment sessions and revises goals when necessary in response to the winding trail of progress.

Although most people would prefer a more predictable process, it is not possible because of the unpredictable nature of habilitation and rehabilitation. People are not machines, and many factors such as attitudes, values, mental functions, and physical geography affect their ability to participate in therapy programs and perform activities. This unpredictability is sometimes unsettling for occupational therapy students and for new practitioners. Clients and family members may have difficulty accepting this unpredictability as well and often view repeating previously learned skills as a step backward. Therefore, the occupational therapy practitioner must reassure clients, families, and others involved that the process is complex and somewhat unpredictable and that movement to a previous step does not signify failure.

Exercise 12.4. John: Performance Continuum

John is a bright 6-year-old with cerebral palsy. He has low tone in his trunk, but after months of therapy, he now can maintain good dynamic balance in long sitting. John's goal is to learn to put on his socks and shoes by himself. Where along the continuum would you begin your occupational therapy intervention and why? Which activities would you select? How would you grade the activity you select?

Suppose you select an activity to teach the concepts of *on* and *off* and to work on dynamic short-sitting balance in which John places large plastic rings on a pole as he sits on a small chair with his feet on the floor. Where on the continuum is this activity? How do you change the activity to bring John to the next level?

(The occupational therapy practitioner would continue by teaching John how to position himself on the chair he would use at home. After John masters the concepts of *on* and *off,* the next activity would address John's short-sitting balance by requiring him to put on his socks and shoes with one foot on the floor. After the practitioner determines that John's balance is sufficient for putting on his socks and shoes in the short-sitting position, she would have him practice putting them on in the long-sitting position.)

As a new practitioner gains more experience, his or her expectations may match the actual outcome more closely, but the expected procedure may still require some modification. The practitioner and the client must accept these facts and adjust the program and expectations to meet the client's current needs and abilities. Occupational therapy will otherwise be less meaningful and less effective. Although the exact process is unpredictable, some trends are evident in the timing and order of the transitions and stages. Figure 12.4 illustrates that the process is not linear; some stages are skipped or take longer to move through, and sometimes certain stages are not attained. The first transition is when someone detects a problem in body function or structure or a problem with participation. At that instant, the client transitions from being a person without a disability to a person with a disability.

Simulation at Each Level of Transition

Simulation of real-life activity plays a crucial role in occupational therapy at each level of transition (see

Figure 12.4. Stages of progression through habilitation and rehabilitation.

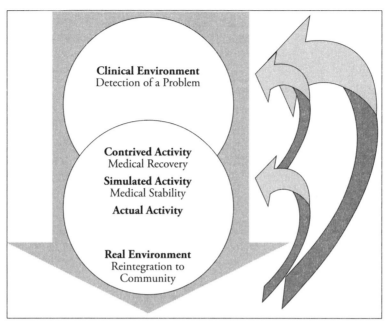

Source. A. Perr. Used with permission.

Figure 12.1). However, the importance of simulation in occupational therapy may not be obvious to clients or their caregivers, especially at the beginning of the process. As therapy progresses, activities resemble real life more closely.

After a traumatic injury or illness, the client has a period of medical recovery in which the primary focus is survival. Even so, initiating occupational therapy, in the form of contrived activities in a clinical environment, may be possible at this point. Because of the client's condition, the occupational therapy practitioner often limits sessions to activities that do not closely resemble real life, and the client may not associate these actions with the accomplishment of an occupation (such as self-feeding) that he or she will perform in the future. For example, the practitioner may ask the client to grasp objects of various shapes and sizes, place and release these objects on various planes, and perform certain movement patterns while sitting or lying in bed. These activities, although contrived, are crucial to promote joint range of motion and muscle flexibility in the upper extremities.

As the person becomes more medically stable, he or she may be better able to participate in therapy. During this stage of transition, in which the client performs simulated activities in a clinical envi-

ronment (see Figure 12.1), learning various skills becomes the focus of occupational therapy. The occupational therapy practitioner may teach the skills individually, and the skills may or may not be related to each other and are sometimes referred to as *subskills.*

After the client masters the subskills to some degree, the practitioner combines them in certain groupings to simulate various real-life activities. Initially, these simulated activities in a client's treatment session may be very different from the expected, eventual occupational performance. Therefore, the client sometimes has difficulty understanding their usefulness in relation to his or her needs and may perform individual skills out of sequence or in awkward ways. The client may also skip some steps or skills altogether at this point.

The treatment sessions are an abstract representation of real life, which can be frustrating for the client and for others involved in the client's progression. Therefore, the occupational therapy practitioner must reassure the client and family that the simulations reflect real-life situations and that the actual activities will eventually be brought into the clinical environment.

During the next stages of transition, the client performs simulations in real environments and real

Case Example 12.3. Betsy: Learning Skills Out of Sequence

Betsy, age 53 years, has bipolar disorder and attends an outpatient mental health clinic. Betsy has learned strategies to control impulsive behavior and foster taking turns, basic money management skills, and how to be appropriately assertive. She eagerly participated in the activities to learn these skills and was able to master them individually. Next, she and the occupational therapist planned a trip to the local supermarket to shop for an upcoming holiday party. During the shopping trip, Betsy had the opportunity to integrate these learned skills into a mostly successful shopping experience in a real environment.

Although Betsy behaved appropriately in the market, the therapist realized that Betsy's approach to shopping was haphazard and inefficient. Therefore, the therapist introduced a smart phone application for shopping list management and shopping strategy. In therapy, they used a department smartphone, but the application was able to be downloaded to Betsy's smartphone.

The therapist designed an activity in which Betsy made a shopping list and organized it according to the categories in the application. They then used a floor plan of the local market to strategize their approach to shopping. They reorganized the shopping list so the categories appeared in the same order as their path through the market. They practiced inputting information with a few more shopping lists that the therapist prepared ahead of time.

Following these clinic-based activities, Betsy and the therapist went back to the market, using the list on the smartphone application to guide their shopping trip. After this successful outing, they discussed the differences between the two shopping trips. Betsy demonstrated good insight and problem solving as they talked about strategies Betsy could implement in her neighborhood market.

activities in simulated environments to prepare for occupational performance in the real environment. As discussed previously, a practitioner may skip steps along this continuum or revisit them until the client achieves maximal performance of the occupation in the real environment. Case Example 12.3 demonstrates that a person may learn skills out of sequence and then later integrate them into an occupation, in this case, first learning skills in a clinic setting, then performing the real-life activity, and then using clinic-based activity simulations to improve that performance.

Simulation to Improve Occupational Performance in Areas Other Than Occupational Therapy

The use of simulation to improve occupational performance is not unique to habilitation or rehabilitation. For instance, everyone can remember practicing each component of a certain skill before putting all the components together and practicing the entire skill in a protected environment and then performing it successfully in the real envi-

ronment. Learning a balance beam routine is one example of this process. A gymnast may begin by practicing each jump and flip on a mat. She may also practice walking on a straight line marked on the floor. For the gymnast, these are subskills, which only distantly resemble the final routine. Once the gymnast masters the individual subskills, she then combines them. The routine is still not exactly the same as the real-life routine; it is a simulation. For example, the gymnast may perform the routine more slowly or on a low or wide beam. Finally, the gymnast performs the routine in its appropriate context, completing the mastery phase of simulation. For the gymnast, real-life performance of the routine occurs during a competition or exhibition. At any time, however, she may return to simulation to refine and practice the individual skills.

Mechanical simulations or mock-ups, computer simulations, visual interactive simulations, physical interactive simulations, virtual online worlds, high-fidelity simulation technology, and virtual interactive gaming technology can provide an accurate representation of the real world. Simulation is commonplace in many areas such as engineering; product design, development, testing, and marketing; industry; and health care. People can analyze ease of use, efficiency, and worker and consumer behaviors through simulations. In marketing, the process of testing a concept, then building and testing a prototype, can measure the viability of ideas long before the product is actually manufactured, thus saving valuable time, effort, and money (Eastlack, 1968).

The value of rigorous testing simulations to determine the durability, effectiveness, usability, and viability of various products and processes cannot be overstated. Industries such as aeronautics and medicine, in which the risk of real-life practice is very high, have long used simulation to train new employees and help veterans hone their skills.

Simulation is a powerful training tool, allowing for multiple practice opportunities, provision of feedback and assessment, and adjustment of environmental demands, all in a safe and controlled learning environment (Brodie, 2005; Grand et al., 2013). However, note that simulation is not a stand-alone training solution but rather a complementary tool to real-world instruction and application.

Physical Interactive Simulation

Physical interactive simulation is used in industry to analyze systems for efficiency and effectiveness. This method of simulation uses models that can be easily changed and with which people can interact. It is also used for hands-on learning. Physical interactive simulation is a dynamic technique that provides a highly accurate representation of the real world and goes beyond *computer simulation,* which lacks physical components and consists of a visual representation of the situation being simulated, or *visual interactive simulation,* which allows users to have some interaction (but because it is only a visual representation, the simulation is not as realistic as with the physical interactive simulation; Winarchick & Caldwell, 1997). Through physical interactive simulation, a person's performance of a task can be simulated and evaluated in a three-dimensional physical model.

For example, Delphi Chassis Systems and Sinclair Community College, both in Dayton, OH, worked together to establish a workplace prototype lab in which analysis of an entire production model saved Delphi Chassis Systems millions of dollars. Users of physical interactive simulation were able to

interact with models before determining their work site setups to maximize productivity and save time and money in development. The models were easy to construct, rearrange, and modify to provide a variety of analyses, including motion economy and ergonomics (Winarchick & Caldwell, 1997).

In the United Kingdom, the National Metals Technology Centre (Namtec) launched an advanced computer design, modeling, and simulation center in 2006 to serve a wide cross-section of manufacturing businesses, metal producers, and engineering firms. Working environments, assembly processes, and product designs are simulated in three-dimensional cinematographic style that allows in-depth scrutiny, thus helping to limit errors early and reduce or eliminate the need for physical prototypes (Barrett, 2007). In this way, the running of a new manufacturing plant can be simulated in its entirety before it is built. In addition, Namtec's virtual reality suite could project computer-generated three-dimensional images of processes and products and allow them to be rotated, zoomed in or out, and modified. As a result, users were able to refine their designs and optimize manufacturing methods and plans before making substantial capital investments to implement them. Computer-aided design and a variety of software programs are available now for everyday users to explore their ideas.

Virtual Online Worlds

Virtual online worlds such as Second Life (www.secondlife.com) exist entirely on the Internet as computer-based, simulated environments in which users interact and live through personally customized human representations of themselves, known as *avatars* (Howarth, 2009). Second Life, the most popular virtual world used by the public, was launched by Linden Lab in 2003. In 2014, Second Life had an estimated 36 million residents. Second Life is an elaborate simulated world, and its program is voice enabled to allow the user to hear and see other avatars, providing real-time social interaction (Hansen, 2008). Included in this virtual three-dimensional universe are universities; libraries; tourist attractions and destinations; social interactive venues for educational, entertainment, and cultural opportunities; and even discussion and support groups.

In one example, a large hospital in California previewed its proposed multimillion-dollar health care complex on Second Life many years before the facility's expected completion. As avatars, staff, patients, and other visitors could tour, experience, and interact with the new technology and with the cutting-edge health care innovation of the (virtual) hospital, including patients' rooms, bedside environmental controls, and surgical suites (Bruck, 2008). This virtual project preview was initially intended as a marketing and staff recruitment tool but could also provide valuable "product testing" and useful feedback to inform the design and use of space in the facility.

Many people access and disseminate health care information through Second Life. Academicians, businesses, not-for-profit organizations, and self-help groups all use Second Life to explore ways in which to leverage their influence (Bruck, 2008). In addition, the Centers for Disease Control and Prevention (CDC) and the National Institutes of Health are active in Second Life. CDC offers virtual health fairs and podcasts and holds virtual meetings on a variety of health topics, with the goal of influencing the real-world health decisions of visitors. Second Life is a boon for many people, including those with social anxiety and autism, who can use the virtual world to socialize, reduce fear, reduce stress, and develop social skills (Bruck, 2008). Avatar dating is popular because it is less threatening to the ego and self-esteem while allowing for personal and physical safety. Some avatar couples in Second Life get married in the real world (Fiorino, 2009; Schechtman, 2012).

Many people use time spent in the virtual world as a temporary escape from a stressful reality. Some universities are using Second Life as a virtual teaching and learning location in which problem-based learning and self-teaching groups can meet and actively interact. By giving students enough time to interact with other avatars (such as patients, staff members, and other professionals) in a safe, simulated environment, it is possible to decrease student anxiety and perhaps increase competence in learning a new skill (Chow, Herold, Choo, & Chan, 2012; Hansen, 2008; Honey, Connor, Veltman, Bodily, & Diener, 2012). Education in the virtual world is not a replacement for face-to-face, real-life, teacher–student interaction but rather an adjunct learning tool—especially in

health care education, where real-life interaction in the natural environment is critical and cannot be simulated. Virtual worlds such as Second Life are a part of our present reality. Online users of all ages can benefit from this technology that offers immersion, simulation, role-playing, and socialization and provides opportunities for creative expression, fun, forming relationships, and learning from and collaborating with others all over the world.

High-Fidelity Simulation Technology

High-fidelity simulation technology refers to simulation that is very close to real life. The industry that trains operators of large tractor trailers, emergency vehicles (such as fire trucks), trains, and specialized heavy equipment can use high-fidelity simulation technology such as the National Advanced Driving Simulator at the University of Iowa (www.nads-sc. uiowa.edu). This simulator, owned by the National Highway Traffic Safety Administration, can recreate the sights and sounds of driving on highways; busy city streets; and narrow, winding country roads. Road conditions, weather conditions, and time of day or night are among the many parameters that can be simulated. In addition, during training, the driver's reaction to a range of environmental distractions (e.g., blown tires, cell phones) are recorded by the simulator's video cameras and sensors (O'Neil, 2001).

Virtual Interactive Gaming Technology

Virtual interactive gaming technology allows players take on various roles and perform various activities in simulated environments. Gaming technologies range from racing to combat to fashion, to name just a few. Industries and organizations such as car dealerships, financial services firms, and business and consulting companies are turning to virtual interactive gaming systems as a way to train their employees. Simulated games, tailored to meet training needs, allow employees to rapidly practice skills, learn new processes, and test their knowledge before they tackle the demands of a real work setting (Brodie, 2005; Cohen, Iluz, & Shtub, 2013; Graafland, Schraagen, & Schijven, 2012).

Simulation in Occupational Therapy

Occupational therapy practitioners use various tools to enhance a client's ability to function in his or her natural environment and to engage more fully in community life. Virtually all practitioners use simulation as a therapeutic modality or tool. It is especially appropriate for use with people who have a variety of functional impairments that affect their participation in daily activities. Simulation can be effective as a therapeutic modality regardless of the client's age, gender, or ethnic or cultural background. In occupational therapy, simulation intervention shares some of the same characteristics and benefits as simulation in other industries and professions. While simulating an activity, occupation, or situation, the practitioner and the client can control the practice intensity, context, and environment of the clinical intervention. The practitioner can also provide feedback to the client and measure the outcome of the intervention.

As in other situations, simulation training by the occupational therapy practitioner is an adjunct to real-world intervention with the client. The client's interaction with the natural setting is crucial to maximizing his or her ability to engage meaningfully and practically in real-life occupations.

Smartphone and Tablet Technology as a Therapeutic Modality

Using smartphone and tablet technology as a therapeutic modality during the occupational therapy process can ease the transition to real life through various levels of simulations. For example, people with disabilities may be able to use smart phones and tablets during their daily lives rather than rely on assistance from another person. In addition to social media, many free or low-cost applications are available that an occupational therapy practitioner can use during intervention and that a client can use in real life. Shopping list, health and wellness, disability aid, and software applications are discussed here.

The use of technology in general has greatly expanded, and several technologies once thought of as specialized, difficult to use, and expensive have become ubiquitous. In addition, technologies originally developed for use by people with disabilities are now being used by people without disabilities, making them easier to find and less expensive to obtain, maintain, and replace.

It is important for practitioners to have a good working knowledge of applications or any other technology, knowing what features are available that can be useful in aiding a client's performance and whether these features can be adjusted to meet a client's increasing abilities.

Social media

Occupational therapy practitioners can use social media to assist the client in transitioning from habilitation or rehabilitation to real life. Practitioners use social media during treatment and as a connection tying the real world back to clinical life. For example, people in rehabilitation programs may communicate with each other over various social media platforms. They may use these platforms to connect with other people who have similar needs and interests, including their disability-related needs.

Shopping lists

Several applications can be used to organize shopping lists by categories and by stores (Figure 12.5; see Case Example 12.3). Some of these applications have ongoing shopping lists so previously listed items can be pulled into new lists. Some also list the cost of the item so the shopper can keep a running tally of money spent. Occupational therapy practitioners can use these applications in several clinical activities, including working on budgeting and money management.

Health and wellness

Several applications focus on the area of health and wellness. For example, medication reminders have visual and auditory alerts that signal the user when it is time to take medications. Some automatically contact a caregiver if the user does not check in, indicating medication was skipped. Some can include reminders for multiple people. Some have refill reminders to alert the user when the prescription is running low (Figure 12.6).

Applications can help people eat nutritious diets. Some identify the contents of ready-made foods

Figure 12.5. A young woman uses a shopping list application to organize her grocery shopping. This type of application can be used to augment a person's cognitive functioning during IADLs.

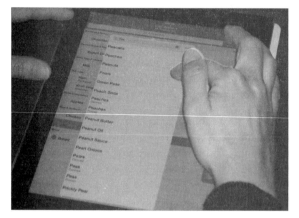

Source. A. Perr. Used with permission.

available in supermarkets (Figure 12.7). Others focus on the ingredients used in cooking. Some provide specific information about dietary needs and can be helpful to people with diabetes or food allergies.

Disability aid

Applications have been developed to aid people with a specific disability. For instance, LookTel developed two identification applications for cell phones for people with visual impairments (Figure 12.8). The first application, Recognizer, can identify an object and say its name out loud when a cell phone lens is aimed at the object. The application can readily identify many objects, and objects not in the application can be added. The second application, Money Reader, can identify denominations of money.

Figure 12.6. Two different functions in pill-monitoring applications can be used to assist people in managing their medications.

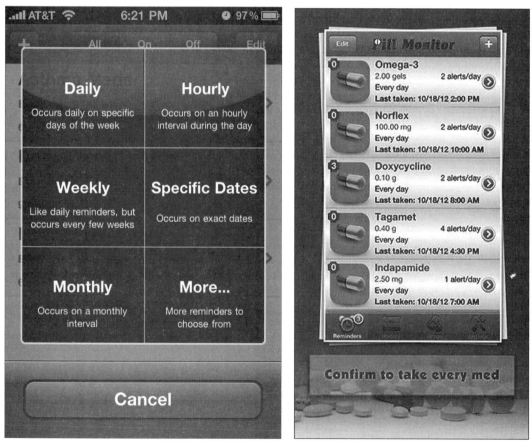

Source. Maxwell Software (www.maxwellapps.com). Used with permission.

Figure 12.7. This application, shown with its various aspects, offers nutritional information on many commercially available products.

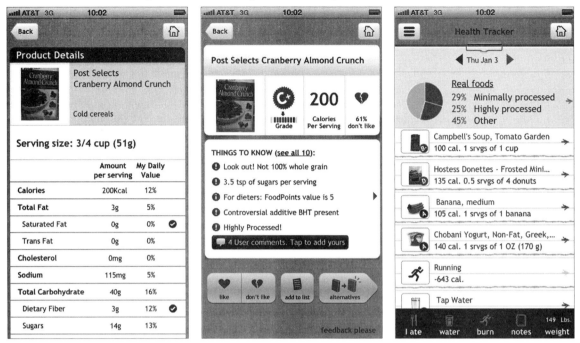

Source. Fooducate, San Francisco, CA. Used with permission.

These applications can also be used to aid people with other disabilities in the real world or in occupational therapy sessions. For instance,

Figure 12.8. When the cell phone is aimed at an object, the application says the name of the item (left). Another application identifies denominations of money (right).

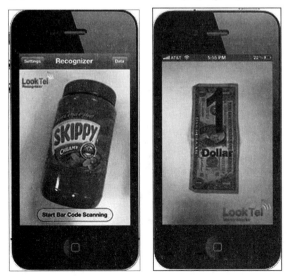

Source. Fooducate, San Francisco, CA. Used with permission.

a person with cognitive or perceptual disabilities could use both applications when supermarket shopping. In the clinic, the occupational therapy practitioner could develop an activity using photographs of objects or the objects themselves and have the client sort them by market department or type of product by using the app. The Recognizer could be used to give multisensory input to the user. Money Reader could be used in therapy for a client with a brain injury who has difficulty differentiating among denominations of paper money.

Software applications in operating systems

Smartphones and tablets are often preloaded with software applications in their operating systems. Such software might include a directory or address book of contacts and a calendar. A client or an occupational therapy practitioner or other professional can customize these and other preloaded applications for people with memory problems or people with other specific disabilities (Figure 12.9). An occupational therapy practitioner might also use software applications in individual and group treatments either for their intended purposes or

Figure 12.9. The client programs his tablet so that the applications he uses meet his specific needs. In this client's case, preprogrammed macros save individual keystrokes as he types.

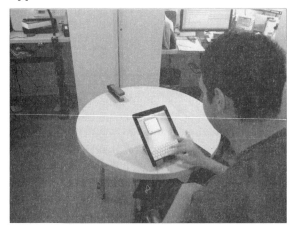

Source. A. Perr. Used with permission.

for many other activities that could focus on various cognitive functions such as planning, problem solving, or following directions.

Many features of smartphones and tablets are adjustable, such as icon and font size, color contrast, and auditory alerts. Additional features labeled "accessibility features" (e.g., color contrasts, speaking text) may be helpful for some people and are available at no additional cost. Specialized applications may also allow people to participate in desired occupations, such as composing music (Figure 12.10). Additional adaptations (not software related) for cell phones and tablets make them easier to use (e.g., a tablet stand; Figure 12.11).

Virtual Reality

For many years, occupational therapy practitioners have used virtual reality as an assessment and treatment tool for clients with physical, cognitive, and psychological impairments. *Virtual reality* is a method of simulation in which visual and auditory input allows the person to experience a location or activity. Sometimes smells are used to make the scene seem more real, or tactile input is used so the person "feels" as though he or she is there. Virtual reality uses interactive computer-based simulations, which can provide the practitioner with a variety of meaningful, motivat-

Figure 12.10. This client uses a cell phone to compose music for multiple instruments.

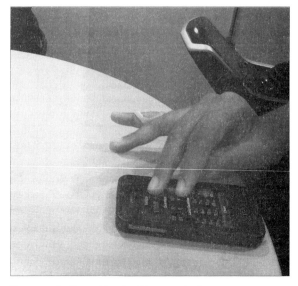

Source. A. Perr. Used with permission.

ing, and fun activities with which to engage the client. These activities, which imitate natural situations, can be individualized, measured, graded, and adapted to facilitate the rehabilitation process (Saposnik, Levin, & Outcome Research Canada [SORCAN] Working Group, 2011; Saposnik et al., 2010; Weiss, Rand, Katz, & Kizony, 2004).

Users of virtual reality interventions can interact with displayed images and manipulate virtual

Figure 12.11. A tablet stand holds the tablet at an angle to optimize the user's abilities and posture.

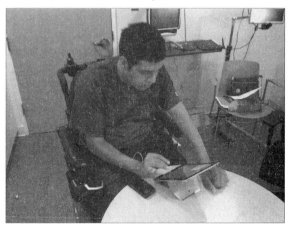

Source. A. Perr. Used with permission.

objects in environments that appear to be similar to those in real life. The essence of reality in virtual interaction is enhanced by the sense of touch (through the field of *haptics*), because a person can feel and manipulate objects in virtual environments. The PHANToM (SensAble Technologies, 2009) is one example of a haptic device that may have applications in occupational therapy. This computer input device allows the user to feel and handle virtual objects as if they were real. The device exerts an external force on the user's fingertips to provide information about the shape and texture of solid virtual objects. By means of this haptic interaction with the virtual environment, a user can improve motor coordination to control a virtual pencil or paintbrush and draw or paint using movements that are free and unimpeded in virtual space.

As the client focuses on the virtual task, he or she may become so immersed in the virtual world that a temporary separation from the real-world environment may occur. The client's interaction with, and sense of presence in, the virtual environment may contribute certain useful information and insights that facilitate improved performance (motor and cognitive) while in the virtual world. A client may transfer newly acquired skills to real-life situations, leading to improved functional ability in the natural environment (Weiss et al., 2004).

Mental health occupational therapy practitioners, as well as psychologists, have successfully used virtual reality therapy to provide interventions for clients with phobias and anxieties (Miller, Silva, Bouchard, Bélanger, & Taucer-Samson, 2012; Rizzo et al., 2011). *Virtual reality therapy* uses computerized simulations of feared situations. For example, a client may have an irrational fear of driving. The equipment used in therapy may consist of a computer monitor with a vibrating platform, steering wheel, and brake and gas pedals; the client wears earphones and wide-range goggles. The computer is programmed with a range of road and weather conditions and with changeable scenery (Ellin, 2003). The client gets a sense of being present and immersed in a fear-inducing and anxiety-provoking driving situation. After repeated practice with the simulated driving experience (i.e., without the risks and danger of a real setting), the client may become more at ease and less fearful of driving. The goal, of course, is to get the client away from the simulation and back behind the wheel, driving safely in the real world with an increased sense of ease.

Gaming tools

Occupational therapy practitioners can use gaming tools as virtual environments in the clinical setting. The Nintendo Wii (Redmond, WA) and Microsoft Xbox (Redmond, WA) have games that are all examples of gaming tools. The Wii is a virtual gaming system that has direct applications as a supplement to other occupational therapy interventions and can be used with clients of all ages to address physical, cognitive, and social interaction deficits. The Wii remote, or Wiimote, is a wand-like motion-sensitive remote control that transmits the motion to the console using short-range wireless communication technology. The console plugs into the television, and the user interacts with Nintendo games on the television screen from up to 10 meters away. The user has a large area in which to make the appropriate body movements required to simulate playing games such as baseball, tennis, golf, and bowling (Connolly, 2008).

The Wii is well suited to address many rehabilitation goals. People can perform real-life movements and exercises to build endurance, strength, and coordination and to stay fit. They can reap these benefits while enjoying participation in virtual leisure and sport activities that impose less physical stress on their bodies. The Wii can play an important role in the rehabilitation of people with neurological (e.g., stroke) deficits and orthopedic and other musculoskeletal injuries (Fung et al., 2010; Saposnik et al., 2010; Tatla, Radomski, Cheung, Maron, & Jarus, 2012; Williams, Doherty, Bender, Mattox, & Tibbs, 2011).

Using the device, a client can move in a safe environment while the occupational therapy practitioner facilitates performance skills such as motor, praxis, sensory, visuospatial orientation, and visual perception. In addition, the practitioner may address cognitive skills (e.g., attention, memory, decision making, judgment) and social skills (e.g., turn taking, assertiveness, fair play) while the client enjoys a virtual game or sport. Improvements in the client's functional abilities gained through the intervention can then be used to address the client's performance of occupations in a natural environment.

The Xbox Kinect allows the user to act as the game controller. Instead of holding and moving a controller, such as with the Wii, the Kinect uses markers on the person, receives information regarding the person's positioning, and translates these positions and movements into game controls. The various games available for the device are controlled by moving body parts and using voice commands. These games can be useful in rehabilitation because they can be extremely fun for some people and encourage movement to operate.

Software has been developed for Kinect for people with various disabilities to address clinical needs. Some open-source software is also currently available to meet various clinical needs. For example, the Kinect can be used to track a person's movements such that he or she may interact with a virtual bubble to move it across the screen. The practitioner may use this to work on balance, reaching, or even attention span.

Role play

In psychotherapy and mental health occupational therapy, occupational therapy practitioners use role play as an educational tool (Bai & Fusco, 2011; Gibson, D'Amico, Jaffe, & Arbesman, 2011). Understanding that role play involves pretend activities, clients are able to act out imaginary scenarios. By participating in this kind of simulation, the client may begin to understand problems, learn other ways of dealing with a situation by observing a variety of solutions, and improve his or her skills and behaviors. Role play provides the participant with simulated examples of how others act in specific situations and how he or she may act (Corsini & Cardone, 1966). Role play also involves the repeated performance of situations in a therapeutic environment, which allows practice while encouraging exploration and spontaneity.

Interventions That Simulate Real Life

Occupational therapy practitioners use client evaluation data to plan treatment by designing interventions that simulate real life. They also use that data to identify the appropriate activities to be simulated, in collaboration with the client if possible. The practitioner then creates an opportunity for the client to engage in those activities in the

---

Exercise 12.5. Jamal: Designing a Simulation

You are working with Jamal, a 14-year-old boy who recently underwent right, below-elbow amputation as a result of a traumatic injury. Jamal was previously right-hand dominant. As a result of the occupational therapy evaluation, you outline goals with input from both Jamal and his parents. One long-term goal is for Jamal to perform activities of daily living and schoolwork using the right upper extremity (which has been fitted with a mechanical prosthesis) as an assist. Another goal is to retrain him to use his left upper extremity as dominant. Describe one simulated activity that you could use to meet the goal of changing dominance. After you have described the activity, answer the following questions:

- How have you set up the treatment environment to replicate the real-life setting in which the activity will take place?
- What are the differences between your simulated environment and the real-life environment?
- How does the activity differ from real life in your simulation?
- How can you change the demands of the activity and the structure of the context to meet Jamal's changing needs as his skills improve?

---

occupational therapy clinic, the classroom, the home, or a community setting. While the client is engaged in the activities, the practitioner uses cues and assistance to allow the client to work through challenges that are useful and that he or she can tolerate to ensure a positive learning experience. These treatments often involve the imagination because the practitioner asks the client to imagine the circumstances and the context in which he or she will perform the occupations.

The client's motivation, interests, and values are key factors to consider before engaging him or her in a simulated activity. For some clients, simulations are motivating and fun. For others, simulations may have no apparent value, and adults may perceive the simulations as children's play. The practitioner should thus endeavor to provide age- and interest-appropriate simulations and should clarify or explain the value of the simulated activity in preparing the client for engaging in an occupation in the real world.

In Exercise 12.5, you were asked to use simulation to target completion of one task that is important to your client. You should have created the context in which the client would play the role of task performer and provided the structure necessary to match the client's abilities and be sufficiently challenging. The task also should have been important and meaningful enough to motivate the client to work hard. These aspects of a simulated activity are controllable by the occupational therapy practitioner, that is, he or she can design the activity to meet the client's needs and abilities at any given time. For example, early in the process, the practitioner may plan the activity so that the client's success is very likely. Later, the client can accept more of the responsibility for success. Case Example 12.4 describes the process of designing simulations to continually meet the increasing abilities of a group

of clients and provides an example of an effective use of simulation in a community setting.

The ways in which an occupational therapy practitioner uses simulations as part of his or her interventions are similar in all areas of practice. The process begins with a comprehensive evaluation, development of specific goals, determination of which performance components need improvement, identification of the occupational performance skills that would benefit from simulated activities, design of simulated activities, and engagement of the client in simulated activities (see Case Example 12.5).

As noted previously, during early recovery from injury or illness is when simulated activities seem abstract and least representative of real life. After mastery, or partial mastery, of the individual components of an activity, the client puts together and

---

Case Example 12.4. Community Center: From Simulation to Job

Clients ages 26 to 66 years in a community center are primarily people who live on the street and do not work. **Brenda, the center's occupational therapist,** collaborates with social workers, psychologists, and vocational rehabilitation counselors in a 3-month work program for the center's clients. One goal of the program is to improve the clients' work habits and skills. Program members start by talking about what they would like to do in the future and what steps are necessary to reach their goals. After the first week, program attendance and participation in group activities become the "job" of program members.

During group meetings, members discuss work behaviors such as grooming, efficiency, and punctuality. During some sessions, Brenda encourages them to role play specific situations (e.g., customer service transaction). Program members then begin to work in the center's gift shop to refine their work skills. As employees, they punch time clocks and meet with their supervisor on a daily basis. In addition to working in the gift shop, members continue to attend group meetings, where they learn interviewing skills, how to write a résumé, and how to complete a job application. They play the roles of the

interviewer and the interviewee to practice their skills. At this point, program members can apply for specific jobs in the center's shop. For example, different people are interested in working in the stockroom, as cashiers, and in management.

For members interested in finding employment outside of the center, center staff work with them to find job listings in newspapers or online or to contact job placement services. In addition, in Brenda's group meetings, members practice developing information for online social and professional networking sites. This information is not posted to any sites until a client's level of function makes it appropriate. Clients go to interviews, sometimes with a job coach or other assistant, and begin their jobs with the help of the job coach. This situation is the highest level of simulation; it is not quite real life because the job coach influences performance and success by assisting, supervising, and encouraging the client.

The job coach continues to work with the client for the required amount of time and then removes himself or herself. At this point, the client is in real life in terms of working. The client may contact the center staff at any time, and the staff often ask graduates of the program to return to talk to new members about the process and the result.

Case Example 12.5. Belle: Toileting

Belle, age 75 years, had a cerebrovascular accident and needed to improve her toileting skills. The initial stage of intervention had Belle participate in tasks and exercises focused on individual steps of toileting. The occupational therapy program included the following:

- Activities in sitting to improve balance and the ability to shift weight
- Activities in sitting that encourage weight bearing through the upper and lower extremities
- Activities requiring a forward weight shift and removing weight from the buttocks
- Fine motor activities and bimanual tasks in preparation for lower-extremity garment management
- Activities in standing to improve balance
- Activities to improve compensation for a visual field cut.

At the next stage of intervention, the occupational therapist addressed transfers to and from the commode, lower-extremity garment management, and toilet paper management and hygiene after toileting in separate occupational therapy sessions. The therapist used one or more sessions to bring Belle to a private bathroom where she could practice transfers to and from the commode.

For garment management, Belle worked on buttoning and unbuttoning buttons and zipping and unzipping zippers on a dressing board. The therapist designed the activity to begin with large buttons and loose buttonholes and move on to progressively smaller buttons and tighter buttonholes. Another treatment session began with large zippers on slippery tracks and moved on to smaller zippers with more resistant tracks.

Once Belle mastered the tasks on the dressing board, the next step was to lay a pair of pants smoothly in her lap. The therapist assisted by holding the pants taut, exposing the zipper, or holding the buttonhole steady. As Belle gained the ability to perform these tasks, the therapist provided less assistance.

The next step in the sequence was to have Belle practice the tasks of buttoning, unbuttoning, zipping, and unzipping on her own pants. After she mastered this step, the therapist and Belle worked on removing and replacing the lower-extremity garments in preparation for toileting.

Other sessions focused on the activities of toilet paper management and hygiene. These interventions followed the same procedure of practice and mastery as the others.

The therapist used different activities to address other areas in which Belle had difficulty. For example, the therapist used paper-and-pencil tasks, bed making, and computer games to increase Belle's awareness of the visual field cut.

As Belle proceeded in therapy, she toileted with assistance at first and then with supervision as she mastered all of the skills required for safe toileting. Eventually, she transitioned all of the simulated activities to the actual performance of toileting. Tasks that were difficult were identified and practiced using simulations. However, unless conditions were optimal, such as when she was already in her wheelchair and wearing supportive shoes with nonslip soles, she sometimes still required assistance. She also required assistance from her husband at home if she was fatigued. Because Belle's long-term goal was to toilet independently regardless of the time of day, the type of clothing worn, or the layout of the bathroom, she will continue with occupational therapy to master this occupation. When she is able to achieve this goal, she will be independent in performing toileting in real life, and her occupational therapy sessions will no longer address this goal.

performs the components in a protected environment. The treatment context is a safe place in which to practice each individual component and many combinations or collections of components. This context allows clients to make mistakes and learn from them, explore alternatives, and develop strategies for improved performance.

Initially, the occupational therapy practitioner sets up the environment to protect the person from distractions and to encourage successful completion of the task. In addition, as illustrated in Case Example 12.5, the practitioner addresses each component of an activity individually. The client practices and masters the tasks and components of each activity and then groups them together until he or she has addressed the entire occupation (in this case, toileting) sufficiently.

Simulations to Ensure That Activities Are Purposeful

Work-centered rehabilitation often uses simulation. Work samples such as Valpar Work Samples (www.basesofva.com) and work simulation and evaluation systems such as the Ergos II Work Simulator (Simwork Systems, Tucson, AZ; Figure 12.12) replicate various job skills. The practitioner can use work samples and work simulations to evaluate a client's functional capacity and abilities; target training of specific work skills; and provide objective, replicable data to measure the progress a client makes toward being able to work.

The practitioner may use a work simulation system to evaluate the client's ability to perform the basic requirements of a specific job as described in the Department of Labor's online resource O*NET (onetonline.org). Job-training simulations include material handling (e.g., lifting, carrying, pushing, pulling) and postural abilities (e.g., climbing, reaching, stooping, bending). Once the simulated work training is completed, the practitioner reassesses client performance to determine whether the client has met the return-to-work goals as indicated by the U.S. Department of Labor job description.

The practitioner may make recommendations for ergonomic adjustments to the client's workspace or modification of the job requirements to allow the client to perform the job. In one Valpar activity, the user must piece together three small metal objects and place them in moving holes on a round track.

Figure 12.12. Ergos work simulator is designed to simulate a variety of work tasks.

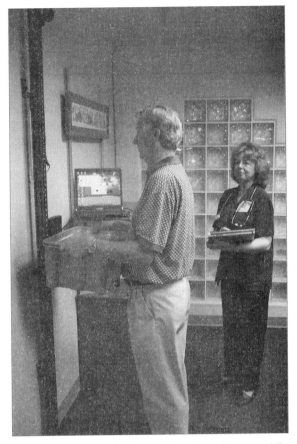

Source. Courtesy of Simwork Systems, Tucson, AZ. Used with permission.

The rate of movement is adjustable so that the holes move faster as the user's fine motor coordination, speed, and planning improve. The practitioner may adjust the time allotted for this activity to meet or challenge the client's abilities and endurance. The practitioner counts the number of sets of objects placed in the holes while the client works. The practitioner and client can track progress in several ways: by the client's ability as the speed increases, the length of time the client participates in the activity, and the number of sets the client completes in a fixed or consistent amount of time.

This Valpar activity simulates the manipulation of small objects and in turn simulates repetitious assembly line work. It is useful for several reasons, including preparing an assembly line worker for return to work, improving a person's fine motor and bimanual coordination, increasing endurance for fine motor tasks, or even increasing tolerance for repetitive work. This tool may be appropriate for people with various disabling conditions, including traumatic hand injury, medical conditions such as diabetes that involve associated sensory impairments, visual impairments in which the purpose of occupational therapy is to improve tactile compensatory strategies, and mental illness that affects a person's concentration and attention span.

Another work-centered simulation involves adults in work rehabilitation using simulated jobs (Ellexson, 1989). In a work-hardening program, activities simulate work skills on which the client must concentrate. Inpatients or outpatients may be contracted by companies to complete work. For example, a cohort of adults with developmental disabilities may work in a program that has a contract to package plastic utensils. This job includes counting the utensils, placing them in bags, sealing the bags, labeling the bags, and placing the bags in boxes. This activity demonstrates how simulation allows the occupational therapy practitioner to organize the environment, break tasks down into components, and offer clients purposeful activity as a treatment tool.

Occupational therapy clinics have long included specially built treatment areas so that the occupational therapy practitioner can provide treatment to clients in settings that simulate their home and community-based environments. Examples include specific areas in the occupational therapy department such as a kitchen, bathroom, bedroom, or living area where clients can practice basic activities of daily living skills and instrumental activities of daily living tasks. These treatment locations are useful when the client has improved to the point at which a more realistic setting than the occupational therapy clinic or laboratory would encourage further progress. A training apartment, for example, may be useful after the client has completed wheelchair transfers in a hospital room and meal preparation in the occupational therapy kitchen area. A client's family members may join him or her in the training apartment so that they can practice caregiving skills before discharge. The training apartment offers a transition between the contrived and simulated activities in the clinic and the performance of activities in real life (in this case, at home).

Occupational therapy practitioners working with children and adolescents often use simulation as part of their interventions. Simulation is frequently the key to engaging young children in a meaningful learning activity. Children use play to explore and learn about their environment by using their imaginations and to receive the sensory stimulation that they need for development. Children with disabilities may be unable to use their imaginations or to participate in play sufficiently to meet these needs. The practitioner's role is, in part, to create an environment where children can use their imaginations to develop new skills or become secure or confident in their abilities (Case Example 12.6).

Jacobs (1991) discussed the importance of introducing various activities that simulate adult roles in making the transition to becoming an adult worker. She discussed the use of *exploratory play* in which children explore objects in the environment to learn about them and master their use and role-playing activities even in preschool-age children. During these role-playing activities, children can explore the physical properties associated with various careers. Children are also able to try out different social skills and behaviors necessary for leadership and teamwork. Throughout school, these skills facilitate the development of work behaviors. For example, behaviors such as punctuality and preparedness are necessary early in a child's schooling, and mastering these skills prepares a child for behaviors that will be necessary later in life at work. Older children may participate in programs in which they develop a mock business and provide some service or product to others.

Several rehabilitation departments across North America use sophisticated, visually appealing, functional simulations of various environments called Easy Street Environments® (Habitat, 1998). These custom environments include more than 30 areas of activity such as a park, restaurant, bank, supermarket, department store, office, theater, and automobile. Easy Street Environments provides convenient, safe, low-risk, weather-free treatment spaces in which occupational therapy practitioners can effectively treat clients of all ages who have a wide range of disabilities. With Easy Street Environments, the practitioner and client may address discharge readiness, community reentry, client and family member training, evaluation of possible

---

Case Example 12.6. Ricardo: Using Play

Ricardo, age 5 years, is a boy in kindergarten who has a learning disability and attention-deficit/hyperactivity disorder. He attends regular classes and has occupational, physical, and speech therapy 3 times weekly. Ricardo switches hand dominance for different activities; he throws a ball with his left hand but writes and uses scissors with his right hand. The occupational therapist observed the following problems during writing activities in the classroom as part of Ricardo's evaluation: impaired fine motor coordination in both hands, associated reactions in the left hand and arm, squeezing the pencil too hard, pressing too hard on the paper, and difficulty releasing the pencil when finished and repositioning it when writing.

The **occupational therapist, Izzy,** determines Ricardo needs a fun way to learn to regulate pressure and to grasp and release the pencil appropriately. Izzy decides to play Blockhead™ with Ricardo. Blockhead is a game in which the players take turns balancing oddly shaped wood blocks on top of one another until one person causes the tower to topple. The person who causes the tower to topple is the "blockhead." Ricardo does not have the attention span, motor skills, or perceptual skills to play Blockhead as it was intended. Therefore, Izzy adapts the game using the same rules and blocks made out of Styrofoam™ and paper. These materials require Ricardo to regulate his grip pressure and use larger gross motor skills.

Izzy has Ricardo play the game while assuming different positions and using both hands. Ricardo plays while seated at a table; while standing; and while lying in a prone position and resting on his forearms, requiring upper-extremity weight bearing. Ricardo's mother reports to Izzy that she bought Blockhead and that Ricardo enjoys playing at home with her and with his older brother. After playing a simulated Blockhead game, Ricardo learned the appropriate rules and developed an adequate attention span and motor skills to play the real game. Izzy notes that Ricardo's improvements carried over to improved writing skills.

---

home adaptations, and assistance needed by the client in the community.

Easy Street Environments is at a level similar to that of the training apartment discussed earlier. These environments introduce the real world and everyday occupations into the clinical setting and fill the gap between the occupational therapy clinic and real life. When a client demonstrates the ability to perform contrived and simulated activities in an occupational therapy clinic but is not yet ready for community reentry, the client may practice addressing environmental, community, and work-related obstacles and challenges in Easy Street Environments. Occupational therapy practitioners who have used these simulated environments have claimed that their clients' confidence in performing instrumental activities of daily

---

Exercise 12.6. Questions About Ricardo

Think about Case Example 12.6, and answer these four questions: (1) What real-life activity does this therapeutic intervention address? (2) How did the occupational therapist use simulation to imitate the real-life activity? (3) What modifications did the therapist make to the environment and the demands of the activity? (4) How do the therapist and the family members provide assistance to make the activity possible?

Exercise 12.7. Questions About Ricardo From an Occupational Therapy Practitioner's Perspective

Take a few minutes to think about more activities that could serve the same purpose for Ricardo. If you were the occupational therapy practitioner, what would you do? How would you set up the environment? How would you alter the assistance given to meet Ricardo's changing needs? How would you help his parents and siblings provide assistance?

living increased and that the practitioner can then use the time more efficiently (Habitat, 1998). The more realistic the simulation is in the controlled setting, as in Easy Street Environments, the easier or smoother the client's transition may be when performing these activities in a natural environment.

Simulation is useful in outpatient settings and can provide an even smoother transition to real life. Clients can work on a certain skill during their therapy sessions and practice the skill at home or in another real-life setting. This homework is actually an advanced form of simulation because although it is still somewhat contrived, it is useful in maximizing a person's ability to perform an activity. When clients try techniques at home, they can bring questions back to therapy, and the practitioner can devise simulated activities to use during treatment that target those specific problems. Each time a client masters a skill in the clinic, he or she can perform the skill at home or in the real-life location as a check.

As the client performs activities satisfactorily at home, the goals for treatment change. The occupational therapy practitioner documents progress and indicates whether occupational therapy should continue after satisfactory performance of the occupation in the real-life situation. Practitioners must not make the mistake of thinking that an excellent simulation supersedes real-life training and application. Simulation, by definition, merely gives the appearance of or imitates what is real. Intense and time-consuming simulation training in occupational therapy may ease the transitioning of skills to real-life performance. Success in simulation, however, does not automatically guarantee success in real life.

Advanced Assistive Technologies and Simulation

As technology advances, simulations also advance, and the distinction between simulation and real life narrows. One particular technology that illustrates this point is the *brain–computer interface (BCI)*, which allows the operation of a computer or computer controller device with brain function. For people with physical disabilities, BCI could mean that a person would not need to move physically to operate a computer. People with conditions such as quadriplegia and locked-in syndrome resulting from spinal cord injury, brain stem stroke, and amyotrophic lateral sclerosis may be able to participate in work, leisure, and self-care when technologies such as BCI are refined and perfected (Cincotti et al., 2007). One BCI system generates computer control by translating the visual evoked potential recorded from the user's scalp over the visual cortex so that the person uses his or her vision for such operations as cursor control. The neurological processing that occurs in the brain's visual cortex is translated to electrical waves that are then used to control the computer.

Another uses electroencephalograph signals generated by the user's intent to define the output (Wolpaw, Birbaumer, McFarland, Pfurtscheller, & Vaughn, 2002). BCI technologies are currently under development and are being used to generate control over computers and other robotic devices, which could lead to increased participation by people with disabilities.

As with BCI, the lines between simulation and real life are merging in other areas. For many years, occupational therapy practitioners have used simulations for evaluation and the training of drivers with disabilities. Vehicle modifications are available so that people with disabilities can drive or ride in vehicles such as cars, vans, and trucks. Developers continue to use and adapt technologies so that people with disabilities can experience and participate in a wide variety of activities. A retired NASCAR racecar, for example, has been configured with a moveable driver's seat to allow transfers into and out of the vehicle (Figure 12.13) and with hand controls (Figure 12.14). Such adaptations allow drivers with disabilities to experience racecar driving—an activity that previously was largely off-limits to people with disabilities. Developers are now working on self-driving cars. In the future, these cars may have uses for people with disabilities. The factors that determine who is able to drive safely may shift as the cars are able to take over some of the tasks of driving.

Real Life

The ultimate goal of occupational therapy is for the client to be successful in his or her occupations in real life. All of the examples in this chapter dem-

Figure 12.13. Racecar with the driver's seat.

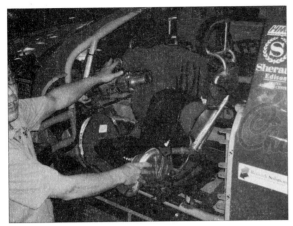

Source. A. Perr. Used with permission.

onstrate how an occupational therapy practitioner uses simulations to prepare clients for real-life activities and occupations, and the transition to real life is the final step in this process. In occupational therapy, the client learns problem-solving skills and other strategies that enable him or her to generalize information to various real-life environments and situations. *Real life* is the usual environment in which any given occupation takes place and includes settings such as the home, workplace, school, places of leisure enjoyment, and private and public transportation. The occupational therapy practitioner can foster the transition to real life by keeping the focus on real life in treatment throughout the habilitation or rehabilitation process.

Figure 12.14. Hand controls for driving.

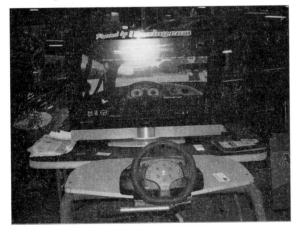

Source. A. Perr. Used with permission.

During therapy, occupational therapy practitioners must address the foundations of performance components and activities that are necessary to engage in real-life occupations. Addressing the psychosocial requirements of an activity is essential, including the appropriateness of the methods and equipment; feelings of embarrassment or pride associated with performance; and support of family members, friends, and others. Real-life occupational performance includes using all of the appropriate activities to engage in an occupation. Real life includes performing activities in the conventional manner, with alternative techniques and compensatory strategies, and with assistive technology. Indeed, when addressing occupational performance in the real-world environment, the practitioner may prescribe and provide adaptive equipment and assistive technology devices. A practitioner may focus on simulations with devices and ensure that clients can use them competently to complete activities in the clinic environment.

Everything changes at home; therefore, a practitioner must address home issues. Phillips and Zhao's (1993) study of *technology abandonment* described patterns of clients' disuse of the devices recommended or provided to them in a physical rehabilitation setting. Four factors influenced technology abandonment: (1) lack of consideration of user opinion, (2) ease of device procurement, (3) poor device performance, and (4) changes in user needs or priorities. The practitioner's role is to address those factors. For example, by ensuring that the device performs as it should, both in the protected therapeutic environment and in the real world, the practitioner can help provide the best possible solution for clients who require assistive technology. The client's home and other real-life environments should be the focus of treatment, and the practitioner should avoid the assumption that if it works in the hospital room, it will work the same at home.

In a related study, Bell and Hinojosa (1995) interviewed 3 participants with spinal cord injuries regarding the effect of assistive devices on their ability to perform their daily routines. They concluded that successful use of these devices in the clinic setting did not necessarily transition to successful use of them at home. Rather, follow-up at home and in-home training were crucial to successfully using assistive devices or compensatory techniques in real life after discharge.

Occupational therapy intervention to prepare a client for real life is limited in scope. Predicting all the environments in which a client may interact is impossible for the practitioner. It is not possible to plan for the unexpected; however, by addressing occupations through simulation in many of the likely environments, it is possible to facilitate, but not guarantee, a successful transition to real life. In addition, note that both the human and the nonhuman contexts in which the client performs any activity influence the realism of the simulation. For example, pretending to lift a heavy object in the proper way in an occupational therapy clinic is different from lifting an object of a similar weight on a busy factory floor. In the latter situation, the context includes noise, the space available, the presence of a supervisor and coworkers, and many distractions. These factors make real-life activity performance much more complex than simulated activity. Again, successful performance in a clinic does not necessarily guarantee success in real life.

Summary

As occupational therapy practitioners become more experienced, identifying clients' long-term goals becomes easier. In turn, planning and organizing simulated activities to address their needs becomes easier. The visualization of the outcome of occupational therapy may not always be accurate because of the unpredictable nature of people, the unpredictability of the setting, and other demands that influence performance. However, usually as a practitioner gains more experience and builds a repertoire of goal-setting and treatment skills, his or her predictions will be more accurate or will more often be accurate.

The practitioner can outline trends in performance and move from contrived to more purposeful real activities in various environments that range from clinical or simulated to real. The ultimate goal is independent activity performance in a real environment; occupational therapy practitioners use simulation in this effort. As in various industries, simulation in occupational therapy allows clients to test and practice techniques in a safe and controlled environment. Practitioners can address problems, gain insights, and explore solutions before attempting real-life performance.

Some practitioners believe that the ultimate setting for providing occupational therapy intervention is the client's work site, home, and community. In these cases, simulation is still used to adapt the activity to the person's ability and the goal of therapy, but the simulations take place in the real environment, fostering a smooth transition to performing the actual activity in the actual environment.

References

American Occupational Therapy Association. (2002). Position Paper—Broadening the construct of independence. *American Journal of Occupational Therapy, 56,* 66. http://dx.doi.org/10.5014/ajot.56.6.660

American Occupational Therapy Association. (2014). Occupational therapy practice framework: Domain and process (3rd ed.). *American Journal of Occupational Therapy, 68*(Suppl. 1), S1–S48. http://dx.doi.org/10.5014/ajot.2014.682006

Bai, X., & Fusco, D. (2011). Enhancing education in the health professions through 3D simulations in a social networking environment. In *Proceedings of Global TIME 2011* (pp. 277–282). AACE. Retrieved from http://www.editlib.org/p/37090.

Barrett, R. (2007). Virtual world. *Metal Bulletin Monthly, 434,* 36.

Bell, P., & Hinojosa, J. (1995). Perception of the impact of assistive devices on daily life of three individuals with quadriplegia. *Assistive Technology, 7,* 87–94. http://dx.doi.org/10.1080/10400435.1995.10132257

Brodie, J. (2005). In the game. *HRMagazine, 50,* 91–94.

Bruck, L. (2008). Second Life: Test-driving real-world innovations. *Hospitals and Health Networks, 82,* 50–54.

Chow, M., Herold, D. K., Choo, T.-M., & Chan, K. (2012). Extending the technology acceptance model to explore the intention to use Second Life for enhancing healthcare education. *Computers and Education, 59*(4), 1136–1144. http://dx.doi.org/10.1016/j.compedu.2012.05.011

Cincotti, F., Mattia, D., Aloise, F., Bufalari, S., Marciani, M. G., Schalk, G., . . . Mattia, D. (2007). Non-invasive brain–computer interface system to operate assistive devices. *Proceedings of the 29th Annual International Conference of the IEEE Engineering in Medicine and Biology Society, 22*(26), 2532–2535.

Cohen, I., Iluz, M., & Shtub, A. (2013). A simulation-based approach in support of project management training for systems engineers. *Systems Engineering.* Advance online publication. http://dx.doi.org/10.1002/sys.21248

Connolly, C. (2008). KUKA robotics open architecture allows wireless control. *Industrial Robot, 35,* 12. http://dx.doi.org/10.1108/01439910810853161

Corsini, R. J., & Cardone, S. S. (1966). *Roleplaying in psychotherapy: A manual.* Chicago: Aldine.

Eastlack, J. O. (1968). New products for the seventies. In J. O. Eastlack & J. Tinker (Eds.), *New product development* (pp. 142–148). Chicago: American Marketing Association.

Ellexson, M. T. (1989). Work hardening. In S. Hertfelder & C. Gwin (Eds.), *Work in progress* (pp. 67–126). Bethesda, MD: American Occupational Therapy Association.

Ellin, A. (2003, April 17). Driving along a virtual road to recovery. *The New York Times,* p. G3.

Fiorino, L. (2009, January 2). Commentary: Need a second life? Have your avatar call my avatar. *The Daily Record.* Retrieved from www.highbeam.com/doc/1P2-19694177.html

Fung, V., So, K., Park, E., Ho, A., Shaffer, J., Chan, E., & Gomez, M. (2010). The utility of a video game system in rehabilitation of burn and nonburn patients: A survey among occupational therapy and physiotherapy practitioners. *Journal of Burn Care and Research, 31,* 768–775. http://dx.doi.org/10.1097/BCR.0b013e3181eed23c

Gibson, R. W., D'Amico, M., Jaffe, L., & Arbesman, M. (2011). Occupational therapy interventions for recovery in the areas of community integration and normative life roles for adults with serious mental illness: A systematic review. *American Journal of Occupational Therapy, 65,* 247–256. http://dx.doi.org/10.5014/ajot.2011.001297

Graafland, M., Schraagen, J. M., & Schijven, M. P. (2012). Systematic review of serious games for medical education and surgical skills training. *British Journal of Surgery, 99,* 1322–1330. http://dx.doi.org/10.1002/bjs.8819

Grand, J. A., Pearce, M., Rench, T. A., Chao, G. T., Fernandez, R., & Kozlowski, S. W. (2013). Going DEEP: Guidelines for building simulation-based team assessments. *BMJ Quality and Safety, 22*(5), 436–448. http://dx.doi.org/10.1136/bmjqs-2012-000957

Habitat. (1998). *Easy Street Environments product literature.* Tempe, AZ: Author.

Hansen, M. M. (2008). Versatile, immersive, creative and dynamic virtual 3-D healthcare learning environments: A review of the literature. *Journal of Medical Internet Research, 10,* e26. http://dx.doi.org/10.2196/jmir.1051

Honey, M., Connor, K., Veltman, M., Bodily, D., & Diener, S. (2012). Teaching with Second Life®: Hemorrhage management as an example of a process for developing simulations for multiuser virtual environments. *Clinical Simulation in Nursing, 8*(3), e79–e85. http://dx.doi.org/10.1016/j.ecns.2010.07.003

Howarth, N. (2009). A whole new world. *e.learning age Magazine, 12.* Retrieved from http://findarticles.com/p/articles/mi_qa5402/is_200812/ai_n31426021/

Jacobs, K. (1991). *Occupational therapy: Work-related programs and assessments.* Boston: Little, Brown.

Miller, L., Silva, C., Bouchard, S., Bélanger, C., & Taucer-Samson, T. (2012). Using virtual reality and other computer technologies to implement cognitive–behavior therapy for the treatment of anxiety disorders in youth. In T. E. Davis III, T. H. Ollendick, & L.-G. Öst (Eds.), *Intensive one-session treatment of specific phobias* (pp. 227–251). New York: Springer.

O'Neil, J. (2001, October 10). Mistakes are measured here, not towed away. *The New York Times,* p. H12.

Phillips, B., & Zhao, H. (1993). Predictors of assistive technology abandonment. *Assistive Technology, 5,* 36–45. http://dx.doi.org/10.1080/10400435.1993.10132205

Rizzo, A., Parsons, T. D., Lange, B., Kenny, P., Buckwalter, J. G., Rothbaum, B., . . . Reger, G. (2011). Virtual reality goes to war: A brief review of the future of military behavioral healthcare. *Journal of Clinical Psychology in Medical Settings, 18,* 176–187. http://dx.doi.org/10.1007/s10880-011-9247-2

Saposnik, G., Levin, M., & Outcome Research Canada (SORCan) Working Group. (2011). Virtual reality in stroke rehabilitation: A meta-analysis and implications for clinicians. *Stroke, 42,* 1380–1386. http://dx.doi.org/10.1161/STROKEAHA.110.605451

Saposnik, G., Teasell, R., Mamdani, M., Hall, J., McIlroy, W., Cheung, D., Bayley, M., . . . Stroke Outcome Research Canada (SORCan) Working Group. (2010). Effectiveness of virtual reality using Wii gaming technology in stroke rehabilitation: A pilot randomized clinical trial and proof of principle. *Stroke, 41,* 1477–1484. http://dx.doi.org/10.1161/STROKEAHA.110.584979

Schechtman, M. (2012). The story of my (second) life: Virtual worlds and narrative identity. *Philosophy and Technology, 25,* 329–343. http://dx.doi.org/10.1007/s13347-012-0062-y

SensAble Technologies. (2009). *Geomagic® haptic devices.* Retrieved from http://www.geomagic.com/en/products-landing-pages/haptic

Tatla, S. K., Radomski, A., Cheung, J., Maron, M., & Jarus, T. (2012). Wii-habilitation as balance therapy for children with acquired brain injury. *Developmental Neurorehabilitation,* 1–15. http://dx.doi.org/10.3109/17518423.2012.740508

United Nations. (2006). *Convention of the rights of persons with disabilities.* Retrieved from http://www.un.org/disabilities/convention/conventionfull.shtml

Weiss, P. L., Rand, D., Katz, N., & Kizony, R. (2004). Video capture virtual reality as a flexible and effective rehabilitation tool. *Journal of Neuroengineering and Rehabilitation, 1,* 12. http://dx.doi.org/10.1186/1743-0003-1-12

Williams, B., Doherty, N. L., Bender, A., Mattox, H., & Tibbs, J. R. (2011). The effect of Nintendo Wii on balance: A pilot study supporting the use of the Wii in occupational therapy for the well elderly. *Occupational Therapy in Health Care, 25,* 131–139. http://dx.doi.org/10.3109/07380577.2 011.560627

Winarchick, C., & Caldwell, R. (1997). Physical interactive simulation: A hands-on approach to facilities improvements. *IIE Solutions, 29,* 34–36.

Wolpaw, J. R., Birbaumer, N., McFarland, D. J., Pfurtscheller, G., & Vaughan, T. M. (2002). Brain–computer interfaces for communication and control. *Clinical Neurophysiology, 113,* 767–791. http://dx.doi.org/10.1016/S1388 -2457(02)00057-3

World Health Organization. (2001). *International classification of functioning, disability and health.* Geneva: Author.

CHAPTER 13.

LEISURE OCCUPATIONS

Laurette Olson, PhD, OTR/L, FAOTA

Leisure is . . . freedom from the necessity of labor. —Aristotle, 1943

Highlights

✧ What is leisure?
✧ Leisure's critical role in human development
✧ Leisure for people with disabilities
✧ Categories of leisure activities
✧ Leisure needs of people with disabilities
✧ Factors affecting leisure participation
✧ Choosing leisure occupations
✧ Leisure occupations across the life span
✧ Barriers to participation in leisure occupations
✧ Leisure for health promotion and prevention of secondary health issues
✧ Expertise of occupational therapy practitioners in leisure development.

Key Terms

✧ Achievement
✧ Balance leisure activities
✧ Casual leisure
✧ Client-centered practice
✧ Communitas
✧ Co-occupations
✧ Coregulation
✧ Core leisure activities
✧ Internal control
✧ Intrinsic motivation

✧ Leisure
✧ Neuropalliative conditions
✧ Play
✧ Playfulness
✧ Relaxed leisure
✧ Self-determination
✧ Serious leisure
✧ Temperament
✧ Timeout
✧ Transitional leisure

This chapter begins by defining leisure occupations and discussing their developmental importance for all people. Next, categories of leisure activities and the characteristics of leisure occupations are presented. In this section, the importance of cognitive, emotional, and physical invigoration is highlighted. A short discussion of leisure occupations specific to people with disabilities follows. The chapter ends with occupational therapy leisure occupations' assessment and intervention. Throughout, evidence-based literature is related to leisure participation to demonstrate the importance and central role that leisure occupations optimally play in supporting a positive quality of life, health, and functioning for persons across the life span. In addition, current literature related to leisure assessment and intervention and to the unique contributions of occupational therapy practitioners is highlighted.

What Is Leisure?

Leisure is what people do in their spare time when they are not engaged in self- or family management, work, or educational activities. By its very nature, what is leisure is subjective; therefore, true leisure is self-determined and autonomous. People are free to participate or not participate without consequences. In leisure occupation, goals and the directions the activity takes come from oneself. Leisure occupations have no external judgment of success or failure imposed on them; only the participants can decide whether their level of participation is adequate for personal enjoyment. Thus, more than any other occupation, leisure affords people with optimal opportunities for developing and sustaining a sense of self-determination.

Current research related to individual persons and families highlights the importance of leisure for health and wellness across the life span (Buswell, Zabriskie, Lundberg, & Hawkins, 2012; Heo, Stebbins, Kim, & Lee, 2013; Zabriskie & McCormick, 2001). Passmore's 2003 study supports the view that leisure occupations promote a sense of competence and self-efficacy through individual achievement or social participation and have a powerful influence on the mental health of adolescents. People who have large amounts of unoccupied time or spend their time in pas-

sive, sedentary, and nonchallenging leisure activities may have negative developmental and health consequences (Barnett & Klitzing, 2006; Conroy, Golden, Jeffares, O'Neill, & McGee, 2010; Oates, Bebbington, Bourke, Girdler, & Leonard, 2011; Zick, 2010).

Leisure's Critical Role in Human Development

It is essential that occupational therapy practitioners and students have a deep appreciation of leisure's critical role in human development, that is, leisure has value for people's health and wellness. In addition, most important for occupational therapy practitioners is an understanding of how people develop and sustain leisure as an occupation. This knowledge causes practitioners to be more likely to explore clients' leisure needs as frequently as they explore self-care, work, or school concerns.

Leisure for People With Disabilities

Current research and articles written by persons with disabilities identify the strong interest of people with disabilities across the life span to be more engaged in physical and community-based leisure activities (Boyce & Fleming-Castaldy, 2012; Shikako-Thomas et al., 2013). Therefore, to be truly client-centered, occupational therapy practitioners must explore and support the development and enactment of clients' leisure roles.

Persons with disabilities, who are the most frequent clients of occupational therapy practitioners, are less likely to be engaged in community-based group activities and are more likely to be inactive and isolated, increasing physical and mental health risks (Dahan-Oliel, Shikako-Thomas, & Majnemer, 2012; Jonsson & Andersson, 2013; Shikako-Thomas et al., 2013; Specht, King, Brown, & Foris, 2002). This exclusion is due in large part to activity-specific, social, and environmental challenges and barriers that limit the motivation; sense of self-efficacy; and participation of persons with disabilities (Alma et al., 2011, Dahan-Oliel, Shikako-Thomas, et al., 2012; Devine & Parr, 2008; Longo, Badia, & Orgaz, 2013; Figure 13.1).

Figure 13.1. This young man with cerebral palsy becomes involved in an arts activity. The activity is developmentally appropriate and enjoyable.

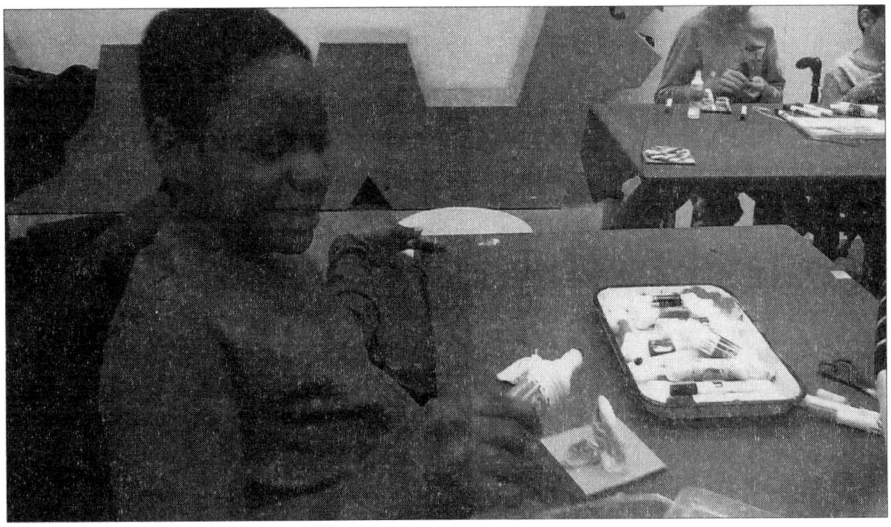

Source. L. Olson. Used with permission.

People with developmental disabilities may have low expectations of their leisure opportunities and their abilities for participation. Students with disabilities engage in fewer activities with peers and family members than their typically developing peers (Leyser & Cole, 2005). They also converse less with their peers about leisure interests such as movies, music, television, food, and pets. Shikako-Thomas et al. (2013) found that adolescents with cerebral palsy were infrequently involved in formal skill-based or self-improvement activities outside of school.

For persons with developmental disabilities, access to community-based support and coaching for leisure participation may be needed to shift sedentary and isolating leisure habits and routines developed over the course of their lives to ones that more fully engage their minds and bodies in individual and social leisure activities (Dahan-Oliel, Shikako-Thomas, et al., 2012; Eriksson, Welander, & Granlund, 2007; Oates et al., 2011).

In addition to being essential for people's quality of life, leisure participation is a powerful tool in supporting adjustment to an acquired disability (Malley, Cooper, & Cope, 2008; Jonsson & Andersson, 2013). Finding ways to participate in what were favored leisure activities before their disability may support the recovery and rehabilitation process beyond leisure participation.

Young adults with physical disabilities may have limited opportunities for socializing and for pursuing leisure activities that interest them. People with disabilities may be limited by the availability of family members for transportation and for their company as they participate in leisure activities outside of their homes. Becoming less engaged with family members and more engaged with peers in leisure pursuits may not be possible or may be much more difficult than it is for young adults without disabilities.

Parents of children with disabilities face challenges in participating in their own leisure activities as well as in facilitating family-based leisure activities. Children with disabilities make greater demands on parents' time because of their greater needs for parental assistance in academic and self-care activities than typically developing children. In addition, gaining access to leisure activities appropriate for children with disabilities may be difficult because of fewer community offerings than are available for typically developing children and the subsequent competition for the opportunities available.

Family members supporting persons with disabilities across the life span may also experience decreased expectations for leisure as a family occupation. They may not have satisfying family leisure activities that support and sustain effective and positive communication, family cohesion, and flexibility (Smith, Freeman, & Zabriskie, 2009; Townsend & Zabriskie, 2010; Wayne & Krishnagiri, 2005).

Services offered within community or health care environments should support persons with disabilities and their families in exploring shared leisure occupations and developing positive family-based leisure habits and routines.

Categories of Leisure Activities

Across people's life spans, leisure can be broadly divided into two types of activities: (1) activities that are personally interesting and engaging and in which a person invests time, energy, and serious attention and (2) activities a person engages in casually or passively to relax or distract himself or herself from the stresses of daily living (Brown, McGuire, & Voelkl, 2008; Fenech & Baker, 2008; Kleiber, Larson, & Csikszentmihalyi, 1986). Both are important but serve different needs. Categorizing a person's leisure activities in this way facilitates understanding how leisure participation supports his or her physical and emotional well-being and personal development.

Some leisure occupations require new learning and provide challenge and intellectual stimulation. Other leisure occupations may resemble adult work, a child's school, or self-care activities. A person who works in business may use leisure time to explore the Internet, write a novel, or refinish old furniture. A high school student may explore astronomy or create a Web site. A retired teacher may volunteer a few days a week in a nursing home. A homemaker may design and make clothing in his or her free time.

Another model for conceptualizing leisure is through the dichotomy of core vs. balance leisure (Hornberger, Zabriskie, & Freeman, 2010; Townsend & Zabriskie, 2010). *Core leisure activities* are routine and home-based leisure activities that draw family members together and support cohesion and stress reduction, such as family dinners, watching television, or playing games as a family unit. When families participate in *balance leisure activities,* they explore new activities together, thus breaking up their routine ways of interacting. These new activities facilitate family members' interacting and collaborating with each other in new situations and in new ways. Families may travel abroad; go on a camping trip; or learn to sail, fish, or ski. This type of family leisure typically requires time, financial resources, and planning.

Leisure Occupations in Which a Person Invests Time, Energy, and Serious Attention

People of all ages participate in leisure occupations for their own personal enjoyment. Throughout life, participation in leisure occupations is a critical safeguard of people's mental health. When the external world of school, work, or everyday living does not seem to offer people affirmation and a sense of mastery, they engage in leisure to fend off depression by reaffirming their abilities, interests, and optimism in their lives. People can also use leisure occupations as a springboard for redirecting their lives in a more satisfying and productive way.

Social control

In modern societies, social control is necessary for people to maintain order and function every day. As members of a society, people need to fulfill certain roles and put aside their own wishes and impulses for immediate gratification. Sometimes people must repress their emotions so that work proceeds harmoniously.

In modern societies, leisure provides opportunities for people to put their commitments aside and experience freedom in activities that satisfy their interests. Moreover, participation in leisure occupations provides people with opportunities to express their desires and their true range of emotions. Such expression of emotions is done with the approval of other people (Neulinger, 1981).

For example, in a creative writing group, an adolescent who writes painfully honest poetry about loss and longing may receive praise from others for the beauty and depth of emotion in his writing. If the adolescent had shared these feelings at his part-time job, coworkers might be nervous or conclude that he is a troubled youth. At football games, the fans cheer loudly while simultaneously feeling an intense camaraderie. In other daily life situations, people would consider this level of emotion inappropriate or deviant.

Needs for belonging and social engagement

All people have a need to belong and to socially engage with others. Throughout people's lives, the activities that help them develop, maintain, or strengthen relationships with others are most often leisure occupations. People plan and share special activities and events with family members and friends so all participants experience pleasure and relaxation (Figure 13.2). When activities have the desired results, people associate the positive experience with those with whom they have interacted, which reinforces those relationships. People will seek out these same people when they are looking for companionship in future activities. They may also come to rely on these people when they need assistance in their daily lives. Further, they would most likely be willing to help them.

People will more likely tolerate and resolve disagreements and frustrations with others when they occur within a relationship that has a strong history of pleasurable interactions. People most often sustain friendships throughout their lives with others with whom they have shared positive experiences that they associate with leisure.

Leisure relationships can be developed or sustained in a variety of ways. For example, Morrison and Krugman (2001) described how the Internet allows for increased interpersonal communication and opens up opportunities to connect with new groups of people. Reich, Subrahmanyam, and Espinoza (2012) reported on the overlap in adolescents' online and offline social networks and how adolescents use instant messaging, e-mail, and social networking to develop friendships. In addition, Gibson, Willming, and Holdnak (2003) described how sharing the experience of being a serious football fan with others can provide a sense of belonging and identity across one's life. Putnam (2000)

Figure 13.2. A grandmother relishes time with her grandchild.

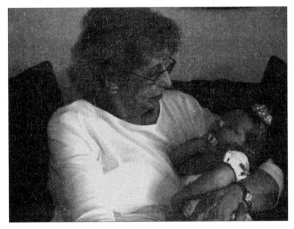

Source. L. Olson. Used with permission.

explored how team sports and communal cultural activities provide opportunities for diverse community members to develop common ground and build positive regard and relationships. Participation in community leisure activities such as bowling or singing in a choir do not require participants to share the same political beliefs or social identity, but these activities can build or deepen relationships among community members.

Smith et al. (2009) examined the ways that core vs. balance family leisure activities facilitate family communication. Townsend and Zabriskie (2010) suggested that overall family leisure involvement predicted positive family functioning. They also found that families that included a child with mental illness tended to rely on balanced leisure activities such as family trips as a way to engage with their children while avoiding conflict. Core leisure activities were less frequent in these families. Buswell et al. (2012) correlated a father's participation in daily family core leisure activities such as family dinner or games with positive family relationships. These research studies on family leisure underline the value of examining the activities that make up clients' family leisure participation. It is important that occupational therapy practitioners include promoting family leisure participation and routines in their intervention plans.

Leisure Occupations to Relax

Often, when people are able to use certain skills to participate in leisure occupations, they consider the occupations relaxing (e.g., reading a novel, knitting, gardening). These occupations fit the definition of *serious leisure* because they enhance quality of life and can provide a person with a sense of achievement, an appreciation of beauty in nature or the arts, a feeling of identification with his or her community, or a sense of fulfillment of his or her potential (Campbell, Converse, & Rodgers, 1976).

Kleiber et al. (1986) labeled a similar category of adolescent leisure as *transitional leisure,* in which the activities prepare an adolescent for the serious aspects of the adult world. These activities promote concentration and challenge and may include extracurricular school activities, individual hobbies such as playing a musical instrument, or developing high-level painting or dancing skills. Passmore (2003), an occupational therapist, labeled this leisure as *achievement* and found that it strongly influenced mental health through enhancing competence. This type of leisure participation correlates with adult occupational prestige and adult civic participation (Putnam, 2000).

Kleiber et al. (1986) identified another category of adolescent leisure called *relaxed leisure,* which encompasses those activities that are pleasurable but not challenging, such as listening to music, watching television, playing videogames, surfing the Internet, interacting on social media sites, or socializing with friends at a local mall or park. Passmore (2003) called this type of leisure *time-out.* These terms are similar to Stebbins's (1997) definition of *casual leisure,* which is "immediately, intrinsically rewarding, relatively short-lived pleasurable activity requiring little or no special training to enjoy it" (p. 18).

Familiar and routine activities help people relax. They allow people to escape from commotion and require little physical or intellectual exertion. Leisure scholars describe this leisure as providing opportunities to rejuvenate oneself from the drudgery and stresses of everyday life (Kraus, 1994; Neulinger, 1981). Some people seek relief by withdrawing from human interactions to read the newspaper. Some may tend to a garden in solitude. Others revive their spirits through enjoying a special meal or drinks with others that create a relaxed mood for conversation and social interaction.

Exercise 13.1. Personal Leisure Activities

Describe your own serious and casual leisure activities. Describe your core and balanced leisure activities with your family members or significant other.

Leisure for Cognitive, Emotional, and Physical Invigoration

People participate in leisure for cognitive, emotional, and physical invigoration. Leisure occupations provide opportunities for people to learn more about themselves, to explore their interests, and to develop skills in the activities that bring them pleasure without concern for their usefulness to others. For example, people may learn to dance, kayak, paint, or play an instrument for no other reason than the pleasure that it brings them. Devel-

oping proficiency in a leisure occupation supports people's sense of mastery and self-efficacy.

Engaging in leisure occupations also has the power to influence people's mood and support a positive perspective about the possibilities of everyday life. For example, adults in Lonsdale and North's (2011) study identified music as a means for managing their moods and increasing their enjoyment while engaged in other activities. Binnewies, Sonnentag, and Mojza (2009) reported that the adults in their study demonstrated improved work performance and outlook on their work after having the time for positive, restful leisure.

Success in a leisure occupation can be an antidote to a negative experience in another part of life. After a successful experience, people may have renewed belief in their capacity to be effective in all parts of their lives. Leisure occupations can be a springboard for people to make real changes in other areas of their lives. Lloyd and Little (2010) found that through learning new physical skills in a supportive, organized physical recreation group environment, female participants reported enhanced physical and emotional well-being, including *self-determination* (i.e., when a person makes a decision for himself or herself without influence from others). The women reported that the experiences increased their optimism and enabled them to set goals to make changes in other areas of their lives.

People also seek leisure for emotional stimulation. Elias and Dunning (1986) stated, "Unless an organism is intermittently flushed and stirred by some exciting experience with the help of strong feelings, overall routinization and restraint . . . are apt to engender a dryness of emotions, a feeling of monotony" (p. 73). During leisure occupations, people can potentially experience the full range of human emotions that they avoid in everyday life. Many children, for example, love to frighten or be frightened on Halloween (Figure 13.3); adults pay high-ticket prices to become engrossed in the pain and suffering of characters in a play. Sloan (1979) reported studies suggesting that the heartbeat and stress level of fans at sporting events can be similar to those of the athletes participating. Although tension and stress increase, these feelings are different from the tension and stress in everyday life and indeed are pleasurable.

Putnam (2000) discussed how the Internet might be part of the solution to the problem with civic engagement in society and with others. He claims

Figure 13.3. Children enjoy the frightening aspects of Halloween by creating scary paintings.

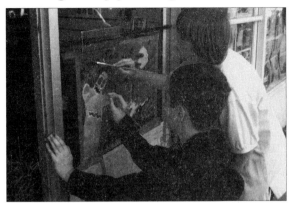

Source. L. Olson. Used with permission.

that the bidirectional communication among people and the exchange of information supports people's engagement. The Internet limits the prejudices that naturally develop among people based on physical attributes. Additionally, virtual communities can be more egalitarian than face-to-face communities. People typically engage in virtual communities differently than they do in real-life communities.

Cyberspace interactions typically develop around one interest about which group members feel passionate and typically remain focused around that issue. Face-to-face communities may begin that way but tend to grow multidimensionally as members observe and interact with others. Putnam (2000) pointed out how interactive video connections such as Skype can decrease the psychological distance and remedy the weak social cues that can be prevalent in Internet communications.

All societies and cultures accept leisure as a social arena for loosening nonleisure restraints. For example, adolescents can express their sexuality more openly in social dance than they can in other environments. A difference, likewise, exists in the openness with which people of different ages show their tension and excitement through bodily movement. Older adults are generally more restrained than teenagers. At a sporting event, a crowd may loudly express very aggressive intentions toward an opposing team that would not be acceptable in a work environment. Roughness and aggression in game play, within the confines of the rules of the game, facilitate enjoyment of watching or playing the game. Aggression guarantees the participants

and the fans a high degree of competitiveness and human drama (Zillman, Sapolsky, & Bryant, 1979).

Spectator sports can ensure a strong emotional bond between members of a team. Spectators can feel a sense of belonging to a larger meaningful group. When the team wins, the spectators get to "bask in reflected glory" (Sloan, 1979, p. 235). Gibson and colleagues (2003) highlighted the sense of group identity in their article "We're Gators . . . Not Just Gator Fans." This title captures the sense of involvement that serious sports fans can have. Although fans cannot attain a direct sense of achievement as can a team player, they can experience a sense of triumph through cheering on their favorite teams. Spectator sports also facilitate social interaction between fans while watching the game or after the event. Without the common focus on sporting events, a group of people may have little to say to each other, yet a shared love of sports can be the basis for days of enjoyment and stimulating conversations for the same group of people (Figure 13.4).

For many people, pets are an important part of their leisure time. Pets fulfill companionship and love needs that people may not get from others in everyday human interactions. A pet is dependent

Figure 13.4. Participation in a soccer game facilitates social interaction for this adolescent, who finds it to be a meaningful leisure occupation.

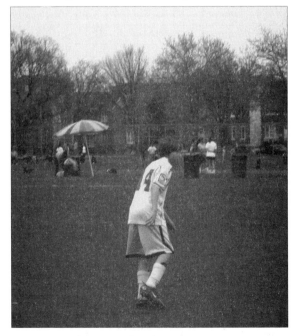

Source. L. Olson. Used with permission.

on its owner for sustenance; the pet's life is centered around its owner. The pet is always present and provides its owner with a routine and companionship; unconditional acceptance; and, potentially, affection. A relationship with a cat or a dog is fraught with fewer complications than relationships with other people. Furthermore, pet owners can lavish attention on a pet in ways that they may not feel comfortable doing with other people.

Leisure as Self-Development

Leisure can be important in self-development. Exploring new leisure activities within a structured group can lessen anxiety for learning and promote camaraderie and friendship that fosters enthusiasm for living and affirmation of the self. Developing the discipline needed to master a new activity is often easier when one participates in a group of like-minded and equally skilled people. When people are in the same situation, they can share small triumphs and give support to each other when they stumble or make mistakes. Joining in with others and working harmoniously fosters engagement and continued interest in a challenging activity.

Independent mastery of solitary leisure occupations also gives people pleasure. In people's solitary time, they may learn to play a musical instrument, write, read, or participate in a range of other activities for their own pleasure. In solitary occupations, people's activity pace is unhurried, and their personal imaginative and creative abilities flourish. Through this process, people get to know themselves more deeply and gain an awareness of what they value and appreciate beyond being with other people. Storr (1988) discussed two opposing human drives: (1) the drive toward closeness and intimacy with other people and (2) the drive toward independence and self-sufficiency. Although love and friendship are essential elements of what makes life worthwhile, solitude has great value. When people learn to make good use of solitude, they have the opportunity to focus on their own desires and interests, separate from the needs and desires of others.

Leisure for Social Consciousness, Altruism, and Service

Leisure can help people cultivate social consciousness, altruism, and service to others. People can fulfill the need to be altruistic through leisure in ways that most work occupations do not meet. Many people use some of their leisure time to help others and in doing so have self-gratifying feelings. Altruistic acts often result in a feeling of invigoration, effectiveness, and control for the doer. For youth, participation in extracurricular activities, both school linked and independent, may lead to increased civic and social involvement in later life. For example, Wood, Larson, and Brown (2009) found that youth reported developing a perspective about themselves as responsible citizens through participating in youth programs.

Leisure Needs of People With Disabilities

Developing play and leisure occupations presents challenges for people with disabilities. For example, Dahan-Oliel, Mazer, and Majnemer (2012) found that children who were born prematurely and who had developmental coordination disorder were restricted in their leisure participation across their lives. Family members and professionals may not explore or consider alternative leisure activities as frequently as they explore alternative methods for work or self-management occupations.

Oates et al. (2011) reported that parents of children with Down syndrome identified leisure participation and friendship as lacking in their children's lives. They stated that these children had infrequent interaction with friends and that the children's recreation was primarily solitary and sedentary. Many of the children used computers for leisure in excess of the 2 hours per day that experts consider healthy (American Academy of Pediatrics, 2013). Oates et al. (2011) found that income status, access to transportation, parental health, time, and family support were either barriers that lessened or supports that increased leisure occupational participation.

Leisure activities are important for everybody, but they may be especially important for people with disabilities. Loy, Dattilo, Kleiber, and Hutchinson (2002) described the positive influence of leisure on the adjustment of adults with recent spinal cord injury. Boyce and Fleming-Castaldy (2012) and Blacker, Broadhurst, and Teixeira (2008) identified the key role of leisure as occupation for self-identity, relationships, and creating meaning in the lives of adults with disabilities.

People with profound intellectual disabilities gained skills as well as positive role identity from volunteering or learning to participate in a sport. Likewise, when these adults participated in these activities, they gained communication skills and improved self-efficacy (Patterson & Pegg, 2009).

Factors Affecting Leisure Participation

Several factors affect the type of leisure activity done throughout the life span, including personal traits, family and cultural factors, and technological factors. The focus of leisure may be different at different points in people's lives. During childhood, engaging parents or other children for fun and stimulation is a primary objective. Children engage others to receive sufficient nurturing, support, and stimulation for healthy development toward adulthood. Children also need physical activity for skill development and physical well-being. Children's participation in leisure occupations (i.e., play) challenges their physical skills without conscious effort and develops their coordination and strength.

Adolescents and young adults may focus on physically exciting leisure occupations that offer the opportunity to meet new people. Participation in some leisure occupations during young adulthood provides a career direction for later life. Children and adolescents often discover lifelong leisure or work interests through their leisure pursuits. For example, a passion for exploring the outdoors may lead to a career as a naturalist or to lifelong participation in hiking and other outdoor activities. Finding a partner and establishing a satisfying adult life separate from the family of origin may be an outcome of leisure pursuits. Dating relationships that develop into marital ones in Western societies typically grow from sharing many positive leisure experiences before marriage.

Throughout adulthood, leisure provides a means to reconnect emotionally to spouses, children, and other adults. Leisure occupations also allow adults respite from work and reaffirm or establish a sense of self that may not be part of everyday routines and responsibilities. In old age, leisure activities may be a means of making connections to others,

defining a sense of identity and purpose, and bringing personal meaning to life.

Personal Traits

Personal traits influence leisure pursuits. For example, *temperament,* the inborn style with which people approach and respond to the environment, affects their activity level, approach and withdrawal tendencies in new situations, adaptability to change, sensory threshold, quality and intensity of mood states, persistence, and attention span (Chess & Thomas, 1984). When people have a low activity level, they tend to seek leisure that is more sedentary. When people have a high activity level and a high sensory threshold, they tend to seek high-intensity pursuits such as skydiving or hunting.

Likewise, personality directs the leisure occupations in which people choose to participate and the extent to which they participate in them. Extraverted people tend to take advantage of many social opportunities and enjoy a variety of group activities. Introverted people may spend more time in solitary pursuits or those requiring the participation of only a few people. Barnett and Klitzing (2006) found that people who were introverted, less social, and high in negative affect were more likely to experience leisure as boredom. They also concluded that when introverted people also exhibited low attention, conscientiousness, and organization skills, they were more likely to experience boredom in their leisure time.

Another personal factor that influences leisure occupation selection is physical stamina and skills. Some people are physically more suited to strenuous physical activities such as skiing, swimming, or tennis. For those with less coordination, skill, or stamina, participation in these activities may feel like work.

Cognitive skill level or interests may determine the leisure occupations in which people are comfortable participating. Those with highly abstract cognitive abilities may choose to play chess, do crossword puzzles, or play word games. People with lower levels of cognitive skills may find these activities boring, confusing, or too demanding or more like work activities. When persons experience a traumatic brain injury, prior leisure occupations that provided self-affirmation and self-efficacy may be not only unsatisfying but also overwhelming and confusing because of awareness of decreased skill or poor executive function capacities such as attention, response inhibition, or ability to monitor performance (Jonsson & Andersson, 2013).

Family and Cultural Factors

Family values and culture greatly affect leisure participation. For example, cultures that value productivity and usefulness, within the family and community, encourage leisure occupations that may revolve around activities related to organized religion or hobbies that produce functional products. In families that believe in the centrality of the family unit, leisure pursuits may be centered around the family (Figure 13.5). In these situations, a family member's free time and creative talents focus on enhancing family life and in celebrating family events. Conversely, when a family believes in each member's self-fulfillment, each family member is encouraged to direct his or her time and energy toward exploring individual interests. This outlook may lead to family members spending more time in solitary activity or in activities with like-minded people outside the family unit.

Cultural beliefs and values also affect how gender or age determines one's leisure occupations. Some cultures delineate appropriate activities by age, gender, or marital status. Some have specific rules about how and when men and women may participate in selected activities. For example, some cultural groups expect married women to spend

Figure 13.5. A father and son spending time together engaged in a mutually enjoyable activity.

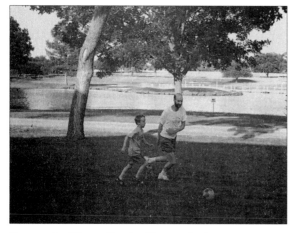

Source. L. Olson. Used with permission.

their leisure time within the family and not in the community at large.

Technological Factors

Technology has had a major effect on social leisure participation of persons across the life span. Adolescents' online social networks support their offline friendships (Reich et al., 2012). Experts also note the importance of adult online social connections for the maintenance and development of friendships. Nimrod (2011) described how online social games engaged senior citizens in their free time. She reported that even lurkers described engagement and enjoyment. Adults with autism spectrum disorders who use social networking sites are more likely to have close friends than their peers who do not participate in online social networks (Mazurek, 2013).

However, social media also presents risks to balanced, healthy leisure participation, including Internet addiction and increased depression when people spend excessive amounts of time updating their own information and viewing what others post, as opposed to engaging in real-life leisure occupations (Lin, Lin, & Wu, 2009; O'Keeffe, Clark-Pearson, & Council on Communications and Media, 2011). According to Litt and Stock (2011), adolescents who spend large amounts of time on Facebook and who view images of alcohol use as normative for their peer group are at greater risk for alcohol abuse.

Internationally, experts have expressed concerns about the amount of leisure time that children and teens devote to passive leisure pursuits such as television and video games. Ivory (2008) reported that the average 8- to 12-year-old plays 13 hours of video games per week and the average 13- to 18-year-old plays 14 hours per week. The American Academy of Pediatrics (n.d.) recommends that parents monitor their children's media diet in light of studies suggesting that excessive media use decreases children's attentional skills and is linked to obesity, sleeping and eating difficulties, and problems in school.

Choosing Leisure Occupations

How people use time outside of leisure occupations may affect how they view and choose leisure time.

Some people view their choice of leisure occupations relative to what they do in their career or vocation. For example, Neulinger (1981) postulated that people choose leisure occupations that are the direct opposite of their daily work routine. A person who works at a desk or a computer may spend his or her free time in physically strenuous outdoor sport occupations (i.e., bike riding or hiking). A mother who spends most of her time tending to the needs of the family may seek out occupations in which she can lose herself, such as jogging, painting, or dancing. When a person's work requires a large amount of solitary time, he or she may actively seek leisure group occupations. However, others may seek leisure occupations related to their chosen career or vocation. Some examples are a person who attends conferences and socializes with members of his or her profession, a high school English teacher who chooses to read novels and attend poetry readings, or a carpenter who builds a boat in his free time.

Social Support

When people feel socially accepted and supported in leisure environments, they are more likely to demonstrate the motivation for participating in available leisure occupations (Devine & Parr, 2008). If they believe they are not likely to receive social acceptance or support, they are more likely to opt out of leisure participation. People with disabilities and their caregivers may be passive or uninvolved in community leisure activities because they experience able-bodied community members as not understanding their needs for accommodations or adaptations for leisure participation. Besides interventions directed at leisure skill development for persons with disabilities and their families, it is important that occupational therapy practitioners consider how to increase their clients' social acceptance and support for leisure participation.

Environmental Considerations

Personal access to leisure environments, materials, and equipment strongly influences how people spend their free time and what leisure occupations they explore. For example, if people live in a rural environment, they are likely to have the opportunity to explore and develop skills in many outdoor activities (Figure 13.6). In a city environment,

Figure 13.6. People who live in a rural environment have more opportunities to explore and engage in outdoor activities.

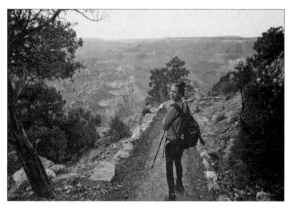

Source. L. Olson. Used with permission.

people have a greater opportunity to participate as a spectator in a range of sporting and creative arts events. Low-income inner city communities may have limited or no resources or facilities for children's afterschool leisure pursuits. In a study of four middle schools in such a community, children reported that they primarily participated in unstructured and passive leisure activities such as watching television and hanging out with their friends when not in school (Shann, 2001). Likewise, when older adults perceived their community environment as unsafe and as lacking in resources, they were less likely to seek out or participate in active leisure occupations (Sallis, King, Sirard, & Albright, 2007).

Environmental barriers greatly hinder the leisure participation of people with disabilities across their life spans. For example, older adults with vision loss participate less in leisure outside of home because of reduced visual cues for negotiating their environment as well as limited understanding from others (Alma et al., 2011). Reduced participation increases risk for functional and cognitive decline. For elderly people, a lack of transportation to their local senior citizens' center severely limits their leisure participation.

Shikako-Thomas and colleagues (2013) discussed how contextual environmental factors have a negative impact on the diversity and intensity of the leisure participation of adolescents with cerebral palsy. Adolescents with cerebral palsy tend to participate in less structured leisure activities that require limited or no environmental modifications. These activities also tend to be more passive and sedentary than those sought by adolescents without disabilities. Not only does this lack of opportunity for varied and active leisure pursuits negatively affect their physical state, it also substantially limits these adolescents' transitional leisure opportunities, which are important for their development of skills for adult life.

Internet

The Internet provides varied leisure opportunities, including online groups, games, and virtual communities, even when physical geography, physical limitations, or economic resources limit a person's leisure participation in his or her real-life communities. For example, people who live in a remote area of the Northwest can participate in a book discussion with like-minded readers through discussion boards or live chats. Second Life, an online virtual world, allows virtual trips to faraway places and access to virtual nightclubs, university lectures, and music concerts at no cost. For persons with disabilities, these resources may provide ready access to a range of leisure activities that would otherwise be unavailable.

However, although many online leisure experiences are positive, others may be negative or may distract persons from pursuing or advocating for community-based leisure participation. It is important that occupational therapy practitioners assist clients and their caregivers in identifying ways that leisure needs may be met through virtual communities and activities and assess the quality of particular virtual leisure environments and activities.

Exercise 13.2. Leisure Pursuits

Think about your leisure pursuits. What factors influence your choice of these leisure activities?

Leisure Occupations Across the Life Span

As people grow and mature, their leisure occupations change. In addition, leisure occupations reflect a person's developmental maturation, developing interests, cultural background, and social peer group.

Infancy and Early Childhood

Leisure in infancy and early childhood include solitary activities and activities with caregivers or peers. A child's first leisure experiences are play. *Play* is a child-initiated occupation that an adult has not structured for teaching specific skills. The child engages in play occupations because he or she wants to and because it is fun (Figure 13.7). The child is free to participate independently or to negotiate sharing the occupation with another. A parent might approach an infant with a busy box, and the infant may bang on it for a few minutes but then crawl away and pick up a pot to bang. The infant is in control of the play occupation. How-

Figure 13.7. This preschool child enjoys dressing and dancing as a ballerina.

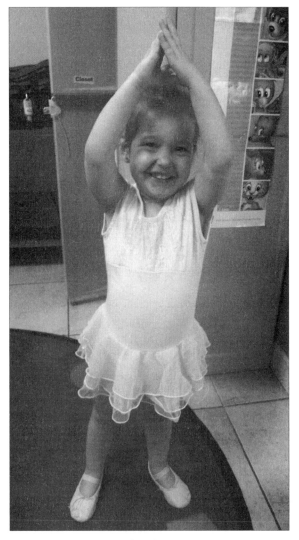

Source. L. Olson. Used with permission.

ever, this same infant may look toward the parent for an indication of when he or she wants the infant to join or move away and when he or she wants the infant to play alone. An older child may build with interlocking plastic bricks or do a puzzle because he or she finds the play occupation interesting rather than because a parent or teacher instructed the child to complete the activity.

Erikson (1963) wrote that children's play "is not the equivalent of adult play . . . it is not recreation. The playing adult steps sideward into another reality, the playing child advances to new stages of mastery" (p. 222). A child's play concerns exploration and discovery in all spheres of human existence. It continuously evolves, and what was once interesting is now boring. A child develops new skills and uses them in novel ways during play. Although building skills is not the purpose of play, through play a child becomes more competent in all areas of human functioning. He or she develops the capacity to cope with his or her environment and develop ego strength and an investment in life (Cotton, 1984).

Playfulness is an important aspect of a child's play. *Playfulness* exists when a child is intrinsically motivated, internally controlled, and able to suspend reality (Bundy, 1997). A child's *intrinsic motivation* drives him or her to participate in particular activities because of the innate rewards experienced in the activity. The child does not participate in play activities because he or she is expecting a reward or praise. The child gets involved to have fun. *Internal control* refers to the child's having primary control over what occurs in the activity. When a child suspends reality, he or she uses objects in new ways to discover new uses for everyday things or to engage in make-believe (e.g., imaginary play or games). A child frames a play occupation by giving cues to others as to how they should act toward him or her. A child, for example, might cue a playmate that they are now going to play house and he or she is going to be the parent. A child who wants to play superheroes and be the "bad guy" may frame the activity so that his or her peers must now fight or run away. These manipulations allow the child to experience life from the perspective of another.

Play begins in infancy when an infant learns to attend to the faces of caregivers. Caregivers smile and make soft sounds at the infant and wait for the infant to respond in kind. Over time, an infant is ready to play peek-a-boo or to imitate facial expressions and sounds that caregivers make. The infant begins to initiate the play, and both he or she and caregivers receive pleasure from the interaction. This mutual interaction evolves to social play by making a different face or sound. Through parent–child play experiences in infancy and early childhood, a child develops the coping skills necessary for play that are more complex. The most important variable in a young child's development of coping skills is the mother's leisure experiences with the child, which is the mother's enjoyment of the play (Murphy & Moriarity, 1976).

Playing and interacting with other children is an important part of the leisure experiences of a child from preschool age onward. When a child shares similar levels of physical activity, exuberance, and open emotional expression with another child, the child becomes more attracted to the child than to adults. The child shares interests with peers, and enthusiasm for activities increases or decreases depending on the reactions of valued peers to those activities. A child is more likely to take chances and participate in new activities when another child is participating. Through leisure play experiences, a child learns the joys of friendship and camaraderie. He or she also learns to negotiate and compromise in the interest of maintaining peer relationships (Figure 13.8).

The supportive guidance of caregivers provides a young child with confidence in his or her capacity to successfully participate in an activity and have

Figure 13.8. Two children interacting in the sand enjoy friendship and camaraderie.

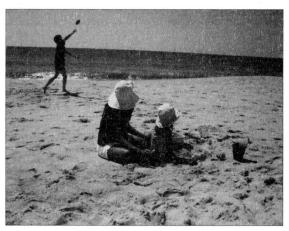

Source. L. Olson. Used with permission.

fun. As a child matures and enters middle childhood, some leisure activities become recreational ones; these activities have playful elements to them, but they are now structured activities that occur as part of a team game or within a club. A child enters these activities having begun to accept rules as necessary for group activity. Without defined rules and some accepted order to activities, little pleasurable activity would occur.

Leisure for a child evolves into more complex games and group activities over time. He or she first masters games of chance and then games requiring strategies. In games of chance, a child learns first to modulate intense excitement related to the process of being in the lead and then to accept losses as "just a game" rather than a statement about his or her competence. The child learns to follow the rules and to inhibit negative emotions that might lead him or her to quit a game prematurely or to become aggressive when a game does not end in his or her favor.

Depending on a child's temperament and innate skills, learning games may initially be challenging to both the child and his or her caregivers. A child may be slow to learn or to acclimate to rules. A younger child often changes the rules and cheats to win until losing becomes less threatening. Once a child understands games and begins to accept rules, his or her animation, physical tension, and excitement in a simple game such as Old Maid can bring almost as much enjoyment to caregivers as it does to the child.

When transitioning to adolescence, a child who participated in structured activities such as hobbies and sports is more likely to be well adjusted (McHale, Crouter, & Tucker, 2001). A child who spends his or her free time just hanging out is more likely to exhibit less adaptive functioning, including poor school grades and more conduct problems. Because leisure occupations are at least partly self-chosen and involve self-control or peer-group control of action and attention, leisure activities can provide opportunities for the development of initiative, self-regulation, and social skills (Larson & Verma, 1999).

Many of the leisure occupations, however, that young people choose may involve little structure or challenge and therefore provide little stimulus for growth. Higher rates of television viewing among children of lower socioeconomic status may be attributable to limited options for other, more rewarding leisure choices. Children often choose television to fill hours of free time. Television watching requires little active self-regulation of attention or behavior from participants; it is also related to obesity and depression. Television can be a default relaxing activity when other occupations are not available, or it may displace functionally similar activities such as attending movies, listening to music, or time spent idling.

Exercise 13.3. Childhood

Think about a child you know well. What activities does that child participate in that you would consider play or leisure? Why? What underlying skills does the child have that support his or her participation? What needs do you think the activities meet for the child? What effect, if any, do you think that the child's participation will have on his or her overall development?

Adolescence

An adolescent's moods are the most positive and his or her activity level is the highest when he or she is engaged in leisure occupations as opposed to work or school activities (Fine, Mortimer, & Roberts, 1990). American adolescents have more time for leisure than they had 30 years ago because of less opportunity or need for employment or participation in housework (Zick, 2010). However, although the ways that adolescents use their leisure time greatly affect their social and cognitive development, American youth are more likely to use their unstructured leisure time for passive leisure activities that are not supportive of life skills development or transition to adulthood (Zick, 2010).

Larson, Hansen, and Moneta (2006) studied the developmental experiences of young people as they participated in different categories of organized leisure activities, including sports, performance and fine arts, and community-oriented and service pursuits. Organized sports stood out as being supportive of adolescents in developing initiative, including setting goals, applying effort, and learning time management. Participation in sports also has the potential for supporting emotional regulation. Service activities were distinguished from other activities by how they connected a young person to adult networks and provided positive relationship experiences. Although unstructured interactions with peers (e.g., hanging out) have the potential to provide young people with rich developmental activities, they reported higher rates of negative influences in their interactions with peers than in organized activities.

Youth programs can be important contexts in which a young person can develop a sense of responsibility (Wood et al., 2009). Youth programs provide opportunities for a participant to develop responsibility in meeting task, role, and time demands as he or she executes meaningful tasks for their groups. Young people feel like active agents in the group's success. In a youth program, a person can identify his or her goals. In a productive group, a person takes ownership of demanding tasks and roles, the expectations of leaders and peers are high, and the consequences associated with the demands are meaningful and important to each participant.

Transitional leisure pursuits can be a sanctuary for an adolescent. These activities most often occur in safe and familiar settings that nurture self-expression and exploration. They may involve visiting the science laboratory or the art room of a favorite teacher after school or they may involve participating in a club or extracurricular class. For example, Wilson (1977, as cited in John-Steiner, 1985) studied the experiences of a group of high school students in art. The art room in a public high school was a retreat from the demands of the school environment. In the room, these adolescents were able to "transcend the limitations of the structure, to engage in acts which are creative or ludic or subversive and to participate in a kind of communitas" (Wilson, 1977, as quoted by John-Steiner, 1985, p. 94). *Communitas* refers to a community in which a strong feeling of equality, solidarity, and togetherness exists.

When an adolescent participates solely in relaxed leisure occupations, he or she is more likely to be less focused and at risk for developing behavior problems that negatively affect development. Without leisure occupations to channel his or her energy positively, the adolescent may seek out adventure through drinking, drug experimentation, or early sexual activity. In contrast, an adolescent who discovers his or her particular talents, and develops habits to cultivate these talents, invests a substantial amount of time in related activities and develops comfort and the ability to use solitude

effectively. As a result, he or she has a stronger grasp on developing self-identity, and peers are less likely to influence him or her negatively. Thus, the adolescent tends to be more open to new experiences and to exhibit higher levels of concentration than do other teens.

Interestingly, an adolescent who spends more time with parents in leisure occupations has a sense of support and consistency. This relationship also encourages intensity and self-direction and enhances his or her attentional capacities for finding and mastering challenges (Csikszentmihalyi, Rathunde, & Whalen, 1993).

Exercise 13.4. Adolescence

Think back to your adolescent years. Describe your participation in leisure activities at that time. What activities were you regularly involved in that might be described as relaxed leisure activities? What activities were you regularly involved in that might be described as transitional leisure activities? How did these activities influence your experiences as an adolescent and your roles as an adult?

Young Adulthood

As people transition from adolescence into adulthood, shifts in leisure activities occur as they continue their education and begin their first real jobs. Many young adults move out of their family homes and enter a different world from that of their childhood and adolescence. This period becomes one of defining oneself outside of one's family of origin. Leisure time may lessen because of work responsibilities or may increase for college students who do not work and who may now live independently with people their own age.

When a young adult becomes a college student, he or she pursues a course of study that expands his or her knowledge into new areas. The student may develop interests in areas about which he or she was previously unaware and may come to find that prior interests are less compelling. The college environment provides numerous new opportunities for leisure activities with new people to befriend. Frequently, a young adult who enters college continues to have a great deal of leisure time. Living independently on a college campus with roommates offers increased opportunities to explore and experiment.

New leisure opportunities may be available at college that were not available in students' communities of origin. A young adult from a large city may find himself or herself in rural areas that provide opportunities for outdoor activities such as bike riding, canoeing, hiking, and skiing. A young adult from a rural area may find himself or herself in a major metropolitan center and discover a love for live music and theater. A new friend may come from a different background and expose the young adult to new social opportunities.

Additionally, activities that were chores during adolescence may now become valued leisure occupations. For example, preparing a meal in one's own apartment for friends may be a way of expressing one's identity and relaxing. Painting and decorating a dorm room or apartment may be a work of self-expression for a young adult.

This time may also involve the loss of treasured leisure occupations because of relocation or the responsibilities of being a college student. During the transition to young adulthood, a young adult may have difficulty coping with changes in tasks and activities. In addition, the young adult may lack opportunities to engage in pleasurable activities and activities in which success is guaranteed. At this time, a young adult may test his or her ability in preparation for the pursuit of a future career.

The leisure occupations of a young adult who enters the workforce may likewise change. Pressure may exist to conform to the culture of the majority, and a young adult must learn to adjust his or her personal values and conduct in the work environment. Leisure occupations are critical for workers to explore so that they may find activities that reaffirm their sense of identity, allow them to develop areas of interest and talent, reaffirm a sense of belonging to specific cultural groups, and rejuvenate the soul and spirit. In the future, workers may continue some of the leisure occupations of their school years, such as participating in local adult sports leagues; playing in music bands; and attending spectator sports, movies, or live music events. An adult who remains in the same geographical area may socialize with the same or similar friends. The major change in an adult's life is when he or she goes to work full-time, which results in a notable decrease in leisure time compared with high school. Leisure time may now be limited to evenings and weekends and days off from work.

For a young adult, a considerable amount of leisure time may focus on establishing a relationship with a significant other, and sharing leisure occupations is a central part of courtship in Western culture. Through leisure occupations, a young person socializes in a nonthreatening, neutral environment in which he or she shares a mutually interesting activity (e.g., dinner, movie, sporting event, bike ride). Such activities allow a relationship to develop in a relaxed manner. When a like-minded person shares leisure activities with another, a bond of friendship may develop. Furthermore, sharing an activity or adventure with another person provides a situation in which one learns about oneself and about the other person.

A person may reflect his or her pleasure in the joint activity by developing a positive regard for the other person and may want to learn more about the other person. As a meaningful relationship with a potential partner develops, a young adult adjusts his or her time commitments to fit the other person's leisure interests. Couples negotiate how much leisure time they will spend together, especially when they have different leisure interests and pursuits. Each person in a couple adjusts leisure expectations in the interest of the relationship: One person may give up socializing in a bar or participating in a league sport to please a partner; another person may adjust to a partner's hobby by developing an interest in that hobby to increase shared leisure time. The couple may take up a new leisure occupation together, such as ballroom dancing, to deepen their bond. Couples begin to share holidays, family traditions, and family events. They begin entertaining friends and family members together. A young wife, for example, may need to accommodate her husband by participating in his traditional Italian family dinner every Sunday.

In healthy young adulthood, a person maintains solitary or group leisure interests that have developed during his or her lifetime. Certain leisure occupations become part of one's persona, support self-esteem, and rejuvenate the participant. A person may have a longstanding love for cars that develops into an interest in restoring vintage cars. Sewing, knitting, or jewelry making may be someone's way of expressing an artistic side, although he or she may work as a store clerk. Others may join adult community sports leagues or coach children's sports teams. A young adult who enjoyed biking as a child and teenager may join a biking club to maintain physical fitness and rejuvenate his or her body. Another adult may become involved in a virtual community or Internet gaming (Nimrod, 2011; Padilla-Walker, Nelson, Carroll, & Jensen, 2010). Internet-based devices such as smartphones may be a primary tool for accessing leisure occupations such as listening to music, making music, playing games, drawing, painting, or participating in photography as a leisure pursuit (Snickars & Vonderau, 2012).

Drinking alcohol during social events is often part of the passage from childhood to adulthood in Western culture. The use of substances such as drugs and alcohol may stem from a search for pleasurable feelings that substances can induce (Kraus, 1994). Alcohol can lower one's inhibitions and make socialization easier; however, when drinking dominates how a person spends his or her leisure time, enjoyment of this occupation (and other activities) diminishes.

Middle Adulthood

Whether an adult chooses to marry or remain single or to have children influences how he or she uses leisure time during middle age. When a person marries, he or she is likely to use some of his or her leisure time to include spouses and extended family. When a person has children, considerable time is usually spent taking care of them and engaging in leisure occupations with them.

Generally, a single adult will continue to seek, establish, and maintain long-term relationships with significant others, but he or she is also likely to pursue and further develop skills from prior hobbies and leisure occupations. A single adult will likely settle in his or her career and adjust to single adulthood; he or she might devote time to enhancing skills in lifelong leisure occupations and pursuing new interests. In the process, he or she would discover more about himself or herself as a person and contribute to society in ways other than caring for children.

In midlife, a single person may become more reflective about community issues or politics and decide that he or she has the personal skills and resources to have a positive effect on the community. Others may turn past hobbies into part-time careers, such as writing, buying and selling antiques, or designing jewelry.

In some ways, single life presents a greater challenge but more opportunity for the development of a rich adult leisure life. Single or childless people may confront expanses of unstructured time unencumbered by responsibilities to a spouse or to children. People may perceive this unstructured time as freedom or as a burden. They can pursue interests without the restraint of the needs of immediate family members. Without an active approach to leisure participation, a single person may experience isolation and discontent. Having solitary leisure interests can be helpful to these adults because others may not be immediately available for interaction.

Finding companions for joint leisure activities is a more active process for single adults. For some, a lack of companionship can present a serious barrier to leisure participation; for others, it is an opportunity to develop new relationships, deepen older relationships, and expand leisure opportunities through varied companions. Single adults are more likely to participate in group travel or adult leisure organizations than are people with families or spouses. Single adults may be more independent and willing to take risks to participate in activities that interest them. Single or married women without children may not experience the retreat from the exploration of their own abilities and personal interests that may occur after having children.

Women's roles notably change when they become parents. Parenting changes a woman's work life or career to a greater extent than it alters a man's, even if a woman continues to work after childbirth. Although men share in child care and home maintenance activities, most mothers fill the role of primary caregiver. Women's former leisure experiences tend to decrease more notably than do their husbands'. Men may share equally in leisure activities with children, but women typically provide more instrumental child care.

Leisure occupations of parents who do not work outside the home are usually home centered. Leisure occupations may include gardening, sewing, home crafts, cooking, and parent–child play. These parents intersperse these occupations among house and child maintenance chores. In families in which both parents work outside the home, family leisure occupations are often limited to evenings and weekends. These occupations are special because the time together is limited. Eating a family meal, reading a book together, and playing a game may be more important than household maintenance activities.

The leisure occupations of a family undergo many transitions as children grow. As infants, children may greatly curtail parents' leisure occupations as parents adjust to parenthood. Leisure may revolve around playful interaction with the infant or sharing parenting experiences with other parents or with older adults who can provide support and guidance to the new parents. Satisfying leisure needs with infants and young children requires effort on the part of the adults (Figure 13.9).

In addition to home-based leisure activities, parents of young children often visit parks and other public places where other parents and children congregate. They may attend religious functions, parent–child drop-in centers, or gym activities designed to facilitate parent–child interaction and interaction with other families. These community activities provide parents with an opportunity to interact with children in the proximity of other parents, which allows adults to share their parenting joys and frustrations. During these activities, children have opportunities to meet other adults and children.

Some parents make connections to their children by sharing their own leisure passions. Parents may teach their children sports, take them to sporting events, and share the experience of cheering for their favorite team. If a child shows an interest in learning a sport that interests a parent, the sport may provide a means through which the parent and child can relate to one another. Positive feelings about the activity become closely associated with positive feelings toward one another, and the sport can bring the two closer together. Parents may return to the leisure occupations of their youth as part of their role as parent. A parent may have loved soccer as a child and now coaches his or her child's soccer team.

When children reach adolescence, family-focused leisure time may occur less frequently. Although adolescents may still participate in selected family, religious, or cultural activities, they tend to begin to move beyond their immediate family for leisure pursuits. Parents may feel loss, abandonment, or a new sense of freedom as their adolescent children's leisure increasingly focuses on activities outside the family unit. Parents may experience jealousy as their teenagers' leisure occupations become more exciting than their own. This change may lead parents to question and reevaluate their own leisure occupations.

When children move on to start their own adult lives, middle-aged adults must refocus their leisure pursuits. Although women are more likely to experience psychological turmoil during their offspring's adolescence before the children leave home, they adjust more easily to the "empty nest syndrome" than do fathers (Steinberg & Steinberg, 1994). Women are more likely to be engaged in exploring new careers, new interests, or community activities than men. Some believe that this change may occur because young women may surrender their own desires in the interest of their husbands and growing families; once their children are grown, women may seek to reclaim their sense of individuality and pursue activities that provide personal satisfaction (Labouvie-Vief, 1994; Niemela & Linto, 1994).

During later middle age, a couple may pursue new joint activities or a parent may reinvest his

Figure 13.9. A mother and son play with Play-doh.® The activity is fun for the child, and the parent values the interaction with her child.

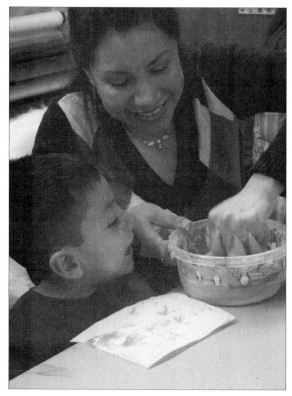

Source. L. Olson. Used with permission.

or her newly acquired time in individual hobbies. Work demands may have lessened, and time previously spent focusing on career building may now be available for leisure pursuits. Leisure travel may become more frequent because children place fewer demands on parents' time and finances. Middle to older adulthood can be a time to do some of the activities that one has always wanted to do but never did.

Adults also begin to see a time limit on their opportunity to participate in those activities. Some people run their first marathons at age 50 years, and others use late middle age to challenge themselves intellectually in ways they wished they had done as younger adults. Some adults reenter education to finish a high school diploma, pursue a college degree for the sake of knowledge, or pursue another career that they expect may be more fulfilling than their first career. For others, late middle adulthood is an opportunity to connect with other adults in ways that were not possible when they were raising children or focusing on their careers. They may develop new or revived passions for occupations such as gourmet cooking, golf, bridge, travel, or book clubs.

This time is when people may have to begin to think about their physical abilities as they become aware that minor physical injuries take longer to heal and affect function longer than in their younger years. People inevitably experience a decrease in visual acuity as they age and perhaps a change in body metabolism that may contribute to weight gain or obesity. Some people in middle adulthood may also develop high blood pressure, diabetes, or high cholesterol. These changes and dysfunctions associated with age may interfere with participation in leisure occupations unless people make accommodations in their routines or activities.

Older Adulthood

Besides avoiding disease and disability, successful aging requires the maintenance of physical and cognitive function and engagement in social and productive activities (Hultsch, Hertzog, Small, & Dixon, 1999; Rowe & Kahn, 1997). The importance of elderly people's establishing or maintaining meaningful occupations was demonstrated in the Well Elderly Research Study (Jackson, Carlson, Mandel, Zemke, & Clark, 1998), which found that identification of and engagement in meaningful

---

Exercise 13.5. Parent Interview

Interview a parent. Discuss the effect of children on his or her participation in leisure activities. What does a parent value in his or her leisure time? How much leisure time does he or she have per day or per week? How does he or she spend it? What leisure activities does he or she participate in alone, with children, and with other adults? Compare his or her leisure experiences with those of a single adult you know.

---

occupations has an effect on the overall well-being of elderly people.

Participating in leisure occupation is the most important predictor of well-being among older adults (Zimmer, Hickey, & Searle, 1997). Carey (2009) reported that older adults who spend 3 or more hours per day in demanding mental activities such as doing crossword puzzles were more likely to maintain their cognitive function and to stave off dementia. Leisure occupations such as playing bridge that combine social connection with strong cognitive demands seem to be the most powerful in maintaining the function of elderly people.

When older adults retire from paid employment, they have a new opportunity to explore their interests, evaluate who they have been during their lifetimes, and think about who they would like to be for the remainder of their lives. If they have maintained some leisure interests throughout their lives, retirement may allow them to expand on those interests and devote more time to the occupations they love.

For others, retirement leads to depression or a crisis as they attempt to adjust to a new way of life. When confronted with unstructured time, these older adults may not have the initiative to pursue new leisure occupations or reconnect with old ones. A grieving process may be related to loss of the previous role. The role of worker is one of the most important roles with which people identify throughout their adult lives.

Past participation in leisure occupations typically determines the activities a retiree seeks. Optimally, people who have neglected developing leisure occupations throughout the earlier part of their lives will begin to explore leisure activities within their community and learn what they really enjoy and value beyond the daily routine of their life's work. Volunteer work in hospitals, schools, or community organizations can provide a structure for daily life similar to that of paid employment and may offer older adults an opportunity to find a new life purpose, enhance self-worth, and increase social contact with others (Morrow-Howell, Hinterlong, Rozario, & Tang, 2003; Singleton, 1996).

People's bodies and minds respond differently to the aging process. Although many elderly people may seek out sedentary activities, many healthy elderly people pursue regular exercise. They may swim a few miles every week, go in-line skating, enter marathons, take Tai Chi or yoga classes, or go biking. Others maintain an interest and regularly participate in outdoor activities. Some older adults actually increase their involvement because they have more discretionary time. Many people retain sedentary interests that have sustained their spirits throughout their lifetimes, including writing, playing an instrument, or painting. As their social obligations lessen, elderly people may focus more on these leisure occupations.

Leisure pursuits may markedly change when adults become grandparents, especially if the grandchildren live nearby. Time spent with family members may now revolve around entertaining and engaging grandchildren. Grandchildren can bring out a relaxed ability to nurture and play that may not have been possible with one's own children. Grandparents may have increased discretionary time and the wisdom of experience to be able to enjoy the time they spend with their grandchildren more. Learning how to play virtual Wii games and activities can support older adults' engagement with their grandchildren. It can also open up older adults to new, productive ways to maintain their physical and mental fitness.

Older adults living alone report fluctuations between extremes of involvement with others and projects and periods of isolation (Siegel, 1993). An issue for these adults is how to find a balance in their time and make the time they have left to live more valuable and meaningful for themselves. Some people may have difficulty managing this life stage; others seek and find inner creative powers they had not recognized during earlier stages in their lives.

For some mature adults, senior citizen centers become important places of social interaction. Regularly attending meetings and activities may provide the structure and support that some older adults

need to deal with the loss of their jobs and former roles at retirement or with the loss of spouses and friends to death. Activities such as bingo, weekly card games, and day trips with local organizations demonstrate a shift from independent occupation to activities that are more interdependent or involve dependence on others. Within the structure of these centers, older adults may find new ways to contribute to their communities; for example, they may make blankets for infants or participate in making products for nonprofit fundraising.

As older adults experience the loss of lifelong partners and close friends, they may find themselves burdened with feelings of isolation and disconnection. Although family members are often key to the physical well-being of elderly people, friends are more consistently related to well-being than are family members (Larson, Mannell, & Zuzanek, 1986). Friends provide unique companionship that transcends the mundane requirements of everyday life; they most typically share similar life experiences and view one another differently than do family members who see the older adult and themselves in their lifelong roles. Although family members are related to lifelong physical well-being, Larson et al. (1986) pointed out how friends influence one's immediate well-being, enjoyment in living, and participation in active leisure activities.

Because many of the daily activities of elderly people are voluntary rather than required work, it is easier to retreat from activity participation. Support groups with adults experiencing similar losses often help them in coming to terms with these experiences and in finding ways to reconstruct meaningful lives. In summarizing the experiences of 56 older women who participated in her qualitative study on aging, Siegel (1993) stated that

[w]ith each death of a loved one, . . . we learn something more about who we are within that relationship and who we are without the presence of that person. With each loss, we also learn more about death and dying and about how to cope and survive. (p. 184)

As people near the end of their lives, they may be unable to participate in some past leisure occupations because of the infirmities of old age. Some may cease participation and not seek new activities that interest them, but many older adults replace physically active pursuits with more passive ones in which they can readily participate (Zimmer et al., 1997). Frequently, as adults get older, they need to shift from occupations that are more active to less active, which is not to imply that people find less satisfaction in these occupations (Parker, 1996). Older adults, who are likely to feel most in control of their lives, will adapt their former interests to their bodies' changes in old age and will work to improve their bodies' functioning for participation in their activities through regular exercise, good nutrition, and mental activity (Baltes & Baltes, 1990; Everard, Lach, Fisher, & Baum, 2000).

Frail elderly people may become homebound and gradually lose interest in many leisure occupations, including social ones. They may spend more time reflecting on the past and become dependent on adult children or community services for social interaction. In some situations, the adult may require adaptations or assistive devices (e.g., a magnifier to read a book or newspaper, adaptations to a telephone to amplify sound) to participate in leisure occupations.

Barriers to Participation in Leisure Occupations

For some people, work and responsibilities seem to fill every waking hour. They may see leisure activities as frivolous. For others, leisure is threatening, frustrating, or a burden. People may be more comfortable with a regular routine made up of required activities than with an expanse of time they must fill with their own planned activities. Engaging in leisure occupations means people need to step outside of their daily routine. It requires people to challenge themselves to participate in activities beyond those required for self- or family maintenance or for work. People have the right not to participate in leisure activities or occupations and to be passive in their free time. This lack of participation, however, can be isolating and may lead to alienation and depression.

In the United States, people have many opportunities to be passive in their leisure time. Although watching television can help fill people's leisure time in a way that makes them feel momentarily better than if they had nothing to do, it can lead people away from learning to truly experience their leisure time. Television is the only leisure activity that seems to inhibit participation in other leisure occupations (Putnam, 2000). Watching television results in people feeling lethargic and passive. Kubey and Csikszentmihalyi (1990) found that heavy television viewing was associated with a great deal of free time, loneliness, and emotional difficulties.

This finding is consistent across cultures. People who engage in do-it-yourself projects at home are more likely to play a sport in their leisure time or to engage in public speaking. People who attend more movies are more likely to attend club meetings or dinner parties or visit friends. People participate in television watching at the expense of nearly every social activity outside of the home (Putnam, 2000). The only activities positively linked to heavy television watching are sleeping, resting, eating, housework, and listening to the radio.

Corporate Influence as a Barrier

When exploring alternative leisure activities, people must recognize that a large amount of corporate profit in Western society is related to mass consumption of leisure equipment and experiences. Corporations barrage people with advertising about the "perfect" use of leisure time that may interfere with the search for personal definitions of ideal leisure. Relentless advertising attempts to convince people that they want what the ads offer. Some people then begin to value only heavily advertised leisure activities. People's social status may be determined by having the "right" pair of running shoes or sports equipment, belonging to the "right" gym, or going on the "right" vacations. People may work more hours to afford leisure versus actually enjoying leisure. Others may participate in fewer leisure activities or passive activities because they believe that participation in leisure activities requires a great deal of money.

Stereotypes as Barriers

Stereotypes can be a barrier to leisure participation, especially for school-age children, teens, and older adults. A group of children may decide that one child is strange and therefore exclude that child in playground activities or in child-initiated clubs. Adolescents identify themselves and each other with crowds who share certain observable behaviors (Brown, 1990). Typical clique identifications in a high school may include "jocks," "brains," or "druggies." Certain cliques have higher social status than others do.

An adolescent who is associated with an unpopular or negative clique may experience rejection and discomfort when trying to participate in leisure activities that are associated with another clique. Devine and Parr (2008) cautioned that unless caregivers monitor how children with severe disabilities are included in leisure activities with nondisabled peers, inclusion can result in reinforcing negative stereotypes of children with disabilities if nondisabled children experience limitation of their own activities and do not experience benefits from their interaction with children with disabilities. A healthy elderly person may feel less included in some community activities that are typically associated with younger adults. He or she may need to prove competence before gaining acceptance in some leisure group activities.

Some people have personal factors that interfere with their ability to engage in leisure activities with others. They may lack the internal resources (e.g., coping skills) or social skills to explore interests or connect with others through personally meaningful and productive activity. Whalen, Jamner, Henker, Delfino, and Lozano (2002) found that adolescents with attention-deficit/hyperactivity disorder (ADHD) symptoms were more likely to spend their time in passive, entertaining leisure pursuits as opposed to hobbies and structured activities. Participants with ADHD in this study were 10 times more likely to have smoked and 4 times more likely to have consumed alcohol than adolescents without ADHD. Adolescents with ADHD may lack the skills to modulate their attention, which is important for skill development in active and productive leisure activities.

Some barriers to participation are caused by a person's negative habits or behaviors such as abuse of drugs or alcohol and participation in gangs, petty crime, or violence, which may inhibit relaxation, excitement, and connecting with others. Even when substance abuse and illegal activities cease, people who have been habitually involved in these activities may lack the skills to find and participate in satisfying leisure activities. Farnworth (2000) found that her sample of adolescent offenders on probation spent 57% of their time engaged in passive leisure activities such as watching television and listening to music. They reported being bored 42% of the time.

Young adults with weaker planning and inhibition control capacities than other young adults are more likely to participate in binge drinking (Mullan, Wong, Allom, & Pack, 2011). In one study, young adults with depression who were also binge drinkers demonstrated reduced visual learning and memory skills compared with persons who were just depressed or were binge drinkers without depression (Hermens et al., 2013).

In determining the leisure needs of these young adults and adolescents, it is important to reflect on how their underlying personality features may interact with their participation in self-destructive leisure activities such as binge drinking and interfere with their development of healthy leisure interests and routines. Barnett and Klitzing (2006) found that the ability to entertain oneself, extroversion, and emotional stability were linked with less boredom and positive leisure participation, whereas negative affect and decreased intrinsic motivation were related to poor use of leisure time.

Exercise 13.6. Interests

Think about leisure pursuits that strongly interest you but in which you do not participate. What are the barriers to your participation?

Leisure for Health Promotion and Prevention of Secondary Health Issues

The occupation of leisure is a critical aspect of life, and developing the occupation of leisure in clients should be a primary concern for occupational therapy practitioners working to prevent secondary disabilities or working with people with disabilities. As described earlier, when people are able to participate fully in leisure occupations, they are more likely to support their mental and physical health.

Across the life span, leisure provides opportunities for personal growth, a sense of competence, physical fitness, positive self-identity, and active social participation and inclusion. It also promotes self-regulation and supports *coregulation* (i.e., when a person acts in response to another person's action) among family members.

Participating in positive leisure occupations prevents secondary health issues that arise from the sedentary behavior, social isolation, or lack of cognitive stimulation associated with boredom. Krane and Orkis (2009) reported that people with disabilities who are physically active are more likely to be employed and more likely to report greater overall life satisfaction, to be more sociable, to have stronger support networks, and to be positive about life prospects than people with disabilities who are not active.

The Well Elderly Study established occupational therapy as an effective preventive treatment of the population of well elderly people (Jackson et al., 1998). This study demonstrated that occupational therapy services focused on the power of occupation and its ability to enhance health through occupation. Participants who were provided with education on a variety of topics relevant to the engagement in meaningful occupations and had opportunities to experience meaningful activities of their choice had more positive gains. Overall, those receiving occupational therapy had gains that were more positive and fewer declines in function than those who took part in a social activity program only.

Expertise of Occupational Therapy Practitioners in Leisure Development

Occupational therapy practitioners have a unique perspective and expertise to offer to educational, community, and health care teams addressing leisure development and participation for persons with or at risk for disabilities and their families, as well as for persons and families marginalized by social and economic adversity. Their knowledge and skills related to assessing the complex array of person-related, task, and environmental barriers to participation are essential for developing and implementing programs that focus on the development of people's leisure skills. They also possess knowledge needed to design evidence-based interventions that facilitate the development of performance skills of individuals and groups for leisure participation. Further, knowledge and skills in activity and environmental analysis, adaptation, and redesign support their creation of interventions that remove barriers to participation.

Occupational Therapy Assessment of Leisure

Occupational therapists evaluate a client's leisure life in a way that captures what the client enjoys doing. *Client-centered practice* has been defined as "an approach to service which embraces a philosophy of respect for, and partnership with, people receiving services" (Law, Baptiste, & Mills, 1995, p. 253). It is critical that occupational therapists develop strong skills in therapeutic communication to engage clients in exploring their leisure occupational interests, values, and challenges. Taylor (2008) provided explicit evidence-based guidance for developing skills in this area that is specific to occupational therapy practice.

The Canadian Occupational Performance Measure (COPM; Law et al., 1994), a client-centered structured interview assessment, provides occupational therapists with a systematic and time-efficient means of gaining information about a client's perceptions of his or her occupational performance and satisfaction. It is used to detect changes in a person's perception of his or her performance and satisfaction with occupational performance. If therapists use the structure of COPM to assess clients' leisure occupations, they should consider adding questions or prompts about the different categories and effects of leisure activities and participation appropriate to clients' stage of life and development.

Some occupational therapy assessments specifically obtain information about clients' range of leisure interests, actual participation, and view of their own participation (Henry, 1997a, 1997b, 2000; Mann & Talty, 1991). Occupational therapy practitioners can use these data to facilitate a focused discussion with clients about their leisure occupations. In the process of exploring clients' stated interests, present participation, and desire for increasing or expanding their participation in specific leisure activities, it is also important to explore how clients' current leisure participation influences their physical and emotional health. Boredom and loneliness are also common leisure concerns for persons with disabilities and are important topics to address in the assessment process.

The Children's Assessment of Participation and Enjoyment and the Preferences for Activities of Children (King et al., 2004) allow therapists to systematically gather and organize information from young people aged 3 to 21 years about their activity preferences, the diversity and intensity of their participation, with whom and where they participate, and their degree of enjoyment of each activity. These assessments explore the participation of children with functional limitations in and out of school activities. The activity items are organized by type to help practitioners guide children and adolescents with disabilities to explore activities similar to ones they have identified as preferred when major barriers exist for success or enjoyment in preferred activities.

Mastery motivation is important for leisure development and participation in serious, achievement-oriented leisure activities. The Perceived Efficacy and Goal Setting System (Missiuna, Pollock, & Law, 2004) is a self-report interview assessment that engages school-age children with disabilities in sharing how they perceive their own competence in everyday activities as well as what they want to work on and what is important to them. With this understanding of children's views of their own competence, the occupational therapist can set collaborative goals for positive leisure development and participation.

The Volitional Questionnaire (de las Heras, Geist, Kielhofner, & Yanling, 1998) and the Pediatric Volitional Questionnaire (Basu, Kafkes, Schatz, Kiraly, & Kielhofner, 1998) are observational assessments that may be helpful when a therapist suspects that motivation is a barrier to a client's leisure development or participation. These assessments are helpful in conjunction with client-centered interviewing or may be used as the key source of information when clients do not possess the verbal or cognitive skills to share their concerns verbally or through written self-reports.

When clients exhibit deficits such as poor attention, inflexibility, poor planning skills, or emotional dysregulation and the therapist suspects these deficits are interfering with leisure participation, it may be helpful to use the Behavior Rating Inventory of Executive Functioning (BRIEF; Gioia, Esquith, Guy, & Kenworthy, 2000). When clients aged 10 or older have the capacity to complete the standardized self-report questionnaire, the results can

be used to facilitate a discussion with them about how their executive functioning affects their leisure participation and then to set goals to develop or strengthen executive functions important for their successful leisure development or participation. The caregiver version of BRIEF provides a different perspective about clients' executive functioning and can also be used to understand perceptions of the executive functions of a child younger than 10 years old or a client who is unable to complete the BRIEF self-report.

Sensory processing assessments such as the Sensory Profile (Dunn, 1999), Sensory Profile School Companion (Dunn, 2006), and the Adolescent/Adult Sensory Profile (Brown & Dunn, 2002) help an occupational therapist understand how clients' responses to everyday sensory input support or interfere with leisure participation. The Barth Time Construction (Barth, 1988), a time chart on which a client pastes colored strips of paper to depict the categories of activities and the amount of time devoted to particular activities over the course of a day and week before a psychiatric hospitalization, is an effective assessment for many clients, especially ones with substance abuse disorders.

The Barth Time Construction provides clients and the therapist with a graphic picture of time use over the course of a week. Clients with substance abuse disorders are frequently struck by the amount of time they have devoted to obtaining and using alcohol or drugs and recovering from the effects of the drugs before seeking treatment. The chart can generate a deep discussion about the lack or minimal amount of meaningful leisure activities in these clients' lives.

Observation-based assessments grounded in the Model of Human Occupation (Kielhofner, 2008) support a occupational therapist's assessment of the impact of client factors, task, and environment on occupational participation. The Short Child Occupational Performance Evaluation (Bowyer et al., 2008) and the Model of Human Occupation Screening Tool (Parkinson, Forsyth, & Kielhofner, 2006) provide therapists with a broad overview of a client's occupational participation, but they can use them to structure observations of factors that facilitate or restrict leisure participation.

When clients have severe physical disabilities, it is important that practitioners provide an in-depth ecological assessment of environmental and activity factors that may restrict leisure participation for these clients. Research on young people and adults with congenital or acquired disabilities identified environmental barriers and insufficient activity modification as the major factors limiting these persons' leisure participation (Berger, 2011; Dahan-Oliel, Shikako-Thomas, et al., 2012; Longo et al., 2013).

Occupational Therapy Interventions

To facilitate change in clients' leisure participation, before intervention, occupational therapy practitioners need to reflect on the change process. Using assessment data, the practitioner and client ideally will have an in-depth understanding of the client's current leisure participation and preferences and challenges to development of leisure occupations.

The first step in the intervention process is to review with or educate clients and their caregivers about the different roles in leisure participation and its importance as an occupation, including ways in which it can facilitate or support development or participation in work and self-care occupations. Without fully understanding the effect of different types of leisure participation on health and wellness, clients and their families may not make leisure a priority in their occupational development or rehabilitation.

Clients and their families may need to make major adjustments in their daily time use, including their daily habits and routines, and invest financial resources in the process of developing meaningful and positive leisure occupations and *co-occupations,* which occur when two or more people physically, emotionally, and intentionally share participation in an occupation. They may also need to expend effort to build new skills, alter their living space, or advocate for the removal of environmental barriers within their communities.

Beyond direct intervention for skill building, optimal service delivery models for supporting clients and families in the process of change are consultation and coaching. These methods focus practitioner interventions on collaborating with clients to decide what skills they need to develop, what task adaptations and strategies are needed and desired to promote activity participation, and what environmental barriers need to be removed.

When consulting, occupational therapy practitioners support clients' participation by sharing observations and strategies with them and their caregivers and then guiding clients in choosing strategies to implement. Practitioners may design or provide materials as well as guide clients through implementation and monitoring of a plan for change. When practitioners use a coaching model for service delivery, they help clients identify what knowledge or skills they need to learn to reach their personally identified goals.

Then, practitioners work to build capacity in clients. Practitioners use questioning to elicit plans and strategies from clients as opposed to the practitioner introducing them. They foster client reflection on and assessment of their own performance before offering their professional views. In this way, clients become aware of how their current behavior and strategy use may be supporting or interfering with their leisure skill development and participation and then learn to refine their behavior or strategies as needed to work toward their own preferred outcomes.

Influence of temperament on interventions

Throughout the intervention process, occupational therapy practitioners should be cognizant of clients' innate temperaments. A clients' temperament affects a practitioners' expectations and style of intervention. People who are generally positive and easily adapt to changes in their physical status or life circumstances are likely to put a practitioner at ease and increase the practitioner's expectation of successful intervention. People who tend to have difficulty persevering, have typically negative states of mind and mood, or are slow to adapt to changes may be frustrating to practitioners, who may then lower their expectations of what the client and practitioner can achieve together. People who are slow to adapt to changes may also need more support at any life stage when they attempt to pursue new leisure activities.

Parent and caregiver interventions

When a child has a learning disability or other cognitive disabilities, parents may struggle with interacting with the child in leisure activities. The child may avoid or be unable to attend to learning the typical leisure activities that parents teach and share with a child. The child may stay focused on familiar and repetitive activities or may be emotionally labile or withdrawn when confronted with leisure experiences that are pleasurable to other children. This circumstance may result in power struggles between parent and child or in a more distant parent–child relationship in which the parent and child are mutually feeling sad, frustrated, and angry.

Occupational therapy practitioners can help parents guide their children in finding pleasurable and engaging individual and family leisure occupations. The practitioner may guide parents in learning how to provide support and assistance to their children so that children build the coping skills to explore unfamiliar activities as well as confront challenges in familiar activities. Parents may learn how to modify and adapt activities to foster their children's participation. Parental engagement in helping children in this way facilitates children's development of attentional and coping capacities that are necessary for future engagement in independent leisure activities. Furthermore, satisfying parent–child leisure interaction has positive effects on both the parents' and the children's sense of competence and mood (Olson, 2006, 2010).

When adult clients have severe physical or cognitive disabilities that seemingly preclude their active engagement in leisure activities, caregivers may assume that these clients are not able to participate in such activities. They may even believe that placing these clients in front of a television or side-by-side with other clients with severe disabilities in a nursing home dayroom is an appropriate and sufficient casual leisure activity. Fenech and Baker (2008) challenged these practices and described the importance of developing sensory diet activities to provide relaxing, casual leisure for adults with *neuropalliative conditions* (i.e., neurological conditions that result in limited life expectancy). Forsblom, Särkämö, Laitinen, and Tervaniemi (2010) identified the impact of music and audiobook listening on relaxation, motor activity, and mood in persons recovering from a stroke.

Adolescent interventions

Adolescents or young adults with disabilities may be isolated from their mainstream peer groups and may have come to believe, accept, and develop comfort with passive, isolating, undemanding leisure pursuits. Adolescents with behavior disorders may have little awareness of their own individual interests, talents, and potential to develop as contributing members of society. They may solely be focused on their role within a negative peer group.

Occupational therapy practitioners may engage adolescents in exploring leisure activities and discovering previously unknown individual interests and talents. For example, an adolescent may find that he really enjoys the solitary experience of baking; baking may give him time to relax away from peers and to think about his own life issues. Baking may lead to more prosocial individual action on the part of the teen at other times of the day. In addition, he may become aware that he has a talent for baking, be motivated to participate in baking activities regularly, and may begin thinking about education or employment in food services or culinary arts.

Adult interventions

Adult clients may also avoid leisure occupations that interest them if they expect to fail because of pain, lack of physical fitness, lack of preparation to undertake the activity, or limited skills. Assisting clients in adjusting their expectations and guiding them in adapting activities or locating adaptive equipment that would allow their participation or help develop the necessary physical skills for participation are important intervention strategies.

Adults with brain injury may lose previous friendships and the ability to participate in some leisure pursuits because of reduced cognitive functioning. Loss of leisure-related occupations can have a major effect on every area of life functioning, and the person may become depressed, passive, and dependent. Participating in a group that focuses on the occupation of leisure may help a person explore potential leisure interests; develop activity, social, and time management skills for leisure participation; learn how to reduce barriers to leisure participation; and build a network of similar people who are interested in joint leisure activities. Creating a personally meaningful leisure life is likely to result in a generalized sense of well-being, independence, and personal control.

Regardless of whether depression is a primary disability or a secondary one related to a physical disability, it can have devastating effects on a person's everyday functioning. Developing leisure interests and experiencing successful participation in them may lessen the negative effects of difficult life situations and give the participant a new perspective on his or her life and the ability to exert control over everyday activities. New interests may reduce a person's sense of alienation and make him or her more available for interaction with others.

Some may need to find leisure outlets to express strong emotions they cannot express in other everyday activities. Actively participating in sports or games or watching spectator sports, for example, may provide a socially acceptable outlet for aggressive impulses. Developing the habit of writing in a journal or composing poetry may provide a means for expressing and working through intense feelings for another person.

Leisure activity analysis in intervention

Over the course of the intervention process, it is important that occupational therapy practitioners teach clients, their caregivers, or both to reflect on how clients' leisure experiences influence their emotional, cognitive, and physical well-being. Developing habits and routines for serious, active, or achievement-oriented leisure occupations may be demanding of time and effort, but active reflection on the positive experiences and outcomes will support continued engagement. Clients or their caregivers may be momentarily happy with leisure time occupied and not cognizant of the long-term effect of unhealthy leisure activities such as excessive television watching, game playing, or drinking of alcohol.

Abuhamdeh and Csikszentmihalyi (2012) reported on how challenge is a strong predictor of enjoyment in intrinsically motivating, goal-directed activities such as sports, games, and serious leisure activities. Occupational therapy practitioners can support clients in finding their appropriate challenge level for individual and group leisure participation. They can also help clients build the coping and executive function skills necessary for mastery motivation and building self-efficacy in leisure participation.

Chronic physical or mental illness in a family may greatly reduce the amount and quality of time and resources available for family leisure activities and thus lessen the emotional support that children receive from their parents or that spouses receive from each other. Joint leisure activities are often the first activities that family members sacrifice as stress increases. Relaxed and joyful interaction may be minimal or nonexistent. Re-experiencing positive family leisure occupations can have a major positive effect on each family member's mood and on the family's overall emotional atmosphere.

Occupational therapy practitioners can help families use core and balance family leisure activities to support their communication, cohesion, and adaptability. When a family member has a disability or a chronic illness, practitioners can guide the family in the redesign of leisure occupations for active and meaningful co-occupation, keeping the contraindications and limitations of the disorder in mind.

Environmental interventions

Guiding clients through the process of altering their physical or social environment so they can readily participate in leisure occupations is an intervention strategy that occupational therapy practitioners regularly use with clients with all levels of disability. Community and home leisure environments can lessen or prohibit leisure participation or enjoyment of persons with disabilities.

Persons with disabilities and their caregivers may need to be educated in ways to create or advocate for needed environmental adaptations. Young people with autism spectrum disorders may feel physically comfortable engaging in family or peer games only when extraneous visual or auditory stimuli in the environment are reduced. Older adults with vision loss may need enhanced visual cues to engage safely in community leisure environments. Persons with congenital disabilities may be unable to traverse or access a local park or museum. Silverman, Bartley, Cohn, Kanics, and Walsh (2012) described the collaborative efforts of some occupational therapy practitioners in working with museums to promote the participation of persons with disabilities.

Occupational therapy practitioners need to guide clients in methods for seeking external resources for regular participation in leisure occupations that interest them. A single adult with a physical disability may be interested in travel, or a senior citizen may be interested in finding partners for playing bridge. Clients may be unaware of how to access free or inexpensive transportation for people with disabilities or may be unaware of how to find community leisure activities or events that offer special rates to persons with disabilities. Helping clients find virtual communities or physical community resources or connecting them to another professional or agency that can find the appropriate external resources are important interventions.

Exercise 13.7. Compare Leisure Values and Experiences

Compare the leisure values and experiences of the people, of all different ages, that you talked to or thought about while reading and studying this chapter. What did you learn about leisure across the life span?

Summary

Although leisure is often a second thought rather than a first, and something that one may consider only after completing the required and routine activities of daily life, it can be a powerful buffer for the stresses and negative events of other occupations. Leisure can facilitate relationships and allow a person to discover a true vocation or life purpose. Through activities that help one express one's full emotional range in socially acceptable activities, one is able to maintain emotional equilibrium. One can experience the benefits of leisure only by truly engaging in activities that capture one's interest and possibly even one's soul.

Leisure is a challenge; it requires as much focus and energy as other human occupations. Without the active pursuit of a leisure life, free time may be a burden instead of a pleasure. It may become a time of passivity, boredom, disconnection, unhappiness, confusion, or loneliness and may thus negatively affect one's engagement and full participation in other daily occupations.

It is critical for occupational therapy practitioners to address clients' leisure needs, despite the pressures to address and meet their other rehabilitation needs and the high demands of the health care system. Helping clients to develop a rich and personally meaningful leisure life may facilitate their

achievement of all other goals of intervention that our society values more than leisure.

References

Abuhamdeh, S., & Csikszentmihalyi, M. (2012). The importance of challenge for the enjoyment of intrinsically motivated, goal-directed activities. *Personality and Social Psychology Bulletin, 38*, 317–330. http://dx.doi.org/10.1177/0146167211427147

Alma, M. A., van der Mei, S. F., Melis-Dankers, B. J. M., van Tilburg, T. G., Groothoff, J. W., & Suurmeijer, T. P. (2011). Participation of the elderly after vision loss. *Disability and Rehabilitation, 33*, 63–72. http://dx.doi.org/10.3109/09638288.2010.488711

American Academy of Pediatrics. (2013). Policy statement: Children, adolescents, and the media. *Pediatrics, 132*(5), 958–961.

American Academy of Pediatrics. (n.d.). *Media and children.* Retrieved from http://www.aap.org/en-us/advocacy-and-policy/aap-health-initiatives/Pages/Media-and-Children.aspx?nfstatus=401&nftoken=00000000-0000-0000-0000-000000000000

Aristotle. (1943). *Politics II: The treatises* (B. Jowett, Trans.). New York: Modern Library.

Baltes, P. B., & Baltes, M. M. (1990). Psychological perspectives on successful aging: The model of selective optimization with compensation. In P. B. Baltes & M. M. Baltes (Eds.), *Successful aging: Perspectives from the behavioral sciences* (pp. 1–34). London: Cambridge University Press.

Barnett, L. A., & Klitzing, S. W. (2006). Boredom in free time: Relationships with personality, affect, and motivation for different gender, racial, and ethnic student groups. *Leisure Sciences, 28*, 223–244. http://dx.doi.org/10.1080/01490400600598053

Barth, T. (1988). Barth time construction. In B. Hemphill (Ed.), *Mental health assessment in occupational therapy: An integrative approach to the evaluative process* (pp. 117–129). Thorofare, NJ: Slack.

Basu, S., Kafkes, A., Schatz, R., Kiraly, A., & Kielhofner, G. (1998). *The Pediatric Volitional Questionnaire Version 2.1.* Chicago: University of Illinois.

Berger, S. (2011). The meaning of leisure for older adults living with vision loss. *OTJR: Occupation, Participation and Health, 31*, 193–199. http://dx.doi.org/10.3928/15394492-20101222-01

Binnewies, C., Sonnentag, S., & Mojza, E. J. (2009). Feeling recovered and thinking about the good sides of one's work. *Journal of Occupational Health Psychology, 14*, 243–256.

Blacker, D., Broadhurst, L., & Teixeira, L. (2008). The role of occupational therapy in leisure adaptation with complex neurological disability: A discussion using two case study examples. *NeuroRehabilitation, 23,* 313–319.

Bowyer, P. L., Kramer, J., Poloszaj, A., Ross, M., Schwartz, O., Kielhofner, G., & Kramer, K. (2008). *The Short Child Occupational Profile (SCOPE), Version 2.2.* Chicago: MOHO Clearinghouse.

Boyce, K. O., & Fleming-Castaldy, R. P. (2012). Active recreation and well-being: The reconstruction of the self-identity of women with spinal cord injury. *Occupational Therapy in Mental Health, 28,* 356–378. http://dx.doi.org/10.1080/0164212X.2012.708603

Brown, B. B. (1990). Peer groups and peer culture. In S. S. Feldman & G. R. Elliot (Eds.), *At the threshold: The developing adolescent* (pp. 171–196). Cambridge, MA: Harvard University Press.

Brown, C. E., & Dunn, W. (2002). *Adolescent/Adult Sensory Profile.* San Antonio, TX: Psychological Corporation.

Brown, C. A., McGuire, F. A., & Voelkl, J. (2008). The link between successful aging and serious leisure. *International Journal of Aging and Human Development, 66,* 73–95. http://dx.doi.org/10.2190/AG.66.1.d

Bundy, A. C. (1997). Play and playfulness: What to look for. In L. D. Parham & L. S. Fazio (Eds.), *Play in occupational therapy for children* (pp. 52–66). St. Louis: Mosby.

Buswell, L., Zabriskie, R. B., Lundberg, N., & Hawkins, A. J. (2012). The relationship between father involvement in family leisure and family functioning: The importance of daily family leisure. *Leisure Sciences, 34,* 172–190. http://dx.doi.org/10.1080/01490400.2012.652510

Campbell, A., Converse, P., & Rodgers, W. (1976). *The quality of American life: Perceptions, evaluations, and satisfactions.* New York: Russell Sage Foundation.

Carey, B. (2009, May 21). At the bridge table: Clues to a lucid old age. *The New York Times.* Retrieved from www.nytimes.com

Chess, S., & Thomas, A. (1984). *Origins and evolutions of behavior disorders: From infancy to early adult life.* New York: Brunner/Mazel.

Conroy, R. M., Golden, J., Jeffares, I., O'Neill, D., & McGee, H. (2010). Boredom-proneness, loneliness, social engagement and depression and their association with cognitive function in older people: A population study. *Psychology Health and Medicine, 15,* 463–473. http://dx.doi.org/10.1080/13548506.2010.487103

Cotton, N. S. (1984). Childhood play as an analog to adult capacity to work. *Child Psychology and Human Development, 14,* 135–144. http://dx.doi.org/10.1007/BF00717321

Csikszentmihalyi, M., Rathunde, K., & Whalen, S. (1993). *Talented teenagers: The roots of success and failure.* New York: Cambridge University Press.

Dahan-Oliel, N., Mazer, B., & Majnemer, A. (2012). Preterm birth and leisure participation: A synthesis of the literature. *Research in Developmental Disabilities, 33,* 1211–1220. http://dx.doi.org/10.1016/j.ridd.2012.02.011

Dahan-Oliel, N., Shikako-Thomas, K., & Majnemer, A. (2012). Quality of life and leisure participation in children with neurodevelopmental disabilities: A thematic analysis of the literature. *Quality of Life Research, 21,* 427–439. http://dx.doi.org/10.1007/s11136-011-0063-9

de las Heras, C. G., Geist, R., Kielhofner, G., & Yanling, L. (1998). *The Volitional Questionnaire Version 4.1.* Chicago: University of Illinois.

Devine, M. A., & Parr, M. G. (2008). "Come on in, but not too far": Social capital in an inclusive leisure setting. *Leisure Sciences, 30,* 391–408. http://dx.doi.org/10.1080/01490400802353083

Dunn, W. (1999). *Sensory Profile: User's manual.* San Antonio, TX: Psychological Corporation.

Dunn, W. (2006). *Sensory Profile School Companion User's Manual.* San Antonio, TX: Psychological Corporation

Elias, N., & Dunning, E. (1986). *Quest for excitement: Sport and leisure in the civilizing process.* New York: Blackwell.

Erikson, E. H. (1963). *Childhood and society* (2nd ed.). New York: W. W. Norton.

Eriksson, L., Welander, J., & Granlund, M. (2007). Participation in everyday school activities for children with and without disabilities. *Journal of Developmental and Physical Disabilities, 19,* 485–502. http://dx.doi.org/10.1007/s10882-007-9065-5

Everard, K. M., Lach, H. W., Fisher, E. B., & Baum, M. C. (2000). Relationship of activity and social support to the functional health of older adults. *Journals of Gerontology, Series B: Psychological Sciences, 55,* S208–S212. http://dx.doi.org/10.1093/geronb/55.4.S208

Farnworth, L. J. (2000). Time use and leisure occupations of young offenders. *American Journal of Occupational Therapy, 54,* 315–325. http://dx.doi.org/10.5014/ajot.54.3.315

Fenech, A., & Baker, M. (2008). Casual leisure and the sensory diet: A concept for improving quality of life in neuropalliative conditions. *NeuroRehabilitation, 23,* 369–376.

Fine, G. A., Mortimer, J. T., & Roberts, D. F. (1990). Leisure, work, and the mass media. In S. S. Feldman & G. R. Elliot (Eds.), *At the threshold: The developing adolescent* (pp. 225–253). Cambridge, MA: Harvard University Press.

Forsblom, A., Särkämö, T., Laitinen, S., & Tervaniemi, M. (2010). The effect of music and audiobook listening on people recovering from stroke: The patient's point of view. *Journal of Music and Medicine, 2,* 229–234. http://dx.doi.org/10.1177/1943862110378110

Gibson, H., Willming, C., & Holdnak, A. (2003). "We're Gators . . . not just Gator fans": Serious leisure and University of Florida football. *Journal of Leisure Research, 34,* 397–425.

Gioia, G. A., Esquith, P. K., Guy, S. C., & Kenworthy, L. (2000). *Behavior Rating Inventory of Executive Functioning (BRIEF).* Lutz, FL: Psychological Assessment Resources.

Henry, A. D. (1997a). *Leisure Interest Profile for Adults (research version 2.0).* Boston: University of Massachusetts Medical Center.

Henry, A. D. (1997b). *Leisure Interest Profile for Seniors (research version 2.0).* Boston: University of Massachusetts Medical Center.

Henry, A. D. (2000). *Pediatric Interest Profiles: Surveys of play for children and adolescents.* San Antonio, TX: Therapy Skill Builders.

Heo, J., Stebbins, R. A., Kim, J., & Lee, I. (2013). Serious leisure, satisfaction, and health of older adults. *Leisure Sciences, 35,* 16–32. http://dx.doi.org/10.1080/01490400.2013.739871

Hermens, D. F., Lee, R. S. C., De Regt, T., Lagopoulos, J., Naismith, S. L., Scott, E. M., & Hickie, I. B. (2013). Neuropsychological functioning is compromised in binge drinking young adults with depression. *Psychiatry Research, 210*(1), 256–262. http://dx.doi.org/10.1016/j.psychres.2013.05.001

Hornberger, L., Zabriskie, R. B., & Freeman, P. (2010). Contributions of family leisure to family functioning among single-parent families. *Leisure Sciences, 32,* 143–161. http://dx.doi.org/10.1080/01490400903547153

Hultsch, D. F., Hertzog, C., Small, B. J., & Dixon, R. A. (1999). Use it or lose it: Engaged lifestyle as a buffer of cognitive decline in aging. *Psychology and Aging, 14,* 245–263. http://dx.doi.org/10.1037/0882-7974.14.2.245

Ivory, J. D. (2008). The games, they are a-changin': Technological advancements in video games and implications for effects on youth. In P. E. Jamieson & D. Romer (Eds.), *Changing portrayal of adolescents in the media since 1950* (pp. 347–376). Grand Rapids, MI: Calvin.

Jackson, J., Carlson, M., Mandel, D., Zemke, R., & Clark, F. (1998). Occupation in lifestyle redesign: The Well Elderly Study occupational therapy program. *American Journal of Occupational Therapy, 52,* 326–336. http://dx.doi.org/10.5014/ajot.52.5.326

John-Steiner, V. (1985). *Notebooks of the mind: Explorations of thinking.* New York: Harper & Row.

Jonsson, C., & Andersson, E. E. (2013). Mild traumatic brain injury: A description of how children and youths between 16 and 18 years of age perform leisure activities after 1 year. *Developmental Neurorehabilitation, 16,* 1–8. http://dx.doi.org/10.3109/17518423.2012.704955

Kielhofner, G. (Ed.). (2008). *A Model of Human Occupation: Theory and application* (4th ed.). Baltimore: Lippincott, Williams & Wilkins.

King, G., Law, M., King, S., Hurley, P., Rosenbaum, P., Hanna, S., & Young, N. (2004). *CAPE/PAC: Children's Assessment of Participation and Enjoyment and Preferences for Activities of Children.* San Antonio, TX: Psychological Corporation.

Kleiber, D., Larson, R., & Csikszentmihalyi, M. (1986). The experience of leisure in adolescence. *Journal of Leisure Research, 18,* 169–176.

Krane, D., & Orkis, K. (2009, February 12). *Sports and employment among Americans with disabilities.* Retrieved from http://www.disabledsportsusa.org/wp-content/uploads/2013/02/Sports-and-Employment-Among-People-With-Disabilities.pdf

Kraus, R. (1994). *Leisure in a changing America: Multicultural perspectives.* New York: Macmillan College.

Kubey, R. W., & Csikszentmihalyi, M. (1990). *Television and the quality of life: How viewing shapes everyday experience.* Mahwah, NJ: Erlbaum.

Labouvie-Vief, G. (1994). Women's creativity and images of gender. In B. F. Turner & L. E. Trol (Eds.), *Women growing older: Psychological perspectives* (pp. 140–165). Thousand Oaks, CA: Sage.

Larson, R. W., Hansen, D. M., & Moneta, G. (2006). Differing profiles of developmental experiences across types of organized youth activities. *Developmental Psychology, 42,* 849–863. http://dx.doi.org/10.1037/0012-1649.42.5.849

Larson, R., Mannell, R., & Zuzanek, J. (1986). Daily well-being of older adults with friends and family. *Psychology and Aging, 1,* 117–126. http://dx.doi.org/10.1037/0882-7974.1.2.117

Larson, R. W., & Verma, S. (1999). How children and adolescents spend time across the world: Work, play, and developmental opportunities. *Psychological Bulletin, 125,* 701–736. http://dx.doi.org/10.1037/0033-2909.125.6.701

Law, M., Baptiste, S., Carswell, A., McCall, M. A., Polatajko, H., & Pollock, N. (1994). *The Canadian Occupational Performance Measure* (2nd ed.). Toronto: Canadian Association of Occupational Therapists.

Law, M., Baptiste, S., & Mills, J. (1995). Client-centred practice: What does it mean and does it make a difference? *Canadian Journal of Occupational Therapy, 62,* 250–254. http://dx.doi.org/10.1177/000841749506200504

Leyser, Y., & Cole, K. B. (2005). Leisure preferences and leisure communication with peers of elementary students with and without disabilities: Education implications. *Education, 124,* 595–604.

Lin, C.-H., Lin, S.-L., & Wu, C.-P. (2009). The effects of parental monitoring and leisure boredom on adolescents' Internet addiction. *Adolescence, 44,* 993–1004.

Litt, D. M., & Stock, M. L. (2011). Adolescent alcohol-related risk cognitions: The roles of social norms and social networking sites. *Psychology of Addictive Behaviors, 25,* 708–713. http://dx.doi.org/10.1037/a0024226

Lloyd, K., & Little, D. E. (2010). Self-determination theory as a framework for understanding women's psychological well-being outcomes from leisure-time physical activity. *Leisure Sciences, 32,* 369–385. http://dx.doi.org/10.1080/0 1490400.2010.488603

Longo, E., Badia, M., & Orgaz, B. M. (2013). Patterns and predictors of participation in leisure activities outside of school in children and adolescents with cerebral palsy. *Research in Developmental Disabilities, 34,* 266–275. http://dx.doi.org/10.1016/j.ridd.2012.08.017

Lonsdale, A. J., & North, A. C. (2011). Why do we listen to music? A uses and gratifications analysis. *British Journal of Psychology, 102,* 108–134. http://dx.doi.org/10.1348/000712610X506831

Loy, D. P., Dattilo, J., Kleiber, D. A., & Hutchinson, S. L. (2002). Dimensions of leisure and depression symptoms after spinal cord injury. *Annual in Therapeutic Recreation, 11,* 43–53.

Malley, D., Cooper, J., & Cope, J. (2008). Adapting leisure activity for adults with neuropsychological deficits following acquired brain injury. *NeuroRehabilitation, 23,* 329–334.

Mann, W. C., & Talty, P. (1991). Leisure Activity Profile measuring use of leisure time by persons with alcoholism. *Occupational Therapy in Mental Health, 10,* 31–41. http://dx.doi.org/10.1300/J004v10n04_03

Mazurek, M. O. (2013). Social media use among adults with autism spectrum disorders. *Computers in Human Behavior, 29,* 1709–1714. http://dx.doi.org/10.1016/j.chb.2013.02.004

McHale, S. M., Crouter, A. C., & Tucker, C. J. (2001). Free-time activities in middle childhood: Links with adjustment in early adolescence. *Child Development, 72,* 1764–1778. http://dx.doi.org/10.1111/1467-8624.00377

Missiuna, C., Pollock, N., & Law, M. (2004). *PEGS: The Perceived Efficacy and Goal Setting System.* San Antonio, TX: Psychological Corporation.

Morrison, M., & Krugman, D. M. (2001). A look at mass and computer mediated technologies: Understanding the roles of television and computers in the home. *Journal of Broadcasting and Electronic Media, 45,* 135–161. http://dx.doi.org/10.1207/s15506878jobem4501_9

Morrow-Howell, N., Hinterlong, J., Rozario, P. A., & Tang, F. (2003). Effects of volunteering on the well-being of older adults. *Journals of Gerontology, Series B. Psychological and Social Sciences, 58,* S137–S145. http://dx.doi.org/10.1093/geronb/58.3.S137

Mullan, B., Wong, C., Allom, V., & Pack, S. L. (2011). The role of executive function in bridging the intention-behaviour gap for binge-drinking in university students. *Addictive Behaviors, 36,* 1023–1026. http://dx.doi.org/10.1016/j.addbeh.2011.05.012

Murphy, L. B., & Moriarity, A. E. (1976). *Vulnerability, coping and growth: From infancy to adolescence.* New Haven, CT: Yale University Press.

Neulinger, J. (1981). *The psychology of leisure.* Springfield, IL: Charles C Thomas.

Niemela, P., & Linto, R. (1994). The significance of the 50th birthday for women's individuation. In B. F. Turner & L. E. Trol (Eds.), *Women growing older: Psychological perspectives* (pp. 117–127). Thousand Oaks, CA: Sage.

Nimrod, G. (2011). The fun culture in seniors' online communities. *Gerontologist, 51,* 226–237. http://dx.doi.org/10.1093/geront/gnq084

Oates, A., Bebbington, A., Bourke, J., Girdler, S., & Leonard, H. (2011). Leisure participation for school-aged children with Down syndrome. *Disability and Rehabilitation, 33,* 1880–1889. http://dx.doi.org/10.3109/09638288.2011.553701

O'Keeffe, G. S., Clarke-Pearson, K., & Council on Communications and Media. (2011). The impact of social media on children, adolescents, and families. *Pediatrics, 127,* 800–804. http://dx.doi.org/10.1542/peds.2011-0054

Olson, L. J. (2006). *Activity group in family-centered treatment: Psychiatric occupational therapy approaches for parents and children.* Binghamton, NY: Haworth.

Olson, L. J. (2010). Social participation frame of reference. In P. Kramer & J. Hinojosa (Eds.), *Frames of reference for pediatric occupational therapy* (3rd ed., pp. 306–348). Baltimore: Lippincott Williams & Wilkins.

Padilla-Walker, L. M., Nelson, L. J., Carroll, J. S., & Jensen, A. C. (2010). More than a just a game: Video game and Internet use during emerging adulthood. *Journal of Youth and Adolescence, 39,* 103–113. http://dx.doi.org/10.1007/s10964-008-9390-8

Parker, M. D. (1996). The relationship between time spent by older adults in leisure activities and life satisfaction. *Physical and Occupational Therapy in Geriatrics, 14,* 61–71. http://dx.doi.org/10.1080/J148v14n03_05

Parkinson, S., Forsyth, K., & Kielhofner, G. (2006). *The Model of Human Occupation Screening Tool (MOHOST) Version 2.0. University of Illinois at Chicago.* Chicago: MOHO Clearinghouse.

Passmore, A. (2003). The occupation of leisure: Three typologies and their influence on mental health in adolescence. *OTJR: Occupation, Participation and Health, 23,* 76–83.

Patterson, I., & Pegg, S. (2009). Serious leisure and people with intellectual disabilities: Benefits and opportunities. *Leisure Studies, 28,* 387–402. http://dx.doi.org/10.1080/02614360903071688

Putnam, R. D. (2000). *Bowling alone.* New York: Simon & Schuster.

Reich, S. M., Subrahmanyam, K., & Espinoza, G. (2012). Friending, IMing, and hanging out face-to-face: Overlap in adolescents' online and offline social networks. *Developmental Psychology, 48,* 356–368. http://dx.doi.org/10.1037/a0026980

Rowe, J. W., & Kahn, R. L. (1997). Successful aging. *Gerontologist, 37,* 433–440. http://dx.doi.org/10.1093/geront/37.4.433

Sallis, J. F., King, A. C., Sirard, J. R., & Albright, C. L. (2007). Perceived environmental predictors of physical activity over 6 months in adults: Activity counseling trial. *Health Psychology, 26,* 701–709. http://dx.doi.org/10.1037/0278-6133.26.6.701

Shann, M. H. (2001). Students' use of time outside of school: A case for after school programs for urban middle school youth. *Urban Review, 33,* 339–356. http://dx.doi.org/10.1023/A:1012248414119

Shikako-Thomas, K., Shevell, M., Lach, L., Law, M., Schmitz, N., Poulin, C., Majnemer, A., & QUALA Group. (2013). Picture me playing—A portrait of participation and enjoyment of leisure activities in adolescents with cerebral palsy. *Research in Developmental Disabilities, 34,* 1001–1010. http://dx.doi.org/10.1016/j.ridd.2012.11.026

Siegel, R. J. (1993). Between midlife and old age: Never too old to learn. In N. D. Davis, E. Cole, & E. D. Rothblum (Eds.), *Faces of women and aging* (pp. 173–185). Binghamton, NY: Harrington Park Press.

Silverman, F., Bartley, B., Cohn, E., Kanics, I. M., & Walsh, L. (2012). Occupational therapy partnerships with museums: Creating inclusive environments that promote participation and belonging. *International Journal of the Inclusive Museum, 4,* 15–29.

Singleton, J. F. (1996). Leisure skills. In C. B. Lewis (Ed.), *Aging: The health care challenge* (3rd ed., pp. 106–125). Philadelphia: F. A. Davis.

Sloan, L. R. (1979). The function and impact of sports for fans: A review of theory and contemporary research. In J. H. Goldstein (Ed.), *Sports, games and play: Social and psychological viewpoints* (pp. 219–262). Hillsdale, NJ: Erlbaum.

Smith, K. M., Freeman, P. A., & Zabriskie, R. B. (2009). An examination of family communication within the core and balance model of family leisure functioning. *Family Relations, 58,* 79–90. http://dx.doi.org/10.1111/j.1741-3729.2008.00536.x

Snickars, P., & Vonderau, P. (2012). *Moving data: The IPhone and the future of media.* New York: Columbia University Press.

Specht, J., King, G., Brown, E., & Foris, C. (2002). The importance of leisure in the lives of persons with congenital physical disabilities. *American Journal of Occupational Therapy, 56,* 436–445. http://dx.doi.org/10.5014/ajot.56.4.436

Stebbins, R. A. (1997). Casual leisure: A conceptual statement. *Leisure Studies, 16*(1), 17–25. http://dx.doi.org/10.1080/026143697375485

Steinberg, L., & Steinberg, W. (1994). *Crossing paths: How your child's adolescence can be an opportunity for your own personal growth.* New York: Simon & Schuster.

Storr, A. (1988). *Solitude: A return to the self.* New York: Ballantine Books.

Taylor, R. R. (2008). *The intentional relationship: Occupational therapy and use of self.* Philadelphia: F. A. Davis.

Townsend, J. A., & Zabriskie, R. B. (2010). Family leisure among families with a child in mental health treatment: Therapeutic recreation implications. *Therapeutic Recreation Journal, 44*(1), 11–34.

Wayne, D. O., & Krishnagiri, S. (2005). Parents' leisure: The impact of raising a child with Down syndrome. *Occupational Therapy International, 12,* 180–194. http://dx.doi.org/10.1002/oti.4

Whalen, C. K., Jamner, L. D., Henker, B., Delfino, R. J., & Lozano, J. M. (2002). The ADHD spectrum and everyday life: Experience sampling of adolescent moods, activities, smoking, and drinking. *Child Development, 73,* 209–227. http://dx.doi.org/10.1111/1467-8624.00401

Wilson, M. (1977). *Passage through communities: An interpretive analysis of enculturation in art education* [Unpublished dissertation]. University Park: Pennsylvania State University.

Wood, D., Larson, R. W., & Brown, J. R. (2009). How adolescents come to see themselves as more responsible through participation in youth programs. *Child Development, 80,* 295–309. http://dx.doi.org/10.1111/j.1467-8624.2008.01260.x

Zabriskie, R. B., & McCormick, B. P. (2001). The influences of family leisure patterns on perceptions of family functioning. *Human Relations, 50,* 281–289. http://dx.doi.org/10.1111/j.1741-3729.2001.00281.x.

Zick, C. D. (2010). The shifting balance of adolescent time use. *Youth and Society, 41,* 569–596. http://dx.doi.org/10.1177/0044118X09338506

Zillman, D., Sapolsky, B. S., & Bryant, J. (1979). The enjoyment of watching sport contests. In J. H. Goldstein (Ed.), *Sports, games and play: Social and psychological viewpoints* (pp. 297–336). Hillsdale, NJ: Erlbaum.

Zimmer, Z., Hickey, T., & Searle, M. S. (1997). The pattern of change in leisure activity behavior among older adults with arthritis. *Gerontologist, 37,* 384–392. http://dx.doi.org/10.1093/geront/37.3.384

CHAPTER 14.

WORK OCCUPATIONS

Jeff Snodgrass, PhD, MPH, OTR, and Jyothi Gupta, PhD, OTR/L, FAOTA

Highlights

✧ History and trends in work, workers, and the workplace
✧ Policy, regulations, and programming in the workplace
✧ Development of worker role and identity
✧ Role of occupational therapy in the workplace.

Key Terms

✧ ADA Amendments Act of 2008
✧ Americans With Disabilities Act of 1990
✧ Discharge planning
✧ Employee Retirement Income Security Act of 1974
✧ Employment laws
✧ Equal Employment Opportunity Commission
✧ Ergonomics
✧ Evaluation
✧ Fair Labor Standards Act of 1938
✧ Family and Medical Leave Act of 1993
✧ Functional capacity evaluation
✧ General Duty Clause
✧ Identity
✧ Individuals With Disabilities Education Act of 1990
✧ Injury prevention
✧ Intervention
✧ Job Accommodation Network
✧ Job demands analysis
✧ Knowledge workers

✧ Labor–Management Reporting and Disclosure Act of 1959
✧ Occupational Information Network (O*NET)
✧ Occupational Safety and Health Act of 1970
✧ Occupational Safety and Health Administration
✧ Outcomes
✧ Person with a disability
✧ Physical demands of work
✧ Referral
✧ Sheltered workshop
✧ Supported employment
✧ Ticket to Work Program
✧ Transition services
✧ Transitional employment
✧ Welfare to Work Program
✧ Work conditioning
✧ Work hardening
✧ Workers' compensation

This chapter provides a broad overview of work as a central occupation, reviews important work policies and programs, and presents the various roles that occupational therapy practitioners fulfill in this area of practice. We begin with a history of work in the United States and how work has changed in response to changes in society. Next, we examine selected policies, regulations, and programming in the workplace. This section presents a historical review of work-related policies and legislation as well as consideration of the most contemporary and relevant policies, regulations, and programming in the workplace that have had the most influence on occupational therapy.

Most of us will spend a considerable part of our lives, nearly 90,000 hours, at work. It is not surprising that in a society that places a high premium on productivity, Americans appear to "live to work" (Okulicz-Kozaryn, 2011, p. 225) and as a "no-vacation nation" take minimal time off from work (Ray & Schmitt, 2007). The benefits of working are evident: It is a source of income, shapes our identity, uses our capabilities in various ways, and challenges and promotes growth, just to mention a few. Despite the benefits of work, according to Deloitte's (2012) Shift Index, 80% of Americans are dissatisfied with their work and on an average will hold 11.3 jobs over their lives (Bureau of Labor Statistics, 2012).

Moreover, 70% of workers are disengaged at work, which costs the United States nearly $500 billion loss per year (Gallup, 2013). U.S. workers experience work-related stress that amounts to billions of dollars in loss of productivity, injuries, and health care costs (Michie, 2002; National Institute for Occupational Safety and Health [NIOSH], 1999). Occupational therapy can influence the well-being of workers and workplaces, and work and industry is one of occupational therapy's area of practice (American Occupational Therapy Association [AOTA], 2007).

History and Trends in Work, Workers, and the Workplace

Work has an esteemed place in most societies and is seen as integral to one's life, contributing to one's identity and self-efficacy (Gupta & Sabata, 2012; Harpaz & Fu, 2002). Work is considered a basic human right because it confers dignity on the person, serves as a means to be a self-sufficient productive member of society, and contributes to the overall economy (United Nations, 1948). Kantartzis and Molineux (2011) attributed the centrality of work and the unquestioned belief in its inherent positive influence on one's identity and health to the Protestant work ethic of many Western societies.

Occupational therapy also subscribes to this view of work, although productivity is viewed across the life course as a continuum, ranging from conventional paid employment to volunteerism (AOTA, 2014). In fact, the historical roots of the profession in moral treatment make clear its intent "to replace brutality with kindness and idleness with occupation" (Gordon, 2009, p. 203). In other words, occupational therapy values productive occupation of time for its positive influences on the health and well-being of people and society as a whole.

The nature of work and the world of work have changed considerably since the beginnings of occupational therapy. The late 19th century was the period of mechanization and the beginnings of mass production of goods in the United States. This era changed not only the way work was done but also the meaning of work to the worker. Prior to this, skilled craftspeople, often working from their homes, had the satisfaction and pride of creating a product from start to finish. In the manufacturing assembly line, however, work was broken down into smaller tasks with each worker contributing in a small way to the larger whole. This breakdown of production to its component tasks meant that work became monotonous, repetitive, and faster paced, and the worker was removed from the final outcome of production (Library of Congress, n.d.).

Modern work also compartmentalized people's daily routines and habits in spatial and temporal terms, ushering in the notions of schedules, planners, and deadlines (Larson & Zemke, 2003). Workplaces demanded increased efficiency and productivity from the workers, sometimes at the cost of worker health and safety. Manufacturing accounted for about 30% of the gross domestic product by the late 20th century (Bureau of Labor Statistics, 2012). Alongside these trends, workplace safety issues and worker activism propelled the need for legislation aimed at equity and nondiscrimination in the workplace. The Equal Employment Opportunity Commission (EEOC) and the field of occupation health and safety (Occupational Safety and Health Administration [OSHA] Act of 1970) came into existence during this time.

In more recent times, two major forces—globalization and technology—transformed the economy and employment. Following the shift of manufacturing overseas, anxiety over outsourcing of jobs to nations with cheaper labor costs prevails in workers in advanced industrialized countries. The nostalgia over the glory days of manufacturing is coupled with concern about an unemployed workforce that do not have the skills to meet the demands of jobs in the current economy. The large numbers of "blue-collar" factory workers led to a lot of physical demands on the workers that did not require a college education or sophisticated training. These jobs are being replaced in large part by the "pink-collar" service sector jobs, performed largely by a female workforce, with less job security and lower wages.

Technology has changed the way goods are manufactured and spawned the information age in the 1970s that continues to the present. The management of information and information systems is an industry that demands "white-collar" workers that Drucker (1999) called the *knowledge workers*. Information is being efficiently packaged with minimal use of materials so workers are manipulating information more than matter, and this is the future of work in advanced economies (Hausmann, 2013). These jobs differ from manufacturing, because the demands on the worker are no longer physical but largely cognitive and psychosocial in nature.

Technology has altered work and workplaces such that anything that can be digitized can be outsourced, and a workday does not need to end. Work can go on around the globe 24 hours a day. This requires that workers be competent in teamwork across multiple cultures; process information at a fast pace; and demonstrate convergent, divergent, and creative thinking (Reinhardt, Schmidt, Sloep, & Drachsler, 2011). Other ways in which workplaces have changed include an increase in telecommuting and the addition of a contingent workforce (e.g., independent contractors, freelancers). Both changes isolate the worker spatially and temporally. Although workers have greater autonomy, they are expected to work independently with little supervision and support. It also blurs the work–life boundaries, and many employers these days expect employees to work outside of the workplace.

Technology, however, when used in conjunction with good communication, time-off through disconnecting, and other best practices at work can be a win-win situation for worker and employer, with increased productivity and creativity and satisfied workers who are better able to maintain a good work–life balance (Perlow, 2012). This change in the nature of work and the way work gets done is important for occupational therapy practitioners to heed, because interventions aimed primarily at physical job demands are less relevant today as cognitive and psychosocial demands are exacerbating stress at workplaces (Gupta, 2008). Work-related stress is associated strongly with workplace injury, musculoskeletal disorders, and chronic pain (Clauw & Williams, 2002).

Besides technology and globalization, the United States, like other industrialized nations, is also experiencing the wave of an aging workforce. Older workers who have to delay their retirement for various reasons are dealing with age-related changes in dynamic workplaces. The nature of work is ever-changing, and workers are expected to adapt quickly, be nimble, and be flexible on the job. Occupational therapy has a lot to offer to older workers and employers, so the transaction can be mutually beneficial (Gupta & Sabata, 2012).

Policy, Regulations, and Programming in the Workplace

Key pieces of legislation and programming have been enacted and implemented over the years to protect employers and employees, to ensure that hiring practices are fair, and to promote safe working conditions. It is imperative for occupational therapy practitioners to be aware of and understand the workplace regulatory and policy environment in which they provide services to effectively serve their clients.

Various work-related legislation has been enacted over the last 100-plus years. Refer to Table 14.1 for an overview of pertinent legislation that has influenced and continues to affect occupational therapy (Library of Congress, 2013).

Table 14.1 Key Work-Related Policies

Policy	Summary Description
Federal Employee Liability Act of 1908	Enacted to protect and compensate railroad workers injured on the job.
Age Discrimination Act of 1967	Prohibits employment discrimination against persons ages 40 years or older.
Rehabilitation Act of 1973	This act and its subsequent amendments were precursors to the Americans With Disabilities Act of 1990 and eliminated discrimination against people with disabilities in programs or activities receiving federal funding.
Americans With Disabilities Act of 1990 (ADA)	Prohibits discrimination and ensures equal opportunity for persons with disabilities in employment, state and local government services, public accommodations, commercial facilities, and transportation.
ADA Amendments Act of 2008	The act places the emphasis on the discrimination at issue instead of an individual's disability. The act retains the ADA definition of a *disability* as an impairment that substantially limits one or more life activities; however, it changes how the statutory terms should be interpreted. This act expands the definition of "major life activities" and clarifies that an impairment that is episodic or in remission is a disability if it would substantially limit a major life activity when active.
Ticket to Work Incentives Improvement Act of 1999	The Ticket to Work Program provides Social Security beneficiaries with disabilities more choices for receiving employment services and increases provider incentives to serve beneficiaries with disabilities who wish to maximize their economic self-sufficiency through work opportunities. These services may be training, career counseling, vocational rehabilitation, job placement, and ongoing support services necessary to achieve a work goal.
Rehabilitation Act Amendments of 1992	The revised act included numerous amendments designed to increase the choice and control of individuals with disabilities over rehabilitation services, both individually and systemically. It emphasized the presumption of ability that people can achieve employment and other rehabilitation goals regardless of the severity of the disability, if appropriate services and supports are made available.
Education of the Deaf Act of 1986	Reauthorized educational programs for deaf people to foster improved educational programs for deaf people throughout the United States.
Omnibus Budget Reconciliation Educational Act of 1987	Gave states the option to offer prevocational and supported employment services to people institutionalized at any time before the waiver program.

Note. Adapted from American Occupational Therapy Association (2011). Used with permission.

The *Americans With Disabilities Act of 1990 (ADA)* was "the most comprehensive legislation for people with disabilities ever passed in the United States" (Karger & Rose, 2010, p. 74). In its broad and inclusive scope to socially integrate people with disabilities, it prohibited discrimination in employment on the basis of disability and required accessibility of state and federal government programs and services, specifically in public accommodations, transportation, and telecommunications. Implementation of the ADA, in the true spirit of its inception, has been a challenge. One reason has been a critique of the definition of *disability* and its interpretation, with arguments spanning from the definition being too restrictive to being too broad. Nonetheless, the ADA defines a *person with a disability* as someone with a recorded physical or mental impairment that substantially limits his or her participation in one or more life activities, such as work.

Employers are prohibited from discriminating against workers with a disability who qualify for employment, as long as they can meet the essential job functions with or without reasonable accommodations in the workplace. Other challenges have been the vagueness of language of "substantially limits," "reasonable accommodation," and perceived hardships on the part of employers in providing accommodation. Karger and Rose (2010) pointed out that employers, fearful of lawsuits, may choose not to hire a person with a disability, which defeats the very intent and purpose of this legislation.

The enactment of the *ADA Amendments Act of 2008* was in response to the narrowing of the definition of disability by the courts and to clarify the language so that courts can consistently apply the broad intent and purpose of the act. Essentially, the focus is on discrimination as it relates to individuals with disabilities rather than their disability.

The *EEOC* is the federal agency that since 1965 has enforced antidiscrimination laws and provided oversight to protect workers from being discriminated against on the basis of their race, color, religion, sex (including pregnancy), national origin, age (40 or older), disability, or genetic information. ADA, for instance, is enforced in the workplace by the EEOC. More recently, when ADA Amendments Act was enacted in 2008, the EEOC was directed to make the necessary changes to the Title I ADA regulations and the interpretive guidance documents (EEOC, 2008). Besides preventing discrimination through community outreach, education, and technical assistance, the EEOC also assesses allegations and complaints; in the event of a clear case of discrimination, the EEOC may in certain instances litigate against employers in the interest of the public good.

Overview of Major Employment Laws

Employment laws include all types of employment protection legislation that cover wages, retirement, unions, and medical leave. The *Fair Labor Standards Act of 1938 (FLSA)* prescribes standards for wages and overtime pay, which affect most private and public employment. Under FLSA, employers must pay covered employees at least the federal minimum wage and overtime pay of at least 1½ times the regular rate of pay. It also restricts the number of hours that children under the age of 16 can work in nonagricultural operations and pro-

hibits the employment of those under the age of 18 in certain jobs considered to be too dangerous (U.S. Department of Labor, n.d.).

The *Employee Retirement Income Security Act of 1974* regulates employers who offer pension or welfare benefit plans for their employees. The *Labor–Management Reporting and Disclosure Act of 1959 (LMRDA;* also known as the Landrum–Griffin Act) deals with the relationship between a union and its members. The LMRDA requires labor organizations to file annual financial reports and reports on certain labor relations practices and sets forth standards for the election of union officers (U.S. Department of Labor, n.d.).

The *Family and Medical Leave Act of 1993* requires employers of 50 or more employees to give up to 12 weeks of unpaid, job-protected leave to eligible employees for the birth or adoption of a child or for the serious illness of the employee or a spouse, child, or parent.

Readers are encouraged to explore the U.S. Department of Labor's (n.d.) Web site for a summary of these and other employment related laws.

Workers' Compensation and Disability Insurance

Workers' compensation is a social insurance program that varies state by state and between federal and state systems. In the United States, most states adopted workers' compensation laws between 1910 and 1920, with Mississippi being the last state to pass a workers' compensation law in 1948 (National Academy of Social Insurance [NASI], 2013a, 2013b). The only other disability benefits programs larger than workers' compensation are the federal Social Security Disability Insurance program and Medicare.

Workers' compensation provides injured workers with four categories of benefits:

1. *Medical care for work-related injuries and illnesses:* 100% of medical costs and cash benefits for lost work time after a 3- to 7-day waiting period.
2. *Temporary disability benefits:* Paid to a worker when a work-related injury or illness temporarily prevents a worker from returning to the job.
3. *Permanent partial and permanent total disability benefits:* Paid to workers who have long-term disabilities as a result of work.

4. *Vocational training:* Covers the costs of services to facilitate a worker's return to gainful employment if he or she is unable to return to a preinjury job. (NASI, 2013b)

Benefits for workers' compensation are paid by private insurance, by state or federal workers' compensation funds, or by self-insured employers. In 2010, private insurance carriers were the largest source of workers' compensation benefits, accounting for approximately 53% of all benefits paid, with self-insured employers covering almost 25% of all benefits paid in 2010 (NASI, 2013b).

Occupational therapy practitioners need to stay abreast of their state workers' compensation laws for legislative changes, which occur on a regular basis. These changes can affect reimbursement in both amount and methods, the types of services that will be covered, who may provide the services, and other issues that may potentially affect the coverage of occupational therapy services (Kornblau & Andersen, 2000).

Occupational Safety and Health Administration

The federal agency responsible for overseeing safe and healthful workplaces is *OSHA,* which operates under the U.S. Department of Labor. The *Occupational and Safety Health Act (OSH Act)* was passed in 1970. The stated purpose of the OSH Act is

> To assure safe and healthful working conditions for working men and women; by authorizing enforcement of the standards developed under the Act; by assisting and encouraging the States in their efforts to assure safe and healthful working conditions; by providing for research, information, education, and training in the field of occupational safety and health; and for other purposes. (OSHA, n.d.-a)

OSHA has a two-pronged mission: (1) to assure safe and healthful workplaces by setting and enforcing standards and (2) to provide training, outreach, education, and assistance to employers and employees. Employers are required to comply with all applicable OSHA standards and must also comply with the *General Duty Clause* of the OSH Act, which stipulates that employers must maintain a safe workplace free of any known and serious hazards.

In addition to the General Duty Clause, OSHA has four primary industry standards that cover the general industry, construction, maritime, and agriculture sectors. The OSH Act encourages states to develop and administer their own job safety and health programs, although OSHA must approve and monitor all state plans. OSHA's jurisdiction covers private sector employers but excludes the self-employed, family farm workers, and government workers except in states that have approved state plans. As of 2013, a total of 27 states operate OSHA-approved state plans (OSHA, 2013b).

As part of the requirements for employers to comply with the OSH Act, employers are required to record and report work-related fatalities, injuries, and illnesses (OSHA, n.d.-b). OSHA normally conducts inspections without advance notice. Although OSHA states that it cannot inspect all 7 million workplaces it covers each year, the agency does focus its inspection efforts on the most hazardous workplaces (Jung & Makowsky, 2012).

According to OSHA (2013a), there are approximately 2,200 inspectors (including state partners) responsible for the health and safety of 130 million workers, which means that the agency has about one compliance officer for every 59,000 workers. Some of the most frequently cited OSHA standards violated include lack of adequate fall protection in the construction industry, poor hazard communication in general industry, electrical wiring hazards in general industry, and improper operation of powered industrial trucks (e.g., forklifts).

Social Security Administration's Ticket to Work Program

The Social Security Administration's (SSA) *Ticket to Work Program* was created in 1999 for people ages 18 through 64 with a disability who receive Social Security Disability Insurance or Supplemental Security Income benefits. According the SSA, the goals of the Ticket to Work Program are to

• Offer beneficiaries with disabilities expanded choices when seeking service and supports to enter, reenter, or maintain employment;

- Increase the financial independence and self-sufficiency of beneficiaries with disabilities; and
- Reduce and, whenever possible, eliminate reliance on disability benefits. (SSA, 2013b)

Eligible beneficiaries with disabilities may voluntarily participate in the program by signing up with an approved provider, which can be an employment network or a state vocational rehabilitation agency. Occupational therapy practitioners may apply to become a designated employment network to provide services to beneficiaries who are enrolled in the Ticket to Work Program. In fact, AOTA has identified the Ticket to Work Program as an emerging practice area (Stoffel, 2010).

The SSA (2013a) publishes a reference source titled *The Red Book,* which provides information about the employment-related provisions of Social Security Disability Insurance and the Supplemental Security Income programs for educators, advocates, rehabilitation professionals, and counselors who serve people with disabilities.

Occupational Information Network (O*NET)

The *Occupational Information Network (O*NET;* http://www.onetonline.org), an important source of occupational information, contains hundreds of standardized and occupation-specific job descriptors. The database also contains an interactive application for searching occupations as well as a set of assessments for workers and students looking to find or change careers.

Occupational therapy practitioners may find the O*NET useful when performing a job analysis or

---

*Exercise 14.1. O*NET Job Search*

Go to the O*NET Web site at http://www.onetonline.org/ and search for an occupation of your choice. Take a few minutes to review the summary of your selected occupation, including the job description, task requirements, knowledge, skills, education requirements, work styles, and values. You will also find information about wage and employment trends. For instance, you can search for Occupational Therapy Assistants (Code: 31–2011.00) and read the summary report.

Exercise 14.2. Job Accommodation Network

Visit the JAN Web site at http://askjan.org/, and navigate to the Searchable Online Accommodation Resource (SOAR) to explore various accommodation options for people with disabilities. For example, an occupational therapy practitioner may have a client who is a butcher with osteoarthritis. Through the SOAR system, you can select "osteoarthritis" and select a limitation that corresponds with the individual needing an accommodation, such as limitations related to fatigue and weakness. The SOAR provides accommodation recommendations, including scheduling periodic rest breaks, providing adjustable workstations, antifatigue matting, and so on.

---

working with a client on vocational exploration activities. For example, a practitioner may use the O*NET to find the occupation-specific descriptors to assist with developing a comprehensive job analysis.

Job Accommodation Network

The *Job Accommodation Network (JAN;* http://askjan.org/) is a resource for guidance on workplace accommodations and disability employment issues. JAN is especially useful for occupational therapy practitioners when working with employers and people with disabilities. A practitioner may be consulting with an employer who is trying to provide reasonable accommodations for an employee who is returning to work after an accident that left the employee with a permanent limitation in upper-extremity dexterity and coordination. JAN would be a good resource to assist both the consulting practitioner and employer with developing appropriate accommodations for the employee.

Development of Worker Role and Identity

One of the most important choices that a person has to make as he or she transitions from adolescence to adulthood is choosing a career. Numerous underlying contextual factors influence and affect choice of career, such as gender, family or group, ethnicity, and socioeconomic status (Fouad & Byars-Winston, 2005). To make an informed choice, a person must consider a complex array of information and data and ultimately choose from many occupational alternatives.

From an occupational therapy perspective, people's occupational choices contribute to their *identity*. In other words, we are what we do, who we are, and who we become. Christiansen (1999) posited that occupational engagement is the means by which people develop and express their identities and have identities conferred on them by others in their context. To be identified as a worker is critical in any society, and more so in American society that places high value on independence and personal responsibility. Working-age adults are expected to work so they can take care of themselves and fulfill their family obligations and responsibility to society as a tax-paying citizen. By doing so, individuals fully participate and experience a sense of belonging in their society.

Earnings partly determine one's socioeconomic status and class identity. Work is also a means to experience self-efficacy and display competence, which contribute to one's overall well-being. The negative consequences of chronic unemployment and underemployment on health are well documented in the literature and are beyond the scope of this chapter (Anderson & Winefield, 2011; Dembe, Erickson, Delbos, & Banks, 2005).

Several career choice and development theories have been introduced over the last century, beginning with the first textbook on vocational choice by Frank Parsons in 1909. Although it is beyond the scope of this chapter to present a comprehensive and detailed examination of all career choice and development theories, a review of the most commonly cited theories are presented in Table 14.2. The table is a synopsis of several of the most commonly cited and used models over the last century that help to explain career development and career choice, including the process and stages of career development and exploration. Although the theories presented in Table 14.2 were not developed by occupational therapists, they are indeed important for occupational therapy practitioners to know and understand in support of work-related practice.

Role of Occupational Therapy in the Workplace

History

The profession of occupational therapy traces its roots to the notion of work as a central occupation in people's lives. The founders of occupational therapy emphasized work-related practice as an integral part of the profession's scope of practice. Prior to the official adoption of "occupational therapy" as the profession's title, the titles "work cure" and "ergotherapy" were entertained as possible titles for the profession. Since the profession's initial founding until the present day, work has been and continues to be an important area of practice.

In 1923, the first educational standards for occupational therapy emphasized the influence of occupation (work) as therapy and the need for occupational therapy practitioners to engage in work-related practice (Jacobs & Baker, 2000). Occupational therapy took a prominent role during World War II as part of the military reconditioning program. Following the war, however, the profession's focus shifted to more physical rehabilitation techniques with less involvement in work-related programming.

During the 1950s and 1960s, vocational rehabilitation services were emphasized because of new federal policies and the overall change in attitudes and treatment of people with disabilities. Federal policies were introduced during the 1950s, such as the Vocational Rehabilitation Act Amendments of 1954 and the Medical Facilities Survey and Construction Act of 1954, which facilitated renewed interest in and emphasis on work-related programming for the profession. In 1959, the Eleanor Clark Slagle lecture was delivered by Lilian Wegg on the "Essentials of Work Evaluation." In her lecture, Wegg outlined essential skills for performing work evaluation that continue to serve as a foundation to contemporary work capacity evaluation (see Wegg, 1960).

By the early 1980s, the profession developed a position paper, *The Role of the Occupational Therapist in the Vocational Rehabilitation Process* (AOTA, 1980), asserting the prominence and importance of work-related practice in occupational therapy. During the 1980s, the need for industrial rehabilitation services grew considerably. This created new and expanded opportunities for occupational therapy

Table 14.2. Vocational Theories of Career Choice and Development

Theory	Overview and Key Points
Parson's Choosing a Vocation Theory (Parsons, 1909)	Widely regarded as the first model developed attempting to explain occupational choice. Parsons viewed occupational choice as something that happened just prior to an individual's entry into the labor market. He asserted that occupational choice involved 3 elements: (1) understanding yourself, (2) understanding the merits of various occupations, and (3) understanding the relationship between these 2 things to make an informed choice.
Holland's Career Typology Theory (modern trait-and-factor theory person–environment model; Chartrand, 1991; Holland, 1973, 1985)	Considers congruence of one's personality, skills, and abilities with the occupational environment. Holland classified personality types into 6 categories: Realistic, Investigative, Artistic, Social, Enterprising, and Conventional. Posits that congruent interactions facilitate stability and incongruent interactions create change in behaviors. This theory serves as the basis for many standardized vocational assessments.
Super's Theory of Vocational Development (life-span, life-space; Super, 1953)	Identifies 6 life and career development stages: • *Crystallization* involves tentative vocational goals (ages 14–18), • *Specification* involves development of focused vocational goals in preparation for adulthood (ages 18–21), • *Implementation* includes training and obtaining gainful employment (ages 21–24), • *Stabilization* is validation of and engaging in one's career choice (ages 24–35), • *Consolidation* is advancing one's career (ages 36–54), and • *Readiness for Retirement* is the preparation for retirement (ages 55 or older). The theorist emphasizes the relationship between self-concept and choice of work and career.
Developmental theory: Ginzberg's Developmental Stages of Vocational Development (Ginzberg, 1952, 1971)	Postulates that career development occurs over an 8- to 10-year period. People search for a fit between their career preferences and opportunities in the job market. Expenditure of time and resources is an important component of career choice that may serve as a deterrent to changing a career.
Social learning theory: Krumboltz's Learning Theory of Career Choice and Counseling (Krumboltz, Mitchell, & Jones, 1976)	Attempts to explain career choice by answering the question: Why do people express various preferences for different occupations at different points in their lives? Examines 4 influencing factors that answer this question: (1) genetic endowment and special abilities, (2) environmental conditions and events, (3) learning experiences, and (4) task approach skills.
Lent, Brown, and Hackett's Social Cognitive Career Theory (Lent, Brown, & Hackett, 1994)	Includes the interactions among personal attributes, external environmental factors, and behavior in career decision making. Other important factors are educational and vocational interests, career-related choices, and performance. This theory proposes 3 models that facilitate career-related interests, including interest development, choice, and performance.
Life Career Development Theory (Gysbers, Heppner, & Johnston, 1987)	Considered more holistic than previous theories, it encompasses all domains of concern to the person and the environment. This theory has many similarities to the basic theoretical underpinnings of occupational therapy. With this theory, people can visualize and plan life careers, referred to as *career consciousness,* by examining future life roles, life settings, and life events while thinking about the effect of gender, ethnicity, religion, race, and socioeconomic status on their development.

Note. Adapted from Braveman and Page (2012) and Kornblau, Lou, Weeder, and Werner (2002).

practitioners in industrial rehabilitation and work hardening.

In 1992, AOTA published an update to the aforementioned position paper titled *Occupational Therapy Services in Work Practice* that has since been revised several times to reach its current edition published in 2011 titled *Occupational Therapy Services in Facilitating Work Performance*. As noted earlier, a major piece of legislation that was enacted in 1990 was the ADA, which continues to the present day to have important implications for work-related practice.

Process of Occupational Therapy in Work

The *Occupational Therapy Practice Framework: Domain and Process* (AOTA, 2014; *Framework*) presents a summary of interrelated constructs that define and guide occupational therapy practice. It describes the various occupations or activities that occupational therapy practitioners consider when working with clients. These occupations include activities of daily living, instrumental activities of daily living, rest and sleep, education, work, play, leisure, social participation, and work. According to the *Framework*, work includes activities needed for engaging in paid employment or volunteer activities and involves

- *Employment interests and pursuits:* Identifying and selecting work opportunities based on assets, limitations, likes, and dislikes relative to work.
- *Employment seeking and acquisition:* Identifying and recruiting for job opportunities; completing, submitting, and reviewing appropriate application materials; preparing for interviews; participating in interviews and following up afterward; discussing job benefits; and finalizing negotiations.
- *Job performance:* Performing the requirements of a job, including work skills and patterns; time management; relationships with coworkers, managers, and customers; leadership and supervision; creation, production, and distribution of products and services; initiation, sustainment, and completion of work; and compliance with work norms and procedures. . . (AOTA, 2014, p. S20)

The process of delivering occupational therapy services includes *evaluation* (i.e., occupational profile and analysis of occupational performance), *intervention* (i.e., intervention plan, intervention implementation, intervention review), and *outcomes*. Occupational therapists work with clients experiencing work dysfunction or promoting workplace health and injury prevention in various and diverse settings, including general hospitals, psychiatric and mental health facilities, outpatient clinics, rehabilitation hospitals, and work sites. The focus of work-related evaluation and intervention is primarily on facilitating the functional and work capacity of the worker to meet the demands of the job (Kaskutas & Snodgrass, 2009).

The process typically begins with a *referral* from a physician. Although some states do not require a physician referral, most settings and third-party payers do. For instance, most workers' compensation insurance carriers will not reimburse for occupational therapy services without a physician referral. Ultimately, the occupational therapy practitioner must adhere to his or her state licensure laws. Referrals, however, are often initiated not just by physicians but also by other professionals, including case managers; employers; and their representatives, such as safety managers, occupational health nurses, workers' compensation carriers, psychologists, and vocational counselors (Kaskutas & Snodgrass, 2009).

Following a referral, the occupational therapist conducts a work-focused evaluation. In addition to the typical assessment methods, the occupational therapist must focus on the worker's capacity to meet the unique demands of the job, such as lifting, pushing, pulling, carrying, time management, stress management, executive functioning, positional tolerances (e.g., overhead work, crouching, bending), endurance, and safety. The occupational therapist may need to conduct a thorough job site analysis to determine the demands of the job.

A unique aspect of a work-focused evaluation is that the occupational therapist must determine the client's potential for returning to work, which is accomplished through work performance testing. The therapist may have the client perform a battery of tests that simulate his or her work or may even observe the client performing the actual work tasks following an evaluation of underlying client factors (e.g., range of motion, strength, endurance, attention to task). Typical questions that need to be answered during the evaluation process include

- Who is the client—person (including family and significant others); population (e.g., workers with musculoskeletal injuries); or organization (e.g., manufacturing plant)?
- Why is the client seeking services, and what are the client's current concerns relative to engaging the occupation of work and ability to return to work?
- What areas of occupation are successful, and is the area of work the primary area causing problems or risks?
- What work contexts and environments support or inhibit participation and engagement in desired occupations?
- Is the client capable of returning to a preinjury job or acquiring the necessary skills to obtain gainful employment?
- What is the client's employment history?
- What are the client's priorities and desired outcomes?

The occupational therapist collaborates with the client and often the referral sources (e.g., physician, case manager, employer's representative) to develop goals and objectives that address targeted work-related outcomes such as return to work and modification of the work (AOTA, 2014; Kaskutas & Snodgrass, 2009). The intervention plan typically has a focus on the client (1) returning to a preinjury job in either a full or limited (restricted) capacity; (2) exploring vocational options, including work skill reacquisition, such as a client who can no longer return to work he or she once performed; or (3) acquiring a work skill, such as a client learning gainful employment skills.

Intervention approaches can be conceptualized as falling into one of five categories or a combination thereof. The intervention approaches include

1. Create or promote,
2. Establish or restore,
3. Maintain,
4. Modify, and
5. Prevent (AOTA, 2014).

In Table 14.3, intervention approaches are described with examples of occupation-based interventions.

To determine success in reaching targeted outcomes (e.g., goals and objectives), occupational therapists use outcome assessment information to plan next steps for the client and to evaluate program delivery (i.e., program evaluation; AOTA, 2014). Typical outcomes that are targeted as part of the occupational therapy intervention process include job acquisition, vocational skill acquisition or reacquisition, unrestricted return to work, or a restricted return to work (e.g., light duty, restricted duty, alternative job duties).

Occupational therapists must possess the knowledge of the job duties and the work environment to understand the context of the client's work (or anticipated work) and the required demands. The mismatch between the client's capacities and the work requirements is the focus of the intervention process and the discharge decision process (Kaskutas & Snodgrass, 2009).

Discharge planning begins at initial evaluation and continues through the delivery of occupational therapy services. It is important to note that part and parcel of measuring outcomes is the need to determine the continuation or discontinuation of services or referral to other professionals and services, including vocational counseling, psychology, physical therapy, and so forth.

Practice Areas: Traditional and Nontraditional

Occupational therapy practitioners are found in diverse settings where work-related services are provided with a wide variety of populations, including people with developmental disabilities, adolescents and younger workers, older workers, and people with mental health illness.

Supported employment

Occupational therapy practitioners contribute expertise and provide skilled services to populations that include clients with developmental disabilities and clients living with mental illness. These services are provided along a continuum of work-related assessment and intervention contexts, including supported employment at sheltered workshops, transitional employment, and supported jobs with one-on-one job coaching (Carrasco, Hermes, & Burgos, 2011).

At a *sheltered workshop,* occupational therapists evaluate the client to determine his or her capacity to meet the demands of work in a structured,

Table 14.3. Intervention Approaches and Examples of Occupation-Based Interventions

Intervention Approach	Examples of Occupation-Based Interventions
Create or promote: An intervention approach designed to provide enriched contextual and activity experiences that will enhance performance for all persons	• Provide barrier-free solutions in the workplace • Deliver an injury prevention course for employees • Assist with design and set-up of computer workstations
Establish or restore: An intervention approach designed to influence client variables such as a skill or ability that has not yet developed or to restore a skill or ability that has been impaired	• Provide vocational exploration activities • Instruct with time management skills • Address lifting and carrying capacity with work simulation
Maintain: An intervention approach designed to provide the supports that will allow clients to preserve current functioning and abilities	• Teach home exercise program for flexibility and strength • Instruct with proper body mechanics while lifting heavy boxes
Modify: An intervention approach that modifies the environment or activity to facilitate performance; includes compensatory techniques	• Provide ergonomic interventions to reduce amount of forceful exertion required • Collaborate with employer to alter work schedule and work tasks • Sequence work tasks for employee with permanent cognitive-processing restrictions
Prevent: An intervention approach designed to reduce or eliminate potential occupational performance problems and barriers	• Collaborate with employer to develop reasonable accommodation policies • Develop a "no lift" policy at the work site to include hydraulic lifting equipment • Create ergonomically designed workstation for all administrative staff in an organization

Note. Adapted from Kaskutas and Snodgrass (2009) and AOTA (2011, 2014).

controlled environment and provide interventions to address the identified mismatches between current capacity and required capacity for the targeted job. The sheltered workshop approach is intended to move the client from simulated or hypothetical situations to real-life work experiences and contexts (Ramsay, Starnes, & Robertson, 2000).

Transitional employment services engage the client in paid positions on a job for businesses or industries on a part-time, limited, and temporary basis while the client continues to receive ongoing training and support from a job coach and others, who may include an occupational therapy practitioner who collaborates with not only the client but also the employer to facilitate the client's engagement in work, modify the job and environment, and teach specific job-related skills (Carrasco et al., 2011).

Supported employment typically engages the client in competitive, gainful employment with support and guidance from occupational therapy practitioners and other team members. Supported employment involves placements in employment settings

that provide fully integrated roles and responsibilities with greater longevity on the job without time restrictions. In other words, these placements offer the greatest chance for the client's long-term success in gainful employment (Carrasco et al., 2011).

Transition services (school to adult life)

Transition services are provided to adolescents who require supportive services to make the transition from childhood to adulthood (Stewart, 2013). Occupational therapy plays an important role in facilitating a person's transition to adulthood as it relates to community participation and employment (Braveman & Page, 2012). Transition services are covered as part of the individualized education program, which was stipulated in the 1997 amendment to the *Individuals With Disabilities Education Act of 1990 (IDEA).* The IDEA defines transition services as

> a coordinated set of activities for a student designed within an outcome-oriented pro-

cess, which promotes movement from school to post-school activities, includes postsecondary education, vocational training, integrated employment (including supported employment), continuing and adult education, adult services, independent living, or community participation. (U.S. Department of Education, n.d.)

Contributions of occupational therapy to the transition process related to work include evaluation of job-related interests and abilities; planning and decision-making regarding job placement; assessing mismatch between job demands and the student's performance; job modifications to accommodate the student's abilities and needs; and job site training of support personnel, including job coaches or coworkers (Stewart, 2013).

Job analysis

Occupational therapy practitioners provide job analysis, often referred to as a *job demands analysis (JDA),* for people who desire to engage in gainful employment or who are returning to the workplace following an injury or illness. A job analysis consists of three major components: (1) the work, (2) the workers, and (3) the workplace. The analysis includes interviews with the incumbent or supervisors regarding the job requirements (Haruka, Page, & Wietlisbach, 2013). In addition to interviews, the occupational therapy practitioner may conduct an on-site JDA that includes observation of the actual job being performed; interviews with supervisors and employees; and direct measurements of tasks, such as lifting, pushing, pulsing, carrying, and positional requirements (e.g., bending, stooping, reaching, standing).

A standardized classification is used to ensure consistency in terminology. The U.S. Department of Transportation (DOT) provides definitions of *physical demands of work,* including the overall level of work, strength demands, and frequencies of the physical demands. For instance, a job that requires lifting, pushing, pulling, or carrying up to 100 pounds on an occasional basis (up to one-third of the day) would be categorized in the "heavy" physical demand category. Table 14.4 provides a snapshot of the DOT physical demand categories of work.

The JDA allows the occupational therapy practitioner to identify the essential functions or tasks of the job. The essential functions of a job are those tasks that all employees must be able to perform with or without reasonable accommodation. The ADA Amendments Act of 2008 has set forth guidelines for determining if a task is essential or marginal (nonessential), including

- Whether the reason the position exists is to perform that function,
- The number of other employees available to perform the function or among whom the performance of the function can be distributed,
- The degree of expertise or skill required to perform the function,
- The actual work experience of present or past employees in the job,
- The time spent performing a function,
- The consequences of not requiring that an employee perform a function, and
- The terms of a collective bargaining agreement.

Ergonomics

Ergonomics is the scientific discipline that deals with the worker; the tools, equipment, and machines that the worker uses; and the environment in which the worker interacts and operates (Annis & McConville, 2012). Ergonomics builds on job analysis by taking what is learned from the JDA and identifying work conditions and job demands associated with the onset of fatigue, overexertion, injuries, and chronic musculoskeletal disorders (Grant, 2012). The literature includes numerous definitions of ergonomics. The International Ergonomics Association (IEA) provides a holistic definition that best captures the broad scope of ergonomics:

> *Ergonomics* (or human factors) is the scientific discipline concerned with the understanding of the interactions among humans and other elements of a system, and the profession that applies theoretical principles, data and methods to design in order to optimize human well-being and overall system performance. (IEA, n.d., p. 1, italics added)

The objective of the application of ergonomics is to fit the work to the worker rather than fit the

Table 14.4. Physical Demand Categories of Work

Physical Demand Level	Occasional (0%–33%)	Frequent (34%–66%)	Constant (67%–100%)
Sedentary	10 pounds	Negligible	Negligible
Light	10–20 pounds	10 pounds	Negligible
Medium	20–50 pounds	10–25 pounds	Up to 10 pounds
Heavy	50–100 pounds	25–50 pounds	10–20 pounds
Very heavy	100+ pounds	50+ pounds	20+ pounds

Note. Adapted from U.S. Department of Labor (1991).

worker to the work. Occupational therapy practitioners use an ergonomic approach with their clients to minimize, if not eliminate, hazards in the workplace. An analogy can be drawn to reducing a person's cholesterol through diet and exercise to reduce, if not eliminate, the hazard of cardiovascular disease. By using a holistic approach incorporating physical, cognitive, and organizational ergonomics, occupational therapy practitioners can work with employees and employers to create a culture of wellness and health that can lead to improved productivity and increased job satisfaction among older workers while reducing operational costs and workers' compensation claims. OSHA (n.d.-a) estimates that employers who implement an injury and illness prevention program will reduce injuries by up to 35%.

The process of ergonomics includes hazard identification and assessment, which requires the occupational therapist to engage in two overarching tasks:

Exercise 14.3. Job Analysis

Referring to Table 14.4, determine the level of work (i.e., Sedentary, Light, Medium, Heavy, or Very Heavy) for each of the following jobs based on the stated requirements:
- *Construction laborer:* Load and unload building materials up to 80 pounds, distributing them to the appropriate locations, according to project plans 3 hours per 10-hour workday.
- *Stocker:* Pack and unpack items up to 25 pounds to be stocked on shelves in stockrooms 5 hours per 8-hour workday.
- *Mail clerk:* Lift and unload containers of mail or parcels of up to 35 pounds onto equipment for transportation to sorting stations for up to 6 hours per 9-hour workday.

---

1. Review of the employer's history of injuries, accidents, and employee turnover, as well as review of injury records (e.g., OSHA log of work-related injury and illness [OSHA 300 log], accident reports, workers' compensation claims, dispensary logs).
2. Assessment of job tasks, processes, tools, and equipment in each work area. (Grant, 2012)

Once ergonomics hazards have been assessed and identified, hazard control and prevention efforts must be undertaken to eliminate or reduce identified hazards, including changes and modifications to the process, work methods and tasks, workstations, equipment, and work organization policies (Bush, 2012). Hazard control and prevention efforts by the occupational therapy practitioner are generally focused on one or more of the following categories:

- *Work practice controls:* Examples include modifications of work methods such as proper body mechanics (e.g., lifting techniques), pacing, employee conditioning (e.g., stretching before and during shift), and job coaching. This category includes education and training of workers with approaches such as continuing education courses to enhance job performance, safety seminars, and on-the-job training.
- *Engineering controls:* This category is considered the most effective hazard control and includes workstation redesign, modification of tools and equipment to better fit the worker, purchase of new equipment, use of hydraulic lifts and rolling carts, suspension of heavy hand tools, and increasing size of tool handles.
- *Administrative controls:* Organizational policies and procedures related to shift work, overtime,

rest breaks, number of employees assigned to a task or job, mandatory retirement age, authority and responsibility, productivity rates, equipment maintenance, incentive pay, light duty, restricted duty, and job rotation.

- *Personal protective equipment:* Although not technically an ergonomic control measure, this category includes various protective equipment such as gloves, respirators, chemical aprons, hard hats, eye protection, earplugs, steel-toed footwear, protection against cold, vibration, and contact stress. (Grant, 2012)

Work hardening and work conditioning

Work hardening is a multidisciplinary rehabilitation program focused on maximizing an individual's work capacity with the overarching goal of returning individuals to work. The typical disciplines involved in a work hardening focused on rehabilitating an injured worker include occupational and physical therapists and assistants, exercise physiologists, vocational counselors, psychologists, licensed counselors, and dieticians (Haruka et al., 2013). AOTA published the *Guidelines for Work Hardening* (Matheson, Ogden, Violette, & Schultz, 1985) that defined and described this area of practice, and the language from these guidelines persists today in current AOTA documents (e.g., AOTA, 2011).

A work hardening program should lay the foundation for a return to work and typically requires the client to be engaged in the program several hours per day, 3 to 5 days per week for 4 to 8 weeks, including a pre- and posttesting such as a functional capacity evaluation (see the next section, "Functional Capacity Evaluations"). The program is focused on simulating the target job with actual equipment from the job, if possible, to create realistic work simulation activities.

Work conditioning, by contrast, is a more generalized approach to rehabilitation, usually consisting of only one discipline (i.e., occupational or physical therapy; exercise physiology) focused on physical conditioning, including strength, endurance, cardiopulmonary fitness, range of motion and flexibility, and coordination. Work conditioning may precede work hardening (Haruka et al., 2013).

Regardless of the approach, the goals of work rehabilitation programs (AOTA, 2012) are as follows:

- Maximize levels of function following injury or illness to maintain a desired quality of life for the worker;
- Facilitate the safe and timely return of people to work following injury or illness;
- Remediate or prevent future injury or illness; and
- Assist individuals in resuming their roles as workers, which can contribute to self-confidence and a view of self as a productive member in society, and prevent deconditioning as well as the negative psychosocial consequences of unemployment.

Functional capacity evaluations

The *functional capacity evaluation (FCE)* is recognized as a comprehensive evaluation that makes use of objective and reliable processes to determine a person's capacity for work and plays an important role in work programs and services. FCEs are typically performed by occupational or physical therapists. Occupational therapists are uniquely qualified to conduct FCEs because of their extensive training in activity and task analysis and focus on function (Haruka et al., 2013).

A study conducted by Soer, van der Schans, Groothoof, Geertzen, and Reneman (2008) sought to achieve consensus for an operational definition of FCE, with the following definition gaining the greatest consensus: "A[n] FCE is an evaluation of capacity of activities that is used to make recommendations for participation in work while considering the person's body functions and structures, environmental factors, personal factors and health status" (p. 394).

An FCE can vary in scope and duration because various FCE approaches and methods are used in practice. Regardless of the approach used, an FCE may be used for, among other purposes, determining work rehabilitation intervention plans and goals, determining return-to-work status, quantifying limitations as part of a disability determination, and resolving a case for purposes of settling a case (Haruka et al., 2013). Questions that can be answered by an FCE regarding a person's work performance and tolerance are as follows:

- Is the client capable of performing his or her pre-injury job?

- What are the client's physical work tolerances?
- Can the client return to work full-time? If not, at what level?
- What limitations will require reasonable accommodation?
- What light duty or job restrictions are necessary?
- What are the client's baseline abilities? (Page, 2012)

The FCE process includes a thorough review of medical, social, and work history; pain assessment and musculoskeletal screening; strength and endurance testing; and evaluation of work simulation and tolerance to work over the course of a day. The FCE matches job demands with actual performance, reliability of subjective reporting, and level of effort (validity) by the client (Kaskutas & Snodgrass, 2009). The occupational therapist must monitor the client's responses and reactions to testing through observation; client reports; and vital signs, including heart rate and blood pressure (Page, 2012). An FCE is typically conducted in 2 to 6 hours, although the evaluation can span 2 days.

Injury prevention programs

Occupational therapy practitioners are concerned with *injury prevention* in work settings. For instance, a client with a diagnosis of carpal tunnel syndrome may be receiving traditional therapy services for splinting, stretching, and work modifications, but a focus on preventing an exacerbation of the condition and future injury (secondary prevention) should always be an important component of the occupational therapy intervention plan.

Injury prevention is an approach that occupational therapy practitioners may use in various work settings. AOTA (2014) states that the ultimate outcome in the occupational therapy process is to support health and participation in life through engagement in occupation. A focus on injury prevention and health promotion aims to "provide enriched contextual and activity experiences that will enhance performance for all persons in the natural contexts of life" (AOTA, 2014, p. S33). Injury prevention has three tiers:

- *Primary prevention:* The goal is to prevent disease or injury from occurring. For example, an individual uses a scissor jack cart to transport 100-pound boxes to prevent the possibility of a low back injury.
- *Secondary prevention:* The goal is to minimize or slow the progression of a disease or injury. For example, someone recently diagnosed with mild carpal tunnel syndrome rearranges the computer workstation to decrease awkward postures of the neck and upper extremity to minimize the progression of carpal tunnel syndrome.
- *Tertiary:* The goals are to manage existing diseases or injuries, prevent further complications, and maximize participation in life. For example, a person with chronic pain participates in a pain management program and implements strategies to minimize pain responses, such as relaxation techniques.

Injury prevention programs often are part of a comprehensive rehabilitation program that includes other interventions discussed in this section, such as work conditioning and ergonomics. A program focused on injury prevention in the workplace delivered by occupational therapy practitioners may include programs and activities focused on improving the worker's fitness and comfort on the job and workplace safety initiatives. On-site injury programs from an occupational therapy perspective typically emphasize education related to health, safety and injury prevention, proper body mechanics, postural awareness, joint protection, ergonomic considerations, symptom awareness, and stress and pain management strategies applicable to work and productive activities (AOTA, 2011). Practitioners may serve as consultants to employers to assist in establishing, implementing, and evaluating injury prevention programs (Haruka et al., 2013).

Welfare to Work and Ticket to Work programs

Nearly 15% of Americans (46.5 million) live at or below the poverty line (U.S. Census Bureau, 2013) and include largely female-headed families on welfare and people with disabilities. Employment is the goal of the *Welfare to Work Program* and the Ticket to Work Program; these programs offer community-based practice opportunities for occupational therapists. Employment will enhance social integration and empower individuals who experience stigma and discrimination and reside on the fringes of society. These people have limited work histories, have experienced chronic unemployment, and may not have completed high school.

Occupational therapists can develop comprehensive community-based programs that address the continuum of seeking, finding, and keeping a job. They can help people match their interests and skills, workplace expectations and behaviors, interpersonal skills, life–work balance, and life skills in general. Services such as these are covered by the Welfare to Work Program (Wilson, 2000, cited in Mowrey & Riels, 2014), and occupational therapists are ideally suited to empower and enable individuals on welfare and individuals with disabilities to participate in work.

In the current economy, many social programs are fiscally strained, which in turn places vulnerable people at further risk. Mowrey and Riels (2014) noted that occupational therapy practitioners are uniquely suited to help these disenfranchised groups and can play various roles from educator consultant to broker–advocate.

Summary

A broad overview of work as a central occupation has been considered, including important work policies and programs and the various roles that occupational therapy practitioners fulfill in this area of practice. Occupational therapy practitioners are found in diverse settings where work-related services are provided with a wide variety of populations, including people with developmental disabilities, adolescents and younger workers, older workers, and people with mental illness.

Work-related services are delivered in various settings, including, but not limited to, sheltered workshops, schools, community settings, industrial environments, and outpatient and inpatient settings (AOTA, 2011). Work as a central occupation has, and always will be, essential to the health and well-being of people and represents an important area of practice for the profession of occupational therapy.

References

Age Discrimination Act of 1967, Pub. L. 90–202, 81 Stat. 602.

American Occupational Therapy Association. (1980). The role of occupational therapy in the vocational rehabilitation process. *American Journal of Occupational Therapy, 34,* 881–883. http://dx.doi.org/10.5014/ajot.34.12.881

American Occupational Therapy Association. (1992). Statement: Occupational therapy services in work practice. *American Journal of Occupational Therapy, 46,* 1086–1088. http://dx.doi.org/10.5014/ajot.46.12.1086

American Occupational Therapy Association. (2007). AOTA's *Centennial Vision* and executive summary. *American Journal of Occupational Therapy, 61,* 613. http://dx.doi.org/10.5014/ajot.61.6.613

American Occupational Therapy Association. (2011). Occupational therapy services in facilitating work performance. *American Journal of Occupational Therapy, 65*(Suppl.), S55–S64. http://dx.doi.org/10.5014/ajot.2011.65S55

American Occupational Therapy Association. (2012). *Work rehabilitation*. Retrieved from http://www.aota.org/About-Occupational-Therapy/Professionals/WI/Work-Rehab.aspx

American Occupational Therapy Association. (2014). Occupational therapy practice framework: Domain and process (3rd ed.). *American Journal of Occupational Therapy, 68*(Suppl. 1), S1–S48. http://dx.doi.org/10.5014/ajot.2014.682006

Americans With Disabilities Act of 1990, Pub. L. 101–336, 42 U.S.C. § 12101 *et seq.*

ADA Amendments Act of 2008, Pub. L. 110–325, 122 Stat. 3553.

Anderson, S., & Winefield, A. H. (2011). Impact of underemployment on psychological health, physical health and work attitudes. In D. C. Maynard & D. C. Feldman (Eds.), *Underemployment: Psychological, economic and social challenges* (pp. 165–185). New York: Springer.

Annis, J., & McConville, J. (2012). Anthropometry. In A. Bhattacharya & J. McGlothlin (Eds.), *Occupational ergonomics: Theory and applications* (2nd ed., pp. 3–54). Boca Raton, FL: CRC Press.

Braveman, B. H., & Page, J. J. (Eds.). (2012). *Work: Promoting participation and productivity through occupational therapy.* Philadelphia: F. A. Davis.

Bureau of Labor Statistics. (2012). *Number of jobs held, labor market activity, and earnings growth among the youngest baby boomers: A longitudinal study* (Report No. USDL-12-1489). Retrieved from http://www.bls.gov/news.release/pdf/nlsoy.pdf

Bush, P. (2012). *Ergonomics: Foundational principles, applications, and technologies.* Boca Raton, FL: CRC Press.

Carrasco, R., Hermes, S., & Burgos, B. (2011). Supported and alternative employment: Developmental disabilities and work. In B. Bravemen & J. Page (Eds.), *Work: Promoting participation and productivity through occupational therapy* (pp. 118–139). Philadelphia: F. A. Davis.

Chartrand, J. M. (1991). The evolution of trait-and-factor career counseling: A person × environment fit approach. *Journal of Counseling and Development, 69,* 518–524.

Christiansen, C. H. (1999). Defining lives: Occupation as identity—An essay on competence, coherence, and the creation of meaning [1999 Eleanor Clarke Slagle Lecture]. *American Journal of Occupational Therapy, 53,* 547–558. http://dx.doi.org/10.5014/ajot.53.6.547

Clauw, D. J., & Williams, D. A. (2002). Relationship between stress and pain in work-related upper extremity disorders: The hidden role of chronic multisymptom illnesses. *American Journal of Industrial Medicine, 41,* 370–382. http://dx.doi.org/10.1002/ajim.10068

Deloitte. (2012). *Shift index.* Retrieved from http://www.deloitte.com/us/shiftindex

Dembe, A. E., Erickson, J. B., Delbos, R. G., & Banks, S. M. (2005). The impact of overtime and long work hours on occupational injuries and illnesses: New evidence from the United States. *Occupational and Environmental Medicine, 62,* 588–597. http://dx.doi.org/10.1136/oem.2004.016667

Drucker, P. F. (1999). *Management challenges of the 21st century.* New York: Harper Business.

Education of the Deaf Act of 1986, Pub. L. 99–371, 100 Stat, 781.

Employee Retirement Income Security Act of 1974, Pub. L. No. 93–406, 88 Stat. 829 (codified as amended in scattered sections of 5 U.S.C., 18 U.S.C., 26 U.S.C., 29 U.S.C., 42 U.S.C.).

Equal Employment Opportunity Commission. (2008, August 1). *The ADA: Your responsibilities as an employer.* Retrieved from http://www.eeoc.gov/facts/ada17.html

Fair Labor Standards Act of 1938, Pub. L. 75–718, ch. 676, 52 Stat. 1060, 1067–68 (codified as amended at 29 U.S.C. § 213, 1982).

Family and Medical Leave Act of 1993, 29 U.S.C. §§ 2601–2654 (2006).

Federal Employee Liability Act of 1908, 45 U.S.C. 51 *et seq.*

Fouad, N. A., & Byars⊠Winston, A. M. (2005). Cultural context of career choice: Meta⊠analysis of race/ethnicity differences. *Career Development Quarterly, 53,* 223–233. http://dx.doi.org/10.1002/j.2161-0045.2005.tb00992.x

Gallup. (2013). *The state of the American workplace: Employee engagement insights for U.S. business leaders.* Retrieved from http://www.gallup.com/strategicconsulting/163007/state-american-workplace.aspx

Ginzberg, E. (1952). Toward a theory of occupational choice. *Occupations: The Vocational Guidance Journal, 30*(7), 491–494.

Ginzberg, E. (1971). *Career guidance: Who needs it, who provides it, who can improve it.* New York: McGraw-Hill.

Gordon, D. (2009). The history of occupational therapy. In E. C. Crepeau, E. Cohn, & B. Boyt Schell (Eds.), *Willard and Spackman's occupational therapy* (11th ed., pp. 202–215). Philadelphia: Lippincott Williams & Wilkins.

Grant, K. (2012). Job analysis. In A. Bhattacharya & J. McGlothlin (Eds.), *Occupational ergonomics: Theory and applications* (2nd ed., pp. 273–292). Boca Raton, FL: CRC Press.

Gupta, J. (2008, June). Promoting wellness at the workplace. *Work and Industry Special Interest Section Quarterly, 22,* 1–4. Retrieved from http://ergonomicsconsulting.wikispaces.com/file/view/SIS_Ergo3.pdf

Gupta, J., & Sabata, D. (2012). Older workers: Maintaining worker role and returning to the workplace. In B. Braveman & J. Page (Eds.), *Work: Promoting participation and productivity through occupational therapy* (pp. 172–193). Philadelphia: F. A. Davis.

Gysbers, N. C., Heppner, M. J., & Johnston, J. A. (1987). *Career counseling.* Alexandria, VA: American Counseling Association.

Harpaz, I., & Fu, X. (2002). The structure and meaning of work: A relative stability amidst change. *Human Relations, 55,* 639–667. http://dx.doi.org/10.1177/0018726702556002

Haruka, D., Page, J., & Wietlisbach, C. (2013). Work evaluation and work programs. In H. Pendleton & W. Shultz-Krohn (Eds.), *Pedretti's occupational therapy practice skills for physical dysfunction* (pp. 337–380). St. Louis: Elsevier.

Hausmann, R. (2013, April 16). The short history of the future of manufacturing. *Scientific American.* Retrieved from http://www.scientificamerican.com/article/manufacturing-short-history-of-future

Holland, J. L. (1973). *Making vocational choices: A theory of careers* (Vol. 37). Englewood Cliffs, NJ: Prentice-Hall.

Holland, J. L. (1985). *Making vocational choices: A theory of vocational personalities and environments.* Englewood Cliffs, NJ: Prentice-Hall.

Individuals With Disabilties Education Act, 1990, Pub. L. 101-476, 104 Stat 1142.

Individuals With Disabilties Education Act, Amendments of 1997, Pub. L. 105–17, 111 Stat 37.

International Ergonomics Association. (n.d.). *What is ergonomics.* Retrieved from http://www.iea.cc/whats/index.html

Jacobs, K., & Baker, N. (2000). The history of work-related therapy in occupational therapy. In B. L. Kornblau & K. Jacobs (Eds.), *Work: Principles and practice* (AOTA Self-Paced Clinical Course, pp. 1–11). Bethesda, MD: American Occupational Therapy Association.

Jung, J., & Makowsky, M. D. (2012). *Regulatory enforcement, politics, and institutional distance: OSHA inspections 1990–2010.* Retrieved from http://www.osha.gov/OshDoc/data_General_Facts/factsheet-inspections.pdf

Kantartzis, S., & Molineux, M. (2011). The influence of Western society's construction of a healthy daily life on the conceptualisation of occupation. *Journal of Occupational Science, 18,* 62–80. http://dx.doi.org/10.1080/14427591.2011.566917

Karger, H., & Rose, S. R. (2010). Revisiting the Americans With Disabilities Act after two decades. *Journal of Social Work in Disability and Rehabilitation, 9,* 73–86. http://dx.doi.org/10.1080/1536710X.2010.493468

Kaskutas, V., & Snodgrass, J. (2009). *Occupational therapy practice guidelines for individuals with work-related injuries and illnesses.* Bethesda, MD: AOTA Press.

Kornblau, B. L., & Andersen, L. T. (2000). Occupational therapy, workers' compensation insurance, and disability insurance. In B. L. Kornblau & K. Jacobs (Eds.), *Work: Principles and practice* (AOTA Self-Paced Clinical Course). Bethesda, MD: American Occupational Therapy Association.

Kornblau, B. L., Lou, J. Q., Weeder, T. C., & Werner, B. (2002). Occupational therapy and theories of career choice and vocational development. In B. L. Kornblau & K. Jacobs (Eds.), *Work: Principles and practice* (AOTA Self-Paced Clinical Course, pp. 1–23). Bethesda, MD: American Occupational Therapy Association.

Krumboltz, J. D., Mitchell, A. M., & Jones, G. B. (1976). A social learning theory of career selection. *The Counseling Psychologist, 6*(1), 71–81. http://dx.doi.og/10.1177/001100007600600117

Labor–Management Reporting and Disclosure Act of 1959, Pub. L. 86–257, 73 Stat. 519-546.

Landrum–Griffin Act of 1959, Pub. L. 86-257, 73 Stat. 519.

Larson, E., & Zemke, R. (2003). Shaping temporal patterns of our lives: The social coordination of occupation. *Journal of Occupational Science, 10,* 80–89. http://dx.doi.org/10.1080/14427591.2003.9686514

Lent, R. W., Brown, S. D., & Hackett, G. (1994). Toward a unifying social cognitive theory of career and academic interest, choice, and performance. *Journal of Vocational Behavior, 45,* 79–122. http://dx.doi.org/10.1006/jvbe.1994.1027

Library of Congress. (2013). *THOMAS.* Retrieved from http://thomas.loc.gov/home/thomas.php

Library of Congress. (n.d.). *Rise of Industrial America: Work in the late 19th century.* Retrieved from http://www.loc.gov.

Matheson, L. N., Ogden, L. D., Violette, K., & Schultz, K. (1985). Work hardening: Occupational therapy in industrial rehabilitation. *American Journal of Occupational Therapy, 39,* 314–321. http://dx.doi.org/10.5014/ajot.39.5.314

Medical Facilities Survey and Construction Act of 1954, Pub. L. 83–482, 68 Stat. 461.

Michie, S. (2002). Causes and management of stress at work. *Occupational and Environmental Medicine, 59,* 67–72. http://dx.doi.org/10.1136/oem.59.1.67

Mowrey, E. W., & Riels, L. A. (2014). Welfare to Work and Ticket to Work Programs. In M. E. Scaffa & S. M. Reitz (Eds.), *Occupational therapy in community-based practice settings* (2nd ed., pp. 257–270). Philadelphia: F. A. Davis.

National Academy of Social Insurance. (2013a). *Trends in workers' compensation benefits, by insurance provider.* Retrieved from http://www.nasi.org/learn/workerscomp/trends-in-benefits

National Academy of Social Insurance. (2013b). *Workers' compensation and disability.* Retrieved from http://www.nasi.org/learn/workerscomp

National Institute for Occupational Safety and Health. (1999). *Stress . . . at work* (NIOSH Publication No. 99-101). Retrieved from http://www.cdc.gov/niosh/docs/99-101/

Occupational and Safety Health Act of 1970, Pub. L. 91–596, 84 Stat. 1590.

Occupational Safety and Health Administration. (2013a). *Commonly used statistics.* Retrieved from https://www.osha.gov/oshstats/commonstats.html

Occupational Safety and Health Administration. (2013b). *State occupational safety and health plans.* Retrieved from https://www.osha.gov/dcsp/osp/index.html

Occupational Safety and Health Administration. (n.d.-a). *OSH Act of 1970: Table of contents.* Retrieved from https://www.osha.gov/pls/oshaweb/owadisp.show_document?p_table=OSHACT&p_id=2743

Occupational Safety and Health Administration. (n.d.-b). *OSHA law and regulations.* Retrieved from http://www.osha.gov/law-regs.html

Okulicz-Kozaryn, A. (2011). Europeans work to live and Americans live to work (Who is happy to work more: Americans or Europeans?). *Journal of Happiness Studies, 12,* 225–243. http://dx.doi.org/10.1007/s10902-010-9188-8

Omnibus Budget Reconciliation Educational Act of 1987, Pub. L. 100–203, 42 U. S. C. § 4211.

Page, J. (2012). Physical assessment of the worker. In B. Braveman & J. J. Page (Eds.), *Work: Promoting participation and productivity through occupational therapy* (pp. 263–282). Philadelphia: F. A. Davis.

Parsons, F. (1909). *Choosing a vocation.* Boston: Houghton-Mifflin.

Perlow, L. A. (2012). *Sleeping with your smartphone: How to break the 24/7 habit and change the way you work.* Cambridge, MA: Harvard Business Review Press.

Ramsay, D., Starnes, W., & Robertson, S. (2000). Work programs for persons with serious and chronic mental illness.

In B. L. Kornblau & K. Jacobs (Eds.), *Work: Principles and practice* (AOTA Self-Paced Clinical Course). Bethesda, MD: American Occupational Therapy Association.

Ray, R., & Schmitt, J. (2007). *No-vacation nation.* Washington, DC: Center for Economic and Policy Research. Retrieved from http://www.cepr.net/documents/publications/2007-05-novacation-nation.pdf.

Rehabilitation Act of 1973, Pub. L. 93–112, 29 U.S.C. § 701 *et seq.*

Rehabilitation Act Amendments of 1992, Pub. L. 102–569, 106 Stat. 4344.

Reinhardt, W., Schmidt, B., Sloep, P., & Drachsler, H. (2011). Knowledge worker roles and actions: Results of two empirical studies. *Knowledge and Process Management, 18,* 150–174. http://dx.doi.org/10.1002/kpm.378

Social Security Administration. (2013a). *The red book: A guide to work incentives.* Retrieved from http://ssa.gov/redbook/

Social Security Administration. (2013b). *Welcome to the work site: Ticket to work.* Retrieved from http://www.ssa.gov/work/

Soer, R., van der Schans, C. P., Groothoff, J. W., Geertzen, J. H., & Reneman, M. F. (2008). Towards consensus in operational definitions in functional capacity evaluation: A Delphi survey. *Journal of Occupational Rehabilitation, 18,* 389–400. http://dx.doi.org/10.1007/s10926-008-9155-y

Stewart, D. (Ed.). (2013). *Transitions to adulthood for youth with disabilities through an occupational therapy lens.* Thorofare, NJ: Slack.

Stoffel, G. (2010). *Leadership and advocacy: Making the centennial vision a reality.* Retrieved from http://www.aota.org/media/Corporate/Files/AboutAOTA/Centennial/Commission/CVandLeadership.pdf

Super, D. E. (1953). A theory of vocational development. *American Psychologist, 8,* 185–190. http://dx.doi.org/10.1037/h0056046

Ticket to Work Incentives Improvement Act of 1999, Pub. L. 106–170, 113 Stat. 1860.

United Nations. (1948). *The universal declaration of human rights.* Retrieved from http://www.un.org/en/documents/udhr/index.shtml#a23

U.S. Census Bureau. (2013). *Poverty highlights.* Retrieved from http://www.census.gov/hhes/www/poverty/about/overview/

U.S. Department of Education. (n.d.). *Building the legacy: IDEA 2004.* Retrieved from http://idea.ed.gov/explore/view/p/%2Croot%2Cstatute%2CI%2CA%2C602%2C34%2C

U.S. Department of Labor. (1991). *The revised handbook for analyzing jobs.* Washington, DC: U.S. Government Printing Office.

U.S. Department of Labor. (n.d.). *Summary of the major laws of the Department of Labor.* Retrieved from http://www.dol.gov/opa/aboutdol/lawsprog.htm

Vocational Rehabilitation Act Amendments of 1954, Pub. L. 83–565, 69 Stat. 652.

Wegg, L. S. (1960). The essentials of work evaluation [Eleanor Clarke Slagle Lecture]. *American Journal of Occupational Therapy, 14,* 65–69, 79.

Wilson, E. (2000). *The role of occupational theapy in Welfare to Work* (Unpublished master's thesis). Ithaca College: Ithaca, NY.

CHAPTER 15.

SELF-CARE OCCUPATIONS

Tsu-Hsin Howe, PhD, OTR, FAOTA, and Anita Perr, PhD, OT, ATP, FAOTA

Highlights

- ✧ What are self-care occupations?
- ✧ Contextual factors
- ✧ Self-care evaluation
- ✧ Self-care intervention
- ✧ Group vs. individual treatment.

Key Terms

- ✧ Activity
- ✧ Activity limitation
- ✧ Attitudinal settings
- ✧ BADLs
- ✧ Behavior theory
- ✧ Body functions
- ✧ Body structures
- ✧ Compensatory frame of reference
- ✧ Context
- ✧ Disability
- ✧ Environmental factors
- ✧ Functioning

- ✧ Habit training approach
- ✧ IADLs
- ✧ Impairment
- ✧ Occupations
- ✧ Participation
- ✧ Participation restriction
- ✧ Personal factors
- ✧ Physical settings
- ✧ Self-care occupations
- ✧ Self-directed learning frame of reference
- ✧ Social settings
- ✧ Strengths-based approach

This chapter defines and describes self-care occupations and their categories, including basic activities of daily living (BADLs) and instrumental activities of daily living (IADLs), and their relationships to occupations. It also explains how BADLs and IADLs are evaluated in the context of occupations.

Because self-care occupations make up a large part of everyone's life, the occupational therapy practitioner's focus on a person's ability to engage in self-care occupations is vitally important. Self-care occupations are fundamental to human existence and affect people's ability to function. By addressing self-care with clients, practitioners shape the daily lives of those they serve. In this chapter, the terms used to organize the discussion of self-care are adopted from the *Occupational Therapy Practice Framework: Doman and Process* (hereafter, *Framework;* American Occupational Therapy Association [AOTA], 2014) and the *International Classification of Functioning, Disability and Health* (*ICF;* World Health Organization [WHO], 2001).

First, the importance of self-care on an individual level is discussed, and then factors that influence the efficacy of self-care are examined. Elements that influence participation in self-care include body function and structure, environmental, and personal factors.

The chapter provides a framework for occupational therapy practitioners to organize a self-care evaluation and to design appropriate interventions for a person who has difficulty with self-care. It emphasizes the importance of addressing a person's self-care occupations when evaluating and designing interventions related to BADLs and IADLs.

Case examples (for Grace and Jon) throughout the chapter demonstrate factors that need to be considered during self-care evaluations and inter-ventions. The case examples also explain how a person's values, priorities, and preferences are taken into consideration during these processes. Grace and Jon lead very different lives and have distinctive patterns of daily living, interests, values, and needs. Their occupational profiles describe various aspects of self-care that practitioners can address.

What Are Self-Care Occupations?

In this chapter, *self-care occupations* are defined as everyday life activities that people do to take care of themselves. BADLs and IADLs in the context of occupation are discussed. *BADLs* are all the tasks a person must engage in or accomplish for personal care and self-maintenance (e.g., bathing, dressing, eating, grooming, toileting; Exhibit 15.1, "Basic Activities of Daily Living") *IADLs* are tasks to support daily life within the home and community that often require more complex interactions than personal care and self-maintenance (AOTA, 2014). Examples of IADLs are care of others, community mobility, financial management, health management and maintenance, and meal preparation (Exhibit 15.2).

Occupations, as defined in Chapter 1, "Occupation, Activities, and Occupational Therapy," are "activities that are personally meaningful to the person who voluntarily engages in them out of personal choice or sociocultural necessity. Thus, occupations are unique to everyone, providing personal satisfaction and fulfillment as a result of engaging in them" (Hinojosa & Blount, 2014, p. 3). Therefore, this chapter includes personal values, preferences, and priorities in the examination of a client's abilities to perform BADLs and IADLs.

Exhibit 15.1. Basic Activities of Daily Living

- Bathing, showering
- Bowel and bladder management
- Dressing
- Eating
- Feeding
- Functional mobility
- Using, cleaning, and maintaining personal care items, such as hearing aids, contact lenses, glasses
- Personal hygiene and grooming
- Sexual activity
- Toilet hygiene

Source. AOTA (2014).

Exhibit 15.2. Instrumental Activities of Daily Living

- Care of others (including selecting and supervising caregivers)
- Care of pets
- Child rearing
- Communication management
- Community mobility
- Financial management
- Health management and maintenance
- Home establishment and management
- Meal preparation and cleanup
- Religious observance
- Safety and emergency maintenance
- Shopping

Source. AOTA (2014).

Self-care occupations are fundamental to human existence and affect peoples' abilities to function. Providing interventions to improve a person's self-care occupations has always been an important part of occupational therapy practice. By addressing self-care occupations with clients, occupational therapy practitioners influence their daily lives. The terms and emphasis of these interventions, however, have shifted over time as populations and the needs of society have changed, and various occupational therapy interventions have gone into and out of vogue.

Early in the profession's history, intervention focused on the mechanics of daily activities, that is, practitioners focused on the acquisition of specific skills. Theoretical rationales and explanations were not used at that time, and interventions were developed through trial and error.

For example, practitioners developed various strategies to establish daily routine skills as evidenced by Eleanor Clarke Slagle's *habit training approach,* which introduces routines to help individuals learn skills to be productive and maintain a balanced daily schedule. Later, during World Wars I and II, interventions became more oriented toward adaptation because of the influence of the medical model and increasing numbers of wounded veterans returning home. In the 1980s, the *compensatory frame of reference* espoused using environmental adaptation, adaptive equipment, and alternative strategies to promote an individual's level of independence. Today, the profession has a renewed emphasis on the importance of activities of daily living (ADLs) and has added new meanings to it.

To explain this further, the importance and scope of ADLs are identified in both the *Framework* (AOTA, 2014) and the *ICF* (WHO, 2001). During the evaluation and intervention process, occupational therapists consider not only a client's activity performance but also the intervention context and its impact on self-care occupations. In other words, occupational therapists include the client's experience and the physical and social contexts when they perform evaluations of and develop interventions for self-care occupations.

A person's specific routines vary by age, culture, ethnicity, gender, and many other factors. Occupational therapy practitioners should address these differences, or preferences, when planning and implementing interventions. Case Example 15.1, Part 1, and Case Example 15.2, Part 1, describe the self-care activities that are important to two occupational therapy clients.

As the field of occupational therapy further explores the definitions of *occupation, activity,* and *task,* it makes sense to think about ADLs in terms of these definitions. At the most basic level, the category of self-care can be considered the occupation. If occupation can be thought of as a collection of activities, then the various components of self-care can be considered activities. In this paradigm, examples of activities are combing hair, expressing sexuality, brushing teeth, toileting, and eating.

The way each person puts the activities of self-care together becomes the occupation and is grounded in personal meanings. Continuing the paradigm, if brushing teeth is the activity, then opening the toothpaste cap, putting toothpaste on the toothbrush, brushing the teeth, and rinsing the mouth are the tasks.

Case Example 15.1, Part 1. Grace: Important Self-Care Activities

Grace is a 45-year-old woman who underwent surgery to repair a brain aneurysm. During the surgery, the aneurysm ruptured, resulting in a hemorrhagic stroke. The result is that Grace is hemiparetic on the right side. She has flaccid paralysis of the right upper extremity. Grace is right-hand dominant. Although the right lower extremity has some areas of abnormal tone and weakness, Grace can ambulate for about 10 feet on level surfaces without using an ambulation aid, such as a cane. She also has slight memory impairment and limited executive cognitive functions.

Upon meeting Grace, her occupational therapist is struck by her precise dressing and grooming. By Grace's report, it is important that she "look well put together." Before her stroke, she wore her hair in long braids, which she braided herself. She jogged 1 to 3 miles at least 3 times a week. She showered each morning before leaving for work. An important occupation was cooking, during which she attended to nutritional advice and enjoyed the challenges of preparing dinner for others.

Case Example 15.2, Part 1. Jon: Important Self-Care Activities

Jon is a 16-year-old boy who broke his right arm while skateboarding. He has compound fractures of the humerus (midshaft) and of the ulna and radius. An external fixator is in place at the humerus. Internal fixators, plates, and screws are in place in the forearm. Jon is right-hand dominant.

Jon is a social teenager who spends a great deal of time getting ready to go out with friends. He works at looking well-groomed and dresses the same as his friends and their role models, mainly hip-hop artists. Jon reports that he has great difficulty putting gel in his hair and getting it to look the way he wants since breaking his arm. Before the injury, Jon showered at school after his gym class 3 times weekly. During his evaluation, Jon revealed that he is uncomfortable dressing and undressing after gym class (both before and since his accident). He worked out about 4 times a week, primarily lifting weights and working to improve his physique before the accident. Regardless of his effort, he still perceives himself as scrawny. He does not want his classmates to see that he is skinny. He thinks he looks like a little kid and does not understand why he is not bulking up like most of the other teens he is friendly with.

Jon has no interest in cooking or preparing meals. His mother prepares meals at home for the whole family. Jon buys lunch in his school cafeteria and says he really does not think about nutrition. He eats pizza for lunch on a nearly daily basis.

Contextual Factors

Everything takes place within a *context,* which is a setting in which an event occurs. Changing the context changes the activity. Contextual factors include two components: (1) environmental factors (external) and (2) personal factors (internal).

Environmental factors are the physical, social, and attitudinal settings in which people live and conduct their lives, and *personal factors* are features that are integral parts of individuals and are brought to situations (e.g., gender, age, coping styles, social background, education, profession, past and current experience, overall behavioral pattern, character). Personal factors influence how a person experiences disability (WHO, 2001).

Contextual factors need to be identified during the ADL evaluation and included during the intervention. Note that for people with disabilities, the impact of contextual factors may be magnified compared with people without disabilities.

Some contextual factors are facilitators and help people perform an activity. For example, for a person with limited hand function, long, lever-style door handles can facilitate performance because the person can open the door just by pushing down the handles. The design of the door facilitates function. Some contextual factors, however, are barriers that limit or prevent performance. Imagine the same person living in an apartment with knob-style door handles. Here, the person is unable to open the doors and needs help, making the door knobs barriers to performance. These examples show that contextual factors affect people's abilities. By understanding each client's contextual factors, occupational therapy practitioners are better able to prioritize treatment and determine what is important for each client.

Environmental Factors

Environmental factors include physical, social, and attitudinal settings. *Physical settings* include the natural or human-made products or systems of products, equipment, and technology in a person's immediate environment. *Social settings* include support and relationships that a person has in his or her own environment. These supports may be physical or emotional in nature. A person may seek support, nurturing, protection, and assistance from others or pets. A person may

establish relationships with other persons at home, work, or school or during play (Schneidert, Hurst, Miller, & Üstün, 2003). *Attitudinal settings* are the observable consequences of customs, practices, ideologies, values, norms, and religious beliefs. Case Example 15.1, Part 2, and Case Example 15.2, Part 2, list these factors as noted by each client's occupational therapist.

Exercise 15.1. Think About Environmental Factors

In the profiles for Grace and Jon, what are the physical, social, and attitudinal facilitators and barriers to participation in daily activities? Think about your own life. What are the environmental facilitators and barriers? How do you use the facilitators? How do you deal with the barriers?

Case Example 15.1, Part 2. Physical, Social, and Attitudinal Settings for Grace

Physical

Grace lives in a studio apartment in a large East Coast city. The apartment is on the second floor, up a flight of 18 steps. The building has no elevator. Grace sleeps on a waterbed that is against the wall at the head and left side. She has a small closet where she keeps the current season's clothing and outerwear. She also has a small dresser for undergarments. Grace's bathroom is very small (5' × 8'). The only storage space she has in the bathroom is a small medicine cabinet over the sink. She has a claw-foot tub with a shower extension attached to the tub spout.

Social

Grace was engaged to be married about 6 months from the time of her surgery. She has no immediate or extended family nearby except for her fiancé, Tony. Grace had 4 or 5 close friends with whom she spoke or spent time about 5 times a week before her stroke. Since then, they have visited regularly in the hospital, and it is expected they will remain supportive and be available to

help Grace. Grace is very pleasant, although somewhat quiet. She has many acquaintances at work, her gym, and church. Grace does not have pets. Before the incident, Grace had never had any medical problems. She saw her physician annually.

Attitudinal

Grace values her social and economic independence. Although she is in love with Tony, they both plan to continue to spend time with their own friends and pursue their own interests in addition to building new friendships and developing new pursuits together. She belongs to a church in her neighborhood, attends services regularly, and participates in other church activities. She met Tony during a fundraising activity sponsored by the church. Graces enjoys yoga and meditation and is learning about Eastern religions. She celebrates her African heritage, celebrates Kwanzaa, and plans to "jump the broom" at her wedding.

Case Example 15.2, Part 2. Physical, Social, and Attitudinal Settings for Jon

Physical

Jon lives in the suburbs, about 2 hours from the city in which Grace lives. He lives in a two-story, four-bedroom house in which all the bedrooms are on the second floor. Jon shares a bedroom with his 14-year-old brother. He sleeps on the bottom bunk. Jon keeps his clothes folded in dresser drawers or hung on hooks or hangers in a closet, but he reports that his room is usually messy, and he usually finds the clothes he wears on the floor or on a chair. The bathroom Jon most frequently uses for his morning routine is shared with his 3 siblings. It has a stall shower. As previously stated, Jon usually showers at school and says it is because if he showers at home, his siblings might not have enough hot water.

Social

Jon lives with his parents and 3 brothers. His extended family lives in nearby states and in Taiwan. The family in the area gets together regularly. He has cousins with whom he is very friendly. Jon has a group of about 15 close friends from school. None of these boys live near Jon because the catchment area for the school is large. John has 1 neighborhood friend: the boy who lives next door and who is about 2 years younger. His school friends do not know about his neighborhood friend because Jon is afraid his friends will tease him for being friends with a younger boy.

Attitudinal

Jon's family is Catholic, but they do not regularly attend church or actively practice religion. His family is generally conservative in their political views. Jon views his family as too traditional and boring. He says that they are sometimes worried about him because he is the "wild" one in the family. Jon and his friends tend to use curse words when they are with each other, but Jon does not curse when he thinks his family members might hear him. Jon's family values education, and they expect him to go to college after graduating from high school.

During intervention, occupational therapy practitioners use environmental facilitators to improve participation in self-care occupations and address environmental barriers to alleviate or lessen their effect. For example, a closet with only a high rod was an environmental barrier for a man in a wheelchair because he could not reach his clothes. A second, lower rod was installed, and now the man can easily reach his clothes (Figure 15.1). If he needs to retrieve an item from the upper rod, he uses a reacher.

Personal Factors

Personal factors comprise the other component of contextual factors aside from environmental factors. They include age, gender, social status, life experiences, and so on. It is easy to see that the daily activities of a 3-year-old differ from those of a teenager, which differ from those of an adult, which further differ from those of an older adult.

Young children may be focusing on learning to dress themselves. Their parents may let them wear clothing with elastic waists or shoes with hook-and-loop closures to minimize hand manipulation and encourage early independence. Most teens have mastered grooming and dressing and focus on conforming to their peer group. Teens may also be more focused on other activities such as learning to drive or shopping. Gender-specific and sexual activities are also important activities and occupations for teenagers. Sex, an often-ignored daily life activity, is extremely important for a person during the developmental stages of adolescence, young adulthood, and adulthood. Once in the adult stage, the focus of daily activities may shift further toward IADLs, such as housekeeping and budgeting. In addition, older adults may have different responsibilities. Depending on the nature of their residence, they may have the responsibility for lawn and garden care if they live in a suburban home;

Figure 15.1. A clothes closet is no longer an environmental barrier; a second rod now makes it an environmental facilitator.

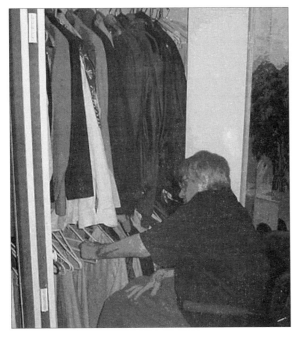

Source. A. Perr. Used with permission.

alternatively, they may choose indoor gardening as a leisure activity if they live in an urban dwelling. Case Example 15.1, Part 3, and Case Example 15.2, Part 3, discuss personal factors for each client.

In the *ICF* (WHO, 2001), "*Functioning* is an umbrella term encompassing all body functions and structure, activities and participation as an umbrella term; similarly, *disability* serves as an umbrella term for impairments, activity limitations or participation restrictions" (p. 3). *Body functions* include physiological and psychological actions of body systems, whereas *body structures* describe anatomical parts of the body such as organs, limbs, and their components. *Impairment* is a problem in body functions or structures. *Activity* and *participation* describe a person's performance at a person or societal level. *Activity limitation* is a difficulty at the person level. *Participation restriction* refers to societal-level impediment. Case Example 15.1, Part 4, and Case Example 15.2, Part 4, describe body structure and function for these clients.

According to the *ICF*, functioning and disability are the outcomes of the interaction between health conditions and the contextual factors (environ-

mental and personal). When a person's interactions result in his or her functioning at less than an optimal level, the person is experiencing a disability or is disabled (Schneidert et al., 2003).

The term *disability* applies in cases in which a person has problems at different levels or problems

---

Case Example 15.1, Part 3. Personal Factors for Grace

At age 45 years, **Grace** cannot believe that she is middle-aged, does not like to think about it, and does not want to think about getting older. She is African American and grew up in a small southern town. She has lived on her own since high school. She earned an undergraduate degree and a master of business administration degree from a prestigious New England university. Her fiancé, Tony, is Brazilian and not yet a U.S. citizen. The couple has been involved for 3 years.

Grace says that before her stroke, their love life was healthy and they had sex regularly. She says that she liked to experiment a little more than he does. Since the stroke, Tony is still caring and compassionate, and they have talked about having intimate relations with each other. Grace currently works for a small business importing gift items from Africa. She loves to travel and has many responsibilities at work that require her to travel to West Africa. She is somewhat concerned about how she will be able to travel once she returns to work.

Case Example 15.2, Part 3. Personal Factors for Jon

Jon is a 16-year-old Asian American high school student. His grade point average is 2.42. He and his male friends often skip school. He has lived his entire life in the same home. He has slept over at friends' houses but not for more than a night. Jon does not have a girlfriend and is extremely hesitant to talk about close personal relationships. Jon says that he is not sexually active. He denies the use of drugs and alcohol.

Case Example 15.1, Part 4. Body Structure and Function Factors for Grace

Body Structure

Grace suffered a left parietal lobe infarct during a planned surgery to clip an aneurysm. She presents with muscle imbalance in the trunk and extremely low tone in the right arm. She has decreased movement in her right leg with less significant changes in tone.

Body Function

Since the neurologic insult, Grace has become quieter and now perceives herself as shy. She does not know how people will react to her new medical condition and is concerned whether she will be able to follow the conversation and understand the nuances. She is somewhat downhearted about her condition and her impending wedding. Her motivation fluctuates from day to day. She tends to be sleepy most of the time and cannot tell whether it is a side effect from her medication. She says she "just feels crummy." She has mild short-term and long-term memory impairment and mild impairment of high-level cognitive functions. Sensory functions are intact. Grace has a mild gait and balance impairment and mild-to-moderate impairment in endurance.

Case Example 15.2, Part 4. Body Structure and Function Factors for Jon

Body Structure

Jon suffered multiple fractures in his right arm and has an external fixator in place for 5 to 7 weeks. He also uses a sling and a bolster to support his arm when standing. Jon's arm should also be raised and supported when he is seated, but he says that he is usually not able to do this. Open wounds exist at the pin sites where the external fixator protrudes from his arm.

Body Function

Jon's mental and sensory functions are intact and age appropriate.

tion) but has difficulty navigating in his community (participation restrictions).

Self-Care Evaluation

Occupational therapists must complete a thorough evaluation to develop an appropriate intervention plan. A comprehensive evaluation identifies areas of limited participation. Further, it identifies how the impairments limit participation. Occupational therapists usually complete an evaluation through the following sequence. They begin the evaluation with an assessment of the client's potential capacity, functional status, and actual abilities. In this part of the evaluation, therapists assess a client's physical, psychological, sensory, perceptual, and cognitive functions. Once therapists have a general understanding of the client's baseline, they conduct a thorough assessment of the client's performance of BADLs. If appropriate, they also assess specific IADLs that are applicable to the client.

Occupational therapists gather information about self-care occupations through self-report, proxy report, direct observation of behavior in settings where clients live, and performance-based measures that use tasks in clinical settings. Each of these methods has strengths and weaknesses. A consensus exists, however, that the best method is

at combined levels. A person can have a problem only at the body level (an impairment) but no activity limitation or participation restrictions; have problems at all three levels of functioning: (1) body (impairments), (2) person (activity limitation), and (3) society (participation restrictions); or have an impairment and activity limitation but no participation restriction, and so forth.

For example, a fourth-finger amputation of the nondominant hand (impairment) does not have any influence on a person's participation at the personal level (no activity limitation) or society level (no participation restrictions). On the other hand, a person who has a double below-knee amputation (impairment) can perform all dressing, bathing, and grooming independently (no activity limita-

direct observation because it depends less on a client's insight and cognitive ability (Kempen, Steverink, Ormel, & Deeg, 1996).

Occupational therapists obtain the most reliable information when the client performs an activity in his or her usual or natural environment. Therapists who work in home-based practice have the advantage of using the client's own environment and materials during evaluations and when developing interventions. However, because most evaluations and interventions occur in a clinic or hospital setting, an alternative is to have the client perform the activity in a closely simulated environment using the real tools, such as his or her own clothing or toothbrush. Care should be taken to bring as much of the usual environment into the evaluation and intervention context as possible, including taking into account the client's values and beliefs and his or her roles and responsibilities.

A person's performance of self-care occupations is a major predictor of his or her dependence, morbidity, and mortality (Millán-Calenti et al., 2010). Estimating the number and characteristics of self-care occupations performed by an occupational therapy client is important because of the increasing number of third-party payers who rely on these measures to determine whether a person qualifies for benefits. Depending on the purpose of the evaluation, therapists may choose to use a standardized assessment or a behavioral checklist (developed either by therapists or by the clinical site) to assist in information gathering. Regardless of the nature of the assessment, it should include information about BADLs, IADLs, and mobility (see Exhibits 15.1 and 15.2) and should provide a reliable and valid way for therapists to quantify the client's performance. Semantic and numeric rating methods can be used to describe self-care performance.

For example, terms such as *independent, moderate assistance,* and *dependent* are used to rate the amount of assistance a client needs during self-care. The *ICF* uses the qualifiers *no problem, mild problem, moderate problem, severe problem,* and *complete problem* to rank the levels of difficulty that a person encounters when performing self-care (WHO, 2001). A numeric scale, such as one ranging from 1 to 7, is also used in some circumstances to delineate levels of independence. The occupational therapist can use any type of rating scale as long as the measures are identified and the descriptions of each

level are clearly defined. The measures should also make sense for the clients being evaluated and for the environment in which they are evaluated.

At times, therapists may rely on reports from the client, the client's family, and others involved in the client's care. Using these methods of self-report or proxy report, therapists gain more understanding of clients' perceived physical competence and learn the coping strategies used in daily activities. These methods, used in conjunction with other evaluation methods, provide a more comprehensive view of the client.

Exercise 15.2. Evaluation

Before moving on to intervention, think about Grace and Jon and perform an imaginary evaluation with them. What areas of self-care are going to be limited? What are the causes for the limitations? Are they body structures? Body functions? Environmental factors? Personal factors?

Self-Care Intervention

Occupational therapy practitioners provide intervention to increase a client's ability to participate in activities, in this case, self-care. Areas of disability should be addressed during goal setting before implementing interventions. Interventions are developed to remedy impairments in body structures and body functions, to maximize facilitating contextual factors, and to eliminate or lessen barriers. The evaluation will help to identify the problem areas. Once an occupational therapist completes the evaluation, the next step is to identify priorities, because it may be impossible to address everything simultaneously. Setting priorities helps the therapist and client focus on the most critical areas to target first.

Client preferences should strongly influence the priorities for intervention, but safety is more important than client preference. Although safety is often the client's highest priority, sometimes the client does not recognize his or her own deficits in judgment and safety awareness. The prevalence of falls in older people, for instance, may be caused in part by an inability to recognize potential hazards. A client may say to a practitioner that the first thing he or she wants to work on is learning to propel his or her wheelchair.

The practitioner, however, recognizes that because of the impairments to body structures, such as those present after a spinal cord injury, the client cannot reach or use the emergency call bell in the hospital room. Every person should be able to call for help if he or she needs it, which means that the first ADL task addressed for most hospitalized patients is using the call system to alert a nurse. The practitioner and the client should have candid, honest discussions when identifying and prioritizing goals.

Exercise 15.3. Priorities of Self-Care for Grace and Jon

What are the self-care priorities for Grace and Jon? Are there safety concerns? First, list as many problems as you can, considering Grace and Jon's conditions. Then put the list in order of priority. Examine your list and think about why you set the priorities as you did and what the rationales are that support your decisions. To do this, you need to use your imagination to fill out the occupational profiles of these individuals. For this exercise, it is fine to fill in the blanks regarding Grace's and Jon's values, priorities, and interests as you develop your rationales for setting priorities. When working with clients, you should ensure that rationales reflect the client's priorities and input.

After completing Exercise 15.3, recall if you identified toileting as a priority. What are the limitations that affect both Grace's and Jon's ability to use a bathroom independently? Read Case Example 15.1, Part 5, and Case Example 15.2, Part 5, and compare your list from the exercise with the priorities in the case examples.

In the case examples, note how communication between client and therapist can lead to mutually agreed-upon goals and priorities. For example, applying hair gel remains a priority for Jon, but both Jon and the therapist agree that they should address wound care and toileting first. In these situations, it is also important for the occupational therapy practitioner to emphasize the connection between improvement in one area leading to improvement in other areas. For instance, the therapist explains

Case Example 15.1, Part 5. Grace's Priorities

Grace is having a difficult time dealing with the changes she is undergoing. The stress of her upcoming wedding and the possibility that she may still have residual disabilities at that time sometimes overwhelm her. Through conversation, Grace and the occupational therapist decide that addressing her depression must start immediately, and intervention strategies specific to depression must be incorporated into every activity they work on.

Other priorities Grace identifies are learning to hold objects in both hands when walking (she wants to be able to carry her bouquet as she walks down the aisle without losing her balance) and being able to dress, bathe, and groom herself so she does not have to rely on others for help. Improving her ability to complete self-care activities independently is especially important to her because she knows how particular she is and she thinks others will be bothered by her idiosyncrasies.

Furthermore, Grace prefers not to change the type of clothing she likes to wear. Therefore, instead of wearing sweat pants with an elastic waist, she learns to use a button aid and zipper pull to fasten her pants after toileting. She is also thinking about what her priorities are for her job and realizes that working on these tasks will be useful in her job as well.

to Jon that working on wound care and toileting would lead to Jon's ability to apply hair gel more easily because they involve improving Jon's coordination using his nondominant hand.

Occupational therapy practitioners may use several theoretical approaches in helping clients choose priorities and make decisions about how to implement intervention. The theoretical base for a *strengths-based approach* postulates that demonstration, practice, repetition, and positive reinforcement are essential elements for increasing the client's competence and mastery of tasks (Deci & Ryan, 1985, 2008).

In this situation, the practitioner begins by using a *self-directed learning frame of reference* (Greber,

Case Example 15.2, Part 5. Jon's Priorities

Jon identifies being able to put gel in his hair as a priority. However, the therapist knows that one ADL task that must be addressed is cleaning the pin sites on Jon's arm. If these sites are not kept clean, infections can develop, which would slow recovery and perhaps lead to further disability. The therapist is not sure whether Jon is mature enough to realize the threat of infection, so one of the first things the therapist does is discuss this potential problem with Jon and his parents, emphasizing the importance of wound care in healing. Jon agrees to make wound care a top priority, which includes washing and drying his right arm, caring for the sling and bolster, and addressing issues of positioning in sitting and standing.

The therapist then discusses toileting with Jon. Jon is embarrassed and admits he does not use the bathroom at school because it is too difficult for him. However, after discussing it with the therapist, Jon agrees that working on toileting is a higher priority than hair care.

Jon's therapist asks about the pants he likes to wear, and Jon decides to put away his button-fly jeans until his arm heals. He chooses to wear sweat pants or loose-fit zipper-fly jeans rather than use an alternative technique such as using a button aid or other adaptive device to help with buttoning. Jon is so happy with the decision he made that he initiates wanting to switch to boxer shorts because briefs are too difficult for him to manage with one hand. If the therapist had not addressed toileting, Jon may not have developed compensatory strategies for this activity.

Hinojosa, & Ziviani, 2013), which involves promoting an individual's self-initiation in identifying his or her learning needs, formulating learning goals, choosing and implementing appropriate learning strategies, and evaluating learning outcomes. This approach was used when the therapist and Jon were deciding on using a button aid or wearing sweatpants. The therapist did not tell Jon that buttons are too difficult; instead, she suggested that many other clients have found that wearing sweatpants is more manageable and comfortable. This approach allowed Jon to make the final decision and increased his sense of competence and control.

The compensation approach to improve occupational performance (Gillen, 2013) involves the practitioner providing the client with various adaptive devices or compensatory strategies to complete a task. For example, Grace was given the opportunity to decide which button aid and zipper pull she felt comfortable using. Once she made the decision, the therapist used the self-directed learning frame of reference to teach her how to use the devices.

Activities are rarely addressed individually. Most activities occur in combinations. For instance, although one focus for both Grace and Jon was toileting, dressing also had to be addressed. This example illustrates a common occurrence in occupational therapy practice settings: Single treatment sessions frequently address multiple problem areas and multiple goals.

Where to Start Intervention

In many instances, it makes the most sense to start intervention at the level of body structures and functions. By improving the status of the body structures, performance of self-care activities improves. In this case, it is important for the occupational therapy practitioner to discuss the relation of the body structure or function to occupational performance, specifically its relationship to self-care. Clients may then be better able to articulate the relationship between specific intervention activities and the goals and activities with which they are associated. This generalization of learning helps the client participate in activities and occupations more fully.

Occupational therapy practitioners base the choice of which treatment approach to use on the client, the limitation, the environment, and all the other factors influencing participation. The treatment process is illustrated in Figure 15.2. The practitioner, after identifying specific problems, develops or selects a sound theoretical rationale for intervention. Included in this rationale is the understanding of how a person develops self-care competencies.

Next, the practitioner identifies a specific theory to facilitate change. This dynamic theory explains

Figure 15.2. Theoretically based intervention.

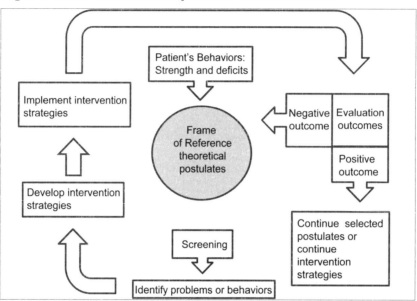

Source. T.-H. Howe. Used with permission.

how change will come about based on validated theories. Learning theories are the most common dynamic theories used to address facilitating ADL competencies. These theories explain how the practitioner should provide instruction to bring about positive outcomes or to shape a specific behavior. For example, the practitioner might use a *behavior theory,* which refers to procedures that change the consequences of behavior (Spiegler & Guevremont, 2010), to guide the shaping of skills for a person who has limited cognitive abilities.

With self-care, the practitioner bases the intervention on some combination of improving function and compensating for a permanent disability. Compensation involves two approaches: (1) changing the strategy used to complete the activity and (2) adding adaptive equipment or technology. In Figure 15.3, the client is using a universal cuff to hold the stylus for her touchscreen smartphone. Because of the paralysis that occurred as a result

Exercise 15.4. Theoretical Rationale for Intervention

Identify a theoretical rationale that you might use to guide your intervention for Jon and Grace. Create an intervention strategy based on the theoretical rationale that would be appropriate for Jon and Grace specific to their self-care goals.

of a spinal cord injury, she is unable to operate her smartphone in the usual way. Although she tried alternate handling methods during treatment, she and her therapist determined that using the universal cuff was the easiest and most effective way for her to hold the stylus. In this example, the therapist guided intervention by using a compensation approach to improve occupational performance. The purpose of this intervention approach is not to change a client's physical abilities but to provide an appropriate tool so the client can perform an occupation.

Addressing Body Structure and Body Function During Intervention

Body structure information tells the occupational therapy practitioner about diagnosis. The anatomical structure, including the presence and extent of impairment, sets the stage for occupational therapy intervention. It is more straightforward to see that a person with missing body parts may have difficulty performing self-care occupations or will need to perform self-care occupations using an alternative technique. The same is true for impairment of any body structure.

During the evaluation, the extent of impairment is identified and the expected recovery is determined. Goals are set according to the anticipated

Figure 15.3. A person with upper-extremity paralysis can access her smartphone with a stylus and a universal cuff.

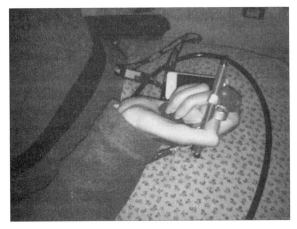

Source. A. Perr. Used with permission.

recovery and the expected ability of the client to compensate for any residual impairment. Related to body structures are body functions. How is the person able to function within the confines of the extent of impairment in any of the body structures?

The occupational therapy practitioner focuses his or her intervention at this level by extracting theoretical rationales from acquisitional frames of reference to guide the intervention. Consistent with the theoretical postulates, the occupational therapy practitioner encourages a client to learn specific skills required for the optimal performance within the client's environment. The practitioner uses purposeful activities to improve body function while maintaining body structures under the best conditions. Case Example 15.1, Part 6, and Case Example 15.2, Part 6, describe clients' interventions.

Guided by the compensation approach to improve occupational performance, both Grace and Jon will use alternative techniques to complete their self-care occupations. Part of the intervention for both clients may include training in upper-extremity range-of-motion exercises. To have the potential for the highest level of independence, both Jon and Grace need to maintain the structural integrity of their arms to allow them to use their arms as fully as possible when they are able to.

As stated earlier, occupational therapy practitioners must gather information about the contextual factors affecting a client's participation in self-care during evaluation by considering how the physi-

cal environment could influence participation. For example, the person pictured in Figure 15.4 has motor impairment secondary to a stroke. He has poor sitting and standing balance, and it is not safe for him to go to the bathroom, especially at night. The practitioner suggested that the commode be placed next to his bed. An additional benefit of placing the commode next to the bed is that he can use the rail for extra support during dressing. He can transfer from the bed to the commode and dress himself independently, without fear of

Figure 15.4. This man has poor sitting balance. He is able to perform lower body dressing while sitting on the bedside commode. Note that the armrests of the commode are available to provide support when he needs it.

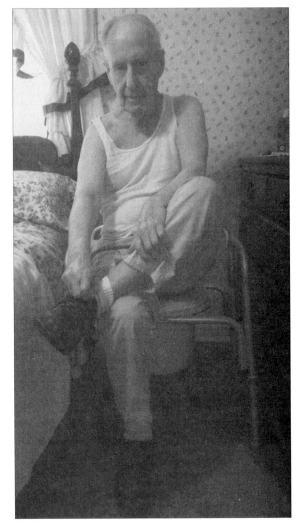

Source. M. Tranquilli. Used with permission.

Case Example 15.1, Part 6. Grace's Intervention

Grace had a hemorrhagic stroke during surgery. At the time of her intervention, she presented with a flaccid right arm. There was some neurological involvement in her right lower extremity and her trunk, but she could stand and walk. Although some cognitive deficits were noted, Grace's overall program was designed to allow medical recovery of body structures to occur, which meant occupational therapy intervention would include purposeful activities to attempt to improve Grace's ability to use her right arm.

Grace's diagnosis is complicated. There is no way to know how much of the blood will be reabsorbed or how much residual damage there will be. The expected recovery of the neurologic system is not known. Brain function may improve as the blood is reabsorbed, and the swelling resolves or the associated areas of the brain may take over for the damaged areas. Because of all these variables, the therapist may have difficulty predicting how much recovery will occur in Grace's flaccid right arm and in her cognitive functioning, so the therapy intervention has to be flexible to address her changing needs.

The theoretical rationale supporting this approach was derived from dynamic system theory and central nervous system plasticity (Sabari, 2008). However, the therapist simultaneously uses another frame of reference to encourage Grace to learn alternative techniques. To guide Grace to use her left arm, the therapist uses postulates from the compensatory frame of reference, which describes using alternative actions to complete tasks and to participate in activities.

For instance, Grace is guided to use her left arm as the dominant arm during activity and to position her right arm to act as a stabilizer. Another example is when a practitioner demonstrates to Grace how to stabilize her toothbrush while applying toothpaste with her left hand. The practitioner then gives Grace time to practice. One-hand techniques are also taught on the chance that she might not recover full function of her right arm. This frame of reference is based on learning theories that highlight the importance of demonstration, practice, and repetition to learn new skills.

As described earlier, Grace is depressed and anxious. A goal of occupational therapy intervention is to address her depression with treatment strategies that are integrated with her other goals. The practitioner uses a frame of reference based on Bandura's (1977) self-efficacy to address Grace's psychosocial functioning. The practitioner applies the theoretical postulates from this theory with the theoretical postulates of the other frames of reference depending on the occupation focused on during therapy. According to Bandura's social learning theory, modeling is an important strategy for learning positive behaviors as a process of improving self-efficacy, so the practitioner helps Grace to express positive expectations which then initiate and model the constructive behavior.

Case Example 15.2, Part 6. Jon's Intervention

Jon has a mostly temporary disability. In all likelihood, the bones will heal. He should recover fully, although a chance exists that he will have limited mobility in his forearm, affecting his ability to supinate and pronate. Jon also is at risk for developing infections at the wound sites. Therefore, the occupational therapy program for Jon focuses on the level of body functions by learning alternative techniques to promote self-care independence while his body structures mend.

falling. The same person is able to perform bed mobility independently after he followed a practitioner's suggestion that he change his bed mattress to a firmer one (Figure 15.5).

The treatment environment influences how the practitioner formulates treatment activities, as shown in Case Example 15.1, Part 7, and Case Example 15.2, Part 7. A discussion of treatment that occurs in simulated and real settings is given in Chapter 12, "Independence: Simulation of Life Activities to Occupations." Occupational therapy practitioners must consider activities' meaningfulness to clients and how to simulate natural environments in the in- or outpatient setting when developing the most optimal interventions for their

Figure 15.5. This man can perform bed mobility after switching to a firmer mattress on the recommendation of an occupational therapy practitioner.

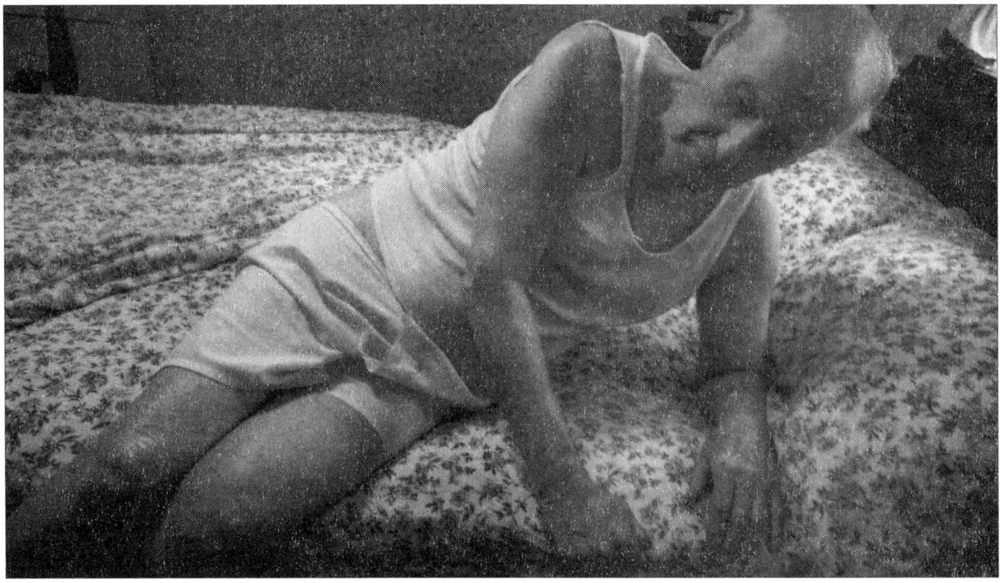

Source. M. Tranquilli. Used with permission.

clients. Many other factors must be considered when developing interventions, including personal factors, such as the client's age and gender, which influence the focus of the treatment, the types of purposeful activities the practitioner brings into treatment, and the client's priorities.

It would be important, for example, to know that a client is a vegetarian so that cooking activities used in therapy include ingredients the client will eat. It is just as important to know whether the person has dietary restrictions related to religion or personal taste and preferences. By tying personal factors to body functions and structures, a practitioner can, for example, see that a client wears dentures or has dysphagia and would prefer soft food that is easy to manage.

Group vs. Individual Treatment

Occupational therapy intervention can be delivered in both individual and group settings. Occupational therapy practitioners work individually with clients when one-to-one attention and assistance are required. Once the client has mastered a certain level of independence in his or her newly acquired skill, he or she can be treated in a group setting with others who have similar goals. Groups also emphasize the social nature of people, fostering physical and emotional supports among clients.

Self-care activities can be addressed effectively in groups. A common example is the existence of self-feeding groups in many settings. A group of clients with dysphagia may eat together, with a speech–language pathologist, an occupational therapy practitioner, or nursing assistant available for cuing

---

Case Example 15.1, Part 7. Grace's Summary

Grace is now on a rehabilitation unit in an acute care hospital and is likely to stay for about 3 weeks before she goes home. This environment is not similar to her home because Grace lives in a small apartment.

Case Example 15.2, Part 7. Jon's Summary

Jon is treated in an outpatient occupational therapy setting. This environment is not similar to his home because Jon lives in a large single-family house.

and assistance. Similarly, routine participation in a grooming group may be effective in helping a client with mental illness resume these activities. This routine group daily life activity uses Slagle's concept of rebuilding routines and allows each participant to develop and refine interpersonal communication skills and appropriate social behaviors (Schwartz, 2003).

Summary

Self-care intervention is central to successful occupational therapy. The occupational therapy practitioner can treat many body structures and body functions by focusing on the activities of daily life. Intervention involves identifying the factors that influence the client's ability to participate in self-care, making the most of the factors that facilitate participation, and lessening or eliminating the effect of barriers. The end result should be the highest level of independence or the highest degree of participation in the self-care that is addressed.

Acknowledgment

The authors thank Michael W. Tranquilli, MA, OTR, for providing photographs for this chapter.

References

American Occupational Therapy Association. (2014). Occupational therapy framework: Domain and process (3rd ed.). *American Journal of Occupational Therapy, 68*(Suppl. 1), S1–S48. http://dx.doi.org/10.5014/ajot.2014.682006

Bandura, A. (1977). Self-efficacy: Toward a unifying theory of behavioral change. *Psychological Review, 84,* 191–215. http://dx.doi.org/10.1037/0033-295X.84.2.191

Deci, E. L., & Ryan, R. M. (1985). *Intrinsic motivation and self-determination in human behavior.* New York: Plenum.

Deci, E., & Ryan, R. (2008). Facilitating optimal motivation and psychological well-being across life's domains. *Canadian Psychology, 49*(1), 14–34. http://dx.doi.org/10.1037/0708-5591.49.1.14

Gillen, G. (2013). Occupational therapy intervention for individuals. In B. A. B Schell, G. Gillen, & M. E. Scaffa (Eds.), *Willard and Spackman's occupational therapy* (12th ed., pp. 322–341). Philadelphia: Wolters Kluwer Health/Lippincott Williams & Wilkins.

Greber, C., Hinojosa, J., & Ziviani, J. (2013). Achieving success: Facilitating skill acquisition and enabling participation. In J. Ziviani, A. Poulsen, & M. Cuskelly (Eds.), *The art and science of motivation: A therapist's guide to working with children* (pp. 123–158). London: Jessica Kingsley.

Hinojosa, J., & Blount, M.-L. (Eds.). (2014). *The texture of life: Purposeful activities in the context of occupation* (4th ed.). Bethesda, MD: AOTA Press.

Kempen, G. I., Steverink, N., Ormel, J., & Deeg, D. J. (1996). The assessment of ADL among frail elderly in an interview survey: Self-report versus performance-based tests and determinants of discrepancies. *Journals of Gerontology, Series B: Psychological Sciences, 51,* 254–260. http://dx.doi.org/10.1093/geronb/51B.5.P254

Millán-Calenti, J. C., Tubío, J., Pita-Fernández, S., González-Abraldes, I., Lorenzo, T., Fernández-Arruty, T., & Maseda, A. (2010). Prevalence of functional disability in activities of daily living (ADL), instrumental activities of daily living (IADL) and associated factors, as predictors of morbidity and mortality. *Archives of Gerontology and Geriatrics, 50,* 306–310. http://dx.doi.org/10.1016/j.archger.2009.04.017

Sabari, J. S. (2008). Optimizing motor skill using task-related training. In M. V. Radomski & C. A. T. Latham (Eds.), *Occupational therapy for physical dysfunction* (6th ed., pp. 618–641). Philadelphia: Wolters Kluwer Health/Lippincott Williams & Wilkins.

Schneidert, M., Hurst, R., Miller, J., & Üstün, B. (2003). The role of environment in the *International classification of functioning, disability and health (ICF)*. *Disability and Rehabilitation, 25,* 588–595. http://dx.doi.org/10.1080/0963828031000137090

Schwartz, K. B. (2003). History of occupation. In P. Kramer & J. Hinojosa (Eds.), *Perspectives in human occupation: Participation in life* (pp. 18–31). Philadelphia: Lippincott Williams & Wilkins.

Spiegler, M. D., & Guevremont, D. C. (2010). *Contemporary behavior therapy* (5th ed.). Belmont, CA: Wadsworth/Cengage Learning.

World Health Organization. (2001). *International classification of functioning, disability and health—Short version.* Geneva: Author.

CHAPTER 16.

CARE OF OTHERS, ACTIVITIES, AND OCCUPATIONS

Kristine Haertl, PhD, OTR/L, FAOTA

Highlights

- ✧ Care and caregiving
- ✧ Caregiving occupations
- ✧ Gender and cultural influences
- ✧ Models of caregiving
- ✧ Parenting
- ✧ Stress, coping, and caregiver burden
- ✧ Role of occupational therapy in caregiving
- ✧ Evaluation
- ✧ Intervention.

Key Terms

- ✧ Authoritarian style
- ✧ Authoritative style
- ✧ Care
- ✧ Caregiver
- ✧ Caregiver burden
- ✧ Caregiving
- ✧ Care receiver
- ✧ Emotional care
- ✧ Evaluation
- ✧ Formal paid caregiving
- ✧ Home-based care
- ✧ Hospice
- ✧ Household care
- ✧ Informal unpaid caregiving
- ✧ Informational care
- ✧ Instrumental care

- ✧ Macro factors
- ✧ Medical care
- ✧ Micro factors
- ✧ Multi-Level Structural Caring Model
- ✧ Noninvolvement
- ✧ Parenting
- ✧ Parenting styles
- ✧ Permissive style
- ✧ Personal care
- ✧ Prevention–intervention continuum
- ✧ Process model
- ✧ Professional caring
- ✧ Role acquisition
- ✧ Role disengagement
- ✧ Role enactment

Caring for others and being cared for by someone are significant occupations. I begin this chapter with an overview of definitions of *care, caregiving,* and *care receiving.* Intrinsic to these definitions are the significant roles and responsibilities of the care providers. I also discuss formal paid caregiving and informal unpaid caregiving, as well as the ever-changing relationship between the caregiver and care receiver as circumstances change.

Next, I present caregiving and caregiving occupations in relation to roles and responsibilities of the people involved. After presenting a brief description of the characteristics of people receiving care, I examine the informal versus formal concept of care.

Two important factors in caregiving and care providing are gender and culture. In the section on gender and cultural influences, I discuss gender and cultural differences within caring roles and explore various parenting and caregiver models (Baumrind, 1967, 1971, 1996; Belsky, 1984), including parenting styles and determinants. I then present Leininger's (1988a) Multi-Level Structural Caring Model, followed by a discussion of the characteristics and consequences of stress and caregiver burden.

The chapter concludes with specific information about the roles and responsibilities of occupational therapy practitioners working with clients and families to assess and develop caregiving skills. Throughout the chapter, readers are encouraged to consider their personal and professional experiences in caregiving. In the exercises provided, readers are given an opportunity to engage in reflection to learn about their specific attitudes and values about caregiving and care receiving.

Care and Caregiving

Humans are social beings who give and receive care throughout life, sharing in daily activities while working to create meaning and satisfaction. From the arrival of a newborn to the passing on of a grandparent, people rely on one another to survive and thrive in the world. Consider a mother raising a toddler, a health practitioner looking after a dying patient, a sister babysitting a brother with a developmental disability, and spouses caring for one another. All these examples encompass acts of care

and caregiving. Our earliest memories often revolve around our parents and caregivers. Our care-receiving memories include when we engaged in playing with a favorite toy and when a parent served a favorite meal or taught us to ride a bike; such experiences shape our development and worldview.

Many in caring positions take on the most significant caregiver roles during the beginning and end of the life span. When relationships shift because of increases in caregiving needs, services from a health care practitioner or educator may be needed to facilitate improved care. Knowledge of care and caregiving is integral to the role of the occupational therapy practitioners in providing holistic services. Occupational therapy practitioners bring expertise to family intervention through their knowledge of physical, psychological, sensory, cognitive, and contextual elements that affect caregiving (American Occupational Therapy Association [AOTA], 2007).

The terms *care* and *caregiving* are often referred to in relation to one person taking care of another, as in a mother caring for a child or a daughter looking after an aging parent. Although the literature often denotes *parenting* as related to the roles and functions of biological or adoptive parents with their children and *caregiving* as the care for someone older (e.g., caring for an aging parent or a spouse with a brain injury), the terms are broader and more complex. *Care* and *caregiving* refer not only to looking after others or the self but also to the tending of and looking after plants and animals.

Definitions for the word *care* often include descriptions such as "concern for" or "anxiety about" others. *Merriam Webster's Online Dictionary* (2014) defines *care* as "suffering of mind"; "a disquieted state of mixed uncertainty, apprehension and responsibility"; "painstaking or watchful attention"; and "regard coming from desire or esteem." Additional descriptions of *care* include words and phrases such as "concern about," "protection," "watchful oversight," and "affection for" (*Collins Essential English Dictionary,* 2013). Thus, definitions of *care* often depend on the context in which the term is used.

Leininger (1988b) differentiated between general care and professional care. She defined *care* and *caring* as "those assistive, supportive, or facilitative acts toward or for another individual or group with evident or anticipated needs to ameliorate or improve a human condition or lifeway" (p. 9). *Professional caring* was defined as "those cognitive and culturally learned action behaviors, techniques, processes or patterns that enable (or help) an individual, family, or community to improve or maintain a favorably healthy condition or lifeway" (Leininger, 1988b, p. 9). Key commonalities in the definitions of *care* and *caring* generally transcend the feelings associated with the terms and focus on the actions required for caregiving.

Caregiving, with the root word *care,* refers to the process of providing care for another. Generally, the concept of *caregiver* refers to the person who provides the primary care and support to a person (Awad & Voruganti, 2008), yet definitions vary on the basis of culture, context, and formal versus informal caregiving. Typically, one person is the caregiver and the other the *care receiver,* but in many instances the role of caregiver may change. For example, a mother and father care for a child, but later in life the roles may change as the child takes care of an aging parent. Caregiving may also occur temporarily during instances of brief illness or disability, such as when a teenager requires extra care for a broken bone sustained in a ski accident or a sibling requires extra care during a bout of the flu.

A review of the literature reveals conceptualizations of caregiving that include both *formal paid caregiving* and *informal unpaid caregiving*. A nurse, home health aide, or occupational therapist may provide formal paid care, whereas a person may take care of a relative or friend in an informal and unpaid context.

Drentea (2007) defined *caregiving* as "the act of providing unpaid assistance and support to family members or acquaintances who have physical, psychological, or developmental needs." She identified three forms of care: (1) instrumental, (2) emotional, and (3) informational. *Instrumental care* includes facilitation of tasks that a person needs to do, such as cooking or providing transportation for a loved one. *Emotional care* involves providing support, emotional assistance, counseling, and emotional companionship. *Informational care,* a key type found in health care, may include education, adaptation of the environment, or training in compensatory techniques.

Despite the differences in types of caregiving, similarities between familial and professional caregiving often include an intense experience with few caregivers providing the care of a person over a 24-hour time period (Lynch & Lobo, 2012), thus supports for both the caregiver and person cared for are important to maximize health and well-being for all in the caregiving relationship.

Although care and caregiving are related concepts, they are not identical. The term *care* is often used primarily to denote emotional feelings, affection for, and concern for the well-being of another. *Caregiving,* however, encompasses the actions and occupations required to meet the daily needs of another. According to Sachs and Labovitz (2004), caregiving may embody aspects of caring, yet one may care for another without providing the actual daily caregiving, as in the instance of an older relative living at a long-term care facility. Similarly, a person may take on a formal caregiving role in a health care setting, yet not have the same affection for the client as would a family member or friend. It is, however, advantageous if the caregiver maintains an unconditional positive regard and has sincere concern for the well-being of the person being cared for.

Exercise 16.1. Caregiver and Care Receiver Roles

Identify the primary roles and activities you have taken on as caregiver and care receiver in your life. Answer these questions:

- How have these roles changed over the course of time?
- Consider your daily schedule and occupational demands. Do the roles of caregiver and care receiver have a prominent place, or do other occupational roles such as being a student require most of your time?
- Do you have competing responsibilities and caregiving roles that create role conflict?
- How can you work to balance your roles?
- How does your participation in the activities influence your daily occupations?
- How did your participation as a caregiver and care receiver influence the person receiving care occupations?
- How will your experiences as a caregiver and care receiver affect you as an occupational therapist?

Caregiving Occupations

Who are caregivers, and what are their roles and functions? Although context greatly influences the nature of caregiving across Western cultures, there are many similarities. Statistics cited by the Caregiver Action Network (2013) indicate that more than 67 million Americans (29% of the U.S. population) care for a family member who has a disability or is ill or aging in any given year. Nationally, of those over age 65 years requiring home health care, more than 80% had a caregiver outside of a formal agency, and men within this cohort were nearly three times as likely as women to have a spouse as their primary caregiver (Jones, Harris-Kojetin, & Valverde, 2012). Among caregivers, it is estimated that unpaid family members will likely continue to be the largest provider of long-term care services (U.S. Department of Health and Human Services, 2003), thus often necessitating education from a health care team including occupational therapy practitioners.

Approximately 66% of caregivers are women (National Alliance for Caregiving & AARP, 2009; Zukewich, 2003); however, people of all ages, genders, and sociocultural backgrounds may be called on to take on caregiving roles. Within Canada, statistics from 2008 to 2009 indicated that about one-third of those over age 45 were caring for someone with a health condition (Statistics Canada, 2012) and that such care involved both emotional tolls and personal satisfaction. In Europe, the familial statistics of caring are even higher; family members provide over 80% of care needs and two-thirds of the caregivers are women (Hoffman & Rodrigues, 2010). Although these statistics reflect the fact that the term *caregiving* is often used in relation to providing assistance for older adults or a person with a disability or temporary illness, caregiving also includes taking care of infants, children, and even plants and animals.

The process of caregiving is relational and involves both those giving care and those receiving care (Figures 16.1). Bumagin and Hirn (2001) identified primary care recipients as including young children, teenagers, persons with temporary or permanent disabilities, and older adults. The authors identified determinants of caregiving to include factors related to who is giving the care, who is receiving the care, how and when the care is given, and the physical and monetary costs.

Although there may be a primary relationship between caregiver and care receiver (e.g., a mother taking care of an infant), caregiving may also

Figure 16.1. Parents should reinforce contributions to daily routines by including children in the completion of household chores.

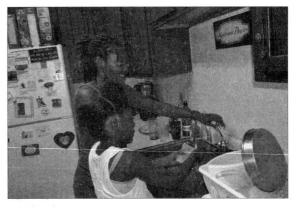

Source. K. Haertl. Used with permission.

involve complex coordination of relationships, such as a child with special needs receiving services from multiple academic and health service agencies (see Case Example 16.1). Within these situations, the role of primary caregiver may change, and communication between caregivers is crucial to provide comprehensive client-centered care.

In the example of John, the nature of caregiving is formal and multifaceted. John has lived in several foster homes and receives care for his basic physical, cognitive, emotional, and academic needs. While it is relatively easy to define the role of pri-

---

Case Example 16.1. John: Identifying Caregivers

John is a 7-year-old child with moderate mental retardation, cerebral palsy, fetal alcohol syndrome, and oppositional defiant disorder. His biological mother was a drug user and abandoned him at birth, and his father's identity is unknown. John has lived in various foster care homes throughout his life. Because of recent assaultive behaviors, he was placed in a crisis home and is currently receiving services through the home, school, and county.

Who are the caregivers in this situation? Are they formal or informal caregivers? What can an occupational therapy practitioner do to facilitate the coordination of care in this instance?

mary caregiver in a parental relationship, it is far more complex in John's situation because the staff members at the crisis home, his case manager, and the special education professionals all have unique roles in John's care.

Caregiving and care receiving may be categorized on the basis of the relationship and the informal versus formal nature of the care provided. Lackey and Gates (2001) classified caregiving for a family member with illness into four broad categories: (1) provision of personal care, (2) provision of medical care, (3) provision of household care, and (4) spending time (emotional care) with the person. *Personal care* includes such tasks as assistance with bathing, grooming, dressing, and feeding. *Medical care* includes the daily activities that assist a person in meeting medical needs, such as wound care or medication administration. *Household care* includes assistance with daily tasks such as cooking and cleaning. *Emotional care* includes providing support by spending time with, talking to, or praying with the care receiver. Drentea's (2007) categorizations differ in broadening the scope to include instrumental, emotional, and informational tasks.

Perhaps one of the most comprehensive conceptualizations of caregiving is that of Sellick (2005), who identified six domains of wellness that are crucial to both the caregiver and the care receiver. Sellick asserted the importance of maintaining wellness within the caregiver–care receiver relationship in these six domains:

1. *Physical:* physical needs, fitness, nutrition, lifestyle, health and medical
2. *Emotional:* expression of feelings, control of stress, problem solving, self-efficacy
3. *Social:* relational; respect for self and others; interaction with the environment, people, pets, and community; social cause
4. *Spiritual:* purpose in life, morals and ethics, self-determination, love, hope, faith
5. *Intellectual:* lifelong learning, cognition, exploration
6. *Vocational:* skill development, work, volunteerism, personal interests.

Consideration of each of these domains of well-being for both the caregiver and the care receiver is crucial to enhancing quality of life (QoL) and the caregiver–care receiver relationship.

Gender and Cultural Influences

Gender and culture heavily influence the roles and functions of caregiving and the development of related skills (Figure 16.2). From our early years, we learn about ourselves and our environment through

Figure 16.2. A child learns to complete complex household activities with the close supervision and assistance of her mother.

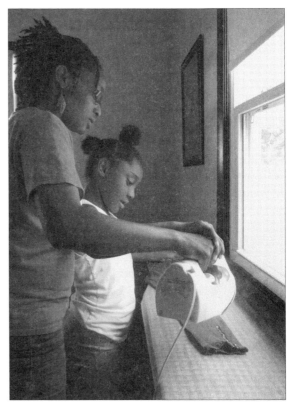

Source. K. Haertl. Used with permission.

our caregivers, often our parents, as the primary role models. The nature of the caregiving relationship may be positive, marked by mutual affection, or it may be strained, as in the instance of a child growing up with an abusive or alcoholic parent.

Regardless of the circumstances, parents are generally the socializing agents for gender roles within society (Leaper, 2002). Whereas primary child-rearing responsibilities traditionally focused on the mother, in recent years fathers have increased their role in child rearing (Riina & Feinberg, 2012). However, differences exist between mothering and fathering, and parents often differentiate how they treat their children on the basis of gender, for example, through the way they dress their children or the toys they give to them (Figure 16.3).

The blending of gender roles has occurred over time, as evidenced, for example, in the increase in numbers of women who are doctors and lawyers and of men taking on significant roles in parenting and child care. In addition, the number of adoptions of children by gay and lesbian couples has increased (Geisler, 2012); thus, the familial and parenting structures have changed over time. Still, Western cultures have maintained distinct differences between genders, as exemplified in the toy aisles of department stores or in television advertisements aimed at audiences of a particular gender.

Generally, caregivers teach girls to care for and nurture dolls, and they give boys trucks, cars, and action figures. Such socialization may lend itself to differing roles for the caregivers: Fathers tend to engage in more physical play with their children,

Figure 16.3. Caregivers can reinforce education goals by becoming involved in their child's homework.

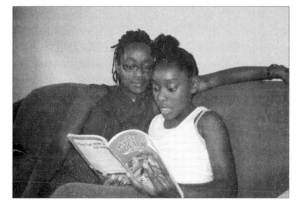

Source. K. Haertl. Used with permission.

whereas mothers engage in more imaginary play (Lindsey & Mize, 2001). Men also are more likely to use more technological approaches in socializing their children, whereas women use creative and pretend forms of play (Abrahamy, Finkelson, Lydon, & Murray, 2003). Gender roles further extend to the socialization of emotion not only in gender differences in emotional expression but also in the responsiveness to emotion based on gender (Root & Denham, 2010), thus influencing gender expression physically, socially, and emotionally.

Gender differences are also noted as people age and take on responsibility for older children, spouses, or parents in relation to tasks, responsibilities, and psychological responses to caregiving (Coutinho, Hersch, & Davidson, 2006; Dahlberg, Demack, & Bambra, 2007; Etters, Goodall, & Harrison, 2008). Some of these caregiving roles may be planned, such as when a couple decides to have children or chooses to assist in caring for a grandchild. Some, however, are unplanned, as in the case of a spouse's traumatic injury or when an aging parent suddenly requires care.

Social behaviors of caring reflect expectations of relationships through the cultural milieu in which the caregiving takes place. The phenomenon of caring is universal, yet it is uniquely expressed across cultures and time. *Culture* includes the beliefs, values, and activities existing within a particular setting or group. Given the many cultural groupings as well as heterogeneity within in-group differences, culture is difficult to universally define (Cardemil, 2010). Although often referred to in relation to ethnic background, the term is far more comprehensive and may include socioeconomic status, geographical locale, gender, sexual orientation, ability status, age, and even a particular professional cohort (Figure 16.4).

Despite the various cultural groupings, much of the literature and research on similarities and differences in caregiving practices is based on ethnic groups. The meaning of caregiving within the familial structure is often ethnocentrically based (Napoles, Chadiha, Eversley, & Moreno-John, 2010); therefore, an understanding of the interface of cultural values and caregiving is essential to providing quality services (McCleary & Blain, 2013). In the United States, older adults from ethnic minority groups are more likely to be taken care of by an extended family network than is true of their European-American counterparts (Yarry, Stevens, & McCallum, 2007), and Latinos and African-Americans are less likely to be taken care of exclusively by a spouse (Sörensen & Pinquart, 2005).

Similarly, Mexican-Americans tend to want to live closer to extended kin than do European-Americans (Burr & Mutchler, 1999). However, integration into U.S. society and socioeconomic factors may also affect the extent to which a person meets financial and personal responsibilities in extended family caregiving (Sarkisian, Gerena, & Gerstel, 2007). Findings have indicated high percentages of Asian-Americans taking care of extended family and aging relatives, but to a slightly lesser extent than other ethnic groups (National Alliance for Caregiving & AARP, 2009).

Figure 16.4. Within the caregiving role, the teaching of basic activities of daily living begins at a young age.

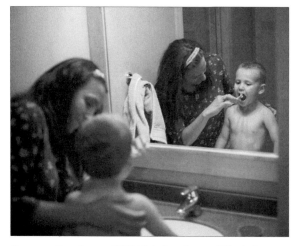

Source. Courtesy of Jill Hotujec (www.jillhotujec-photography.com). Used with permission.

Despite these differences, common variables exist across cultures. Some commonalities include the learning of caregiving roles from parents and kin during the developmental years; personal and cultural beliefs about the responsibility for taking care of one's family or kin; and the development of unique cross-cultural beliefs about caregiving, incorporating personal and familial beliefs, attitudes, and behaviors (Ayalong, 2004).

Models of Caregiving

Although a comprehensive presentation of models of caregiving is beyond the scope of this chapter, a general understanding is important for occupational therapy practitioners. Just as the *Occupational Therapy Practice Framework: Domain and Process* (AOTA, 2014) addresses clients at the level of people, organizations, and populations, caregiving theories apply to all levels of service delivery. Conceptually, caregiving models vary in their focus from a global perspective on the systems and structures that support and govern caregiving to a more individualized emphasis on practitioner care and the relationship between caregivers and care receivers. Authors have described micro factors and macro factors that affect caregiving at all levels (e.g., Leininger, 1988a; Mak, 2005).

The *Multi-Level Structural Caring Model* proposed by Leininger (1988a) is a hierarchical model used to conceptualize the scope, nature, and structures of caring. This model's highest level is a worldwide multicultural societal focus of caring. Leininger (1988a) asserted that study within this level can generate information regarding broad views and theoretical underpinnings of care. At the midlevel, specific cultures and systems are emphasized, providing information about the systemic aspects of culture that influence care, such as legal, political, health care, and economic systems. At the lowest level are the individual or group foci, conceptualizing caring structures and functions within family or small interpersonal groups.

In contrast to large groupings, authors have also identified multilevel factors that influence caregiving on an interpersonal level. Mak (2005) identified *macro factors* affecting individual caregivers, including sociocultural factors (e.g., ethnicity, age, gender, income); interpersonal factors, such as marital factors and kinship ties; structural factors, such as managed care and health care systems; and clinical factors, such as the health of the caregiver and care receiver. *Micro factors* that influence caregiving include the individual experiences, day-to-day encounters, and occupational patterns within the caregiving relationship.

A caregiving relationship may have strengths in certain factors, such as a close caring relationship, yet be negatively affected by lack of resources, exacerbation of illness, role strain, or limited health care coverage. To provide holistic client-centered services, health practitioners must plan evaluation and interventions taking all levels of caregiving into consideration.

Parenting

Parenting includes familiar activities of daily living (ADLs) and the development of performance patterns that incorporate the addition of a child into the family's daily life (Giese, 2010). Adding a child to a family is always an adjustment. When there are added complexities of the disability of a child or parent, the process may need the service of a health care team, including an occupational therapy practitioner.

In recent years, parenting models emphasize an ecological theoretical framework that acknowledges multiple factors that influence parenting and child development (Farnfield, 2008). Research on parenting and subsequent theories and models are often focused on the relationship between parent and child based on attachment theory (Bowlby, 1982), styles of parenting (Baumrind, 1967, 1971, 1996), and parental processes (Belsky, 1984). A comprehensive description of attachment styles and temperament may be found in the psychology literature; for the purposes of this chapter, the works of Baumrind (1967, 1971, 1996) and Belsky (1984; Belsky, Pasco Fearon, & Bell, 2007; Belsky, Vandell, et al., 2007) are discussed. Consideration of these prominent models should include a bioecological perspective that acknowledges individual factors and the interactions of the parent, child, and environment (Kiff, Lengua, & Zalewski, 2011; Figure 16.5).

Baumrind's Presentation of Parenting Styles

In her seminal work, Baumrind (1967, 1971) found that parents differ in their expressions of maturity,

Figure 16.5. Occupational engagement within the home enables children to learn daily family routines and habits.

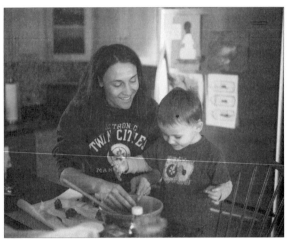

Source. Photograph courtesy of Jill Hotujec (www. jillhotujecphotography.com). Used with permission.

communication, discipline, and warmth. On the basis of these dimensions, she identified distinct *parenting styles*, including permissive, authoritative, authoritarian, and noninvolvement.

The *permissive style* of parenting governs children in an accepting, affirmative, and nonpunitive manner. In this style, parents generally make few demands of the child and maximize child input, yet do not seek to model antisocial behaviors, behaviors that result in disobedience, or low tolerance for challenge. Over time, a child with permissive parents may lack self-control and may struggle with the firm demands later placed on him or her in school.

An *authoritative style* of parenting emphasizes autonomy and self-will; values the child's gifts, talents, and individuality; and yet sets clear expectations for standards. This type of parenting leads to a well-adjusted child with the ability to regulate emotion and positive social skills. In this style of parenting, parents value the child's individuality but continue to maintain their parental authority and their role in setting limits.

An *authoritarian style* of parenting seeks to shape the child's behaviors through discipline, firm expectations, and a set code of conduct. This type of parent is often strict and may use external forces and rules, such as those derived from religion, specific philosophies, or an external set of beliefs to help guide parenting. Some people equate authoritarian styles with more control and less flexibility, which may lead to children with anxious and withdrawn demeanors and poor frustration tolerance.

A final style of parenting includes *noninvolvement,* which may result in low responsiveness, low involvement, and low demands. In extreme cases, a parent may neglect the child or leave him or her without the necessary care. Over decades of research, Baumrind (1967, 1971, 1996) concluded that the authoritative parenting style, which seeks to use warmth and guidance through listening and shaping the child's behaviors, is most effective and results in a happier, better-adjusted child than the other parenting styles.

Although contextual cultural variations occur in parenting styles, Sorkhabi's (2005) work concluded that Baumrind's (1967, 1971) four parenting styles are applicable to both individualistic and collectivist cultures. She asserted, however, that the manifestations of parenting styles may not result in similar outcomes in collectivist cultures and that more research is needed to confirm this assertion. Recent research on youth from a diverse cultural representation suggests that parenting styles influence adolescent development and response to conflict, yet multiple variables must be taken into account, including the dynamics of the relationships within the family, the environment, the nature of conflict, and the presence of psychological difficulties (McKinney & Renk, 2011).

Thus, although Baumrind's work applies to diverse populations, care must be taken to apply holistic client-centered practices to working with families. Baumrind's seminal work on parenting styles continues to be upheld and used in various studies to investigate the effects of parenting practices (e.g., Brenner & Fox, 1999; Dehyadegary, Yaacob, & Juhari, 2012; Woolfson & Grant, 2006).

Belsky's Process Model

Research has revealed a link between the quality of parenting and subsequent child development (Belsky, Vandell, et al., 2007). Whereas Baumrind (1967, 1971) emphasized parenting styles, Belsky (1984) developed a *process model* that sought to explain the determinants or factors that influence parenting and their subsequent effects on child development. Belsky's (1984) model asserts that

"parents' developmental histories, marital relations, social networks, and jobs influence individual personality and general psychological well-being of parents and, thereby, parental functioning and, in turn, child development" (p. 84).

Belsky identified three domains or determinants influencing the parental process: (1) personal and psychological resources of the parents, (2) characteristics of the child, and (3) contextual sources of stress and support. He determined that the most powerful determinants in supporting parental function and child development were parental personality and psychological well-being. This model assumes that parenting is influenced by forces both internal and external to the parent and child, along with the contextual factors in which the parenting takes place. Marital relationship, social network, and work are major contextual influences on stress and support. Belsky asserted that many factors influence parenting; however, these factors do not equally influence the parenting process. Personality and developmental history indirectly shape the parenting process through a broader context.

Subsequent to Belsky's original research and model, Belsky, Vandell, et al. (2007) found that although parenting is most influential in determining child development, the quality of early childcare experiences external to the home also affects development, performance, and behavior. In addition, there seem to be cultural differences in some of the determinants of parenting. Cardoso, Padilla, and Sampson (2010) found that patterns of parental maternal stress in non-Hispanic White and non-Hispanic Black populations were consistent with Belsky's model, yet for Mexican-American mothers, social support rather than spousal support helped ameliorate parental stress. Therefore, determinant factors of parenting should include a cultural lens, and through an understanding of the determinants of parenting and caregiving, therapists should work to teach skills designed to enhance the relationship between caregiver and care receiver (Figure 16.6).

Stress, Coping, and Caregiver Burden

With respect to care of an older adult or an ill person, models differ in their approach from the

Figure 16.6. Fathers play an integral role in the development of the child.

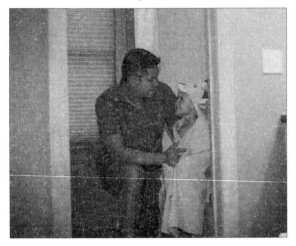

Source. Photograph courtesy of Jill Hotujec (www.jillhotujecphotography.com). Used with permission.

parenting models discussed earlier. Many of the models of caring for people with an illness or a disability focus on the stress, coping demands, and caregiver burden of the caregiving situation. The term *caregiver burden* refers to the emotional, financial, and physical strains resulting from a caregiving situation. However, some researchers have argued that models of caregiving that focus only on stress and burden are inadequate given the complexity of caregiving situations (Upton & Reed, 2006). They proposed that models of care for someone with an illness or disability must take into account the caregiver, care receiver, and context in which the caregiving takes place.

Care for an ill, infirmed, or older person occurs in many environments, including institutionalized settings, small group homes, health care facilities, and within the family home. With numbers of older adults increasing globally, many nations have reemphasized aging in place and family-based care (Bhattarai, 2013). *Home-based care* may include specialized in-home services in addition to education of the caregiver and family to maximize QoL for all and to decrease caregiver and care receiver stress.

A caregiver's stress increases when a person considers additional external demands. Many contextual variables influence caregiver stress and burden, yet researchers have emphasized the importance of the subjective perceptions of family members and caregivers in determining levels of caregiver burden

(Bumagin & Hirn, 2001; Murray, Tarren-Sweeny, & France, 2011). Given similar illnesses and family situations, differences occur in perceived stress. Variability results from familial relationships, external supports, and attitudes toward the caregiving situation. Some families and people are more resilient to the stressors resulting from caregiving roles, whereas others struggle to meet their daily obligations along with caregiving demands.

Positive coping strategies, caregiver mastery, social support, and education have been shown to mediate the stress caused by caregiver burden (Ergh, Rapport, Coleman, & Hanks, 2002; Murray et al., 2011; Pakenham, 2001; Pioli, 2010; Wells, Dywan, & Dumas, 2005). A sense of coherence or a perceived ability to respond to stress by using effective coping strategies is important in maintaining caregiver health and decreasing caregiver burden (Chumbler, Grimm, Cody, & Beck, 2003; Gallagher, Wagenfeld, Baro, & Haepers, 1994). Perceived self-efficacy and ability to handle caregiver situations also influence caregiver burden (Riley, 2007).

Within occupational therapy, practitioners emphasize skill building and creating a client–environment fit (Dooley & Hinojosa, 2004) to maximize occupational performance and reduce stress. Everyday occupation and co-occupational involvement between caregivers and care receivers have been found to create meaning and help mitigate disruption and stress in caregiving situations (Abelenda & Helfrich, 2003; Hasselkus & Murray, 2007). Occupational therapy practitioners working with caregivers may emphasize providing family supports to reduce stress and maximize QoL for both caregivers and care receivers. Thus, a family perspective and clear understanding of the complexities of the occupational therapy practitioner–family relationship are integral to maximizing health and QoL (Klein & Liu, 2010).

In addition to servicing families within the hospital and home settings, occupational therapy practitioners are instrumental in the facilitation of care transition (moving from one setting to another). Families may have to cope with caregiving at home with guilt and ambivalence should a child with disabilities have to be placed in a group home or an older spouse or family member in a nursing home. Kellett (1999) identified five themes common to family caregivers after nursing home placement:

1. A perceived loss of control
2. A feeling of disempowerment
3. A perceived sense of failure
4. Feelings of simultaneous sadness, guilt, and relief
5. The feeling of being forced to make a negative choice.

A person may experience such feelings of ambivalence and loss when having to place a child with disabilities in a group home. It is important for occupational therapy practitioners to support the family through such transitions and to include the family members in decisions regarding the extent and nature of their involvement after placement. Practitioners can support families and caregivers by maintaining contact and staying involved with their family member's care in several ways through visits, involvement with the care team, and ongoing communication.

In recent years, specialists have placed additional emphasis on encouraging research and models of care that provide support for family caregivers and emphasize the preservation of meaning and QoL for both caregiver and care receiver (e.g., Sellick, 2005; Vellone, Piras, Talucci, & Cohen, 2008). Within home-based care, Corcoran and Gitlin (2001) examined 100 caregivers and occupational therapy strategies used within the home. They found that caregivers were receptive to environmental and social strategies to improve care and that 81% of them followed through and used suggested intervention strategies. The use of such

---

Exercise 16.4. Long-Term Care Facility or Group Home

Have you ever had a friend or family member placed in a long-term care facility or group home? What was the influence on the family and on the person placed in the long-term care facility or group home? As an occupational therapy practitioner, what strategies can you use to facilitate family involvement after placement? How can the family still maintain meaningful occupational and social engagement with the person placed in the long-term care facility or group home? How will you, as the occupational therapy practitioner, support the family in working through these transitions?

---

strategies appeared to enhance overall personal and family health.

In addition to home-based care, *hospice* models designed for people at the end of life focus on dignity, comfort, and QoL throughout the dying process. Although experts initially designed hospice care for end-of-life issues, many of its goals are applicable to all caregiving situations. Four key values identified by Lattanzi-Licht (2001) within the hospice model are the worth of the person, the importance of choice and self-determination, provision for whole-person care, and family-centered care.

Hospice stresses the importance of support to the dying person, his or her family members, and his or her loved ones in areas including QoL, self-worth, individuality, security, and autonomy (Lattanzi-Licht, 2001). Hospice also aims to enhance dignity through holistic, individualized approaches that focus on comfort, pain management, and care. This support continues for the family after the loved one's death, with grieving, recognition of the loss, and a period of mourning being part of the process. Such care may also include the community, neighbors, and those who care about the person to provide education and support throughout the entire hospice experience (e.g., Poroch, 2012).

During the transition into hospice, daily patterns and activities may shift, yet the preservation of self-worth, dignity, and meaning is imperative. In studying people in hospice, Jacques and Hasselkus (2004) found that throughout the dying process, occupational engagement takes on new meaning even in ordinary and familiar everyday activities. Provision for daily routines that support meaningful occupational engagement and co-occupation between caregivers and care receivers throughout all phases of care appear to mediate stress brought on by daily requirements of caregiving and the transition to hospice or other caregiving facilities.

The role of rehabilitation practitioners in the hospice environment includes working to maintain function in the end-of-life process and serving to preserve and enhance overall QoL for the entire family (Javier & Montagnini, 2011). Thus, practitioners serving all client populations may benefit from consideration of the goals and values of the hospice model in supporting QoL throughout all phases of habilitation, rehabilitation, and caregiving.

Role of Occupational Therapy in Caregiving

As the demographic profiles of many industrialized nations shift toward increasing numbers of older adults, the occupational therapy profession must work to meet the needs of increasing numbers of families who are informal caregivers for those with illness and disability. Although many health professions adhere to models of caregiving, occupational therapy practitioners hold a unique viewpoint in their emphasis on the use of meaningful activities and occupation in the intervention process. A comprehensive review of the need for occupational therapy services in caregiving families revealed key themes, including

- Importance of emphasizing meaning and motivation in the caregiving relationship;
- Emphasis on caregiver–care receiver occupations and the use of meaningful activities in therapy;
- Acknowledgment of gender roles that often influence occupational engagement;
- Importance of developing positive caregiving–care receiving routines and habits;
- Management and development of environmental structures and modifications to support occupation performance and improve outcomes; and
- Use of models (e.g., Person–Environment–Occupation Model; Law, 1998) to facilitate positive adaptation (Coutinho et al., 2006).

The AOTA (2014) *Framework* cites an overarching assertion of occupational therapy's domain in "promoting the health and participation of persons, groups, and populations through engagement in occupation" (p. S1). Within the realm of caregiving, occupational therapy practitioners work with families to maximize client participation, meaning, and engagement in occupations and related activities that support the development of caregiving skills. The primary client may include the caregiver (e.g., a client with mental health concerns who is learning parenting skills), the care receiver (e.g., a client with dementia whose family must be educated in the client's caregiving needs), or an entire system (e.g., facilitating positive environments for seniors).

When considering environmental and caregiver supports to maximize occupational engage-ment, Haertl (2011) emphasized the importance of including the family and the extended care network (additional people involved with a client's care and daily activities) throughout the evaluation and intervention process. For family, key questions identified by Haertl include

- What is the role of the family in the client's life?
- Are there conflicts within the family, and what is the client's view of the family?
- To what extent is the family involved in the therapy process?
- Will the client return to live with the family (or spouse)? If not, where will the client live?
- Is there agreement regarding the course of intervention among the family, health professionals, and other care providers? and
- What are the family's strengths, resources, and needs? How can the strengths be most effectively used, and how can the needs be most successfully met?

Key questions for the extended care network include

- Who are the important people in the client's life, and how will the extended care network be involved in the therapy process?
- Are the caregivers adequately trained, prepared, and willing to follow through with the intervention plan? What are the training needs?
- What extended care network resources are available, and how can they best be used?
- What are the strengths and needs of the extended care network; how are they used?

Family and caregiver occupational therapy services should bolster social supports and enhance family strengths and function (Jaffe, Humphry, & Case-Smith, 2010). Such support may include the use of direct models of intervention, education, and adaptation or home modification. An occupational therapist might evaluate or intervene at the client, family, or systems level.

Evaluation

Evaluation is learning about clients' needs and strengths and involves the use of various methods and strategies. Some evaluations are nonstandardized and involve observation and interviews, and others involve the use of standardized assessments. Although the AOTA's (2014) *Framework* lists care of others and care of pets as instrumental activities of daily living (IADLs) within occupational therapy's domain of practice, limited options are available pertaining to direct occupational therapy–standardized assessments for parenting and caregiving. Most of the formalized instruments designed for the assessment of ADLs and IADLs focus on self-care skills rather than care of others.

Sachs and Labovitz (2004) identified the use of interviews, ethnography, and the Canadian Occupational Performance Measure (COPM; Law et al., 1994) as client-based tools that an occupational therapist might use to identify caregiver needs and priorities. An occupational therapist might use the updated COPM with both clients and families to identify priorities, goals, and client–caregiver perceptions of change over time (Law et al., 2005). A newer family-based tool in occupational therapy, the Life Participation for Parents (Fingerhut, 2013), assesses parental satisfaction and participation in daily occupations. Therapists may also use formal and informal occupation-based self-reports, interviews, and observations to assess the caregiver relationship and to identify strengths and needs related to priorities for therapy.

Outside the field of occupational therapy, several interdisciplinary tools exist related to parenting and caregiving. From an interdisciplinary perspective, Gordon (2012) identified the use of questionnaires, observation, clinical expertise, and interviews as integral to the parenting evaluation process. Evaluations may focus on determining actual skills in parenting or, for court-related purposes, determining whether a person is fit to parent. Often these types of assessments focus on observation and self-report.

The Parenting Stress Index (PSI; Abidin, 1995) is a self-report instrument often used in high-risk families to identify parents' stress levels. The PSI is designed for parents of children with physical and emotional problems, for families at risk of failing to promote normal development, and for parents who may be at risk for dysfunctional parenting. Measurements are rated on a Likert-type 5-point scale that ranges from *strongly agree* to *strongly disagree* in relation to child characteristics, parent personality, and contextual variables.

In recent years, the PSI has had increased international use, including in China (Yeh, Chen, Li, & Chuang, 2001), Japan (Tachibana et al., 2012), and India (Gupta, Mehrota, & Mehrota, 2012). Therapists also use the short form for assessing parents of a child with autism (Zaidman-Zait et al., 2010). When used with alternative populations, a therapist should be cautious because studies suggest that certain items may not fully replicate psychometric properties when used to compare families without children with disabilities (Zaidman-Zait et al., 2010).

For families who have a child with autism spectrum disorder, the Autism Parenting Stress Index effectively identifies parents who need extra supports (Silva & Schalock, 2012). Similar to other tools, the instrument has parents self-report on a Likert scale ranging from 0 (*not stressful*) to 5 (*so stressful we cannot cope*). Recent research indicates that two other questionnaires, the Parent Behavior Importance Questionnaire–Revised (Mowder & Shamah, 2011a) and the Parent Behavior Frequency Questionnaire–Revised (Mowder & Shamah, 2011b), appear to have sound psychometric properties and may be useful measures before, during, and after parental training programs.

Another interview-based tool, the Structured Problem Analysis of Raising Kids (Staal, van den Brink, Hermanns, Schrijvers, & van Stel, 2011), has been shown to be effective in identifying risks and needs in families of toddlers. Another widely used tool in research, the Alabama Parenting Questionnaire (Frick, 1991), includes both child and parent versions to assess five dimensions of parenting: (1) positive involvement with children, (2) supervision and monitoring, (3) use of positive discipline, (4) consistency with discipline, and (5) use of corporal punishment. Although it has been used fairly extensively in research (e.g., Elgar, Waschbusch, Dadds, & Sigvaldason, 2007; Hawes & Dadds, 2006; Scott, Briskman, & Dadds, 2011), the questionnaire has practical application in both clinical and research settings.

In addition to self-questionnaires, observation and task assessment are helpful in parenting and caregiving situations. The Keys to Interactive Parenting Scale (Comfort & Gordon, 2005) is an observational tool designed to measure parent behaviors with children 2 months old through preschool age. The evaluator conducts a videotaped observation in a familiar environment and rates parents on 12 behaviors in areas such as sensitivity, involvement in child activities, reasonable expectations, and responsiveness to the child. Informal play and parent–child interaction observations are also used to determine strengths and needs for planning intervention.

Evaluation of caregivers for older adults and for people with disabilities often includes a survey of the strengths and needs in the caregiving situation and a review of the caregiving environment. Instruments fall into both general and illness-specific categories. Several tools, including the Carers' Checklist (Hodgson, Higginson, & Jefferys, 1998), Caregiver Burden Inventory (Novak & Guest, 1989), Caregiving Activity Survey (Davis et al., 1997), and Caregiver Reaction Assessment (Given et al., 1992), are specifically designed to assess caregiving situations for older adults and people with cognitive disorders and dementia (Figure 16.7).

The Carers' Checklist is designed for people with dementia and their caregivers; it assesses the

Figure 16.7. Over time, caregiving roles may shift. In this setting, a well 92-year-old is assisted by her daughter for transportation needs.

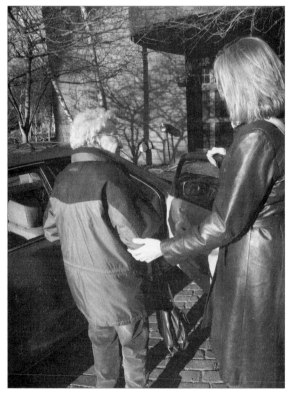

Source. K. Haertl. Used with permission.

caregiving situation, the symptoms of dementia, the burden of care, the strengths and needs of the caregiving situation, and the impact of services. A therapist can use this tool to facilitate intervention planning and monitor change over time. The Caregiving Activity Survey monitors use of time within the daily occupations of the caregiving relationship, including communication, transportation, dressing, eating, appearance and grooming, and supervision. An updated version (McCarron, Gill, Lawlor, & Beagly, 2002) includes bathing, toileting, housekeeping, and nursing activities.

The Caregiver Burden Inventory (Novak & Guest, 1989) reviews five dimensions of burden: (1) time-dependent, (2) developmental, (3) physical, (4) social, and (5) emotional. The Caregiver Reaction Assessment examines and measures caregiver reaction to caring for an older relative with an illness. Dimensions measured include esteem; lack of family support; and impact on schedules, finances, and health. A Chinese version of the instrument was recently found to have sound psychometrics (Ge et al., 2011).

Another tool, the American Medical Association's Caregiver Self-Assessment, has been shown to be useful in improving health services to families and in early identification of caregiver depression (Epstein-Lubow, Gaudiano, Hinckley, Salloway, & Miller, 2010). Additional general tools, such as the Appraisal of Caregiving Scale (Oberst, 1991; Oberst, Thomas, Gass, & Ward, 1989), the Caregiver Burden Scale (Elmståhl, Malmberg, & Annerstedt, 1996), the Caregiving Self-Efficacy (Zeiss, Gallagher-Thompson, Lovett, Rose, & McKibbin, 1999), and the modified version of the Caregiving Appraisal Scale (Hughes & Caliandro, 1996), may be used to assess perceived burden, self-efficacy, and personal satisfaction in various caregiving situations.

In addition to surveys and interviews, it is advantageous if the caregiver evaluation process involves observation and a review of the environment. The occupational therapist identifies strengths and barriers in the environment in which the daily routine typically occurs. The occupational therapist should give consideration to occupational engagement in the environment and to adaptations that may be needed to enhance occupational performance. Formal tools such as the Home Observation for Measurement of the Environment (Caldwell & Bradley, 1984) and the Environmental Rating Scales (Burgess & Borowsky, 2010; Harms, Clifford, & Cryer, 1998; Harms, Cryer, & Clifford, 2003, 2007; Harms, Jacobs, & White, 1996) are useful in pediatric populations to assess environmental factors that support healthy development.

For adults and seniors, an occupational therapist might use the Home Assessment Profile (Chandler, Duncan, Weiner, & Studenski, 2001), a newer version of the Functional Environment Assessment (Chandler, Prescott, Duncan, & Studenski, 1991), and the Safe at Home (Anemaet & Moffa-Trotter, 1997, 1999) to assess environmental needs in the home and to identify resources needed for the client and caregiver to maximize occupational performance and to provide opportunities for meaningful engagement in daily activities. These assessments provide a review of the home environment in which caregiving takes place and identify the extent to which assistance is needed and barriers to performance exist and give suggestions for resources and equipment. Formal assessments in conjunction with informal observations are used to develop an occupational profile and priorities for intervention (see Figure 16.8).

After the evaluation process is completed, the creation of an occupational profile results in a greater understanding of the client's past and current occupational performance, patterns of daily living, strengths, and needs (AOTA, 2014). The development of an occupational profile in a caregiving relationship should include client and contextual factors pertaining to the caregiver, the care receivers, and the systems that influence the provision of care. The resulting analysis of occupational performance should identify key priorities and outcomes for intervention.

Intervention

Therapeutic interventions to caregiving should be client centered and occupation based. Within the context of the caregiving relationship, the client may include the caregiver and care receiver, along with additional family members and service practitioners (e.g., a personal care attendant) involved in the care. AOTA (2014) emphasizes the importance of guiding the intervention plan through the client's goals, values, interests, and occupational needs; health and well-being; performance skills and patterns; context and client factors; and the best available evidence. Within the therapist–client relationship, the emphasis is placed on maximizing QoL for the caregiver and care receiver while fostering occupational performance and participation throughout the lifespan (Figure 16.9).

General Recommendations for Intervention

Working with caregivers and families in a client-centered model may be a challenge because of the

Figure 16.8. Within the same relationship, this mother cared for her daughter during a recent illness.

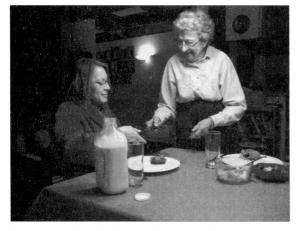

Source. K. Haertl. Used with permission.

Figure 16.9. Although caregiving is often taken on by women, men also take on caregiving roles. Wayne (middle) often took care of his son, who had a brain injury and epilepsy, and his 90-year-old aging father.

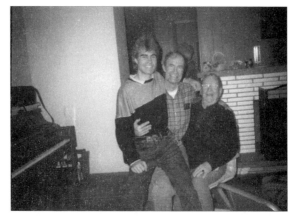

Source. K. Haertl. Used with permission.

potential for disagreement regarding priorities for intervention. Family members and primary caregivers may question health professionals' decisions regarding care (Bowers, 1988; Hasselkus, 1988). Communication and discussion of priorities are critical before the onset of intervention.

To move beyond the therapist's priorities and work toward a collaborative relationship, the therapist may have to suspend personal ideals and beliefs to fully discover the occupational patterns, values, and beliefs of the client and family (Gitlin, Corcoran, & Leinmiller-Eckhardt, 1995). Partnerships in therapy should engage "parents, families and other paid/formal and unpaid/informal caregivers to develop strategies that support occupational engagement and participation, health, and well-being, as well as support caregivers as they cope with the complex demands inherent in the caregiving role" (Gray, Horowitz, O'Sullivan, Behr, & Abreu, 2007, p. CE1).

Within the occupational requirements of caregiving, Hasselkus (1988) outlined three broad goals identified by caregivers: (1) getting things done, (2) promoting the care receiver's health and well-being, and (3) maintaining the caregiver's health and well-being. To achieve these goals, the occupational therapy practitioner uses intervention strategies that include education, skill training, adaptation, and modification. Determining the specific requirements for intervention involves understanding the dynamic interaction of the caregiver and care receiver while taking into account the contextual factors of the environment, occupational routines and requirements, and priorities.

Schumacher, Stewart, Archbold, Dodd, and Dibble (2000) and Schumacher, Beidler, Beeber, and Gambino (2006) identified nine core skills important in the caregiving process:

1. *Monitoring*—ensuring that everything is going well
2. *Interpreting*—making sense of observations
3. *Making decisions*—considering options for the best course of action
4. *Taking action*—carrying out daily caregiver tasks and requirements
5. *Providing hands-on care*—ensuring safety and comfort while providing care
6. *Making adjustments*—considering the best strategies

7. *Accessing resources*
8. *Working together* with the person who is ill and considering the personhood of both the caregiver and the care receiver
9. *Negotiating* the health care system.

For occupational therapy practitioners, application of these core skills includes working through these processes while maximizing QoL and enhancing opportunities for meaningful engagement in daily activities. Initial stages involve identification of the client's current state, the contextual influences of the setting in which the caregiving takes place, assessment of the relationship between care receiver and caregiver, and identification of the role of the occupational therapist throughout the evaluation and intervention process.

Sachs and Labovitz (2004) adapted four stages as outlined by Gitlin et al. (1995) in planning for caregiver intervention. The first stage involves identification of the primary caregiver and the current strategies and practices used in the caregiving relationship. The second stage involves coming to an understanding of the caregiver's perspective, daily routines, values, and beliefs. In the third stage, the therapist self-questions the knowledge gained and considers the congruency of the practitioner's and caregiver's priorities and values. The final stage involves designation of the intervention. In this process, it is important to identify to what extent the caregiver and care receiver agree on priorities. For instance, a wife may be the primary caregiver for a husband newly diagnosed with Alzheimer's disease. As his illness progresses, she may believe that it is unsafe for him to drive, yet he may identify his return to driving as a priority. The occupational therapy practitioner's communication skills in therapeutic interactions are crucial in working to find common agreement on priorities for intervention.

Cohn and Henry (2009) categorized occupational therapy services to caregivers as including

• *Skill training*—facilitating education in relation to the condition of the care receiver, helping organize schedules and ensure meaningful personal and family occupations, teaching parenting and caregiver skills, and facilitating communication within the caregiving relationship;
• *Adaptations*—compensatory techniques and environmental adaptation; and

- *Support services*—support groups and connecting clients to needed community and health service support.

Exercise 16.5. George With Alzheimer's Disease: Caregiver and Care Receiver

Consider this situation: You have been working with George, a 61-year-old real estate agent diagnosed during the past year with Alzheimer's disease. Over time, George's wife has had to take on some of the higher-level daily occupations such as managing finances and paying the bills. George has continued to place high importance on his work of selling homes. His position requires him to drive clients around town, yet his wife claims he frequently gets lost and at times disobeys traffic laws. She has expressed sincere concern about the safety of his driving.

As George's wife gradually takes on a caregiving role, how would you as an occupational therapy practitioner support the two of them in this process? How would you address the disagreement about driving? What strengths and barriers do you see in this situation? What would be your role as an occupational therapy practitioner?

An important area of consideration in this scenario is clarification of the occupational therapy practitioner's role in working with the caregiver. Often, the practitioner's primary therapeutic relationship is with the care receiver or person in need. Thus, client privacy and the needs of the family and all those involved in the client's care must be balanced. In addition, a newly formed caregiver situation will likely require a period of transition for both the caregiver and the care receiver. The therapist serves the client by using appropriate strategies to address the identified needs while simultaneously working with the family to implement occupational adaptations and environmental modifications that will maximize occupational performance and enhance the caregiver–care receiver relationship. In this scenario, a therapist might be asked questions related to a person's competency to continue with work, transportation alternatives, available resources, and plans for the future.

In George's case, in order for a therapist to apply the key questions presented earlier in the chapter,

the therapist would need to consider the relationship of George and his wife, the context in which he will be discharged, and the current and future prognosis. A comprehensive evaluation of George's current cognitive status and ability to complete ADLs is important, along with an evaluation of his discharge environment. The use of the COPM (Law et al., 2005) may provide valuable input from both George and his wife related to priorities, current routines and habits, and areas of meaningful engagement.

For those in the middle to late stages of Alzheimer's disease, driving is often contraindicated, because although the client may continue to remember how to turn on and steer the car, navigating signs, safety situations, and unfamiliar environments requires higher level cognitive skills. If George continues to have some level of knowledge related to his vocation, a therapist might suggest meeting with his employer and being prepared to suggest consideration of alternatives. For clients who have to adapt to transition out of work, the addition of meaningful activities in the daily routine promotes QoL.

Additional questions related to the family's resources and needs should be addressed, along with the health and well-being of George's wife and her ability to meet her own and George's daily needs in the caregiving role. Therapists for a family with someone with Alzheimer's disease should address prognosis and caregiving concerns along with any home modifications or any daily programs (e.g., adult day care) or in-home services that are advised. Preservation of meaning and family education is also important, as is close work with the multidisciplinary team.

The role and interactions of occupational therapy practitioners within the caregiving relationship shift over time. In earlier stages, practitioners serve to educate the care receiver and caregiver and facilitate adaptation to roles and responsibilities in the caregiving relationship. Perkinson, La Vesser, Morgan, and Perlmutter (2004) outlined the roles and responsibilities of the practitioner and family through application of Aneshensel, Pearlin, Mullan, Zarit, and Whitlatch's (1995) three stages of caregiving: (1) role acquisition, (2) role enactment, and (3) role disengagement. Within each stage, the practitioner and family interact in a unique manner on the basis of the situation's contextual needs.

In the initial stage of *role acquisition,* given the challenge of a newly acquired illness, the family has to adjust to new roles, functions, and routines. During this stage of caregiving, the practitioner serves as an educator regarding the illness, helps the family identify resources, and anticipates future needs. In the *role enactment* stage, the family may need additional training related to direct care skills and advice about resources available to them. Particularly in cases of progressive illness or disease, this stage may also involve discussion of future environmental or housing needs. During this phase, the occupational therapy practitioner may need to expand skills training in use of special devices, home modification, and consideration for community placement.

For those with a terminal illness, or perhaps a child with disabilities who reaches adulthood, the final stage of *role disengagement* involves major transition. Although this model was originally patterned around older adults and coping with death, it can also be applied to deal with the emotional stresses associated with placing a grown child in a residential facility or a grown child's decision to move away from home. During this stage, caregivers often have to work through grief, loss, and bereavement. An occupational therapy practitioner's role is to facilitate support for the family members in coping with loss and transition. Families may require assistance to find support groups, to identify new roles should the loved one move into a community facility or group home, and to deal with grief in times of death and loss. Throughout each of these stages, the practitioner works with the family to promote skills and routines that preserve time for meaningful activity and promote QoL for all people in the caring relationship (Figure 16.10).

Caregiving for Those With Illness and Special Needs

The concern of much of the literature on caregiving is caring for people with illness or disability, yet often it is the caregiver who has the special needs or conditions. Parents with disabilities and populations unaccustomed to providing caregiving (e.g., children) may require training and support to fulfill caregiving roles. Questions surrounding a person's competence to provide parenting or to take on a caregiving role may arise, particularly in

Figure 16.10. Preservation of meaningful occupations is important within the caregiving relationship.

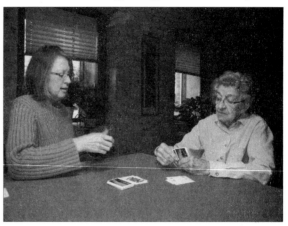

Source. K. Haertl. Used with permission.

instances of cognitive or psychological impairment such as major mental illness or a severe traumatic brain injury. Similarly, caregivers may themselves develop challenges, such as an older woman caring for her spouse who later has a stroke or a parent who becomes physically disabled after an illness or severe injury.

Although the number of people with major cognitive issues in caregiving roles has increased, services to these populations have not increased correspondingly (Kirkpatrick, 2008). A family systems approach to working with all people involved in the caregiving situation takes into account caregivers' and care receivers' needs. Programs such as those evolving from the United Kingdom's Combined Skills Model emphasize the rights of people with special needs to serve in caregiving roles but also focus on providing services to the entire family unit (Young & Hawkins, 2006).

The Social Care Institute for Excellence (2007) identified general principles of good practice for services to parents with special needs, and these principles are furthermore applicable to all caregiving situations:

- It is important to address needs arising from people who have special needs or considerations before making judgments about capacity for caregiving.
- The rights of the caregivers and the responsibilities of service organizations should be clear and transparent.

- There should be positive working relationships among service organizations, service disciplines, and the people receiving services.
- There should be a *prevention–intervention continuum,* in which provided services range from preventing dysfunction to intervention for dysfunction.

For occupational therapy practitioners, considerations of daily occupational patterns in caregiving situations, current skills and resources, and barriers to performance facilitate a foundation for the therapeutic relationship. The practitioner generally works with an interdisciplinary team to develop strategies to ensure that caregivers' and care receivers' needs are met.

Occupational therapy practitioners' roles and functions when working with caregivers who have special needs may include evaluation of skill and competence and intervention for the purposes of training, modification, and procurement of resources. People with changes of caregiving roles caused by a traumatic event have differing needs from those with chronic conditions (Fasoli, 2008). Techniques to prevent the decline of caregiving roles, such as in the case of an older adult with decreasing physical function, may include the implementation of daily physical tasks or group activities designed to bolster physical, cognitive, and social capacities (Jackson, Carlson, Mandel, Zemke, & Clark, 1998). Services for children or teens assisting in the caregiving of a parent or sibling should include not only skills training but also consideration of their disrupted roles as students, friends, and leisure participants (Lackey & Gates, 2001).

People with mental illness have often found providing care and maintaining a parenting role to be a motivating factor in agreeing to services because maintaining such roles provides a connection to the community and a way to acknowledge themselves as "normal" (Bassett & Lloyd, 2005; Gewurtz, Krupa, Eastabrook, & Horgan, 2004). For those with cognitive issues, given potential difficulties with generalization, often it is best for evaluation and intervention to occur in the natural environment (Cohn & Henry, 2009).

Finally, people with major physical and motor impairments often need adaptive strategies and home modification to facilitate caregiving. The use of ergonomic techniques to facilitate lifting and carrying, energy conservation techniques to minimize fatigue, and environmental modification such as adaptive cribs and changing tables help preserve the parent–child bond and facilitate maximal occupational performance in the parenting role (Fasoli, 2008).

When a client is unable to fully carry out caregiving roles, the occupational therapy practitioner, multidisciplinary team members, client, and family work together to identify available supports. The addition of in-home care and supportive services may be advantageous. When possible, the professional should extend efforts to facilitate the bond between the caregiver and care receiver amid the presence of external supports.

Summary

This chapter provides an overview of the definitions of *care* and *caregiver,* a description of gender and cultural influences on caregiving, a review of current models, and discussion of the roles and functions of occupational therapy practitioners. Occupational therapy serves a unique and vital role in providing services to caregivers and care receivers. Using a client-centered, occupation-based evaluation and intervention, occupational therapy practitioners work to enhance meaning and QoL for the caregiver and the care receiver.

Service provision includes the micro (i.e., individual–family) approach and the macro (i.e., systems) approach. Unique to the profession, occupational therapy evaluates and plans intervention through assessment of the client–environment fit; the daily caregiving occupational patterns; the strength and barriers to health, well-being, and daily occupational performance; and development of strategies to enhance quality of life for both caregiver and care receiver.

Acknowledgments

Special thanks to those who participated in the photographs for this chapter: Linda Buxell; Estelle Buxell; Jocelyn (Jazz) and Jada Smith; Jill, Mickey, and Kaden Hotujec; and in honor of my father Wayne Keplinger, in memory of my grandfather

Horace "Kep" Keplinger, and in memory of my brother Brian Keplinger.

References

Abelenda, J., & Helfrich, C. (2003). Family resilience and mental illness: The role of occupational therapy. *Occupational Therapy in Mental Health, 19,* 25–39. http://dx.doi.org/10.1300/J004v19n01_02

Abidin, R. R. (1995). *Parenting Stress Index* (3rd ed.). Lutz, FL: Psychological Assessment Resources.

Abrahamy, M., Finkelson, E. B., Lydon, C., & Murray, K. (2003, Spring). Caregivers' socialization of gender roles in a children's museum. *Perspectives in Psychology,* pp. 19–25.

American Occupational Therapy Association. (2007). AOTA's statement on family caregivers. *American Journal of Occupational Therapy, 61,* 710. http://dx.doi.org/10.5014/ajot.61.6.710

American Occupational Therapy Association. (2014). Occupational therapy framework: Domain and process (3rd ed.). *American Journal of Occupational Therapy, 68*(Suppl. 1), S1–S48. http://dx.doi.org/10.5014/ajot.2014.682006

Anemaet, W. K., & Moffa-Trotter, M. E. (1997). *The user friendly home care handbook.* McLean, VA: LEARN.

Anemaet, W. K., & Moffa-Trotter, M. E. (1999). Promoting safety and function through home assessments. *Topics in Geriatric Rehabilitation, 15,* 26–55. http://dx.doi.org/10.1097/00013614-199909000-00005

Aneshensel, C. S., Pearlin, L. I., Mullan, J. T., Zarit, S. H., & Whitlatch, C. J. (1995). *Profiles in caregiving: The unexpected career.* San Diego: Academic Press.

Awad, A. G., & Voruganti, L. N. (2008). The burden of schizophrenia on caregivers: A review. *PharmacoEconomics, 26,* 149–162. http://dx.doi.org/10.2165/00019053-200826020-00005

Ayalong, L. (2004). Cultural variants of caregiving or the culture of caregiving. *Journal of Cultural Diversity, 11,* 131–138.

Bassett, H., & Lloyd, C. (2005). At-risk families with mental illness: Partnerships in practice. *New Zealand Journal of Occupational Therapy, 52,* 31–37.

Baumrind, D. (1967). Child care practices anteceding three patterns of preschool behavior. *Genetic Psychology Monographs, 75,* 43–88. http://dx.doi.org/10.1037/h0024919

Baumrind, D. (1971). Current patterns of parental authority. *Developmental Psychology Monograph, 4,* 1–103. http://dx.doi.org/10.1037/h0030372

Baumrind, D. (1996). The discipline controversy revisited. *Family Relations, 45,* 405–414. http://dx.doi.org/10.2307/585170

Belsky, J. (1984). The determinants of parenting: A process model. *Child Development, 55,* 83–96. http://dx.doi.org/10.2307/1129836

Belsky, J., Pasco Fearon, R. M., & Bell, B. (2007). Parenting, attention and externalizing problems: Testing mediation longitudinally, repeatedly and reciprocally. *Journal of Child Psychology and Psychiatry, and Allied Disciplines, 48,* 1233–1242. http://dx.doi.org/10.1111/j.1469-7610.2007.01807.x

Belsky, J., Vandell, D. L., Burchinal, M., Clarke-Stewart, K. A., McCartney, K., Owen, M. T., & NICHD Early Child Care Research Network. (2007). Are there long-term effects of early child care? *Child Development, 78,* 681–701. http://dx.doi.org/10.1111/j.1467-8624.2007.01021.x

Bhattarai, L. P. (2013). Reviving the family model of care: Can it be a panacea for the new century? *Indian Journal of Gerontology, 27,* 202–218.

Bowers, B. J. (1988). Family perceptions of nursing home care: A grounded theory study of family work in a nursing home. *Gerontologist, 28,* 361–368. http://dx.doi.org/10.1093/geront/28.3.361

Bowlby, J. (1982). *Attachment and loss: Vol. 1. Attachment* (2nd ed.). New York: Basic Books.

Brenner, V., & Fox, R. A. (1999). An empirically derived classification of parenting practices. *Journal of Genetic Psychology, 160,* 343–356. http://dx.doi.org/10.1080/00221329909595404

Bumagin, V. E., & Hirn, K. F. (2001). *Caregiving: A guide for those who give care and those who receive it.* New York: Springer.

Burgess, A. L., & Borowsky, I. W. (2010). Health and home environments of caregivers of children investigated by child protective services. *Pediatrics, 125,* 273–281. http://dx.doi.org/10.1542/peds.2008-3814

Burr, J. A., & Mutchler, J. E. (1999). Race and ethnic variations in norms of filial responsibility among older adults. *Journal of Marriage and the Family, 61,* 674–687. http://dx.doi.org/10.2307/353569

Caldwell, B., & Bradley, R. H. (1984). *Home observation for measurement of the environment* (rev. ed.). Little Rock: University of Arkansas.

Cardemil, E. V. (2010). The complexity of culture: Do we embrace the challenge or avoid it? *Scientific Review of Mental Health Practice, 7,* 41–47.

Cardoso, J. B., Padilla, Y. C., & Sampson, M. (2010). Racial and ethnic variation in the predictors of maternal parenting stress. *Journal of Social Service Research, 36,* 429–444. http://dx.doi.org/10.1080/01488376.2010.510948

Caregiver Action Network. (2013). *Caregiving statistics.* Retrieved from http://caregiveraction.org/statistics/

Chandler, J. M., Duncan, P. W., Weiner, D. K., & Studenski, S. A. (2001). Special Feature—The Home Assessment Profile—A reliable and valid assessment tool. *Topics in Geriatric Rehabilitation, 16,* 77–88. http://dx.doi.org/10.1097/00013614-200103000-00010

Chandler, J. M., Prescott, B., Duncan, P. W., & Studenski, S. (1991). Reliability of a new instrument: The Functional Environment Assessment. *Physical Therapy, 71*(Suppl.), 574.

Chumbler, N. R., Grimm, J. W., Cody, M., & Beck, C. (2003). Gender, kinship and caregiver burden: The case of community-dwelling memory impaired seniors. *International Journal of Geriatric Psychiatry, 18,* 722–732. http://dx.doi.org/10.1002/gps.912

Collins Essential English Dictionary. (2013). Care. Retrieved from www.thefreedictionary.com/care

Cohn, E. S., & Henry, A. D. (2009). Caregiving and childrearing. In E. B. Crepeau, E. S. Cohn, & B. A. Schell (Eds.), *Willard and Spackman's occupational therapy* (11th ed., pp. 579–591). Philadelphia: Lippincott Williams & Wilkins.

Comfort, M., & Gordon, P. (2005). *Keys to Interactive Parenting Scale.* Cheyney, PA: Comfort Consultants.

Corcoran, M. A., & Gitlin, L. R. (2001). Family caregiver acceptance and use of environmental strategies provided in an occupational therapy intervention. *Physical and Occupational Therapy in Geriatrics, 19,* 1–20. http://dx.doi.org/10.1080/J148v19n01_01

Coutinho, F., Hersch, G., & Davidson, H. (2006). The impact of informal caregiving in occupational therapy. *Physical and Occupational Therapy in Geriatrics, 25,* 47–61. http://dx.doi.org/10.1080/J148v25n01_04

Dahlberg, L., Demack, S., & Bambra, C. (2007). Age and gender of informal carers: A population-based study in the UK. *Health and Social Care in the Community, 15,* 439–445. http://dx.doi.org/10.1111/j.1365-2524.2007.00702.x

Davis, K. L., Marin, D. B., Kane, R., Patrick, D., Peskind, E. R., Raskind, M. A., & Puder, K. L. (1997). The Caregiver Activity Survey (CAS): Development and validation of a new measure for caregivers of persons with Alzheimer's disease. *International Journal of Geriatric Psychiatry, 12,* 978–988. http://dx.doi.org/10.1002/(SICI)1099-1166(199710)12:10<978::AID-GPS659>3.0.CO;2-1

Dehyadegary, E., Yaacob, S. N., & Juhari, R. B. (2012). Relationship between parenting style and academic achievement among Iranian adolescents in Sirjan. *Asian Social Science, 8,* 156–160. http://dx.doi.org/10.5539/ass.v8n1p156.

Dooley, N. R., & Hinojosa, J. (2004). Improving quality of life for persons with Alzheimer's disease and their family caregivers: Brief occupational therapy intervention. *American Journal of Occupational Therapy, 58,* 561–569. http://dx.doi.org/10.5014/ajot.58.5.561

Drentea, P. (2007). Caregiving. In G. Ritzer (Ed.), *Blackwell encyclopedia of sociology.* Retrieved from www.blackwellreference.com/public/tocnode?id=g9781405124331_chunk_g97814051243319_ss1–7

Elgar, F. J., Waschbusch, D. A., Dadds, M. R., & Sigvaldason, N. (2007). Development and validation of a short form of the Alabama Parenting Questionnaire. *Journal of Child and Family Studies, 16,* 243–259. http://dx.doi.org/10.1007/s10826-006-9082-5

Elmståhl, S., Malmberg, B., & Annerstedt, L. (1996). Caregiver's burden of patients 3 years after stroke assessed by a novel caregiver burden scale. *Archives of Physical Medicine and Rehabilitation, 77,* 177–182. http://dx.doi.org/10.1016/S0003-9993(96)90164-1

Epstein-Lubow, G., Gaudiano, B. A., Hinckley, M., Salloway, S., & Miller, I. W. (2010). Evidence for the validity of the American Medical Association's Caregiver Self-Assessment Questionnaire as a screening measure for depression. *Journal of the American Geriatrics Society, 58,* 387–388. http://dx.doi.org/10.1111/j.1532-5415.2009.02701.x

Ergh, T. C., Rapport, L. J., Coleman, R. D., & Hanks, R. A. (2002). Predictors of caregiver and family functioning following traumatic brain injury: Social support moderates caregiver distress. *Journal of Head Trauma Rehabilitation, 17,* 155–174. http://dx.doi.org/10.1097/00001199-200204000-00006

Etters, L., Goodall, D., & Harrison, B. E. (2008). Caregiver burden among dementia patient caregivers: A review of the literature. *Journal of the American Academy of Nurse Practitioners, 20,* 423–428. http://dx.doi.org/10.1111/j.1745-7599.2008.00342.x

Farnfield, S. (2008). A theoretical model for the comprehensive assessment of parenting. *British Journal of Social Work, 38,* 1076–1079. http://dx.doi.org/10.1093/bjsw/bcl395

Fasoli, S. E. (2008). Restoring competence for homemaker and parent roles. In M. V. Radomski & C. A. Trombly (Eds.), *Occupational therapy for physical dysfunction* (6th ed., pp. 854–874). Baltimore: Lippincott Williams & Wilkins.

Fingerhut, P. E. (2013). Life Participation for Parents: A tool for family-centered occupational therapy. *American Journal of Occupational Therapy, 67,* 37–44. http://dx.doi.org/10.5014/ajot.2013.005082

Frick, P. J. (1991). *Alabama Parenting Questionnaire.* Birmingham, AL: Author.

Gallagher, T. J., Wagenfeld, M. O., Baro, F., & Haepers, K. (1994). Sense of coherence, coping and caregiver role overload. *Social Science and Medicine, 39,* 1615–1622. http://dx.doi.org/10.1016/0277-9536(94)90075-2

Ge, C., Yang, X., Fu, J., Chang, Y., Wei, J., Zhang, F., . . . Wang, L. (2011). Reliability and validity of the Chinese version of the Caregiver Reaction Assessment. *Psychiatry and Clinical Neurosciences, 65,* 254–263. http://dx.doi.org/10.1111/j.1440-1819.2011.02200.x

Geisler, M. (2012). Gay fathers' negotiation of gender role strain: A qualitative inquiry. *Fathering, 10,* 119–139. http://dx.doi.org/10.3149/fth.1002.119

Gewurtz, R., Krupa, T., Eastabrook, S., & Horgan, S. (2004). Prevalence and characteristics of parenting among people served by Assertive Community Treatment. *Psychiatric Rehabilitation Journal, 28,* 63–65. http://dx.doi.org/10.2975/28.2004.63.65

Giese, T. (2010). Infant, toddler, and young child development. In B. E. Chandler (Ed.), *Early childhood: Occupational therapy services for children birth to five* (pp. 41–75). Bethesda, MD: AOTA Press.

Gitlin, L. N., Corcoran, M., & Leinmiller-Eckhardt, S. (1995). Understanding the family perspective: An ethnographic framework for providing occupational therapy in the home. *American Journal of Occupational Therapy, 49,* 802–809. http://dx.doi.org/10.5014/ajot.49.8.802

Given, C. W., Given, B., Stommel, M., Collins, C., King, S., & Franklin, S. (1992). The Caregiver Reaction Assessment (CRA) for caregivers to persons with chronic physical and mental impairments. *Research in Nursing and Health, 15,* 271–283. http://dx.doi.org/10.1002/nur.4770150406

Gordon, P. (2012). *Choosing the right parenting assessment tool to delight your funders.* Retrieved from http://comfortconsults.com/blog/bid/243638/Choosing-the-Right-Parenting-Assessment-Tool-to-Delight-Your-Funders

Gray, K., Horowitz, B. P., O'Sullivan, A., Behr, S. K., & Abreu, B. C. (2007). Occupational therapy's role in the occupation of caregiving. *OT Practice, 12,* CE-1–CE-8.

Gupta, V. B., Mehrota, P., & Mehrota, N. (2012). Parental stress in raising a child with disabilities in India. *Disability, CBR, and Inclusive Development, 23,* 41–52. http://dx.doi.org/10.5463/DCID.v23i2.119.

Haertl, K. H. (2011). Strategies for adults with developmental disabilities. In C. H. Christiansen & K. M. Matuska (Eds.), *Ways of living: Adaptive strategies for special needs* (4th ed., pp. 171–205). Bethesda, MD: AOTA Press.

Harms, T., Clifford, R., & Cryer, D. (1998). *Early Childhood Environment Rating Scale–Revised (ECERS–R).* New York: Teachers College Press.

Harms, T., Cryer, D., & Clifford, R. (2003). *Infant Toddler Environment Rating Scale–Revised (ITERS–R).* New York: Teachers College Press.

Harms, T., Cryer, D., & Clifford, R. (2007). *Family Childcare Environment Rating Scale (FCERS–R).* New York: Teachers College Press.

Harms, T., Jacobs, E. V., & White, D. R. (1996). *School Age Care Environment Rating Scale.* New York: Teachers College Press.

Hasselkus, B. R. (1988). Meaning in family caregiving: Perspectives on caregiver/professional relationships. *Gerontologist, 28,* 686–691. http://dx.doi.org/10.1093/geront/28.5.686

Hasselkus, B. R., & Murray, B. J. (2007). Everyday occupation, well-being, and identity: The experience of caregivers in families with dementia. *American Journal of Occupational Therapy, 61,* 9–20. http://dx.doi.org/10.5014/ajot.61.1.9

Hawes, D. J., & Dadds, M. R. (2006). Assessing parenting practices through parent-report and direct observation during parent-training. *Journal of Child and Family Studies, 15,* 555–568. http://dx.doi.org/10.1007/s10826-006-9029-x

Hodgson, C., Higginson, I., & Jefferys, P. (1998). *Carers' checklist: An outcome measure for people with dementia and their carers.* London: Mental Health Foundation.

Hoffman, F., & Rodrigues, R. (2010). Informal carers: Who takes care of them? *European Centre Policy Brief.* Retrieved from http://www.euro.centre.org/data/1274190382_99603.pdf

Hughes, C. B., & Caliandro, G. (1996). Effects of social support, stress, and level of illness on caregiving of children with AIDS. *Journal of Pediatric Nursing, 11,* 347–358. http://dx.doi.org/10.1016/S0882-5963(96)80079-0

Jackson, J., Carlson, M., Mandel, D., Zemke, R., & Clark, F. (1998). Occupational lifestyle redesign: The Well-Elderly Study Occupational Therapy Program. *American Journal of Occupational Therapy, 52,* 326–336. http://dx.doi.org/10.5014/ajot.52.5.326

Jacques, N. D., & Hasselkus, B. R. (2004). The nature of occupation surrounding dying and death. *Occupation, Participation and Health, 24,* 44–53.

Jaffe, L., Humphry, R., & Case-Smith, J. (2010). Working with families. In J. Case-Smith (Ed.), *Occupational therapy for children* (6th ed., pp. 108–140). Maryland Heights, MO: Elsevier.

Javier, N. S., & Montagnini, M. L. (2011). Rehabilitation of the hospice and palliative care patient. *Journal of Palliative Medicine, 14,* 638–648. http://dx.doi.org/10.1089/jpm.2010.0125

Jones, A. L., Harris-Kojetin, L., & Valverde, R. (2012). Characteristics and use of home health care by men and women aged 65 and over. *National Health Statistics Report, 52,* 1–7.

Kellett, U. M. (1999). Transition in care: Family carers' experience of nursing home placement. *Journal of Advanced Nursing, 29,* 1474–1481. http://dx.doi.org/10.1046/j.1365-2648.1999.01035.x

Kiff, C. J., Lengua, L. J., & Zalewski, M. (2011). Nature and nurturing: Parenting in the context of child temperament. *Clinical Child and Family Psychology Review, 14*, 251–301. http://dx.doi.org/10.1007/s10567-011-0093-4

Kirkpatrick, K. (2008). Working with parents with a learning disability. *Learning Disability Today, 8*, 8–11.

Klein, J., & Liu, L. (2010). Family–therapist relationships in caring for older adults. *Physical and Occupational Therapy in Geriatrics, 28*, 259–270. http://dx.doi.org/10.3109/02703181.2010.494822

Lackey, N. R., & Gates, M. F. (2001). Adults' recollections of their experiences as young caregivers of family members with chronic physical illnesses. *Journal of Advanced Nursing, 34*, 320–328. http://dx.doi.org/10.1046/j.1365-2648.2001.01761.x

Lattanzi-Licht, M. (2001). Hospice as a model for caregiving. In K. J. Doka & J. D. Davidson (Eds.), *Caregiving and loss: Family needs, professional responses* (pp. 19–31). Washington, DC: Hospice Foundation of America.

Law, M. (Ed.). (1998). *Client-centered occupational therapy.* Thorofare, NJ: Slack.

Law, M., Baptiste, S., Carswell, A., McColl, M. A., Polatajko, H., & Pollock, N. (1994). *Canadian Occupational Performance Measure* (2nd ed.). Toronto: CAOT Publications.

Law, M., Baptiste, S., Carswell, A., McColl, M. A., Polatajko, H., & Pollock, N. (2005). *Canadian Occupational Performance Measure* (4th ed.). Ottawa: CAOT Publications.

Leaper, C. (2002). Parenting girls and boys. In M. H. Bornstein (Ed.), *Handbook of parenting: Vol. 1. Children and parenting* (2nd ed., pp. 189–225). Mahwah, NJ: Erlbaum.

Leininger, M. (Ed.). (1988a). Cross-cultural hypothetical functions of caring and nursing care. In M. Leininger (Ed.), *Caring—An essential human need: Proceedings of the three National Caring Conferences* (pp. 95–102). Detroit, MI: Wayne State University Press.

Leininger, M. (Ed.). (1988b). The phenomenon of caring: Importance, research questions and theoretical considerations. In M. Leininger (Ed.), *Caring—An essential human need: Proceedings of the three National Caring Conferences* (pp. 3–16). Detroit, MI: Wayne State University Press.

Lindsey, E. W., & Mize, J. (2001). Contextual differences in parent–child play: Implications for children's gender role development. *Sex Roles, 44*, 155–176. http://dx.doi.org/10.1023/A:1010950919451

Lynch, S. H., & Lobo, M. L. (2012). Compassion fatigue in family caregivers: A Wilsonian concept analysis. *Journal of Advanced Nursing, 68*, 2125–2134. http://dx.doi.org/10.1111/j.1365-2648.2012.05985.x

Mak, W. W. (2005). Integrative model of caregiving: How macro and micro factors affect caregivers of adults with severe and persistent mental illness. *American Journal of Orthopsychiatry, 75*, 40–53. http://dx.doi.org/10.1037/0002-9432.75.1.40

McCarron, M., Gill, M., Lawlor, B., & Beagly, C. (2002). A pilot study of the reliability and validity of the Caregiver Activity Survey–Intellectual Disability (CAS–ID). *Journal of Intellectual Disability Research, 46*, 605–612. http://dx.doi.org/10.1046/j.1365-2788.2002.00437.x

McCleary, L., & Blain, J. (2013). Cultural values and family caregiving for persons with dementia. *Indian Journal of Gerontology, 1*, 178–201.

McKinney, C., & Renk, K. (2011). A multivariate model of parent–adolescent relationship variables in early adolescence. *Child Psychiatry and Human Development, 42*, 442–462. http://dx.doi.org/10.1007/s10578-011-0228-3

Merriam Webster's Online Dictionary. (2014). Care. Retrieved from www.merriam-webster.com/dictionary/care

Mowder, B. A., & Shamah, R. (2011a). Parent Behavior Importance Questionnaire–Revised: Scale development and psychometric properties. *Journal of Child and Family Studies, 20*, 295–302. http://dx.doi.org/10.1007/s10826-010-9392-5

Mowder, B. A., & Shamah, R. (2011b). Test–retest reliability of the Parent Behavior Importance Questionnaire–Revised and the Parent Behavior Frequency Questionnaire–Revised. *Psychology in the Schools, 48*, 843–854. http://dx.doi.org/10.1002/pits.20593

Murray, L., Tarren-Sweeny, M., & France, K. (2011). Foster carer perceptions of support and training in the context of high burden of care. *Child and Family Social Work, 16*, 149–158. http://dx.doi.org/10.1111/j.1365-2206.2010.00722.x

Napoles, A. M., Chadiha, L., Eversley, R., & Moreno-John, G. (2010). Developing culturally sensitive caregiving interventions: Are we there yet? *American Journal of Alzheimer's Disease, 25*, 389–406. http://dx.doi.org/10.1177/1533317510370957

National Alliance for Caregiving & AARP. (2009). *Caregiving in the U.S. in 2009.* Bethesda, MD: Author.

Novak, M., & Guest, C. (1989). Application of a multidimensional Caregiver Burden Inventory. *Gerontologist, 29*, 798–803. http://dx.doi.org/10.1093/geront/29.6.798

Oberst, M. T. (1991). *Appraisal of Caregiving Scale: Manual.* Detroit, MI: Wayne State University.

Oberst, M. T., Thomas, S. E., Gass, K. A., & Ward, S. E. (1989). Caregiving demands and appraisal of stress among family caregivers. *Cancer Nursing, 12*, 209–215. http://dx.doi.org/10.1097/00002820-198908000-00003

Pakenham, K. I. (2001). Application of a stress and coping model to caregiving in multiple sclerosis. *Psychology Health and Medicine, 6,* 13–27. http://dx.doi.org/10.1080/13548500125141.

Perkinson, M. A., La Vesser, P., Morgan, K., & Perlmutter, M. (2004). Therapeutic partnerships: Caregiving in the home setting. In C. H. Christiansen & K. M. Matuska (Eds.), *Ways of living: Adaptive strategies for special needs* (3rd ed., pp. 445–461). Bethesda, MD: AOTA Press.

Pioli, M. F. (2010). Global and caregiving mastery as moderators in the caregiving stress process. *Aging and Mental Health, 14,* 603–612. http://dx.doi.org/10.1080/13607860903586193

Poroch, N. C. (2012). Karunpa: Keeping spirit on country. *Health Sociology Review, 21,* 383–395. http://dx.doi.org/10.5172/hesr.2012.21.4.383

Riina, E. M., & Feinberg, M. E. (2012). Involvement in childrearing and mothers' and fathers' adjustment. *Family Relations, 61,* 836–850. http://dx.doi.org/10.1111/j.1741-3729.2012.00739.x

Riley, G. A. (2007). Stress and depression in family carers following traumatic brain injury: The influence of beliefs about difficult behaviours. *Clinical Rehabilitation, 21,* 82–88. http://dx.doi.org/10.1177/0269215506071279

Root, A. K., & Denham, S. A. (2010). The role of gender in the socialization of emotion: Key concepts and critical issues. *New Directions for Child and Adolescent Development,* 1–9. http://dx.doi.org/10.1002/cd.265

Sachs, D., & Labovitz, D. R. (2004). Range of human activity: Care of others. In J. Hinojosa & M. Blount (Eds.), *Texture of life: Purposeful activities in occupational therapy* (2nd ed., pp. 414–436). Bethesda, MD: AOTA Press.

Sarkisian, N., Gerena, M., & Gerstel, M. (2007). Extended family integration among Euro and Mexican Americans: Ethnicity, gender and class. *Journal of Marriage and the Family, 69,* 40–54. http://dx.doi.org/10.1111/j.1741-3737.2006.00342.x

Schumacher, K. L., Beidler, S. M., Beeber, A. S., & Gambino, P. (2006). A transactional model of cancer family caregiving skill. *Advances in Nursing Science, 29,* 271–286. http://dx.doi.org/10.1097/00012272-200607000-00009

Schumacher, K. L., Stewart, B. J., Archbold, P. G., Dodd, M. J., & Dibble, S. L. (2000). Family caregiving skill: Development of the concept. *Research in Nursing and Health, 23,* 191–203. http://dx.doi.org/10.1002/1098-240X(200006)23:3<191::AID-NUR3>3.0.CO;2-B

Scott, S., Briskman, J., & Dadds, M. R. (2011). Measuring parenting in community and public health research: Using brief child and parenting reports. *Journal of Child and*

Family Studies, 20, 343–352. http://dx.doi.org/10.1007/s10826-010-9398-z

Sellick, J. (2005). *Traditions: Improving quality of life in caregiving.* State College, PA: Venture.

Silva, L. M., & Schalock, M. (2012). Autism Parenting Stress Index: Initial psychometric evidence. *Journal of Autism and Developmental Disorders, 42,* 566–574. http://dx.doi.org/10.1007/s10803-011-1274-1

Social Care Institute for Excellence. (2007). *The adult services resource guide 9: Working together to support disabled parents.* London: Author.

Sörensen, S., & Pinquart, M. (2005). Racial and ethnic differences in the relationship of caregiving stressors, resources, and sociodemographic variables to caregiver depression and perceived physical health. *Aging and Mental Health, 9,* 482–495. http://dx.doi.org/10.1080/13607860500142796

Sorkhabi, N. (2005). Applicability of Baumrind's parent typology to collective cultures: Analysis of cultural explanations of parent socialization effects. *International Journal of Behavioral Development, 29,* 552–563. http://dx.doi.org/10.1080/01650250500172640.

Staal, I. I., van den Brink, H. A., Hermanns, J. M., Schrijvers, A. J., & van Stel, H. F. (2011). Assessment of parenting and developmental problems in toddlers: Development and feasibility of a structured interview. *Child: Care, Health and Development, 37,* 503–511. http://dx.doi.org/10.1111/j.1365-2214.2011.01228.x

Statistics Canada. (2012). *Informal caregiving for seniors.* Retrieved from http://www.statcan.gc.ca/pub/82-003-x/2012003/article/11694-eng.htm

Tachibana, Y., Fukushima, A., Saito, H., Yoneyama, S., Ushida, K., Yoneyama, S., & Kawashima, R. (2012). A new mother–child play activity program to decrease parenting stress and improve child cognitive abilities: A cluster randomized controlled trial. *Plos One Journal, 7,* e38238. http://dx.doi.org/10.1371/journal.pone.0038238

Upton, N., & Reed, V. (2006). The influence of social support on caregiver coping. *International Journal of Psychiatric Nursing Research, 11,* 1256–1267.

U.S. Department of Health and Human Services. (2003). *The future supply of long-term care workers in relation to the aging baby-boom generation: Report to Congress.* Washington, DC: Author.

Vellone, E., Piras, G., Talucci, C., & Cohen, M. Z. (2008). Quality of life for caregivers of people with Alzheimer's disease. *Journal of Advanced Nursing, 61,* 222–231. http://dx.doi.org/10.1111/j.1365-2648.2007.04494.x

Wells, R., Dywan, J., & Dumas, J. (2005). Life satisfaction and distress in family caregivers as related to specific behavioural changes after traumatic brain injury. *Brain Injury, 19,* 1105–1115. http://dx.doi.org/10.1080/02699050500150062

Woolfson, L., & Grant, E. (2006). Authoritative parenting and parental stress in parents of pre-school and older children with developmental disabilities. *Child: Care, Health and Development, 32,* 177–184. http://dx.doi.org/10.1111/j.1365-2214.2006.00603.x

Yarry, S. J., Stevens, E. K., & McCallum, T. J. (2007). Cultural influences on spousal caregiving. *Generations, 31*(3), 24–30.

Yeh, C. H., Chen, M. L., Li, W., & Chuang, H. L. (2001). The Chinese version of the Parenting Stress Index: A psychometric study. *Acta Paediatrica (Oslo, Norway), 90,* 1470–1477. http://dx.doi.org/10.1111/j.1651-2227.2001.tb01615.x

Young, S., & Hawkins, H. (2006). Special parenting and the combined skills model. *Journal of Applied Research in Intellectual Disabilities, 19,* 346–355. http://dx.doi.org/10.1111/j.1468-3148.2006.00276.x

Zaidman-Zait, A., Mirenda, P., Zumbo, B. D., Wellington, S., Dua, V., & Kalynchuk, K. (2010). An item response theory analysis of the Parenting Stress Index–Short Form with parents of children with autism spectrum disorders. *Journal of Child Psychology and Psychiatry, and Allied Disciplines, 51,* 1269–1277. http://dx.doi.org/10.1111/j.1469-7610.2010.02266.x

Zeiss, A. M., Gallagher-Thompson, D., Lovett, S., Rose, J., & McKibbin, C. (1999). Self-efficacy as a mediator of caregiver coping: Development and testing of an assessment model. *Journal of Clinical Geropsychology, 5,* 221–230. http://dx.doi.org/10.1023/A:1022955817074

Zukewich, N. (2003). Unpaid informal caregiving. *Canadian Social Trends, 70,* 14–18.

CHAPTER 17.

OCCUPATIONS IN THE CONTEXT OF SPIRITUALITY

Barbara J. Hemphill, DMin, MS, OTR, FAOTA

Highlights

✧ Self, mind, and spirituality
✧ Occupation and spirituality
✧ Spirituality, religion, and faith
✧ Spirituality, activity, and occupation
✧ Occupational therapy's focus on occupational performance
✧ Treatment plans and intervention
✧ Boundaries and ethical considerations.

Key Terms

✧ Activity
✧ Boundaries
✧ Brain
✧ Compassion
✧ Consent
✧ Expressive media
✧ Health
✧ Holism
✧ Journaling
✧ Meditation
✧ Mind
✧ Occupational performances

✧ Patient
✧ Profession
✧ Quality of life
✧ Religion
✧ Religious coping
✧ Self
✧ Soul
✧ Spiritual assessments
✧ Spiritual coping
✧ Spirituality
✧ State of mind

Occupational therapy is uniquely positioned to address the needs of the whole person in treatment. From its very origins, the profession has embraced notions of rehabilitation that address not only a physical injury or a mental difficulty but also the value of activity and occupation to give an individual a sense of purpose and fulfillment, a renewed sense of wellness that gives deeper meaning to life. Thus, it is reasonable, and valuable, to consider how occupation and purposeful activity contribute to an improved spiritual condition.

This chapter defines spirituality and distinguishes it from faith, belief systems, and religious practice. I examine the importance of a healthy spiritual condition to overall wellness and the concept of holism as a way to examine the multidimensional needs of the individual in treatment.

I also take the concepts and apply them to practice. The chapter explores ways to assess spiritual conditions and how to develop interventions that address every level and each goal a client and practitioner identify, working together in a mutually supportive environment. From there, I discuss various activities that can specifically enhance the spiritual experience in treatment. I also examine the boundaries and limits of an occupational therapy practitioner's competency and discuss them in relation to ethical considerations of the profession.

Adolf Meyer, the principal founder of occupational therapy, was guided by a humanistic philosophy that originated out of the Zwinglian tradition "that recognized the full complexity of the individual and the therapeutic process that would enable patients to adapt to the problems of living" (Schwartz, 2003, p. 26). From the humanistic model, a core principle of *holism* emerged. This principle emphasizes a multidimensional view of people from the social, physical, and spiritual factors that influence occupational behavior. Scholars and researchers have written about the social and physical aspects of occupational therapy. They have, however, neglected spirituality until recently. From the latter part of the 20th century until now, research has emerged that has shown a relationship among religion, spirituality, and health. According to Koenig (2011), there have been nearly 3,000 relevant published quantitative studies, and nearly all of them show a positive relationship between spiritual/religious health and mental and physical health.

Fundamentally, occupational therapy is about the value of occupation to the whole person: the physical body, the mind, and the spirit. Purposeful activities not only provide ways to engage the body and mind but also provide a sense of satisfaction and improve *state of mind*—a sense of fulfillment that improves the spirit; it is intangible yet understood. Thus, the role of purposeful activities in a therapeutic setting is a crucial aspect of care for the total person, providing opportunities to a client to once again feel hopeful, useful, and fulfilled. It can therefore be useful to consider more carefully the role of occupational therapy beyond simply practical applications to the role it can play as part of spiritual healing.

Some of the ways of looking at spirituality can seem strange or new in this context, but the theories and ideas that animate occupational therapy overall are familiar touchstones that guide the principles under discussion here. My goal—in addition to providing ways to think about spirituality, include it in existing approaches to practice, and improve overall outcomes—is to foster a continued conversation about the best practices that can be adopted across the field of occupational therapy that address every client need, including improved state of mind and an enhanced sense of wellness. Further research and study offer the potential to broaden the impact of therapeutic intervention and to make the improved spiritual condition a fundamental part of the overall therapeutic experience.

Self, Mind, and Spirituality

Within each person, there is an inner personal awareness, a freestanding observant *self*, comprising brain, soul, and mind. Newberg, D'Aquili, and Rause (2001) defined *brain* as a "collection of physical structures that gather and process sensory, cognitive and emotional data: the *mind* is the phenomenon of thoughts, memories, and emotions that arise from the perceptual processes of the brain" (p. 33). The mind is "something separate from the brain, a free-floating consciousness that could be considered a 'soul'" (p. 34). The self is not the same as the mind; the mind exists before the self and makes possible memories, emotions, and affect associated with caring, meaningfulness, and other essential parts of the self.

In other words, there is a hierarchy, beginning with the brain at its base, the physical place where cognition begins. The mind is at the second order and functions because of brain function. The mind is present at birth, and a person's true self (observant self) derives from the mind. Without the mind, the observant self cannot develop and a person cannot distinguish himself or herself from the outer world. The brain and mind have to function to recognize the observant self. The *soul* is the highest order, and the mind can be the same as the soul. It is through the observant self that there is a connection with the soul, and, therefore, a person may experience spirituality, thinking about the state of the mind.

Within the cerebral cortex are association areas that correspond to the various regions of the brain. One is the orientation association area, which is located near the parietal lobe. It helps distinguish the self from the rest of the world and orients the self in space. If this area loses function, a person is unable to find the boundaries of his or her body, and the mind is no longer able to perceive a sense of self at all. There is no ego, no sense of a defined person. *Spirituality* includes having a relationship with oneself and others as well as having a world view that affects and defines quality of life (QoL).

Occupation and Spirituality

What QoL is to one person may be something different to another. A person's *QoL* is defined by a perspective on individual performance in four areas: (1) physical and occupational function, (2) psychological state of mind, (3) social interaction, and (4) somatic or bodily state (Christiansen & Baum, 1997). Spirituality is a part of each of those areas.

Occupations restore doing in people with disabilities or maintain doing in people who are well. Researchers study what people do in life, and the central tenet of the science of occupation is the idea that people adapt to situations in the environment through occupation; that is, they adapt through deliberate, mindful, organized action. Being able to adapt within one's environment can improve state of mind, which serves to address the spirit. Occupational therapy emphasizes adapting while engaging in an activity, resulting in improved QoL (Zemke & Clark, 1996).

Spiritual QoL is achieved through relationships that promote interconnectedness among individuals, the world, and a transcendent entity—a higher power outside of the self; in occupational therapy, this means interconnectedness among the client, the practitioner, and some higher power. *QoL* is "a state of well-being and functioning that includes a level of comfort, enjoyment, and the ability to participate in meaningful activities or occupations" (Crepeau, Cohn, & Schell, 2003, p. 1033). What provides meaning in human spirituality happens in the mind (Newberg et al., 2001).

In thinking about the concept of a "higher power outside of the self," one can consider the example of Alcoholics Anonymous (AA) and other programs for drug and alcohol addictions, in which members (or clients in treatment settings) are encouraged to see beyond themselves, to understand and admit that addiction—a mental obsession—cannot be solved alone. A higher power can be called "God" out of any religious tradition one chooses; in the AA program, a higher power can be "your own conception of God" (AA World Service, 1993, p. 47) or indeed, another concept that is defined primarily as outside of the self. That is, a higher power is defined, individually, as something other than and outside of the person. Working backward, then, a sense of spirituality—understanding the quality in one's life—has to include a sense of one's place and relationship to the world.

A person lives his or her spirituality in the context of the self and the outer world. Health care services are carried out in intervention settings and are influenced by clients' beliefs, perceptions, and culture. Spirituality, whether conscious or unconscious, is expressed through action in the world. The clients' culture and customs are seated in the external world and influence how services are delivered (American Occupational Therapy Association [AOTA], 2014).

Spirituality, Religion, and Faith

A definition of *spirituality* as state of mind allows for a more generalized, universal application. Limiting spirituality to a discussion of religious belief and expression excludes a range of possibilities and a variety of nonreligious, but spiritual, experiences. Although expression of religious belief or faith may be important to an individual, it is important for health care providers to respect all faith traditions or the decision to avoid one altogether. Focusing on spirituality is one way to broaden the discussion.

In our context, then, *religion* refers to a specific faith or set of beliefs. There may be faith in a spiritual being and reliance on religious texts. Religion can proscribe certain codes of behavior, believers, or their religious community. There may be expectations around expressions of faith, such as prayer, and specific dietary prohibitions or modes of dress.

Expressions of religious faith can be extremely important and meaningful to a client, even in a therapeutic setting. Failing to respect or honor these faith-based expectations may not only limit the efficacy of an intervention but also may be detrimental to a client's state of mind, limiting the benefits and affecting overall outcomes. Seeing a client fully in all his or her human dimensions, including state of mind, leads to greater improvement to overall function. Respecting religious faith, or the absence of it, is one way to address a client's spiritual needs.

Nevertheless, it remains important to distinguish between the spiritual and the religious. Improving the spirit can be helpful and therapeutic in various settings. Changing or counseling a religious belief is the function of faith-based professionals and organizations. Although spirituality may have a religious or faith-based component, in a health care setting the focus is on what affects the spirit, not what addresses the faith. Respecting religion and faith does not mean imposing one externally.

AOTA's (2014) *Framework* distinguishes between religion and spirituality. It states that *religious activities* are participating in religion as "an organized system of beliefs, practices, rituals, and symbols designed to facilitate closeness to the sacred or transcendent (Moreira-Almeida & Koenig, 2006, p. 844) (p. S20)," whereas *spirituality* is the "aspect of humanity that refers to the way individuals seek and express meaning and purpose and the way they experience their connectedness to the moment, to self, to others, to nature, and to the significant or sacred" (Puchalski et al., 2009, p. 887) (p. S 22).

Spirituality, Activity, and Occupation

Because spirituality is a state of mind, in itself it is not an *activity*; however, the practice of spirituality, or trying to influence state of mind, surely is. Some activities may influence state of mind as a corollary result; for example, endorphins released through physical activity, such as swimming, can be seen this way. Similarly, seeing a process through to a successful outcome, such as cooking a meal, can result in a sense of accomplishment and therefore improve state of mind.

There are some activities in which influencing the spirit is a goal unto itself. Meditating, studying literature, and even something as simple as listening to music can be used primarily to influence a state of mind, or spiritual outcome.

An occupation need not be a ritual or include special objects or symbols to have spiritual meaning. When a person pays particular attention to the way an occupation is done and the context in which it is performed, that occupation becomes an opportunity for meaning. Kabat-Zinn (1994) suggested that any occupation can be an activity of spirit if attention is given to its style and context. Hasselkus (2002) stated that

> We think of occupation as a vehicle by which our internal world [or spiritual self] is expressed in our external world [or outer self], i.e., by which our spiritual consciousness is given expression in our daily lives. Occupation opens the door between the inside room and the outside room; occupation unites the internal and external dimensions of our selves. (p. 112)

Occupational Therapy's Focus on Occupational Performance

In occupational therapy, through meaningful activities, each person expresses his or her spiritual occupation through *occupational performances* or skills in the outer world. Occupational therapy practitioners use occupation to allow the client to express his or her spirit in everyday life through form, function, and meaning.

In the intervention process, occupational therapy practitioners perform the occupations that are specific to the role of a health care provider. They can and may use activities to make conscious that which is unconscious and to help the client express his or her spiritual needs in the outer world. A cli-

Figure 17.1. Spirituality as an occupation.

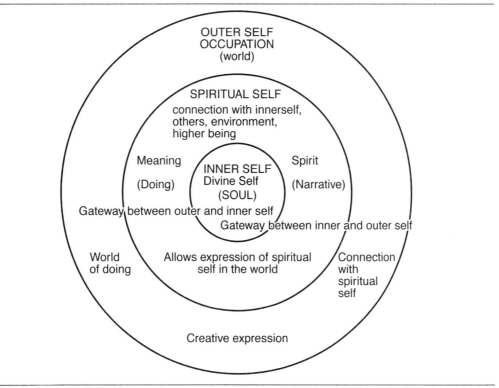

Source. From "Spirituality as an Occupation," by B. J. Hemphill, 2008, AOTA Annual Conference & Expo, Long Beach, CA. Adapted with permission.

ent will express and repeat spiritual activities that have meaning. The practitioner's goal is to achieve balance through the therapeutic relationship. The relationship between the occupational therapy practitioner and the client involves the soul and spirit of both persons. This interaction, in the context of the treatment setting, can be a spiritual experience when each person is receptive to the other's soul and spirit.

Occupation acts like a vehicle through which the soul can communicate with the spirit (see Figure 17.1). For example, an occupational therapy practitioner might use the occupation of projective media to help a client express an imbalance between the soul (inner world) and spirit (outer world). Through painting, the client is able to express this imbalance in the outer world, where it has meaning.

Spiritual Assessment

For occupational therapy practitioners, the process of approaching the spiritual condition is similar to other areas (e.g., mental, physical). To identify needs and provide therapeutic intervention, a pro-

cess of evaluation and assessment serves as a necessary first step.

Exhibit 17.1 lists elements that might be included in a spiritual assessment. Koenig (2007) suggested 6 reasons why practitioners should be concerned about a client's spirituality:

1. Many patients are religious or spiritual and would like it addressed in their health care.
2. Religion influences the patient's ability to cope with illness.
3. Patients, particularly when hospitalized, are often isolated from their religious communities.
4. Religious beliefs affect medical decisions and may conflict with medical treatments.
5. Religious involvement is associated with both mental and physical health and likely affects health outcomes (one way or another).
6. [Religion] influences health care in the community. (p. 15)

A client may depend on religion to cope with personal and health-related issues. *Religious coping* is "the use of religious beliefs or practices to reduce the emotional distress caused by loss or change" (Koenig, 2007, p. 19). The client may engage in practices such as praying, meditating, reading from sacred literature, attending worship services, or engaging in spiritual rituals. The client may want to have support from clergy or familiar members of a church, synagogue, mosque, or temple. When a client is isolated from his or her religious community, a minister is not always available to visit. Therefore, the client does not have access to religious recourses as he or she would in his or her own environment. It is important that health practitioners provide a way to identify a client's spiritual needs and resources and make referrals to pastoral care professionals who are trained to address these needs.

Religious coping is the most important factor in recovery from illness (Koenig, 2007), which can be more broadly defined as *spiritual coping*. According to Koenig, "during the twentieth century, more than twelve hundred studies examined the relationship between religion and health" (p. 22). Various methodologies may produce varying results, but they generally support a positive relationship between religion and health. For our purposes, it will help, again, to broaden the religious perspective to a more general sense of spirituality. The research demonstrates that spirituality is important in the recovery from such illnesses as heart disease, arthritis, kidney disease, cystic fibrosis, diabetes, cancer, gynecologic cancer, HIV/AIDS, chronic pain, and terminal illness.

Since 2000, The Joint Commission requires that a professional take and document a spiritual history when a client is admitted to an acute care hospital, nursing home, or home health care agency. The spiritual history usually falls on the nurse to administer, because of the The Joint Commission's requirement.

Because religion is the vehicle through which many people express their spirituality, most of the spiritual assessments collect data from a religious perspective (Pargament, 1997). Generally, there are four reasons a practitioner might conduct a spiritual assessment (Hodge, 2003):

1. *To provide effective, client-centered services:* A therapist must have an unbiased, culturally sensitive understanding of clients' spiritual worldviews.

2. *To understand the importance of respect for client self-determination:* "In order to integrate sclients' spiritual beliefs and values into the therapeutic process, helping professionals must have some knowledge of what those beliefs and values are. Spiritual assessment provides a means to elicit clients' spiritual beliefs and values so that they can be integrated into the therapeutic process" (p. 7).

3. *To meet the growing interest in using clients' strengths to address problems.*

4. *To follow professional code of ethics:* "Professional codes of ethics typically suggest that helping professionals are ethically obligated to engage in spiritually competent practice" (p. 7). An example is the National Association of Social Workers (NASW; 2008) code.

Exhibit 17.1. Spiritual Assessment Questions

Examples of elements that could be part of but are not required in a spiritual assessment include the following questions directed to the patient or his or her family:

- Who or what provides the patient with strength and hope?
- Does the patient use prayer in his or her life?
- How does the patient express his or her spirituality?
- How would the patient describe her or his philosophy of life?
- What type of spiritual/religious support does the patient desire?
- What is the name of the patient's clergy, minister, chaplain, pastor, or rabbi?
- What does suffering mean to the patient?
- What does dying mean to the patient?
- What are the patient's spiritual goals?
- Is there a role of church/synagogue in the patient's life?
- How does your faith help the patient cope with illness?
- How does the patient keep going day after day?
- What helps the patient get through this health care experience?
- How has illness affected the patient and his/her family?

Note. From *Standards FAQ Details: Spiritual Assessent* by The Joint Commission. Copyright © 2013, by The Joint Commission. Used with permission.

The most widely used spiritual assessments are quantitative measures or pen-and-paper questionnaires. Spirituality seems better served by qualitative assessment methods. Qualitative approaches tend to be holistic, open-ended, individualistic, ideographic, and process oriented (Franklin & Jordan, 1995). Spiritual histories are commonly a series of questions. Supplements to spiritual histories are diagrammatic instruments, such as paper-and-pencil drawings, and projective instruments, such as painting.

A spiritual history could be administered at different times but at some point early on in the intake process, for example,

1. *During admission to the health facility:* The professional who conducts the medical history would obtain a spiritual history.
2. *During the initial occupational therapy evaluation:* The occupational therapist conducts a spiritual history during the initial evaluation and integrates relevant questions while obtaining an occupational profile.
3. *During a health maintenance visit as part of a well-person evaluation:* The occupational therapist obtains information about the environment and support system, such as family, job, and sources of stress, that would enhance desired outcomes. (AOTA, 2014)

If the intake professional does not administer a spiritual history during the admissions process, the occupational therapist may administer one during his or her initial occupational therapy evaluation. A therapist may repeat a spiritual history after several months or years, if appropriate. Changes in a client's condition and current medical, social, or environmental status would be indicators that a therapist should review or update a client's spiritual history. A therapist might consider other types of assessments for the reevaluation in addition to a spiritual history.

Guidelines for Selecting Spiritual Assessments

Fitchett (2002) suggested seven issues to consider when selecting a spiritual assessment:

1. *"Is the model's concept of spirituality explicit or implicit?"* (p. 90). Most assessments in this area

of occupation are implicit, meaning they are objective.

2. *"Is it substantive or functional?"* (p. 91). A substantive assessment focuses on the client's beliefs and values, whereas a functional assessment focuses on how the client practices his or her beliefs and values.
3. *"Does it include one or more dimensions of spiritual life?"* (p. 91). A one-dimensional assessment is asking one question, such as "What is your denomination?" A multiple dimension looks at several questions that explore spiritual life in several ways and may provide more depth and insight.
4. *"Is it static or developmental?"* (p. 92). Does the assessment expect change? A developmental assessment expects change in spiritual development. Fowler's (1981) stages of spiritual development are an example.
5. *"Does it have a dynamic perspective?"* (p. 93). The therapist needs to "know what people say, what they believe and feel as well as observations of unconscious attitudes and emotions that might or might not be consistent with those that are consciously held" (p. 93).
6. *"Is the context for spiritual assessment holistic?"* (p. 93). The client's spirituality should not be isolated from her or his religious practices, culture, personality, family, and health. The therapist needs to be alert to ideations about religion that may be caused from a brain injury, medication reactions, or reaction to a stressful situation, or a new religious insight related to health.
7. *"Is the spiritual dimensions [sic] distinct from the psychosocial one?"* (p. 94). In other words, does the assessment assess spirituality and not psychosocial aspects? To put it another way, do not substitute a psychological test for a spiritual one.

The 7 × 7 model described by Fitchett (2002) is the closest to meeting all seven guidelines. This model provides the language that a therapist can use to assess the nonbeliever. It is for people who describe themselves as spiritual but not religious. The FICA Spiritual Assessment Tool (Puchalski, 1999) asks only five questions. There are other assessments that meet some of the guidelines:

- HOPE Questions (Anandarajah & Hight, 2001)
- Spiritual history (Koenig, 2004; Maugans, 1996; Puchalski & Romer, 2000)

- Spiritual Intelligence Assessment (Yaacov & Kravitz, 2007)
- Multidimensional Measurement of Religious/ Spirituality for Use in Health Research (Fetzer Institute and National Institute on Aging Working Group, 2007)
- Spiritual assessment guidelines (Schnorr, 2005)
- OT–Quest Assessment (Schulz, 2008)
- Daily Spiritual Experience Scale (Underwood & Teresi, 2002).

After reviewing several assessments, a practitioner can determine which assessment is best for the context of practice.

Treatment Plans and Intervention

Developing a plan of intervention for the occupational therapy client is not vastly different when spiritual factors are taken into account. Holism and client-centered practice tell us that the goals of a therapeutic intervention should address every aspect of the person, meaning physical and mental rehabilitation should be accompanied by addressing spiritual goals as well. The assessment process allows occupational therapy practitioners to understand the client's needs on each of these levels, and a practitioner's treatment plan should similarly develop interventions that address the needs of the whole client.

Clients are appreciative when their health professional inquires and is knowledgeable about spiritual issues and values their beliefs (Koenig, 2008). They feel supported when the practitioner attempts to integrate their spiritual beliefs into the health care plan. A nonreligious client may resist these attempts, and the practitioner needs to respect avoidance of such discussions.

At the same time, as with a client who may be reluctant to admit to a physical limitation, a client's discomfort with identifying spiritual needs should not be the end of an intervention. Taking a spiritual history in itself is an intervention because it leads to discussion and openness about the client's values and beliefs. It is also important for the practitioner to establish relationships with the faith community, especially its faith leaders. Establishing a relationship with the ministers, priests, rabbis, and imams

---

Exercise 17.1. Spirituality Assessment

- Administer a spiritual history assessment to a client, acquaintance, or another student.
- Develop spiritual questions from the guidelines that could be used in a clinical setting.

---

in the community promotes support and care and shows respect for different approaches to faith.

Healing the whole person is central to the practice of occupational therapy. Kramer, Hinojosa, and Royeen (2003) defined *holism* as "the importance of considering the physical, social, cognitive, psychological, and spiritual dimensions of each person" (p. 40). It is considered a core principle of the practice of occupational therapy. "A holistic, multidimensional view includes full consideration of physical, social, cognitive, psychological, and spiritual factors as shaping behavior" (p. 40). It is the combination of these factors that makes up the profile of a person (AOTA, 2014). *Health*, in a holistic sense, was defined by Kass (1981) and was discussed by Kramer et al. (2003) "as the well working of the organism as a whole and as a state of being revealed in activity relative to each species as a standard of bodily exercise or fitness" (p. 40).

The goals for therapeutic care are client centered. Occupational therapy practitioners should think holistically when developing an intervention plan and determining intervention goals in collaboration with the client and, if appropriate, his or her family. It can be therapeutic for the client to identify and prioritize those items that are distressing based on the assessment. Also, it will help the client realize that he or she has been heard and that the concerns will be integrated into the intervention plan (Puchalski & Ferrell, 2010). The goals should be measurable, be specific, and use various modalities. The client determines what is important. Measurable goals should be thorough and address every aspect of treatment, including physical accomplishments, mental improvements, and enhancements to state of mind.

Occupational therapy practitioners should identify the client's spiritual strengths and use them to enhance outcomes. Hodge (2003) identified five spiritual strengths that have some degree of empirical validation:

1. [Having a] relationship with the Ultimate is a key strength
2. Facilitating coping
3. Defeating loneliness
4. Promoting a sense of mission and purpose
5. Instilling a sense of personal worth and value, and providing hope for the future. (p. 23)

It is important that practitioners maintain a balance between developing spiritual strengths and keeping vigilance on the task at hand.

Practitioners should also develop an intervention plan that is culturally sensitive. Galanti (2008, p. 78) offers the following 7 suggestions:

1. Honor patient requests for same-sex providers whenever possible.
2. Provide spiritual directors when necessary. It must be remembered that clergy may not be available. Hospitals are reducing their pastoral services and combining their services with social services to achieve budgetary cuts.
3. Respect patient's religious beliefs, even when they conflict with your own.
4. Allow patients privacy for prayer.
5. Be aware that different religions have different holy days. (e.g., Friday for Muslims, Saturday for Jews, Sunday for Christians).
6. Allow patients to make informed choices regarding risks when medical procedures conflict with their religious beliefs.
7. Learn what symbols are sacred to those that are treated, and respect them. (p. 87)

When developing the intervention plan, occupational therapy practitioners should use the modalities that are functional to the client's needs. For example, use the client's sacred text to increase hand dexterity to turn the pages. Reading religious literature can help with stress and a feeling of hope. Be aware of the client's dietary needs when teaching feeding and food preparation, and respect cultural expectations and traditions.

Koenig (2008) also has suggestions of what not to do. First, practitioners should never prescribe religion to a nonreligious person. "This involves coercion and possibly represents an ethical and human rights violation" (p. 169). Second, practitioners should stop the spiritual history if the client appears uncomfortable. This means that the spiritual history is client centered and providing it is the client's choice.

Third, it is important to clearly distinguish spirituality and spiritual practice and religion and religious practice. For example, the spiritual history may allow a religious client to express a desire to pray regularly. This can aid the practitioner in addressing a spiritual need, but the expression of a belief or cultural tradition should come from the client. The practitioner's beliefs and cultural traditions should ideally remain private and outside the treatment setting.

Practitioners should never mention prayer before the spiritual history is taken. Clients may be offended if practitioners are not of the same denomination or religion. Remember, the health professional has an authority status and the client may want to please the therapist, so a suggestion to pray together may seem like a requirement, rather than a suggestion, undermining trust and a client's sense of a safe personal space. Fourth, practitioners should either have religious training to provide spiritual counsel or advice to a client or should refrain from such counseling without this advanced training. Addressing a faith-based need is a complex issue, and occupational therapy practitioners should refer such matters to trained faith-based counselors.

Finally, never argue about religious beliefs, even when those beliefs interfere with the medical procedures. It is best to learn about the values and beliefs of the client. Seek to understand and adapt the environment to accommodate religious rituals.

Expressive Media

One intervention modality is to use *expressive media,* such as color pencil drawing, painting, or magazines for collage, and other objective media that can be used to help the client achieve the need for spiritual expression. When a client does not know what to do with the media, the occupational therapy practitioner should direct the client to just plunge into the material and draw, paint, or cut and paste. The purpose is to communicate the client's spiritual journey rather than to assess his or her talent. The goal is to help the client tell his or her story while nurturing the client-centered relationship (Hodge, 2003; Reynolds, 2008). The client interprets the final product and the practitioner simply accepts what the client shares.

Meditation

Meditation is another modality that occupational therapy practitioners could use that would allow the client to express his or her spirituality and promote relaxation (Koenig, 2008). Meditation can facilitate feelings of personal balance and harmony, relaxation, and increased awareness of oneself and one's environment. Meditation practices can also assist with the development of intuition, self-insight, and greater self-trust. An expansion of consciousness often occurs from meditation that replaces feelings of isolation, provides greater personal security, and creates a sensation of being in communion with the universe. Gawain and King (2011) offered the following steps that describe a beginning-level meditation exercise. An occupational therapy practitioner can use this process at the beginning of a therapy session to help a client relax.

1. Ask the client to lie in a comfortable position with eyes closed and breathe deeply, relaxing the mind and body.
2. Instruct the client to "imagine a very powerful presence within and all around that is totally loving, strong, and wise and is nurturing, protecting, and guiding."
3. Have the client "relax and enjoy the feeling that he or she is being totally taken care of by the universe" (p. 12). Conclude the meditation with the following affirmation: "I feel and trust the presence of the universe in my life." (p. 12)

The practice of daily meditation in the therapeutic environment may facilitate both personal and spiritual growth. There are many references that explore options for guided meditation in general ways, which can provide ideas for the practitioner and for the client who wishes to make a regular practice of meditation on his or her own.

Journaling

Occupational therapy practitioners can use journaling as an assessment (Haertl, 2008). Haertl defined *journaling* as "a form of personal writing that expresses perceptions, experiences, dreams, and creativity from the perspective of the self" (p. 61). She also stated, "the use of journal writing is often instrumental in developing insight and work-ing on personal goals, and may be used as a therapeutic tool in rehabilitation" (p. 61).

There are several approaches to journal writing to address spirituality. However, a common approach used by an occupational therapy practitioner is to ask the client to write about his or her spiritual journey. The practitioner instructs the client to use the journey as a metaphor to describe a lifetime of activities that are significant to the client. When the client shares the journal with the practitioner, the practitioner could explore the spiritual nature of the journey by asking the question, "What changed?" This requires the client to begin his or her story with a clear picture of who he or she was at the start of their journey.

When an occupational therapy practitioner gives the client the task of journaling, he or she gives the client a notebook and a writing instrument. The practitioner then discusses with the client the time of day that would be convenient for the client to write. This will help the client develop a writing habit. The practitioner should not care about the client's grammar, spelling, or sentence structure.

It does not matter if the writing occurs daily like a diary or only when the client has something to say. Sharing the content of the journal should not be done in a way that can make the client uncomfortable, and the practitioner should be clear about respecting personal, private aspects of a spiritual journey. Care should be taken as well not to judge content or suggest that there is a "right way" to reflect on spiritual matters, nor should the practitioner feel compelled to share his or her own personal information.

Another important point is that the client needs to understand that the writing is never done and he or she always has something to add or subtract. The therapeutic goal is for client growth, perhaps have an epiphany about his or her spirituality, reduce spiritual distress, and express his or her illness experience.

Boundaries and Ethical Considerations

Occupational therapy practitioners must practice within the *boundaries* of their competence. If the needs of the client exceed the spiritual competence of the occupational therapy practitioner, it is the

Exercise 17.2. Goal and Journal Writing

- Write 5 goals that are measurable and have specific outcomes that improve spiritual strengths.

- Write 5 goals that use the modalities discussed in this section that will demonstrate client spiritual needs.

- Write a question that you wish you knew the answer to. Then write a memory that helps explain the origin of the question.

- Write a memory that you cherish. Reflect on how this memory continues to nourish you.

- Reflect on a discrepancy between what you believe and how you live. Without judgment, write what it feels like to live with this dichotomy.

- Describe in detail the items in your coat pocket or purse. What meaning have you already given them? What else might they symbolize about you or about your life?

- Make a list of people who have contributed to your spiritual development in simple and profound ways.

- Recall a small journey you have taken. As you write the story of this journey, be aware of how the external journey mirrored your soul's journey.

- Choose a place that carries emotional potency for you and have a dialogue with it. What do you have to say about this place?

- Choose a memory that is emotionally loaded. Without ever addressing the event itself, write in the negative space.

Note. Adapted from *Writing the Sacred Journey: The Art and Practice of Spiritual Memoir*, by E. Andrew, 2005. Boston: Skinner House Books. Copyright © 2005, by Skinner House Books. Used with permission.

practitioner's responsibility to recognize the limits of his or her skills and refer the client to a spiritual counselor. It is important that the practitioner obtain client consent before referring to clergy. In all cases, the client should have full control of any communication with a spiritual counselor and must approve any contact or communication.

Some pitfalls for occupational therapy practitioners to consider when addressing spiritual issues in the clinical setting are (1) "stepping beyond the boundaries of competency by addressing issues that lie in the expertise of professional religious caregivers or does not follow up on spiritual needs to ensure that they are adequately addressed" (Koenig, 2007, p. 100); (2) establishing a relationship with a client without taking a spiritual history; (3) providing spiritual advice; (4) being unaware of their own religious beliefs and how they can interfere in the treatment process; and (5) viewing conservative views as "regressive or Victorian" (Koenig, 2007, p. 101).

Pellegrino (1979), who has written extensively about professional roles in medicine, developed a model that uses four words: (1) *profession,* (2) *patient,* (3) *compassion,* and (4) *consent.* First, she proposed that the therapist must be competent in the knowledge and skills of the profession; the professional's knowledge must be grounded in theory and be evidence based. Second, she recognized that the patient is in a vulnerable position and the therapist has power to influence the patient's decision making. Third, *compassion* means that the therapist must be empathetic and relate to the patient's suffering. Fourth, *consent* means that the client-centered relationship should exist with the absence or perception of coercion.

These boundaries and ethical considerations are part of the ethical codes of health care professions such as nursing, social workers, physical, and occupational therapy. Ross (2010) stated that "the spiritual principles of social justice, human dignity and worth are at the heart of codes—either implicitly or explicitly—of most disciplines in health care" (p. 11). When it is explicitly stated in the ethical codes, such as in nursing and social work, the word *spirituality* is mentioned as an obligation or a duty to address the spiritual concerns of the client.

Respect for the religious and spiritual beliefs of a client is also central to the code of ethics. For example, the NASW (2008) Code of Ethics states that a social worker must include a spiritual assessment when evaluating a client and must educate himself or herself in the area of cultural diversity and religious beliefs.

The Reference Guide to the Occupational Therapy Code of Ethics and Ethics Standards does not explicitly include a principle about spiritual practice (Slater, 2011). In the section titled "Patient Abandonment," the code accepts the position on spirituality from the *Comprehensive Accreditation*

Manual for Hospitals (JCAHO & Joint Commission Accreditation Hospital, 2007), which states, "in the delivery of health care there should be respect for a health care practitioner's cultural values, ethics, and religious beliefs and the impact these may have on patient care" (p. HR–21). In Principle 4, "Social Justice," the code states,

> Occupational therapy personnel shall provide services that reflect an understanding of how occupational therapy service delivery can be affected by factors such as economic status, age, ethnicity, race, geography, disability, marital status, sexual orientation, gender, gender identity, religion, culture, and political affiliation. (JCAHO, 1998, p. 12)

Spirituality is implied and couched in various other sections of the code. It is mentioned in the section titled "Am I Facing an Ethical Dilemma?" in which self-interest and social roles are addressed. There are no standards for continuing education to develop knowledge and skills in the delivery of spiritual health care. Perhaps this is for the future.

Summary

Spirituality refers to a part of individuals that can be very private, intensely personal, even hidden away. It is natural and understandable that there has been a social and cultural discomfort in some settings, especially public ones, for looking at and addressing spiritual needs as part of helping one another in difficult circumstances. Respect for personal freedoms and individual choices, a sense of "do your thing," and social permissiveness can also make it seem as if there is a barrier to sharing spiritual insights with one another, a failure to respect differing belief systems, or judging another's experiences and conclusions.

However, we know that a person's spirit and state of mind are integral elements to the whole person's health and ability to recover from adverse events, well beyond simply an intuitive sense that wellness is as much a state of mind as a physical sensation. Addressing the spiritual needs of those in treatment should not seem optional or an interesting afterthought, no more than suggesting that

a wound, simply by looking visibly healed, needs no more treatment. Understanding and addressing all of the needs of a person in treatment and defining wellness in the broadest and most holistic terms help everyone.

The work of understanding and addressing spiritual needs is ongoing and continues to develop. Research should continue that will perhaps demonstrate the value of treating the spiritual condition as an aspect of health. Occupational therapy practitioners should carefully assess clients' spiritual needs and state of mind; occupational therapy is uniquely situated to combine therapeutic, purposeful activities that can address all of a client's needs and goals.

Using some of the suggested assessments and activities listed in this chapter and making spiritual wellness part of the ongoing treatment conversation are all useful steps toward ensuring the spiritual component of health is addressed. Sharing best practices, ideas, and insights with others ensures that the practitioner conversation continues. Publishing carefully researched studies adds to the body of knowledge.

It is possible to have this conversation about spiritual concerns in public, while respecting differences and respecting people's personal and private boundaries, and make progress in addressing spiritual health. The conversation is vital. Seeing rehabilitation as a process of interacting with the whole person—by adding spiritual health and improving state of mind to treatment goals—is central to occupational therapy.

References

Alcoholics Anonymous World Service. (1993). *Alcoholics Anonymous: The story of how many thousands of men and women have recovered from alcoholism* (4th ed.). New York: Author.

American Occupational Therapy Association. (2010). Occupational therapy code of ethics and ethics standards (2010). *American Journal of Occupational Therapy, 64*(Suppl.), S17–S26. http://dx.doi.org/10.5014/ajot.2010.64S17

American Occupational Therapy Association. (2014). Occupational therapy framework: Domain and process (3rd ed.). *American Journal of Occupational Therapy, 68*(Suppl. 1), S1–S48. http://dx.doi.org/10.5014/ajot.2014.682006

Anandarajah, G., & Hight, E. (2001). Spirituality and medical practice: Using the HOPE Questions as a practical tool for spiritual assessment. *American Family Physician, 63,* 81–89.

Andrew, E. (2005). *Writing the sacred journey: The art and practice of spiritual memoir.* Boston: Skinner House.

Christiansen, C., & Baum, C. (Eds.). (1997). *Enabling function and well being* (2nd ed.). Thorofare, NJ: Slack.

Crepeau, E. B., Cohn, E., & Schell, B. A. B. (Eds.). (2003). *Willard and Spackman's occupational therapy* (10th ed.). Philadelphia: Lippincott Williams & Wilkins.

Fetzer Institute and National Institute on Aging Working Group. (2007). *Multidimensional measurement of religious/spirituality for use in health research.* Retrieved from http://www.fetzer.org/resources/multidimensional-measurement-religiousnessspirituality-use-health-research

Fitchett, G. (2002). *Assessing spiritual needs: A guide for caregivers.* Lima, OH: Academic Renewal Press.

Fowler, J. (1981). *Stages of faith.* San Francisco: Harper.

Franklin, C., & Jordan, C. (1995). Qualitative assessment: A methodological review. *Families in Society, 76,* 281–293.

Galanti, G. A. (2008). *Caring for patients from different cultures.* Philadelphia: University of Pennsylvania Press.

Gawain, S., & King, L. (2011). *Living in the light: Follow your inner guidance to create a new life and a new world* (25th ed.). New York: New World Library.

Haertl, K. (2008). Journaling as an assessment tool in mental health. In B. Hemphill (Ed.), *Assessments in occupational therapy mental health: An integrative approach* (pp. 61–80). Thorofare, NJ: Slack.

Hasselkus, B. (2002). *The meaning of everyday occupation.* Thorofare, NJ: Slack.

Hemphill, B. J. (2008, April). *Spirituality as an occupation.* Paper presented at the AOTA Annual Conference & Expo, Long Beach, CA.

Hodge, D. (2003). *Spiritual assessment: Handbook for helping professionals.* Botsford, CT: North American Association of Christians in Social Work.

The Joint Commission for the Accreditation of Hospital Organizations. (1998). *Comprehensive accreditation manual for hospitals.* Oak Brook, IL. Author.

The Joint Commission. (2007). *2008 Comprehensive accreditation manual for hospitals: The official handbook.* Oak Brook, IL: Joint Commission Resources.

The Joint Commission. (2013). *Standards FAQ details: Spiritual assessment.* Retrieved from http://www.jointcommission.org/standards_information/jcfaqdetails.aspx?StandardsFaqId=290&ProgramId=47

Kabat-Zinn, J. (1994). *Wherever you go, there you are: Mindfulness meditation in everyday life.* New York: Hyperion.

Kass, J. (1981). Regarding the end of medicine and the pursuit of health. In A. R. Caplan, J. T. Engelhardt, & J. J. McCart-

ney (Eds.), *Concepts of health and disease: Interdisciplinary perspectives* (pp. 3–30). Reading, MA: Addison Wesley.

Koenig, H. G. (2004). Taking a spiritual history. *JAMA, 291,* 2881. http://dx.doi.org/10.1001/jama.291.23.2881

Koenig, H. (2007). *Spirituality in patient care: Why, how, when, and what.* West Conshohocken, PA: Templeton Press.

Koenig, H. (2008). *Medicine, religion, and health: Where science and spirituality meet.* West Conshohocken, PA: Templeton Press.

Koenig, H. (2011). *Spirituality and health research.* West Conshohocken, PA: Templeton Press.

Kramer, P., Hinojosa, J., & Royeen, C. B. (Eds.). (2003). *Perspective in human occupation: Participation in life.* Philadelphia: Lippincott Williams & Wilkins.

Maugans, T. A. (1996). The SPIRITual history. *Archives of Family Medicine, 5,* 11–16. http://dx.doi.org/10.1001/archfami.5.1.11

Moreira-Almeida, A., & Koenig, H. G. (2006). Retaining the meaning of the words religiousness and spirituality: A commentary on the WHOQOL SRPB group's "A Cross-Cultural Study of Spirituality, Religion, and Personal Beliefs as Components of Quality of Life" (62: 6, 2005, 1486–1497). *Social Science and Medicine, 63,* 843–845. http://dx.doi.org/10.1016/j.socscimed.2006.03.001

National Association of Social Workers. (2008). *Code of ethics.* Retrieved at https://www.socialworkers.org/pubs/code/code.asp

Newberg, A., D'Aquili, E., & Rause, V. (2001). *Why God won't go away.* New York: Ballantine.

Pargament, K. (1997). *The psychology of religion and coping: Theory, research, practice.* New York: Guilford Press.

Pellegrino, E. D. (1979). Toward a reconstruction of medical morality: The primacy of the act of profession and the fact of illness. *Journal of Medicine and Philosophy, 4,* 32–56. http://dx.doi.org/10.1093/jmp/4.1.32

Puchalski, C. (1999). *Spiritual History Tool–FICA®.* Retrieved from http://www.hpsm.org/documents/End_of_Life_Summit_FICA_References.pdf

Puchalski, C., & Ferrell, B. (2010). *Making health care whole: Integrating spirituality into patient care.* West Conshohocken, PA: Templeton Press.

Puchalski, C., Ferrell, B., Virani, R., Otis-Green, S., Baird, P., Bull, J., . . . Sulmasy, D. (2009). Improving the quality of spiritual care as a dimension of palliative care: The report of the Consensus Conference. *Journal of Palliative Medicine, 12,* 885–904. http://dx.doi.org/10.1089/jpm.2009.0142

Puchalski, C., & Romer, A. L. (2000). Taking a spiritual history allows clinicians to understand patients more fully. *Journal of Palliative Medicine, 3,* 129–137. http://dx.doi.org/10.1089/jpm.2000.3.129

Reynolds, F. (2008). Expressive media used as assessment in mental health. In B. Hemphill (Ed.), *Assessment in occupational therapy mental health* (pp. 81–100). Thorofare, NJ: Slack.

Ross, L. (2010). Why the increasing interest in spirituality within healthcare? In W. McSherry & L. Ross (Eds.), *Spiritual assessment in healthcare practice* (pp. 5–16). Keswick, England: M&K.

Schnorr, M. A. (2005). *Spiritual assessment guidelines.* Retrieved from https://old.fgcquaker.org/quaker-library/fosteringmeetings/0229

Schulz, E. (2008). OT–Quest Assessment. In B. Hemphill-Pearson (Ed.), *Assessments in occupational therapy mental health* (pp. 263–289). Thorofare, NJ: Slack.

Schwartz, K. B. (2003). History of occupation. In P. Kramer, J. Hinojosa, & C. B. Royeen (Eds.), *Perspectives in human occupation: Participation in life* (pp. 18–31). Philadelphia: Lippincott Williams & Wilkins.

Slater, B. Y. (Ed.). (2011). *Reference guide to the occupational therapy code of ethics and ethics standards, 2010 edition.* Bethesda, MD: AOTA Press.

Underwood, L. G., & Teresi, J. A. (2002). The Daily Spiritual Experience Scale: Development, theoretical description, reliability, exploratory factor analysis, and preliminary construct validity using health-related data. *Annals of Behavioral Medicine, 24,* 22–33.   http://dx.doi.org/10.1207/S15324796ABM2401_04

Yaacov, R., & Kravitz, J. (2007). *Spiritual Intelligence Assessment.* Retrieved from http://www.spiritualintelligence.com.

Zemke, R., & Clark, F. (1996). *Occupational science: The evolving discipline.* Philadelphia: F. A. Davis.

CHAPTER 18.

OCCUPATIONS, ACTIVITIES, AND EMPOWERMENT

Rita P. Fleming-Castaldy, PhD, OTR/L, FAOTA

Highlights

- ✧ Disempowerment of people with disabilities
- ✧ Myths about disability
- ✧ Impact of disempowering myths on rehabilitation practice
- ✧ Empowerment theory, the empowerment process, and disability
- ✧ Guidelines for empowering practices in occupational therapy
- ✧ Developmental considerations for empowering practice
- ✧ Challenges to empowering practice
- ✧ Resources and supports for empowerment
- ✧ Ensuring future empowering practices in occupational therapy.

Key Terms

- ✧ Budgetary cutbacks
- ✧ Centers for independent living
- ✧ Clinical reasoning
- ✧ Conditional reasoning
- ✧ Dependence
- ✧ Developmental continuum
- ✧ Disability rights organizations
- ✧ Disability studies
- ✧ Disempowerment
- ✧ Empowerment theory
- ✧ Exceptionality
- ✧ Fear of disability
- ✧ Interactive reasoning
- ✧ Networks

- ✧ Occupational profile
- ✧ Online resources
- ✧ Outcomes
- ✧ Narrative reasoning
- ✧ Personal care assistance
- ✧ Personal tragedy
- ✧ Paternalistic approaches
- ✧ Predisability life
- ✧ Procedural reasoning
- ✧ Processes
- ✧ Recovery
- ✧ Resources and supports
- ✧ Transition planning
- ✧ Values

The contributors to this textbook consistently emphasize the capacity of occupations and their related activities to empower people to attain well-being and live a desired life; however, professionals often do not actualize this potential in practice (Honey, 1999; McCormack & Collins, 2010; Redick, McClain, & Brown, 2000). Occupational therapy practitioners can use empowerment theory to guide their development of effective partnerships with the people with whom they work, thus enabling them to become active agents in their lives. *Empowerment theory* provides practitioners with guidance on how to advance the empowerment process and facilitate the development of the knowledge, skills, and attitudes that build personal power, increase choice, and enable control.

In this chapter, I provide foundational information about empowerment theory and describe the theoretical congruence between empowerment and occupational therapy. I examine the relationships between empowering practices, the therapeutic use of purposeful activity, and engagement in meaningful occupations that enable participation. My focus is on the empowerment of persons with disabilities because these are the people with whom occupational therapy practitioners most typically work (American Occupational Therapy Association [AOTA], 2010b). This emphasis is solely because of space constraints and is not meant to imply that occupational therapy practitioners cannot engage in empowering practices with other oppressed cohorts, such as people who are illiterate, unemployed, impoverished, homeless, imprisoned, or refugees or survivors of war and natural disasters (Kronenberg & Pollard, 2006; Moyers & Dale, 2007). The information I present can be (and should be) applied to any person who is disempowered.

I examine beliefs and practices that disempower and confront the historical and continued acquiescence to approaches that are inconsistent with empowerment. Because there are real challenges to the use of empowering practices, I make specific suggestions to promote the empowerment of all who engage in occupational therapy. Throughout this chapter, I emphasize giving voice to the lived reality of persons with disabilities who experience empowerment and disempowerment every day. I include learning activities to raise consciousness about disempowerment and to develop the knowledge, skills, and attitudes needed to work with people in an empowering manner.

Disempowerment of People With Disabilities

Many people with disabilities have the characteristics inherent to an empowered life. However, people with disabilities also disproportionately share some of the following major disempowering characteristics with other marginalized groups (Kielhofner, 2005; World Health Organization [WHO], 2011) that contribute to their *disempowerment:*

- *Unemployment.* Less than half (41%) of people ages 21 to 64 with a disability are employed, compared with 79% in this age group without a disability (Brault, 2012). The proportion of employed noninstitutionalized civilian persons older than 16 is 18% for persons with disabilities and 67% for persons without disabilities (U.S. Bureau of Labor Statistics, 2012).
- *Inadequate education.* The high school graduation rate (including certificates and special or equivalency diplomas) for students with disabilities varies greatly by state from a low of 20% to a high of 90%, with 57% attaining a regular diploma in states that report these data (National Dropout Prevention Center for Students With Disabilities, 2012). Transition planning and services are often inadequate for preparing students with disabilities for their postsecondary lives (WHO, 2011).
- *Poverty.* People with disabilities have lower incomes and are more impoverished than people without disabilities. Adults ages 18 to 64 with disabilities have a poverty rate that is twice the poverty rate of those without disabilities (28% vs. 13.7%; U.S. Census Bureau, 2011).
- *Scarce housing.* Adequate, accessible, and affordable housing is scant in the United States. The average rent for a modest apartment is higher than the monthly income of most people with disabilities. Housing discrimination against people with disabilities is prevalent (WHO, 2011; see Figure 18.1).

Myths About Disability

The mere fact of having a disability can be disempowering to people with disabilities because of prevailing myths about disability, which I discuss here.

Figure 18.1. Despite the passage of federal legislation such as the Fair Housing Act of 1968 and the Americans With Disabilities Act of 1990, activism is still needed to increase the availability of accessible and affordable housing for persons with disabilities.

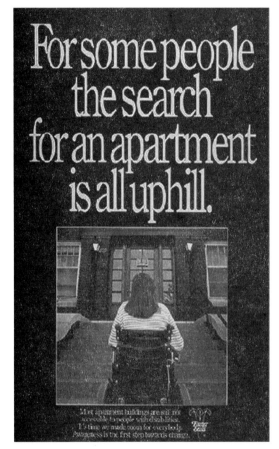

Source. Photo courtesy of Easter Seals. Used with permission.

Disability Is an Abnormal Pathology

The view of disability as pathological has a long-standing history, with one of the most disturbing examples being the display of people with disabilities as circus sideshow freaks (Longmere & Umansky, 2001). Although these public displays are obsolete, the view that disability is not normal still prevails (WHO, 2011). This stance denies the reality that more than 56.7 million noninstitutionalized Americans have a disability (Brault, 2012). This statistic does not include the millions of people in residential programs, nursing homes, correc-

tional facilities, and psychiatric institutions. Can a characteristic be considered abnormal when almost 1 in 5 people residing in the community share it and it has the potential to be incurred by any person at any moment? The disability group is the one minority group that anyone can join at any time.

Disability Is a Personal Tragedy

The perspective that people with disabilities are to be pitied is firmly established in Western culture. Dickens's portrayal of Tiny Tim, the 1960s telethon parades of children struggling to walk while strapped to full leg braces, and biographies authored and movies produced to evoke sympathy have all contributed to the view of disability as a misfortune and *personal tragedy* (Kielhofner, 2005; Snow, 2006; see Figure 18.2).

Contrary to this pitiful view, disability rights activists celebrate their differences and affirm that their personal attributes are not innately disabling. They challenge people without disabilities to stop feeling sorry for them and instead join in the fight against social inequities and inaccurate stereotypes, which are the true source of disability (McCormack & Collins, 2010; Snow, 2006). In the narra-

Figure 18.2. The view of disability as a tragic occurrence that makes life unbearable has strong roots in American culture.

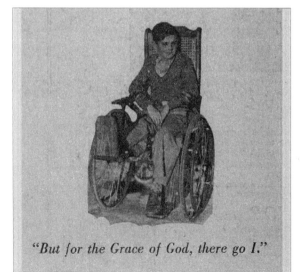

Source. Courtesy of Roosevelt Warm Springs Archive, Warm Springs, GA. Used with permission.

tion to his award-winning short film titled *Thumbs Down to Pity*, Snow, an independent young adult with cerebral palsy, confronts Hollywood's "pity portrayals" of people with disabilities. He describes his life as productive, satisfying, and "nothing like" Hollywood typecasting.

Disability Is to Be Feared

The possibility of incurring a disability is frightening to many. This *fear of disability* is evident in the prenatal testing for conditions such as spina bifida and Down syndrome. Although exploring the moral complexity of these practices is beyond the scope of this chapter, Neville-Jan (2005), an occupational therapist with spina bifida born before these technological advances, raised thought-provoking questions when she asked, "Would I exist today? Is there a value to having spina bifida?" (p. 528). These questions have been raised by many disability activists (Longmere & Umansky, 2001).

The devaluation of life often escalates with intellectual disorders and mental illnesses. Because the mainstream media equates these disorders with irrational thought, impulsivity, and violence, stigmatizing fear reigns. The disempowering impact of fear is accentuated when communities do not confront stigma and fail to protect the rights of persons with disabilities or provide opportunities for participation (Corrigan, 2002; WHO, 2011).

A Person With a Disability Must Rise Above Limitations to Have a Satisfactory Life

Typically, people with disabilities portrayed as successful in the mainstream media are extraordinary (e.g., a mountain climber with paraplegia, a marathon wheelchair runner), yet people do not expect *exceptionality* of people without disabilities. When people apply this expectation of exceptionality to persons with disabilities, then the quality of their lives is perceived as compromised by their disability, and disempowerment occurs.

Contrary to this myth, a routine life can be satisfying, even when assistance is required to complete daily tasks. People with disabilities who self-direct their lives are often satisfied with its quality, regardless of their functional limitations (Fleming-Castaldy, 2011). Disability activists contend that

Figure 18.3. Keith Williams, community organizer for the Northeast Pennsylvania Center for Independent Living, asserts, "Contrary to popular belief, people with disabilities multitask like everyone else." Basic adaptive equipment and community-based personal care assistance enable Keith (who has arthrogryposis) to live, work, and play where he chooses.

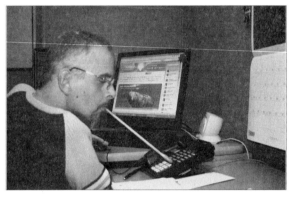

Source. Photo by Nicole Spaldo, who worked with Keith as his personal care attendant for 5 years. Used with permission.

having autonomy, choice, and control in managing services results in increased power over one's life, thus increasing its quality (Morris, 1997; WHO, 2011). A self-determined life (even one viewed as ordinary) can be as satisfying to a person with disability as it is to a person without one (Figure 18.3).

The Intelligence and Rational Decision-Making Capacity of People With Certain Disabilities Should Always Be Questioned

This myth is prevalent in the approaches used by professionals who work with persons who have mental health, cognitive, or developmental disabilities. Professionals are biased when they assert that all decisions that differ from their opinion are symptomatic and should be questioned (Honey, 1999). Assuming that persons who have disabilities are not intelligent because their disability hinders their learning is false. Also erroneous is the assumption that someone with communication deficits resulting from developmental disabilities (e.g., autism, cerebral palsy) is mentally retarded

(Shoener, Kinnealey, & Koenig, 2008). The impact of these invalid assumptions and diagnoses is beyond disempowering; it is harmful. As discussed in Shoener et al. (2008) and as poignantly described by David, a teen assumed to be mentally retarded, misdiagnosis can result in never daring to have dreams.

Professionals Hold the Key to a Person's Recovery From Disability

Recovery is the ability of a person to live a satisfying life of choice while managing the effects of illness on his or her life (Corrigan, 2006). Although professional services can support and facilitate recovery, the assumption that a person cannot recover without these services is false. This belief is inherently disempowering because it removes power from the person with the disability (Bishop, 2001; McCormack & Collins, 2010). A person with a disability can and does recover without (and in some cases in spite of) professional intervention (WHO, 2011). Consumer-operated services can effectively enable recovery and empowerment (Corrigan, 2006). Children with developmental delays can progress, even if families decide not to implement all suggested professional interventions (Holzmueller, 2005).

The Desired and Anticipated Outcome of Rehabilitation Is Acquiring Skills to Perform Activities That Enable the Continuation of a Person's Predisability Life

Although some can and do reach the goal of continuing their *predisability life,* resuming previous life activities is not attainable for many persons with disabilities (Toal-Sullivan & Henderson, 2004; WHO, 2011). If the expected outcome of rehabilitation is to resume a former lifestyle and it does not occur (as is often the case), then the person and professional perpetuate unrealistic expectations. When previous functional levels are not achieved, a person with a disability may experience emotional distress that impedes a postdisability life (Toal-Sullivan & Henderson, 2004).

When persons with disabilities must rely on others to complete daily activities, unanticipated dependency that occurs may foster feelings of personal helplessness (Charlton, 1998). How a person with a disability perceives his or her dependence on others can influence the quality of his or her life (Fleming-Castaldy, 2011; Morris, 1997). For example, does he or she view the need for services as a contributor to independence and personal empowerment or as a sign of personal inefficacy? Thus, the independent resumption of activities should not be the desired outcome of rehabilitation (Charlton, 1998; Toal-Sullivan & Henderson, 2004). Rather, the outcome of occupational therapy should be active engagement in meaningful and desired occupations in a personally satisfying and self-determined manner (AOTA, 2014). I discuss methods to achieve this end in the section "Guidelines for Empowering Practices in Occupational Therapy."

A Person With Significant Disabilities Cannot Live Independently

Although the functional limitations associated with many disabilities result in the need for *personal care assistance (PCA)* to complete tasks, *independent living* is not reliant on activity performance. People are independent when they self-determine how and when their desired activities are performed (AOTA, 2002; Charlton, 1998; WHO, 2011). Adherence to the myth that disability precludes independent living has historically led to the institutionalization of people with disabilities. Currently, public funding significantly limits community-based PCA, resulting in many people with disabilities remaining institutionalized (WHO, 2011). Institutionalization hinders participation in life and increases dependency. The resulting diminished autonomy and decreased quality of life (QoL) are disempowering (Magasi & Hammel, 2009).

It is important to recognize that providing PCA in the community does not ensure that the independence of the care recipient is acknowledged, respected, or facilitated. Many community-based programs adhere to the belief that having adequate PCA requires professional oversight and agency staff management. These paternalistic policies and practices disempower people with disabilities by restricting their choice of and limiting their control over service delivery and fostering dependence.

Charmaz (1983) described the disempowering experience of "being bathed and dressed by strangers with rough hands and patronizing attitudes" (p. 186). He concluded that arrangements made to "aid" the person with a disability can "underscore fears of incapacity or incompetence" (p. 186) when they are not self-determined. Conversely, when persons with disabilities self-select and self-direct their services, they have a satisfactory life and increased autonomy (Fleming-Castaldy, 2011; WHO, 2011). These effects enable independent living results that are highly congruent with empowerment.

Impact of Disempowering Myths on Rehabilitation Practice

The perpetuation of the above-mentioned myths contributes to the prevalence of disempowering practices by rehabilitation professionals (Kielhofner, 2005). Stigmatization and fear of disability undermine the establishment of trusting collaborative relationships (Corrigan, 2002), which are the foundation of empowering practices. Professionals who pity people with disabilities typically adopt a protective maternal approach, which makes forming an empowering partnership impossible. Unhealthy *dependence* is fostered when professionals and other care providers do not give people with disabilities opportunities to take chances, do not give them the right to fail, and do not allow them to make mistakes. This infantilizes them, because personal growth, maturity, and resilience (all of which are essential for empowerment) are developed by taking chances, learning from mistakes, and recovering from failures.

Some professionals believe that they are essential for the recovery of a person with a disability and place themselves in the role of expert. They do not seek the opinions of the person with the disability about his or her preferred life course (Honey, 1999; McCormack & Collins, 2010). A disturbing example of this is the finding of Johnson and Sharpe (2000) that 92% of the special education administrators surveyed would be least likely to facilitate a student-led individualized education plan meeting.

When persons with disabilities express personal goals, professional feedback is often tokenistic, unsupportive, or demeaning (Knox, Parmenter, Atkinson, & Yazbeck, 2000). Rehabilitation pro-

fessionals often tell persons with disabilities (or their families) that successful adaptation requires them to give up many aspirations because they are unrealistic (Holzmueller, 2005; Wehmeyer, 2004).

For example, my brother, Kevin, was told by many that attending college was a waste of time because his Friedrich's ataxia was progressive. They could not envision what Kevin hoped to gain from this experience. Professionals consistently viewed Kevin's resistance to accepting these imposed limitations as maladaptive and clear evidence of his denial of the terminal nature of Friedrich's ataxia. Fortunately, one vocational counselor partnered with Kevin to achieve his goal. The benefits derived from this empowering experience were far greater than the bachelor's and master's degrees earned. Kevin's student role provided him with a satisfying, self-directed life, including meaningful activities and valued occupations, plus partying on spring break! Table 18.1 includes other practice site–specific considerations that occupational therapy practitioners must address, because they affect empowerment.

Practitioners who view themselves as experts further undermine the autonomy and control of people with disabilities when they adopt *paternalistic approaches* (Charlton, 1998; McCormack & Collins, 2010). These disempowering practices diminish the self-efficacy and perceived capabilities of people with disabilities. People need to believe their efforts have the potential to be successful (Bandura, 1977). When professionals treat people with disabilities in a manner that diminishes their internal locus of control, they may have difficulty seeing the point of any efforts to alter their situation. The resulting inability to self-determine desired goals and engage in self-directed behaviors is disempowering (Fleisher & Zames, 2001).

Even if a practitioner does not adopt a paternal or expert stance, possessing professional expertise automatically establishes a separation from nonprofessionals and infers a hierarchical relationship (Gaitskell, 1998). This imbalance of power in the therapeutic relationship can produce feelings of disempowerment (Franits, 2005). Because occupational therapy practitioners often perceive their role as helpers who fix functional limitations, they can be disempowering (Abberley, 1995; Taylor, 2001). When academic and clinical education stresses the profession's focus as attain-

Table 18.1. Practice Considerations for Infusing Empowerment Into Occupational Therapy

Practice Setting	Issues and Concerns That Can Affect Empowerment	Case Example
Early intervention	Sociocultural stigma of parental responsibility for disability. Parents' grief for an anticipated child. Need to emotionally adjust and chart an alternative story for the family. Practitioner's emphasis on developmental norms and milestones, not uniqueness of child.	The parents of a toddler with significant developmental delays report that they have not initiated several of the practitioner's "homework" suggestions because they are too disruptive to the family's routine. The family includes 2 older children, ages 4 and 12 years.
Schools	Noncompliant educational systems that do not obtain parents' or students' voices for individualized education and transition plans. Participation restrictions that limit engagement and perpetuate segregation.	During a transition planning meeting, a 14-year-old describes goals for his postsecondary life, which his parents state are not possible given their child's functional limitations. Several team members concur.
Acute care hospital	Short lengths of stay limit the focus of rehabilitation to the most critical need. Productivity demands and documentation requirements contribute to reductionist practices dominating care.	A 53-year-old concert pianist incurred a concussion and multiple fractures to her dominant hand. She is a part-time student pursuing a music therapy degree. Length of stay is likely 3 days.
Psychiatric partial hospital	Staff mistrust of the rational thinking capabilities of people with mental illness and discomfort with relationships based on equality. Stigma limits opportunities for participation in educational, work, leisure, and living environments.	A 28-year-old with an 18-year history of schizophrenia begins his first day at a partial hospitalization program after a 5-day hospitalization. He is living in a proprietary home and is unemployed. He states he wants to move into his own apartment, finish his college degree, and get a job.
Skilled nursing facility	Residency is most often not a personal choice. Diminished community participation. Loss of control over daily life routines. Restricted occupational roles, limited purposeful activities, and social isolation.	An 87-year-old new resident is referred to occupational therapy for poststroke rehabilitation. The person refuses to participate in the initial evaluation because "life is over" now that her home is "lost" and all friends are "gone."

ing functional independence in performance, the disempowering nature of occupational therapy is reinforced (Taylor, 2001).

Exercise 18.1. Setting the Stage for Empowering Partnerships

Consider how you approach a first session with people you will be working with in occupational therapy. Is your approach empowering or disempowering? Compose a 2- to 3-sentence approach that you would use in the practice scenarios provided in Table 18.1 to introduce yourself as an occupational therapy practitioner who is willing to partner with the person (or his or her caregiver) to facilitate self-directed participation.

Empowerment Theory, the Empowerment Process, and Disability

Empowerment theory integrates theories of control and personal identity with an understanding of sociopolitical contexts to propose that people with disabilities are competent and can proactively participate in life. Empowerment theory focuses on involving persons with disabilities in self-determining and controlling their lives (Charlton, 1998). Zimmerman and Warschausky (1998) proposed that empowerment occurs when persons have perceived control, collaborate with others to attain goals, and are cognizant of supports and barriers to efforts to self-direct life. They described this personal empowerment according to three dimensions: (1) values, (2) processes, and (3) outcomes.

Values

The *values* underlying empowerment theory represent core beliefs that govern how persons with disabilities work with professionals and vice versa. These values include the belief that disability is not synonymous with illness and incompetence; rather, persons with disabilities are valued as capable of wellness and competence. Consequently, person-directed collaboration between people with disabilities and professionals is respected and expected (Zimmerman & Warschausky, 1998). These values of empowerment are congruent with occupational therapy's core values of equality, freedom, justice, dignity, and truth (AOTA, 2010a). They are evident in the profession when practitioners believe that persons with disabilities are competent and often fully capable of independently self-managing their service delivery (Figure 18.4).

Processes

Empowering *processes* are the mechanisms through which persons with disabilities work with each other, professionals, agencies, and communities to gain control over their lives. These involve the

Figure 18.4. Mutual respect is the foundation for empowerment. Michael Auberger talks with a police officer at an ADAPT rally.

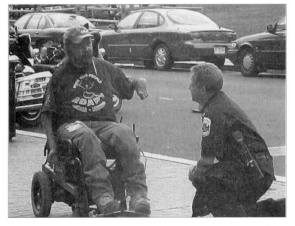

Source. Kathleen Klienmann. Copyright © 2000 by TRIPIL. Used with permission.

Exercise 18.2. Self-Assessment of Values Regarding Power

Fidler (1993) observed that "the capacity to empower self and others is greatly shaped by our values and beliefs about our self and others" (p. 584). Thus, for self-knowledge and personal growth, it is essential to examine one's empowering and disempowering personal views and attitudes. The following questions ask you, as an occupational health practitioner, to reflect on perspectives and issues that can influence your implementation of empowerment principles in practice.

What does power mean to you? What is the difference between control and power? Is it acceptable for a practitioner to be uncertain about a preferred course of action? Consider the cases in Table 18.1. How do you balance the desired empowerment outcome for each person to live a self-determined life with legitimate concerns about the person's realistic chances for success vs. failure? Does the person's diagnosis or age influence your perceptions of his or her ability to decide to self-direct his or her services?

provision of opportunities to help people acquire the knowledge and skills needed to make decisions, self-advocate, and access and manage resources to become self-reliant in the existing sociopolitical environment. Overcoming obstacles that prevent full community participation and changing conditions that present barriers to living a self-directed life are essential empowering processes (Zimmerman & Warschausky, 1998).

In occupational therapy, these empowering processes begin with the attainment of the person's perspective during evaluation (AOTA, 2014). Subsequent empowering processes include the development of self-determined goals; the provision of person-centered interventions, consumer education, and training in personal advocacy skills; and effective management of resources and opportunities to develop and practice leadership skills.

Outcomes

The effects of empowering values and processes include *outcomes* related to increased awareness, control, and participation. Empowered persons with disabilities understand their sociopolitical context. They are motivated to use their acquired knowledge and skills to influence their environment and participate fully in society. Empowered individuals perceive themselves as competent and actively engage in behaviors to exert control over their lives, resulting in an increased sense of autonomy and perceived control (Zimmerman & Warschausky, 1998). These empowerment outcomes are evident at the conclusion of occupational therapy when clients successfully attain self-determined goals for participation, live self-directed lives, and self-advocate to obtain needed services to engage in desired occupations.

Guidelines for Empowering Practices in Occupational Therapy

Occupational therapy based on empowerment promotes and maximizes opportunities and supports for disenfranchised people to gain internal and external control over their environments, actualize their potential for self-direction, and attain self-determined lives (Redick et al., 2000). Practice focused on the knowledge, skills, and attitudes needed to effect change and determine QoL is empowering (Loft, McWilliam, & Ward-Griffin, 2003; Townsend, 1996).

Overall Guidelines

To counter the disempowering effects of disability and facilitate empowerment, the following principles should guide occupational therapy practice.

1. Establish partnership relationships that respect the expertise of each participant

Empowering practice requires client-centered and family-centered approaches grounded in an equitable distribution of power (Honey, 1999; Knox et al., 2000; Kyler, 2008). The practitioner should share realistic and accurate information that offers possibilities rather than pathologizing the situation (Holzmueller, 2005; Knox et al., 2000; Moghimi, 2007). The client's or caregivers' intimate knowledge of the unique effects of disability on current and envisioned occupational performance combined with the practitioner's professional competencies can lead to the attainment of self-determined goals (AOTA, 2014; Wehmeyer, 2004). Acknowledging the expert status of the person supports his or her autonomy, internal locus of control, and self-efficacy—characteristics essential for empowerment (Franits, 2005).

2. Presume intelligence and the potential for competence

Shoener et al. (2008) described the experience of David, who people assumed had an intellectual deficit because of his inability to verbally communicate. It was not until David's professional team used an approach that respected him as an individual and trusted his capacity at the age of 14 years that the validity of this assumption was discredited. As a result, a comprehensive, nonjudgmental occupational therapy evaluation provided an accurate determination of David's capabilities, and he subsequently acquired effective communication, which he said "freed my little voice to be heard" (Shoener et al., 2008, p. 547).

David's vivid and insightful description of living with autism spectrum disorder provides a powerful and highly intelligent voice, which gives testament to the importance of assuming the intellectual capability of all persons with disabilities.

3. Adopt a multitrack mind to apply all types of clinical reasoning

Rogers (1983) identified clinical reasoning as essential for helping persons with disabilities live "the good life." *Clinical reasoning* can be defined as "the process used by practitioners to plan, direct, perform, and reflect on client care" (Schell, 2003, p. 131). Occupational therapy practitioners use complex mental processes of thinking about the individual; the disability; the uniqueness of the situation; and the personal, social, and cultural meanings the individual gives to the disability (Fleming, 1991).

Novice practitioners tend to emphasize *procedural reasoning* because it is concrete (Gaitskell, 1998). Although procedural reasoning is required to identify abilities and challenges to performance, its technical emphasis can be disempowering (especially if used exclusively). Practitioners must put procedures into the context of the client's valued roles and meaningful occupations (AOTA, 2014).

Going beyond the singular use of procedural reasoning to the multifaceted use of clinical reasoning facilitates empowerment. Using *interactive reasoning* to develop a collaborative, trusting therapeutic relationship; *conditional reasoning* to consider the unique developmental, social, and cultural aspects of a client's life (Fleming, 1991); and *narrative reasoning* to listen to an envisioned story (Mattingly, 1991) can have the desired empowerment outcome of enabling the client to engage in a self-determined intervention program. Pragmatic reasoning can ensure that the practitioner considers the influence of personal and practical constraints on service delivery (Schell & Cervero, 1993).

Practitioners must acknowledge that neither disability nor its resulting functional limitations are inherently disempowering; rather, external factors are often the cause of disempowerment (Abberley, 1995). Consequently, the conscious application of pragmatic reasoning helps occupational therapy practitioners understand the social, political, and economic realities of practice and negotiate the pragmatic contextual issues that can hinder or facilitate empowerment.

Evaluation Guidelines

Occupational therapy practice standards emphasize that the focus of evaluation and the type of tools used should always consider clients' occupational roles, concerns, perspectives, and expectations (AOTA, 2014; Moyers & Dale, 2007). These fundamental principles enable empowering practices. Moreover, engaging the clients or their caregivers in an open discussion about the evaluation process and its outcomes can facilitate rapport and the development of a collaborative relationship (Hinojosa, Kramer, & Crist, 2010; Moghimi, 2007). The result for the client who is receiving services is an empowering partnership. Conversely, disempowerment of the client occurs when the therapist does not apply the core principles of collaboration, self-determination, client-centered practice, or family-centered practice during occupational therapy evaluation.

The *occupational profile* is a person-centered occupational therapy evaluation (AOTA, 2014). However, some constraints may preclude the profile from being used (e.g., in a setting with a short

Exercise 18.3. The Empowering Application of Clinical Reasoning

Review the case examples outlined in Table 18.1. Identify the evaluation methods and intervention approaches typically used in these practice situations. Reflect on the technical explanations of these methods and approaches (procedural reasoning). Describe how you can explain these procedures to the client (or caregiver) to engage him or her in the occupational therapy process (interactive reasoning) while considering the uniqueness of the client's situation (conditional reasoning). How can you proactively deal with each setting's challenges and existing constraints to facilitate empowering practices? Identify resources and supports that you can use to address existing barriers to empowerment (pragmatic reasoning).

length of stay; when a person's primary focus is pain relief; Gutman, Mortera, Hinojosa, & Kramer, 2007). Hinojosa et al. (2010) proposed that when practice realities constrain the completion of a full occupational profile, the therapist should focus on the process aspects of this evaluation. Because a comprehensive understanding of a client is the ultimate goal of the occupational profile, using the occupational profile as only an initial evaluation is not the most effective use of this tool; rather a therapist should use the occupational profile throughout service delivery to inform intervention (AOTA, 2014; Hinojosa et al., 2010). The ongoing collaboration that can result from following this suggestion can ensure that the therapist is engaging with the client (an empowering stance), not doing things to or for the client (a disempowering approach).

In addition to the occupational profile, an occupational therapist has many other tools available to support the integration of empowerment principles into the evaluation process. These include, but are not limited to, the Canadian Occupational Performance Measure (Law et al., 1998), Occupational Self-Assessment (Baron & Kielhofner, 2006), Role Checklist (Barris, Oakley, & Kielhofner, 1988), and Test of Playfulness (Law, Baum, & Dunn, 2005). The Self-Assessment of Role Performance and Activities of Daily Living Abilities (SARA™; Lounsbury, 2010) and the Reflective Staircase described in Chapter 11, "Redesigning Lifestyles:

Table 18.2. Empowerment Guidelines for Approaches Used in Occupational Therapy

Occupational Therapy Approach and Empowering Characteristics	Empowerment Guidelines
Health promotion Does not assume disability. Focuses on natural contexts. Aims to create and promote enriched experiences.	Consider all persons as capable of health and wellness, even those with a diagnosed condition. Provide multiple in vivo opportunities for performance of desired activities and meaningful occupations. Create equal opportunities for people with disabilities to engage in natural activities for health and wellness (e.g., wheelchair yoga classes for stress reduction, play groups for new parents and their children).
Remediation or restoration Addresses limitations that hinder performance. Develops and restores new or impaired skills and abilities.	Collaborate to determine person's priorities for skill development. Provide interventions to develop the abilities needed to engage in desired occupational roles (e.g., driver rehabilitation to enable resumption of soccer mom role; strength, endurance, and mobility training to facilitate assumption of the new role of quad rugby player).
Compensation or adaptation Modifies the demands or context of activity to enable performance in natural contexts.	Partner with people to establish their priorities for activity performance. Provide adaptations and compensations that enable performance of people's desired activities in their natural settings (e.g., adaptive play equipment in a barrier-free playground; a personal digital assistant programmed to give cues that help organize work and school tasks).
Maintenance Provides supports that enable the retention of performance abilities. Focuses on meeting occupational needs to preserve quality of life.	Recognize the disempowering impact of limited supports and scant resources for maintaining persons with disabilities in their environments of choice. Network with available services to provide needed and desired supports (e.g., service coordination services to enable a young adult with an intellectual disability to live independently in his or her own apartment).
Disability prevention Addresses risk factors for difficulties in occupational performance. Prevents the development of contextual barriers to occupation.	Assess the person's contexts to identify risks for disempowering disability (e.g., poor ergonomics at work, unrelenting stress due to intense caregiving demands). Provide consultation and referrals to prevent the exacerbation of risks into dysfunction (e.g., consult to ergonomically adapt work sites; refer the parent of an infant with multiple complex medical needs to a home-based, family-care respite program).

Note. Adapted from *Occupational Therapy Practice Framework: Domain and Process, 3rd Edition,* 2014, *American Journal of Occupational Therapy, 68*(Suppl. 1), S1–S48. Copyright © 2014 by the American Occupational Therapy Association. Adapted with permission.

Using Activities to Meet Occupational Needs," are also measures supportive of an empowering evaluation process.

Evaluation tools from other fields (e.g., Consumer Constructed Empowerment Scale [Rogers, Chamberlin, Ellison, & Crean, 1997]; Quality of Life Inventory [Frisch, 1994]) can also provide relevant information to gain subjective perspectives and establish an intervention plan focused on personal empowerment to attain desired goals. When using any assessment, a therapist must be careful not to let the task-oriented nature of the evaluation process hinder his or her ability to hear the client's story (Merryman & Riegel, 2007). Active listening to discern the meaning of disability to the person is essential to empowering practice (Franits, 2005; McCormack & Collins, 2010).

Intervention Guidelines

The *Occupational Therapy Practice Framework: Domain and Process* (AOTA, 2014) describes five approaches used in intervention. Table 18.2 highlights the empowering characteristics of each approach and provides guidelines for using them in an empowering manner.

During implementation of these intervention approaches, the application of the core principles of collaboration, self-determination, client-centered practice, and family-centered practice facilitates empowerment. Empowering interventions provide experiences based on choice that facilitates meaningful involvement (AOTA, 2014; Honey, 1999). To be fully empowering, occupational therapy practitioners must focus on outcomes beyond the clinic, home, or school walls. Intervention must move beyond simulated activities to include in vivo activities.

Practitioners must provide persons with disabilities multiple opportunities to acquire the knowledge and skills needed to become self-reliant and self-determined and to participate fully in their desired environments (Townsend, 1996). Effective interventions are based on, or work toward, a match between the client's abilities and expectations. A practitioner applies his or her activity and occupational performance analysis and synthesis skills to provide clients with the "just-right" challenge to achieve desired goals (AOTA, 2014). Without the analysis of performance in activities, a practitioner cannot effectively help clients develop meaningful occupational roles (Gutman et al., 2007).

A practitioner's use of activities provides a context in which clients learn what they are capable of achieving. Moreover, when a practitioner skillfully adapts activities so that they naturally become an occupation as the clients performs them in their own natural environment, the clients are afforded the opportunity to identify barriers and experience challenges that may not be evident in a simulated experience (Pierce, 2001).

Using this knowledge, the practitioner and client can develop solutions to enable desired occupational performance in the client's typical contexts. Educating a person with disabilities, his or her caregivers, or family members in the principles and methods of activity and environmental analysis, gradation, and modification can provide effective strategies that enable the postrehabilitation performance of desired activities and meaningful occupations in diverse settings (AOTA, 2014). Knowing how to handle future situations can strengthen a family's control, which sustains the client and family members as a family (Knox et al., 2000).

Throughout the occupational therapy process, the development of self-advocacy skills should permeate all interventions. Practitioners can support clients' confident identification of assets, limitations, aspirations, legal rights, and personal responsibilities. If needed, practitioners can provide skills training in communication, assertiveness, and personnel management to help clients become effective self-advocates for living life as they choose (AOTA, 2002, 2014).

Developmental Considerations for Empowering Practice

All of the aforementioned principles and approaches can be applied across the *developmental continuum*. Their effective implementation, however, requires an understanding of development. Failure to consider the client's or caregiver's life stage can contribute to disempowerment. For example, when working with infants and young children, a occupational therapy practitioner typically supports the child's development but may not be cognizant of his or her influence on the family's and child's unfolding identity (Holzmueller, 2005).

To balance disempowering messages of a hopeless future, a practitioner needs to examine the possibilities unique to the child's evolving story and provide pragmatic advice when hope wanes. An occupational therapist should balance a summary of standardized developmental assessments (which commonly identify lags in development) with assessment data that measure gains from the child's and family's perspective about existing and potential strengths (Holzmueller, 2005).

When a child reaches adolescence, a practitioner can facilitate the transition of decision-making power from the parents to the adolescent. A practitioner can help adolescents develop the knowledge, skills, and attitudes needed for self-determined independent living, postsecondary education, or employment in adult life (Gulati, Paterson, Medves, & Luce-Kapler, 2011; Wehmeyer, 2004). Effective *transition planning* must include active collaboration with parents, especially if they have difficulty seeing their child assuming adult roles and occupations that the child has chosen. Supporting the self-determination of adolescents can result in more positive outcomes in adult life (Wehmeyer, 2004;

WHO, 2011). To accomplish this, a practitioner must review the practice models he or she uses to ensure that the approach is effectively meeting the adolescent's goals for living a self-directed life.

School-based practice traditionally emphasizes the use of sensorimotor and developmental models, which are insufficient for the acquisition of the living skills needed to live a self-determined life post-secondary education. Interventions are needed to help an adolescent negotiate the multiple intense changes that occur during this life stage, develop a positive stable role identity, acquire self-efficacy, learn essential life skills, and achieve autonomy (Chinman & Linney, 1998). Gulati et al. (2011) described a conceptual framework using enabling group occupations informed by the adolescents to empower them to attain desired roles.

When working with an adult, the practitioner must counter the disempowering effects of the medical model with the implementation of person-directed approaches to ensure that the client's life stage is considered in formulating a self-directed intervention plan (e.g., beginning a career, establishing a household, raising a family, planning a career change or retirement). To empower an older adult, the practitioner must confront stereotypical and ageist views that equate age with incompetence and loss of control (Loft et al., 2003). The practitioner should use a balanced negotiated approach to decision making based on partnership and shared power when working with an older adult (Moats & Doble, 2006). The disempowering structures that are often inherent in long-term care facilities must be recognized, and concerted efforts must be made to engage the resident, family members, and primary care providers (e.g., nurses' aides) in service care planning (Ingersoll-Dayton, Schroepfer, Pryce, & Waarala, 2003).

Challenges to Empowering Practice

Although concepts congruent with empowerment permeate the literature of occupational therapy and infuse theoretical frameworks, there is no documented evidence that these beliefs have infused actual practice. In contrast, the literature identifies many constraints to the implementation of empowerment into practice (Kyler, 2008; Redick et al., 2000). Anecdotal information received from

students after fieldwork also reflects a lack of integration of these values and beliefs. Several of the major challenges to empowering practices and strategies to address these follow.

Budget Cutbacks and Capped Reimbursement

Empowerment is often a low priority in the current system of care. *Budgetary cutbacks* that lead to decreased services and fewer sessions limit the opportunities to solicit, hear, and act upon the voiced opinions of clients (Redick et al., 2000). Ironically, these constraints can support the use of empowering practices.

In acute care, partnership relationships help people view the provided services as the first step in their rehabilitation (Belice & McGovern-Denk, 2002). A client's investment in the rehabilitation process is enhanced when an occupational therapist implements evaluation focused on the client's goals. Lounsbury (2010) reported that the use of the SARA (which asks clients to identify what they expect from their rehabilitation) enabled person-directed goal setting, promoted client-centered services, and effectively measured functional outcomes to meet reimbursement requirements (Aherne, 2002). Educating clients with disabilities, their caregivers, or family members in the self-management of the clients' postrehabilitation life facilitates recovery (Belice & McGovern-Denk, 2002; Loft et al., 2003; WHO, 2011).

Personal Adjustment and Identity Concerns

People with a new disability may require time to adjust to the reality of their altered lives. They may share many of the stigmatizing myths of disability previously discussed. The resulting disempowering personal identity may limit their ability to engage in rehabilitation (Kielhofner, 2005; Merryman & Riegel, 2007). Occupational therapy practitioners must be careful not to label this disengagement as evidence of poor motivation. Rather, they should partner with the client to identify the social, cultural, physical, economic, and political obstacles to engagement (Abberley, 1995; WHO, 2011).

Intervention should focus on the removal of these barriers and the provision of supports that enable the development of a positive self-identity as a person with a disability capable of living a full and satisfying life (Kielhofner, 2005). Moreover, practitioners should endorse the client's potential for recovery (Corrigan, 2002). The development of positive self-efficacy can mediate the disempowering effects of stigma (Vauth, Kleim, Wirtz, & Corrigan, 2007).

Lack of Faith or Trust

Many persons with disabilities have extensive histories of disempowerment. Often, they are the recipients of services that offer them no choices or control. Consequently, they may consider attempts to self-direct services as futile because experience has taught them that no one will listen and nothing will change (Honey, 1999; Merryman & Riegel, 2007). An occupational therapy practitioner's consistent approach in partnering with the client in an honest and respectful collaboration can renew faith and build trust that the desire for participation is not "just talk" (Honey, 1999, p. 264). Practitioners can also use interactive reasoning to actively seek the client's voice and support his or her development as an expert who is capable of self-determination.

Residual Symptoms and Functional Limitations

Occupational therapy practitioners must judiciously consider a client's capabilities when there are safety concerns. Empowerment does not require endangerment. Peer advocates and support networks can provide a balance between autonomy and safety (Honey, 1999). An important point in recovery is recognizing that the client's symptoms of mental illness typically require systemic monitoring and planned management (Merryman & Riegel, 2007). Programs such as the Wellness Recovery Action Plan effectively promote wellness (Copeland, 2001). Recognizing that exacerbated symptoms can compromise rational independent decision making, people with disabilities can complete advance directives about how they want their intervention to proceed and designate a health proxy. This acknowledges diagnostic realities without disempowering the person (Copeland, 2001).

People may differ in their inclination for control over different aspects of life or their ability to

assert this power (Fleming-Castaldy, 2011; Honey, 1999; Loft et al., 2003). Practitioners should not interpret this disinterest as symptomatic of a deficit in motivation or a weakness in will. A client's desire for control and comfort level of self-direction should be determined and respected. Together, the client and the practitioner should make sure that resources (e.g., a peer advocate, a service coordinator) support self-determination at the client's comfort level.

Practitioners' Attitudes

The vestiges of the previously discussed myths of disability remain to influence how practitioners approach people with disabilities. Practitioners may be hesitant to share power, have paternal or maternal views toward the client, or have stereotypical expectations (Kielhofner, 2005; Merryman & Riegel, 2007). Each practitioner must confront these disempowering beliefs with active self-reflection, honest self-critique, proactive use of supervision, and open dialogues with peers and the client. Assertive use of the resources listed below can help practitioners develop the attitudes needed to infuse empowerment into their practices effectively.

Resources and Supports for Empowerment

Occupational therapy practitioners seeking to enact empowering practices must recognize that support from multiple sources helps counter the challenges mentioned earlier. Pragmatically, an individual practitioner cannot feasibly meet all of a client's needs; however, community and national resources can facilitate goal attainment and enable participation. I strongly believe that it is an ethical responsibility for each practitioner to proactively acquire and assertively share knowledge about *resources and supports* that foster empowerment.

Disability Studies

Disabilities studies provide practitioners with an appreciation of the longstanding disempowerment of people with disabilities, the evolution of the disability rights movement, and the lived experience of disability. The knowledge gained from these studies can facilitate practitioners' commitment to advocating for enduring societal changes that can prevent history from repeating itself. First-person narratives of living with a disability enhance practitioners' understanding of the uniqueness of persons with disabilities and the consequences of empowering and disempowering practices and policies (Franits, 2005; Kielhofner, 2005; McCormack & Collins, 2010). One growing body of knowledge is narratives that give voice to the occupational experiences of persons with disabilities (Kielhofner, 2005).

Integrating the knowledge gained with the latest literature on effective evaluation and intervention approaches enables occupational therapy practitioners to provide best practice that is inclusive of the person's subjective experience (Franits, 2005). Sharing current information with service recipients provides an empowering level of control and is an essential foundation for informed decision making (Knox et al., 2000; WHO, 2011)

Professional Networks

Empowering practices require openness to diverse opinions, a commitment to innovation, and the attainment and maintenance of excellence (WHO, 2011). Joining with colleagues to listen to concerns, share challenges, and celebrate successes can facilitate the development of personal and professional networks of participants (e.g., Metropolitan New York District [MNYD], 2009a). An exemplar of the empowering effects of a professional network is the MNYD Mental Health Task Force, whose regular meetings have provided its participants with the benefits of professional networks for over a decade.

Disability and Consumer Organizations

Practitioners can support empowering practices by participating in organizations committed to the full participation of persons with disabilities. Partnering with members of *disability rights organizations* (e.g., National Alliance for the Mentally Ill [NAMI], American Association of People With Disabilities, ARC for People With Intellectual and Developmental Disabilities [ADAPT]) and parent, caregiver, and consumer groups (e.g., clubhouse members) can help a practitioner move from an

insular view of the effects of disability on participation to a broader perspective of living with a disability.

A practitioner who establishes partnerships with disability rights groups can share his or her expertise about the empowering effects of occupation to enable participation. Together, a practitioner and nonpractitioner can work toward obtaining the societal changes needed for full participation by all members of society (Swarbrick & Pratt, 2006). For example, the aforementioned MNYD Mental Health Task Force partnered with a mental health consumer group to present an annual conference focused on recovery and with the local chapter of NAMI to provide programs supportive of the annual NAMI antistigma empowerment walk (MNYD, 2009a, 2009b). These partnership activities clearly epitomize the values and realize the goals of empowerment.

Occupational therapy practitioners should encourage their clients to join empowering organizations (WHO, 2011). For example, *centers for independent living (CILs)* are primary sources that provide links for persons with all types of disabilities to multiple services that enable empowerment (e.g., peer advocates; no-interest and low-interest loans for home modifications). Membership in CILs and other disability rights and consumer-driven organizations introduces people to an empowerment culture that can foster a positive identity as persons with disabilities. Clubhouse programs based on the recovery model are particularly empowering for people with mental illness, because they do not distinguish between professional staff and nonprofessional consumer members (Swarbrick & Pratt, 2006). Both CILs and clubhouses provide self- and peer advocacy training that can further support personal empowerment.

Online Resources

All of the national disability rights organizations and many local ones maintain excellent websites and *online resources* dedicated to the empowerment of persons with disabilities. Several of these organizations send free e-blasts to inform subscribers about current issues, practices, and policies that support empowerment. In addition to informing the practitioner, these resources should be shared with all service recipients because "information equals power" (Honey, 1999, p. 262). The power of information technology should be harnessed to disseminate knowledge, build partnerships, and advocate for societal change (Baker, 2000; Cottrell, 2005, 2007; WHO, 2011).

The disempowering effects of practices that do not use available resources versus the outcomes of empowering practices that integrate additional supports became strongly evident during my doctoral research. While conducting my study of the QoL for persons with disabilities who use PCA, almost no participants who had received or were currently receiving occupational therapy shared information that reflected that their practitioner had informed them of key resources (Fleming-Castaldy, 2011).

For example, Jim, a young adult who experienced a stroke at age 19 years, stated he was not told about any supports for resuming college and independent living. His rehabilitation focused solely on the return of sensorimotor function and independent performance of basic activities of daily living (ADLs). Jim did not attain complete sensorimotor return and remained dependent in several basic ADLs. He was discharged to live with his family and receive basic ADL assistance from aides employed by a home health agency. As a result, he "felt like a baby" and was "all dressed up with nowhere to go." Jim lived this "nonexistence" until after his second stroke at the age of 22 "saved his life."

Although the functional outcome of this second rehabilitative stay did not differ from the first, the QoL outcome Jim subsequently achieved was its polar opposite. Although Jim continued to require assistance for basic ADLs, he reported that he was highly satisfied with his life. Jim hired people he likes "who can adapt their schedule around mine" and "who know I'm not an idiot just because I need help." At the time of the study, he was a college senior living independently in an off-campus apartment ("I felt too old for a dorm"), working as a peer advocate, and deciding which graduate program best suited his interests and whether he should first take time off to travel Europe with friends. As Jim summed up, "Life is good." What enabled Jim to move from a life of despondency to one of satisfaction and potential?

Jim attributed this substantial change to his second occupational therapist, who used the Role Checklist to identify his past, present, and future valued roles. Together, they discussed the reality that Jim did not identify any current valued role except as a family member (which was compromised because he felt "like a burden") and that he saw no future roles for himself. The therapist effectively applied narrative reasoning and asked Jim to envision and describe his optimal future. She and Jim collaborated to develop goals for the resumption of his previously valued roles. The occupational therapist structured all sessions (even those focused on sensorimotor return) toward role acquisition. These included multiple sessions to develop Jim's ability to self-direct his PCA and self-advocate.

At discharge, the therapist provided Jim with a referral to his area CIL. Although this center was an hour's drive from his home, Jim partnered with CIL staff via Internet communications and targeted in-person meetings to obtain consumer-directed PCA and vocational services that enabled him to attain the future he had imagined. By using all types of clinical reasoning and looking beyond the clinic walls, this occupational therapist provided Jim with the knowledge, skills, and attitudes he needed to live an empowered, self-determined life.

However, Jim's experience with an occupational therapy practitioner committed to empowering practices was unique. In my dissertation, participants were more likely to share the disempowering practices of practitioners. These included a woman with multiple sclerosis who reported that her life was not as satisfying as it had been in the past because her declining vision made reading too difficult. Her occupational therapy practitioner advised her to buy recorded books, but she could not afford them. Apparently, the practitioner was not aware that public libraries loan these for free and that the Library of Congress has a free home delivery recorded book program for persons with visual impairments and physical disabilities.

Similarly, uninformed practitioners did not tell a person who missed driving about programs that fund automobile adaptations. Nor did the person frustrated by his inability to schedule agency-provided PCA at times that enabled him to attend his children's school functions learn that consumer-directed PCA was available to give him this desired control. These findings troubled me greatly because I knew supports external to traditional services could empower people to lead self-directed lives and be engaged in meaningful activities and desired occupations.

Exercise 18.4. Community Resources for Empowerment

Find out what resources are available in your community to support the empowerment of people with disabilities and other disenfranchised groups. Key resources to track down are CILs; adult education programs; one-stop career centers; and consumer, family, and caregiver support and advocacy groups. Identify national resources that can be accessed to supplement local ones. Because it is important to determine the efficacy of services before recommending them, contact each resource as a potential consumer. Review the resource's policies, service usefulness, and personnel availability to assess whether they comply with empowering practices.

Ensuring Future Empowering Practices in Occupational Therapy

For occupational therapy to become a profession recognized as one of empowerment, practitioners must individually and collectively articulate the relationship between occupation and the ability to lead a self-determined life. Empowering practices must infuse the process of occupational therapy across the developmental continuum and in all practice settings. Those committed to empowerment must recognize that the attainment of subjective power does not equate the achievement of objective power. A person may have the capacity to self-direct his or her life, but efforts may be thwarted by systemic barriers (e.g., no transportation to get to work). Objective power occurs when structures, systems, and policies exist that enable and support subjective empowerment (Charlton, 1998; Honey, 1999). Consequently, occupational therapy practitioners must proactively and assertively work with others outside the profession to ensure that clients can fully participate in society as they choose.

To help make this elusive aim a reality, I propose that occupational therapy practitioners take the following action steps:

1. *Revitalize a commitment to the founding principles and core values of occupational therapy.* The ethos of occupational therapy is inherently congruent with empowerment (Peloquin, 2005). Steadfast dedication to this heritage and enduring spirit strongly supports occupational therapy practitioners' engagement in empowering practices.

2. *Use the* Occupational Therapy Code of Ethics and Ethics Standards (AOTA, 2010a) *as the bridge from disempowering practices to empowering ones.* AOTA's ethical codes provide an effective moral guide for rejecting the disempowerment of people and for working vigilantly toward the empowerment of all. Table 18.3 describes how these ethical principles can provide a conceptual bridge to empowerment. Consistent and honest personal reflection is required to ensure the actualization of these connections in daily practice.

3. *Design research that is fully inclusive of people with disabilities or other marginalized groups.* Research based on empowerment recognizes the validity of the mantra, "Nothing about us, without us." The external examination of disenfranchised people is disempowering. Empowering research seeks to learn from participants. Thus, researchers must actively seek people to be the primary informants about their lived experiences (Block, Skeels, & Keys, 2006: Hammell, Miller, Forwell, Forman, & Jacobsen, 2012). Although this aim is best attained through qualitative inquiry, quantitative studies can also be designed to obtain participants' voices. Contemporary definitions of evidence-based practice include the integration of clients' values, beliefs, and priorities with established research and theories (Ilott, 2012).

Gutman (2008) proposed that occupational therapy research should address concerns that clients identify as most important. Consequently, the examination of the impact of disability experiences on participation should be a research priority (Gutman, 2008), and research agendas should be informed by participants' priorities (Hammell et al., 2012). Participatory action research (PAR) and participatory intervention research (PIR) can be used to examine participation (Block et al., 2006; Knox et al., 2000).

These approaches assertively apply empowering practices to research design and implementation. Multiple PAR and PIR exemplars exist to guide occupational therapy researchers in their development of projects that are inclusive of the voices of persons with disabilities and their caregivers; sensitive to social, cultural, and political

Table 18.3. Occupational Therapy Code of Ethics and Ethics Standards and Empowerment

Ethical Principle and Key Attributes	Principle's Bridge to Empowerment
Beneficence: Concern for the well-being of service recipients, defense of the rights of others, and concerted advocacy for needed services.	Well-being is attained when people have choice and control over their lives; advocating for services and policies that enable self-directed lives for all is expected.
Nonmaleficence: Imposition or infliction of harm to service recipients must be avoided.	Harm is imposed and inflicted when people are deprived of free choice, receive insufficient services, or are given prescriptive options; confronting policies and practices that demean people and deny basic human rights is required.
Autonomy: Respect for service recipients' personal values, beliefs, preferences, and decisions.	Independence is realized through collaborative partnerships as led by the person; policies and practices that enable autonomous self-direction and honor people's rights to self-determination (e.g., Individuals With Disabilities Education Improvement Act of 2004) are necessary.
Duty: The competence of practitioners must be attained and maintained, a commitment to lifelong learning is a mandate.	Empowering practice requires the development of proficiencies beyond professional specialization; the assertive pursuit of knowledge about policies and practices supportive of people's empowerment and the development of advocacy skills are vital.
Social justice: The assurance that services and resources are distributed fairly, equitably, and appropriately.	Just practitioners must address the impact of social inequities on health and well-being, confront injustices that limit opportunities for full participation in society, and advocate for the fair and just treatment of all.
Procedural justice: Compliance with laws, institutional standards, and AOTA policies to ensure that rules about professional services are applied consistently, impartially, and fairly.	The just rendering of services compels practitioners to be astute about all laws and policies that support empowerment; ignorance of the law does not excuse disempowering practices (e.g., poor transition planning).
Veracity: Practitioners must accurately represent themselves and fully disclose information about their services that may affect outcomes.	Truthful practice, which enables trust; informed awareness and honest acknowledgment of personal, professional, institutional, social, or political biases are required.
Fidelity: Relationships with clients, colleagues, and other professionals must be respectful, fair, and discreet; integrity is required for good-faith relationships.	A shared and unwavering commitment to moral action requires practitioners to confront ethical breeches; being silent when observing or learning of disempowering practices is the same as personally engaging in this practice.

Source. From "Occupational Therapy Code of Ethics and Ethics Standards," 2010a, *American Journal of Occupational Therapy, 64,* S18–S26. Copyright © 2010 by the American Occupational Therapy Association. Adapted with permission.

contexts; improve the QoL of disenfranchised groups as a community and as individuals; and achieve "a shared vision for social change" (Block et al., 2006, p. 5).

4. *Integrate empowerment theory into occupational therapy educational curricula.* To help a future practitioner develop the knowledge, skills, and attitudes needed for empowering practice, occupational therapy curricula must broaden their scope to include the disability rights perspective (WHO, 2011). Educators must foster the belief

that the desired outcome of occupational therapy is a person's ability to lead a self-directed, occupationally meaningful life, not independent activity performance. Moreover, each student needs to become more astute about the economic, social, and political barriers to full community participation faced by marginalized populations. Thibeault (2006) urged occupational therapy educators to stop training students in "a vacuum of the rich" and to "train students to be responsible global citizens" (p.

Exercise 18.5. Advocating for Empowerment

Reflect on the challenges to empowering practices in the different practice situations described in Table 18.1. What policy changes are needed to remediate societal barriers to empowerment? Complete an Internet search to identify a professional association (e.g., AOTA) or disability rights organization (e.g., ADAPT, NAMI) that is actively working to change disempowering policies. Review the advocacy options available. Identify ones that you can act on to further these efforts to enact empowering policies (e.g., write a letter to your state or federal representative, participate in the NAMI walk, join a rally).

160). Confronting each student's attitudes about disability, power, control, choice, and independence may contribute to a reflective practitioner who is committed to empowering practices (Taylor, 2001).

5. *Partner with disability rights organizations and other activists representing disenfranchised groups.* An occupational therapy practitioner can join with advocates, policymakers, and lobbyists to remove social, economic, and political barriers to participation (Cottrell, 2005, 2007; Lohman, Gabriel, & Furlong, 2004; WHO, 2011). I believe that we have a moral obligation to confront social inequities that disempower people, because not to act is to acquiesce.

6. *Inform clients in occupational therapy about empowering options for their lives.* AOTA's (2014) *Framework* includes self-advocacy as both an intervention method and an outcome of occupational therapy. However, if a person is not cognizant of the resources available to him or her, these goals may be difficult (or impossible) to achieve. Consistent with my research, Magasi and Hammel (2009) described the disempowerment of adult women forced to live in nursing homes because they were unaware of community-based alternatives.

Redick et al. (2000) found that few occupational therapists used available resources to inform clients about the ADA even though the majority (90%) acknowledged the importance of these mandates for the participation of people with disabilities. Only 1% to 5% reported implementing ADA-related activities with their clients, and only 14% used a CIL as an ADA resource. Each occupational therapy practitioner must assert his or her commitment to participation and actualize this viewpoint. Practitioners must move beyond token statements of support for participation to serve as informational and organizational liaisons to persons with disabilities. Increased knowledge about choices that enable self-determination and participation is essential for the achievement of empowerment (Magasi & Hammel, 2009; Redick et al., 2000; Wehmeyer, 2004).

Summary

It was not my intention (nor was it feasible) to describe the full range of ideas, theoretical principles, and actions that constitute empowerment in this chapter. Rather, I sought to increase awareness of the potential for occupational therapy to serve as a vehicle for empowerment. The congruence between empowerment and occupational therapy's foundational principles, core values, and ethics is clear, but each practitioner must realize that beliefs alone cannot empower. He or she must recognize the multifacets of people and the complexities of their contexts. Each practitioner must acknowledge that external disempowering barriers often stymie the real gains made in occupational therapy. Consequently, a practitioner must be prepared to confront myths, services, and policies that limit rather than promote empowerment.

I hope that the learning exercises in the chapter sparked active reflection, raised critical consciousness, and engendered a personal commitment to the development and promotion of empowering practices and policies. By partnering with a person with a disability and other marginalized people and their families and caregivers, occupational therapy practitioners can help service recipients develop the knowledge, skills, and attitudes needed to enable subjective power and to advocate for the systemic changes required for objective power. These empowerment outcomes, combined with the empowering potential of purposeful activity and meaningful occupation, can enable participation long after occupational therapy services have ceased. This end result empowers a person to be his or her own agent of change to live a self-determined life in environments of choice and fulfills the promise and purpose of occupational therapy to enable participation for all.

Acknowledgments

I thank former University of Scranton graduate assistant Kristin Leccese and former University of Scranton work-study student Katherine Regimbal for their research assistance with this work, as well as Jenna Osborn, former University of Scranton graduate assistant, for her editorial assistance with the previous edition of this chapter. I also thank Allison Amole, Allison Kearney, Colleen Scannell, Lauren Siconolfi, and Nicole Spaldo (former members of my graduate faculty-mentored research group) for their research contributions to the previous edition of this chapter, stimulating discussions about the actualization of empowerment in occupational therapy, and helpful editorial critiques.

Dedication

I dedicate this work to my brother, Kevin Michael Fleming (1954–1989). Although Kevin could not win his battle with Friedrich's ataxia, his tenacious fight to live a self-directed life remains my inspiration.

References

Abberley, P. (1995). Disabling ideology in health and welfare: The case of occupational therapy. *Disability and Society, 10,* 221–232. http://dx.doi.org/10.1080/09687599550023660

Aherne, A. M. (2002). *Testing the validity of the Self-Assessment of Role Performance and Activities of Daily Living Abilities (SARA) using other standardized assessments.* Albany, NY: Sage Colleges.

American Occupational Therapy Association. (2002). Broadening the construct of independence. *American Journal of Occupational Therapy, 56,* 660. http://dx.doi.org/10.5014/ajot.56.6.660

American Occupational Therapy Association. (2010a). Occupational therapy code of ethics and ethics standards. *American Journal of Occupational Therapy, 64*(Suppl.), S18–S26. http://dx.doi.org/10.5014/ajot.64.1.18

American Occupational Therapy Association. (2010b). *Occupational therapy workforce and compensation study.* Bethesda, MD: Author.

American Occupational Therapy Association. (2014). Occupational therapy practice framework: Domain and process (3rd ed.). *American Journal of Occupational Therapy, 68*(Suppl. 1), S1–S48. http://dx.doi.org/10.5014/ajot.2014.682006

Americans With Disabilities Act of 1990, Pub. L. 101–336, 42 U.S.C. § 12101.

Baker, M. (2000). Patient care (empowerment): The view from a national society. *British Medical Journal, 320,* 1660–1662. http://dx.doi.org/10.1136/bmj.320.7250.1660

Bandura, A. (1977). Self-efficacy: Toward a unifying theory of behavioral change. *Psychological Review, 84,* 191–215. http://dx.doi.org/10.1037/0033-295X.84.2.191

Baron, K., & Kielhofner, G. (2006). *A user's manual for the Occupational Self Assessment (OSA), Version 2.2.* Chicago: University of Illinois, Model of Human Occupation Clearinghouse, Department of Occupational Therapy, College of Applied Health Sciences.

Barris, R., Oakley, F., & Kielhofner, G. (1988). The role checklist. In B. J. Hemphill-Pearson (Ed.), *Mental health assessment in occupational therapy: An integrative approach to the evaluative process* (pp. 73–91). Thorofare, NJ: Slack.

Belice, P., & McGovern-Denk, M. (2002). Reframing occupational therapy in acute care. *OT Practice, 7*(8), 21–22, 24–26.

Bishop, M. (2001). The recovery process and chronic illness and disability: Applications and implications. *Journal of Vocational Rehabilitation, 16,* 47–52.

Block, P., Skeels, S. E., & Keys, C. B. (2006). Participatory intervention research with a disability community: A practical guide to practice. *International Journal of Disability, Community and Rehabilitation, 5.* Retrieved from http://www.ijdcr.ca/VOL05_01_CAN/articles/block.shtml

Brault, M. (2012, July). *Americans with disabilities: 2010 household economic studies* (Current Population Reports Series P-70-131). Retrieved from http://www.census.gov/prod/2012pubs/p70-131.pdf

Charlton, J. (1998). *Nothing about us without us.* Berkeley: University of California Press.

Charmaz, K. (1983). Loss of self: A fundamental form of suffering in the chronically ill. *Sociology of Health and Illness, 5,* 168–195. http://dx.doi.org/10.1111/1467-9566.ep10491512

Chinman, M., & Linney, J. (1998). Toward a model of adolescent empowerment: Theoretical and empirical evidence. *Journal of Primary Prevention, 18,* 393–413. http://dx.doi.org/10.1023/A:1022691808354

Copeland, M. (2001). Wellness Recovery Action Plan (WRAP): A system for monitoring, reducing and eliminating uncomfortable or dangerous physical symptoms and emotional feelings. *Occupational Therapy in Mental Health, 18,* 127–150.

Corrigan, P. W. (2002). Empowerment and serious mental illness: Treatment partnerships and community opportunities. *Psychiatric Quarterly, 73,* 217–228. http://dx.doi.org/10.1023/A:1016040805432

Corrigan, P. W. (2006). Impact of consumer-operated services on empowerment and recovery of people with psychiatric disabilities. *Psychiatric Services, 57,* 1493–1496. http://dx.doi.org/10.1176/appi.ps.57.10.1493

Cottrell, R. P. (2005). The Olmstead decision: Landmark opportunity or platform for rhetoric? Our collective responsibility for full community participation. *American Journal of Occupational Therapy, 59,* 561–568. http://dx.doi.org/10.5014/ajot.59.5.561

Cottrell, R. P. (2007). The New Freedom Initiative—Transforming mental health care: Will OT be at the table? *Occupational Therapy in Mental Health, 23,* 1–25. http://dx.doi.org/10.1300/J004v23n02_01

Fair Housing Act of 1968, Pub. L. 100–420, 42 U.S.C. 3601–3619.

Fidler, G. S. (1993). The quest for efficacy. *American Journal of Occupational Therapy, 47,* 583–586. http://dx.doi.org/10.5014/ajot.47.7.583

Fleisher, D., & Zames, F. (2001). *The disability rights movement: From charity to confrontation.* Philadelphia: Temple University Press.

Fleming, M. H. (1991). The therapist with the three-track mind. *American Journal of Occupational Therapy, 45,* 1007–1014. http://dx.doi.org/10.5014/ajot.45.11.1007

Fleming-Castaldy, R. P. (2011). Are satisfaction with and self-management of personal assistance services associated with the life satisfaction of persons with physical disabilities? *Disability and Rehabilitation, 33,* 1447–1459. http://dx.doi.org/10.3109/09638288.2010.533246

Franits, L. E. (2005). Nothing about us without us: Searching for the narrative of disability. *American Journal of Occupational Therapy, 59,* 577–579. http://dx.doi.org/10.5014/ajot.59.5.577

Frisch, M. B. (1994). *QOLI: Quality of Life Inventory.* Minneapolis: Pearson Assessments.

Gaitskell, S. (1998). Professional accountability and service user empowerment: Issues in community mental health. *British Journal of Occupational Therapy, 61,* 221–222.

Gulati, S., Paterson, M., Medves, J., & Luce-Kapler, R. (2011). Adolescent group empowerment: Group-centred occupations to empower adolescents with disabilities in the urban slums of North India. *Occupational Therapy International, 18,* 67–84. http://dx.doi.org/10.1002/oti.294

Gutman, S. (2008). From the Desk of the Editor—Research priorities of the profession. *American Journal of Occupational Therapy, 62,* 499–501. http://dx.doi.org/10.5014/ajot.62.5.499

Gutman, S. A., Mortera, M. H., Hinojosa, J., & Kramer, P. (2007). Revision of the *Occupational Therapy Practice Framework. American Journal of Occupational Therapy, 61,* 119–126. http://dx.doi.org/10.5014/ajot.61.1.119

Hammell, K. R., Miller, W. C., Forwell, S. J., Forman, B. E., & Jacobsen, B. A. (2012). Sharing the agenda: Pondering the politics and practices of occupational therapy research. *Scandinavian Journal of Occupational Therapy, 19,* 297–304. http://dx.doi.org/10.3109/11038128.2011.574152

Hinojosa, J., Kramer, P., & Crist, P. (Eds.). (2010). *Evaluation: Obtaining and interpreting data* (3rd ed.). Bethesda, MD: AOTA Press.

Holzmueller, R. L. (2005). Therapists I have known and (mostly) loved. *American Journal of Occupational Therapy, 59,* 580–587. http://dx.doi.org/10.5014/ajot.59.5.580

Honey, A. (1999). Empowerment versus power: Consumer participation in mental health services. *Occupational Therapy International, 6,* 257–276. http://dx.doi.org/10.1002/oti.101

Ilott, I. (2012). Evidence-based practice: A critical appraisal. *Occupational Therapy International, 19,* 1–6. http://dx.doi.org/10.1002/oti.1322

Individuals With Disabilities Education Improvement Act of 2004, Pub. L. 108–446, 118 Stat. 36471.

Ingersoll-Dayton, B., Schroepfer, T., Pryce, J., & Waarala, C. (2003). Enhancing relationships in nursing homes through empowerment. *Social Work, 48,* 420–424. http://dx.doi.org/10.1093/sw/48.3.420

Johnson, D., & Sharpe, M. (2000). Results of a national survey on the implementation of the transition service requirements of IDEA. *Journal of Special Education Leadership, 13,* 15–26.

Kielhofner, G. (2005). Rethinking disability and what to do about it: Disability studies and its implications for occupational therapy. *American Journal of Occupational Therapy, 59,* 487–496. http://dx.doi.org/10.5014/ajot.59.5.487

Knox, M., Parmenter, T., Atkinson, N., & Yazbeck, M. (2000). Family control: The views of families who have a child with an intellectual disability. *Journal of Applied Research in Intellectual Disabilities, 13,* 18–28. http://dx.doi.org/10.1046/j.1468-3148.2000.00001.x

Kronenberg, F., & Pollard, N. (2006). Political dimensions of occupation and the roles of occupational therapy. *American Journal of Occupational Therapy, 60,* 617–625. http://dx.doi.org/10.5014/ajot.60.6.617

Kyler, P. (2008). Client-centered and family-centered care: Refinement of the concepts. *Occupational Therapy in Mental Health, 24,* 100–120. http://dx.doi.org/10.1080/01642120802055150

Law, M., Baptiste, S., Carswell, A., McColl, M. A., Polatajko, H., & Pollock, N. (1998). *The Canadian Occupational Performance Measure* (3rd ed.). Ottawa: CAOT Publications.

Law, M., Baum, C., & Dunn, W. (2005). *Measuring occupational performance: Supporting best practice in occupational therapy.* Thorofare, NJ: Slack.

Loft, M., McWilliam, C., & Ward-Griffin, C. (2003). Patient empowerment after total hip and knee replacement. *Orthopedic Nursing, 22,* 42–47. http://dx.doi.org/10.1097/00006416-200301000-00012

Lohman, H., Gabriel, L., & Furlong, B. (2004). The bridge from ethics to public policy: Implications for occupational therapy practitioners. *American Journal of Occupational Therapy, 58,* 109–112. http://dx.doi.org/10.5014/ajot.58.1.109

Longmere, P., & Umansky, L. (2001). *The new disability history: American perspectives.* New York: New York University Press.

Lounsbury, P. A. (2010, November 13). T*he SARA™ outcome measurement system: Simple and effective.* Paper presented at the New York State Occupational Therapy Association Annual Conference, New York.

Magasi, S., & Hammel, J. (2009). Women with disabilities' experiences in long-term care: A case for social justice. *American Journal of Occupational Therapy, 63,* 35–45. http://dx.doi.org/10.5014/ajot.63.1.35

Mattingly, C. (1991). The narrative nature of clinical reasoning. *American Journal of Occupational Therapy, 45,* 998–1005. http://dx.doi.org/10.5014/ajot.45.11.998

McCormack, C., & Collins, B. (2010). Can disability studies contribute to client-centred occupational therapy practice. *British Journal of Occupational Therapy, 73,* 339–342. http://dx.doi.org/10.4276/030802210X12785840213328

Merryman, M., & Riegel, S. (2007). The recovery process and people with serious mental illness living in the community: An occupational therapy perspective. *Occupational Therapy in Mental Health, 32,* 51–73. http://dx.doi.org/10.1300/J004v23n02_03

Metropolitan New York District, New York State Occupational Therapy Association. (2009a, January). MNYD Mental Health Task Force. *NYSOTA News,* p. 12.

Metropolitan New York District, New York State Occupational Therapy Association. (2009b, January). NAMI NYC Metro Walk May 9, 2009. *NYSOTA News,* p. 13.

Moats, G., & Doble, S. (2006). Discharge planning with older adults: Toward a negotiated model of decision making. *Canadian Journal of Occupational Therapy, 73,* 303–311. http://dx.doi.org/10.1177/000841740607300507

Moghimi, C. (2007). Issues in caregiving: The role of occupational therapy in caregiver training. *Topics in Geriatric Rehabilitation, 23,* 269–279. http://dx.doi.org/10.1097/01.TGR.0000284770.39958.79

Morris, J. (1997). Care or empowerment? A disability rights perspective. *Social Policy and Administration, 31,* 54–60. http://dx.doi.org/10.1111/1467-9515.00037

Moyers, P., & Dale, L. (2007). *The guide to occupational therapy practice* (2nd ed.). Bethesda, MD: AOTA Press.

National Dropout Prevention Center for Students With Disabilities. (2012). *An analysis of states FFY annual performance report data for indicator B1 (graduation).* Retrieved from http://www.ndpc-sd.org/documents/Analysis_of_State_Reports/NDPC-SD_FFY_2010_Indicator_B1_summary.pdf.

Neville-Jan, A. (2005). The problem with prevention: The case of spina bifida. *American Journal of Occupational Therapy, 59,* 527–539. http://dx.doi.org/10.5014/ajot.59.5.527

Peloquin, S. M. (2005). Embracing our ethos, reclaiming our heart. *American Journal of Occupational Therapy, 59,* 611–625. http://dx.doi.org/10.5014/ajot.59.6.611

Pierce, D. (2001). Occupation by design: Dimensions, therapeutic power, and creative process. *American Journal of Occupational Therapy, 55,* 249–259. http://dx.doi.org/10.5014/ajot.55.3.249

Redick, A. G., McClain, L., & Brown, C. (2000). Consumer empowerment through occupational therapy: The Americans With Disabilities Act Title III. *American Journal of Occupational Therapy, 54,* 207–213. http://dx.doi.org/10.5014/ajot.54.2.207

Rogers, E. S., Chamberlin, J., Ellison, M. L., & Crean, T. (1997). A consumer-constructed scale to measure empowerment among users of mental health services. *Psychiatric Services, 48,* 1042–1047.

Rogers, J. C. (1983). Clinical reasoning: The ethics, science, and art [1983 Eleanor Clarke Slagle Lecture]. *American Journal of Occupational Therapy, 37,* 601–616. http://dx.doi.org/10.5014/ajot.37.9.601

Schell, B. A. B. (2003). Clinical reasoning: The basis of practice. In E. B. Crepeau, E. Cohn, & B. Schell (Eds.), *Willard and Spackman's occupational therapy* (10th ed., pp. 131–139). Philadelphia: Lippincott Williams & Wilkins.

Schell, B. A., & Cervero, R. M. (1993). Clinical reasoning in occupational therapy: An integrative review. *American Journal of Occupational Therapy, 47,* 605–610. http://dx.doi.org/10.5014/ajot.47.7.605

Shoener, R. F., Kinnealey, M., & Koenig, K. P. (2008). You can know me now if you listen: Sensory, motor, and communication issues in a nonverbal person with autism. *American Journal of Occupational Therapy, 62,* 547–553. http://dx.doi.org/10.5014/ajot.62.5.547

Snow, B. (2006). *Thumbs down to pity.* Retrieved from http://www.disabilityworld.org/01_07/video.shtml

Swarbrick, P., & Pratt, C. (2006). Consumer-operated self-help services: Roles and opportunities for occupational therapists and occupational therapy assistants. *OT Practice, 11,* CE-1–CE-8.

Taylor, M. (2001). Independence and empowerment: Evidence from the student perspective. *British Journal of Occupational Therapy, 64,* 245–252.

Thibeault, R. (2006). Globalisation, universities, and the future of occupational therapy: Dispatches for the majority world. *Australian Occupational Therapy Journal, 53,* 159–165. http://dx.doi.org/10.1111/j.1440-1630.2006.00608.x

Toal-Sullivan, D., & Henderson, P. R. (2004). Client-Oriented Role Evaluation (CORE): The development of a clinical rehabilitation instrument to assess role change associated with disability. *American Journal of Occupational Therapy, 58,* 211–220. http://dx.doi.org/10.5014/ajot.58.2.211

Townsend, E. (1996). Enabling empowerment: Using simulations versus real occupation. *Canadian Journal of Occupational Therapy, 63,* 113–128. http://dx.doi.org/10.1177/000841749606300204

U.S. Bureau of Labor Statistics. (2012). *Persons with a disability: Labor force characteristics. 2011.* Retrieved from http://www.bls.gov/news.release/disabl.nr0.htm.

U.S. Census Bureau. (2011). *Income, poverty, and health insurance coverage in the United States: 2010.* Retrieved from http://www.census.gov/prod/2011pubs/p60-239.pdf.

Vauth, R., Kleim, B., Wirtz, M., & Corrigan, P. W. (2007). Self-efficacy and empowerment as outcomes of self-stigmatizing and coping in schizophrenia. *Psychiatry Research, 150,* 71–80. http://dx.doi.org/10.1016/j.psychres.2006.07.005

Wehmeyer, M. (2004). Self-determination and the empowerment of people with disabilities. *American Rehabilitation, 28,* 22–29.

World Health Organization. (2011). *World report on disability.* Geneva: Author.

Zimmerman, M. A., & Warschausky, S. (1998). Empowerment theory for rehabilitation research: Conceptual and methodological issues. *Rehabilitation Psychology, 43,* 3–16. http://dx.doi.org/10.1037/0090-5550.43.1.3

CHAPTER 19.

REFLECTIONS FOR THE FUTURE: OCCUPATION, PURPOSEFUL ACTIVITIES, AND ACTIVITIES

Marie-Louise Blount, AM, OT, FAOTA; Jim Hinojosa, PhD, OT, BCP, FAOTA; and Paula Kramer, PhD, OTR, FAOTA

Highlights

✧ Resolve ambiguity of terminology
✧ Published research based on the question(s) that underlie the study
✧ Published research based on research methodology
✧ Future research on occupation-based intervention
✧ Creating the future of occupational therapy.

Key Terms

✧ Activity as a means
✧ Functional goals
✧ Meaning
✧ Occupation as an end
✧ Occupational performance

✧ Occupational synthesis
✧ Purposeful activities
✧ Qualitative research
✧ Quantitative research

In this chapter, we discuss our reflections on the therapeutic use of occupations and activities, and we discuss the implications of this scholarly work for the future of the profession. Our objective is to link this work with our vision for the profession into the next decade. The profession's valuing of and perspectives on occupation and activity as foundational concepts will continue to shape future occupational therapy research and practice.

We have not attempted to critique all the research related to occupational therapy. In fact, we have carefully selected publications to illustrate questions about theory and frames of reference, choosing relevant, researchable questions; issues of efficacy; and both qualitative and quantitative approaches that provide basic information you can use to develop and refine your own ideas.

The chapter discusses the development of the critical concepts of the profession in terms of occupation and activity. Occupation-based intervention is presented as a major part of the occupational therapy process. An examination of the evolution of occupation-based intervention is explored. As time goes on, the profession may revise and clarify the use of particular terminology, and scholars will continue to debate how to use and interpret key terms. Some terms may emerge as critical to the development of the profession and others may disappear from our lexicon. Society and technology change and occupational therapy practice will change, but this chapter demonstrates that we tend to absorb the most valuable content of our past and blend it with the emerging content of the future.

Resolve Ambiguity of Terminology

Historically, occupational therapy practitioners have used the terms *occupation* and *activity* at different times and sometimes interchangeably. As reported by Bauerschmidt and Nelson (2011), the term *occupation* was initially used by practitioners, but then its use declined rapidly until the 1980s. In the 21st century, the term *occupation* has been used more frequently within the occupational therapy literature (Bauerschmidt & Nelson, 2011). During this same period, occupational therapy practitioners rarely have used the terms *activity* and *purposeful activity*. Yet, together, these terms define the

basic tenets of the profession, having been equated with *occupation* for years, consistent with the profession's philosophical base (American Occupational Therapy Association [AOTA], 1979). Not long ago, the 2011 AOTA Representative Assembly (2012) changed this situation by adopting a revised philosophical base in the *AOTA Policy Manual* that uses only the term *occupation,* having removed the term *purposeful activity.* The document refers to *activity* only once. The *Occupational Therapy Practice Framework: Domain and Process* (*Framework;* AOTA, 2014) and the Accreditation Council for Occupational Therapy Education (2012) use the terms *occupation* and *activity.*

In the past decade, many occupational therapy practitioners have described their interventions as *occupation-based interventions,* linking occupation with purposeful activities. Interventions are said to be based on occupations selected by the client. This terminology avoids the use of the term *activity* and reinforces the foundational importance of occupation. As written in a 2005 report to the AOTA Executive Board from the Ad Hoc Workgroup on Implementing Occupation-Based Practice (Nielson et al., 2005):

> The isolated use of preparatory or purposeful activity is not [occupation-based practice]. The use of these approaches must be explicitly explained with the relationship to occupation clearly evident and occupation ultimately introduced as primary to the intervention process. Linkage requires that the therapist integrate their technical skill base with their understanding of occupation and consistently use their integrated knowledge to address all of the complex aspects of occupational performance. Lastly, linkage means making sure that the client understands the purpose of our intervention and why and how participation in occupation is therapy. (pp. 2–3)

In this report, the authors described occupation-based practice as client-centered and one in which intervention begins with the occupational therapy practitioner explaining *occupation* to the client. Based on the client's occupational needs, assessment and intervention address the client's present needs and future goals and roles. Occupation-based intervention "ends with getting them back into those life activities and infuses occupation into the intervention phase through activity selection, analysis and modification" (Nielson et al., 2005, p. 3). Finally, occupation-based practice "culminates with documentation that illustrates the client's status or progress in his/her ability to actively and meaningfully participate in the activities of his/her life" (Nielson et al., 2005, p. 3). Although using the term *occupation-based* avoids using the term *activities,* in the end, the authors of this report recognized the fundamental importance of participating in meaningful life activities.

The move to occupation-based interventions requires occupational therapy practitioners to explore the theoretical constructs that underlie this shift in terminology. Theoretically, practice and education of the public should be linked; however, two different types of terminology seem to be needed: one for the profession to develop knowledge and constructs and another to explain to the public what we do. Today, the profession and many practitioners predominantly use *occupation,* yet the World Health Organization (2001) uses the terms *activity* and *participation.* We believe that occupational therapy must reconcile its language with that of the rest of the world and of the layperson to aim at better understanding and recognition of occupational therapy. We suggest that, although as a profession, occupational therapy continues to use the term *occupation,* it should clarify that this term is interchangeable with *activity* and that occupational therapy practitioners should use *activity* with the public, because it is more understandable. Using language that is more generally understood will lead to greater understanding of occupational therapy.

We believe that in addition to focusing on occupation and activities, occupational therapy practitioners need to highlight the importance of participation. Although participation is implied in saying that someone engages in an activity, the crucial importance of participation is not obvious. When a person participates in the occupation or activity, the practitioner has selected a therapeutic medium that is relevant to the person. Without participation, the occupation is just a desire or idea to a person. Active participation requires that the person be actively involved in and self-motivated to complete the occupational performance necessary for the occupation. Participation also involves the person as an active arbiter of his or her environ-

ment. A person who participates in an occupation is making choices and, by doing so, becomes involved in his or her life. Participation does not imply that an occupation must be done with another person; it means a person engages in something that he or she values and finds meaningful. For example, for some people going grocery shopping alone is an occupation. Further, the ability to participate in an occupation ultimately allows the person to participate with others and participate in society.

As we edited these chapters and read scholarly publications, we concluded that the terms *occupation, activity,* and *occupation-based* are all useful to the profession. Further, we believe it is critical that occupational therapy practitioners use these terms within the context of participation. Specifically, first, we propose the term *occupation* is most appropriate when used within the context of the profession and to guide its research and practice. Second, we propose that occupational therapy practitioners use *activity* associated with *participation* when communicating externally to the public.

We must link participation to the use of activities in a way that promotes the public's understanding of occupation. Activity as a valuable construct should not be dropped from our lexicon, and proposing internal and external language will make it clearer what we do. Third, we advocate using the term *occupation-based* to describe the interventions within the profession and with other professionals. We believe that *occupation-based* clearly describes the profession's unique perspective concerning the link between activities and occupation, an area unique to occupational therapy practice.

Examining *Occupation* and *Activity* as Distinct Concepts

Occupational therapy scholars have proposed that occupation and purposeful activities are two distinct concepts—their definitions in publications and research studies are not precisely alike. Yet, confusion is often evident when authors claim the two concepts are interrelated or connected in some way. For example, as stated in the *Framework,* "Sometimes occupational therapy practitioners use the terms *occupation* and *activity* interchangeably to describe participation in daily life pursuits" (AOTA, 2014, p. S6). In the *Framework,* the term *occupation* "denotes life engagements that are constructed of multiple activities"

(AOTA, 2014, p. S6). This statement would imply that occupation is a broader or higher level concept than activity. It is our opinion that occupation and activities are two interrelated concepts. As stated in Chapter 1, "Occupation, Activities, and Occupational Therapy," we believe that occupation is the broader concept and includes activities.

Occupational therapy practitioners are ultimately concerned with human occupation. Occupations are grounded in personal meaning, are goal directed, are personally satisfying, and reflect clients' cultural backgrounds (Hinojosa, Kramer, Royeen, & Luebben, 2003). Practitioners must recognize that occupations are made up of activities and tasks. Some activities are purposeful because they are meaningful or have a meaningful outcome for the person engaged in the activity. Other activities occupy time and may not have personal meaning; they just need to be done. Practitioners must use activities within the configuration of occupation-based intervention. As eloquently quoted by Polatajko and Davis (2012), occupation-based enablement involves "the full range of enablement, from the specialized therapeutic use of activity for impairment reduction, to the use of advocacy to promote greater occupational inclusion and justice" (Polatajko et al., 2007, p. 180).

We support the use of language most appropriate for the situation, depending on what occupational therapy practitioners are trying to communicate and to whom they are trying to communicate. We have frequently observed that practitioners and scholars preface a word with *occupation* or *occupational* to indicate it is a unique term or concept for them and the profession. For example, a common term such as *engagement* is referred to as *occupational engagement*. This use of language to indicate ownership of a concept or the uniqueness of a concept can be misleading to the consumer and other practitioners and scholars, therefore limiting the ability to communicate effectively. We believe the attachment of the word *occupation* or *occupational* to other concepts does not strengthen practitioners' and scholars' commitment to the construct of occupation and results in misunderstandings. Can our uniqueness be illustrated in another way?

Occupation and Activity as a Means

Many occupational therapy practitioners believe occupation can be both the means and the ends of occupational therapy. These practitioners believe they can use occupations in their interventions with clients to bring about change. They also believe the outcome of intervention is the client's ability to engage in his or her occupations. In this book, we have proposed that occupations can be defined only by the person who is engaged in them. *Occupational synthesis* takes place when the client who has received occupational therapy spontaneously and unconsciously engages in activities that are personally meaningful and that support his or her ability to function.

From our perspective, occupational therapy practitioners use activities. When possible, they use activities that are meaningful to the client, that is, *purposeful activities.* The goal of intervention and the outcome is that the client integrates these purposeful activities into his or her occupations and continues to engage in them as part of everyday life. The engagement in activities within the context of intervention is *activity as a means.* When the client integrates activities into his or her daily occupations, it becomes *occupation as an end* (see Chapter 6, "Activity Synthesis as a Means to Structure Occupation").

Qualitative basic research has begun to produce a body of theoretical information about occupation (Gewurtz, Stergiou-Kita, Shaw, Kirsh, & Rappolt, 2008; Lindström, Sjöström, & Lindberg, 2013; Teitelman, Raber, & Watts, 2010). Researchers should continue this work with increased focus on establishing a sound body of theoretical knowledge about the construct of occupation as it relates to people and society.

Establishing the effectiveness of specific occupational therapy interventions requires that occupational therapy practitioners and researchers examine the treatment modalities they use within the context of a frame of reference or guidelines for intervention that specify their application. Applied researchers must examine treatment guidelines within the theoretical rationale that underlies them and be concerned with practical answers about whether a theoretically based intervention (e.g., frame of reference, conceptual model of practice, guidelines for intervention) has the outcome that it predicts (Dirette, 2013; Mosey, 1996). From this perspective, activities are one tool that practitioners use to bring about change. As a tool, researchers must examine activities within their theoretical context. For example, dressing activities may be used with children to develop body awareness, imaginary play skills, or activities of daily living (ADL) skills. For an adult, dressing may be an activity used in the context of an occupation-based intervention to develop socially appropriate self-care skills. When providing occupational therapy, one therapeutic tool is rarely used alone. Most often, on the basis of the intervention's theoretical base, a practitioner uses several tools in specified manners as therapeutic media.

Although we suggest examining the use of activities within the context of the frame of reference used, much occupational therapy research has focused on establishing the efficacy of using activity. In these studies, purposeful activities or occupations are the independent or treatment variable (e.g., cause, treatment, controlled factor, manipulated variable). Many of these studies have supported the basic belief that therapeutic activities are more effective if they have meaning to the person (Gewurtz et al., 2008; Lyons, Orozovic, Davis, & Newman, 2002; Yoder, Nelson, & Smith, 1989).

Importance of Meaning

While writing Chapter 4, "Occupation and Activity Analysis," Karen A. Buckley raised the following questions with the editors: Is meaning the important dimension of an activity that makes it purposeful to the person participating in it? Is meaning adequately addressed in discussions of purposeful activities and occupation? These questions led to a provocative conversation about the importance of meanings in determining whether an activity was purposeful. By definition, all occupations have meaning to the person engaged in them. The subjective meaning a person gives to an activity determines whether it is an occupation. As Hasselkus (2002) observed, occupations are a source of meanings and give meaning to people's lives.

Hammell (2004) wrote, "Doing of self-care, productive and leisure activities, is inadequate to address issues of meaning in people's lives" (p. 296). *Meaning* is the essence of what makes an activity purposeful and critical for an occupation-based intervention. Although occupational therapy practitioners often give more attention to the goal directedness of an activity, the activity's meaning to the participant is probably more important.

Note that this meaning is not always positive. For example, a person may find an activity humiliating (Hammell, 2004). Examples might be using stacking cones as a treatment activity when the person does not see any meaning in stacking cones or having an engineer used to working with complex machinery screwing nuts onto bolts. Perhaps in the end, the meaning an activity has for a person will determine its therapeutic potential. If a person realizes that participating in an activity he or she thinks is boring or useless may result in improvement, then the person's thoughts about the activity might change. When he or she adds subjective meaning to the activity, the activity then becomes meaningful and the intervention occupation-based. The issue of meaning requires further research and philosophical examination.

Published Research Based on the Questions That Underlie the Study

Many occupational therapy practitioners may think they do not need to learn about research because they are only interested in being clinicians. Evidence-based practice, however, demands that all practitioners have a basic understanding of research and its influence on practice. With support from research literature, practitioners can provide better services. When practitioners read published research, it is important they first understand the research questions, which are the foundation of research. Identifying research questions is the first step to conducting useful research. Before selecting appropriate research methods, the researcher needs to answer the question "What exactly do you want to find out?" (Punch, 1998). Once the researcher has a clear research question, he or she then needs to determine the kind of data necessary to answer the question and whether and how the data can be collected and analyzed.

Students often ask where research questions come from. As intelligent creatures, people constantly ask questions and search for the answers. Researchers use systematic methods to investigate questions to explain behavior and understand people's lives. In fact, finding interesting research questions is not difficult; they emerge as practitioners observe their environment and actions. Questions come from practitioners' practices, everyday observations, and reading. In this section, we present only a few examples to illustrate how research is based on research questions.

Occupational therapy practitioners often ask questions related to their daily practice, such as "Are the occupation-based interventions effective for achieving the goals?" For example, Paul and Ramsey (1998) asked whether music-making activity as a form of occupationally embedded exercise improves active shoulder flexion and elbow extension in people with hemiplegia. Practitioners need to add to their understanding about the meaning of occupation. To improve the quality of services, some people may ask what the nature of occupations is for their clients. Lyons et al. (2002) investigated what the occupational experiences of people with life-threatening illness are while they are attending a day hospice program. Other practitioners have examined the relationships between purposeful activities and performances and behaviors. For example, Yoder et al. (1989) conducted a randomized group experiment to examine whether differences are elicited by the purposefulness of activities as they compared the duration and frequency of rotatory arm movement in elderly female nursing home residents. Recently, Bravi and Stoykov (2007) examined the use of an upper-limb training protocol that involved task-oriented training. Research questions such as these determine what research is done in occupational therapy, and most important, these questions and their answers eventually determine what practitioners learn.

Although many occupational therapy researchers have collected much information about the application of activities and occupations, occupational therapy practitioners still need more research to substantiate practice. According to AOTA and the American Occupational Therapy Foundation's (2011) occupational therapy research agenda, the profession's research priority is conducting research related to occupational therapy interventions.

Gutman (2008), editor-in-chief of the *American Journal of Occupational Therapy,* noted that the *Centennial Vision* (AOTA, 2007) urged the profession to provide evidence supporting the efficacy of occupational therapy in six broad practice areas: (1) children and youth; (2) productive aging; (3) mental health; (4) health and wellness; (5) work and industry; and (6) rehabilitation, disability, and participation. In accordance with occupational

therapy's societal contract and in an effort to fulfill the mission of the *Centennial Vision*, the profession must strive to meet five specific research priorities:

1. Provide evidence for the efficacy of clinical practice.
2. Test the reliability and validity of our assessment instruments.
3. Examine how engagement in occupation can promote developmental milestones, health and wellness throughout the lifespan, and productive aging.
4. Provide fundamental or basic research information regarding how specific disability experiences affect community and social participation—with the intent to ultimately use this information to develop clinical guidelines that can be tested for efficacy.
5. Explore topical questions (i.e., current issues) whose answers will provide direction for the profession's continued growth and evolution. (p. 499)

This list provides directions for researchers to ask questions concerning different aspects of occupational therapy practice, from specific factors to broad models and from the individual level to the societal level.

Just asking questions is not enough, however. Occupational therapy researchers need to ask important, relevant, and answerable questions clearly stated in a straightforward manner. Occupational therapy practitioners work in many different settings by applying various therapeutic modalities with a wide range of populations. The potential for research is unlimited. With an increased demand for practitioners to provide evidence and to grow bodies of knowledge to support practice, occupational therapy researchers should focus on investigating occupational therapy effectiveness and developing theories about the nature of human occupations and relationships between health and occupation (Gillette, 1991). Once a person has a research question, he or she needs to develop a comprehensive outline that describes the implementation of the study.

Published Research Based on Research Methodology

Both quantitative and qualitative methodologies are important to occupational therapy. Choosing to use either a quantitative approach or a qualitative approach does not make research good or bad. Whether a study uses the most appropriate approach to investigate the problem under study is crucial. Whatever design is used, it must be appropriate to the research questions being studied. The appropriate approach and the rigor of the study is what make the research valuable or not.

Specific research questions dictate the most appropriate approach, and different research questions will lead to different methods (Plante, Kiernan, & Betts, 1994; Punch, 1998). In this section, our intention is not to educate readers about details of quantitative and qualitative methods but to provide a few examples of each method to illustrate how they can be used in occupational therapy research.

Quantitative Research

Briefly stated, a *quantitative research* approach focuses on examining preselected variables that have been thought to be pertinent, on the basis of either existing theoretical statements or the researcher's own interpretation, to determine measurable and causal relationships among them. The investigators manipulate the numerical data through statistical analysis to seek an explanation of the causes and determinants of the phenomenon (Tamhane, 2009; Velleman & Bock, 2008). The current trend in occupational therapy emphasizes the importance of quantitative research using systematic reviews. The long-range goal is to increase the amount of research using randomized controlled trials.

An occupational therapy researcher who uses quantitative designs typically uses experimental, quasi-experimental, or nonexperimental (i.e., descriptive or single-subject) designs or identifies and isolates specific variables and then uses specific measurement instruments to collect information on these variables. To support and justify therapeutic use of occupations and activities, occupational therapy researchers have been greatly concerned with supporting occupational therapy's value to society by presenting the efficacy of occupational therapy intervention. Researchers can replicate studies with quantitative research designs to verify the findings and add them to the existing knowledge. For example, Schepens, Sen, Painter, and Murphy (2012) conducted a meta-analysis comparing falls in community-dwelling older adults related to activities and participation. They used 20 cross-sectional and prospective studies. Fall-related efficacy was strongly related to active participation and engagement in activity.

Moreover, some have suggested that quantitative research methods provide better communication with other professions in the scientific community. With numerical comparisons, quantitative research findings can strengthen the evidence for the efficacy of occupational therapy intervention. In the seminal study of the well elderly, Clark et al. (1997) evaluated the effectiveness of occupational therapy preventive services for well elderly people in a randomized controlled trial. With 361 participants, they compared the differences in several outcome measurements elicited by the occupational therapy group, the social activity control group, and the nontreatment control group. Clark et al. found statistically significant findings across various domains, providing strong support for the effectiveness of preventive occupational therapy services.

As we stated earlier, a quantitative method that is frequently used in occupational therapy is the systematic review. In 2007, Legg et al. did a systematic review to assess whether occupational therapy focused explicitly on personal ADLs enhances recovery for patients after stroke. On the basis of inclusion criteria, they identified nine randomized controlled trials with a total of 1,258 participants and concluded that occupational therapy can improve performance and reduce the risk of deterioration. Howe and Wang (2013) reviewed 34 studies on feeding interventions with infants and young children. Three broad intervention themes were identified: (1) behavioral, (2) parent-directed and educational, and (3) physiological. A synthesis of the studies showed that various approaches result in positive outcomes in feeding performance, feeding interaction, and feeding competence of parents and children.

Although manipulating independent variables and obtaining a control group is difficult, many occupational therapy researchers choose to approach their questions by using descriptive or one-group design. In 2013, O'Toole, Connelly, and Smith examined 15 participants with chronic diseases, providing a weekly occupation-based self-management group over 6 weeks. They found that such programs may be effective in improving perception of and satisfaction with occupational performance after intervention. White, Mulligan, Merrill, and Wright (2007) used a quasi-experimental design to determine whether 68 children with possible sensory-processing deficits performed less well on an occupational performance measure. They found statistically significant differences and concluded that children who identified with sensory-processing deficits are likely to experience some challenges in performing everyday occupations.

With limited sources of samples, many researchers use single-subject or case study designs. Single-subject designs compare each participant's performance across a timeline under different conditions. Such designs enable researchers to examine the efficacy of intervention with people who have some specific characteristics. Through careful inspection of data, they can provide information about why an intervention is effective for one client but not for others (Dunn, 1993). Skubik-Peplaski, Carrico, Nichols, Chelette, and Sawaki (2012) designed a single-subject study involving a 55-year-old man after a stroke with upper-extremity impairment. He participated in 15 sessions of occupation-based intervention, designed to imitate a home environment. Data were collected at baseline and periodically throughout the intervention. Occupation-based intervention led to increased functional changes and use of the upper extremity, thus improving occupational performance. In another single-subject study, Dickerson and Brown (2007) investigated the use of constraint-induced movement therapy for a 24-month-old child with hemiparesis. Daily measures of hand use on eight gross and fine motor activities supported the finding that the child maintained improvements after the splinting phases of the treatment and after overall completion of the treatment.

Qualitative Research

A researcher chooses to use a *qualitative research* approach when exploration and participant-centered detail concerning a phenomenon are needed. The approach is holistic in its context. Qualitative research helps researchers obtain a better understanding of a social phenomenon from the participants' perspective (Creswell, 2012). Qualitative data are useful for developing theories and understanding natural behaviors.

Qualitative research methods can be used to develop theories by generating a systematic knowledge base and understanding about participation in occupations. They can also be used to investigate the effect of occupational therapy intervention on quality of life, health, and wellness. Qualitative researchers believe that a focus on participants' perspectives and experiences and what these experiences mean to them provides the most meaningful data. Moreover, many researchers believe that qualitative research methods have a goodness of fit with searching for viable information about clients' performance in a natural context (Dunn, 1993; Yerxa, 1991).

Many qualitative approaches can be applied in occupational therapy research. They provide new knowledge to the profession by exploring complex, multilevel human qualities (Yerxa, 1991). In a qualitative study, Lindström et al. (2013) conducted qualitative interviews and field observations with 16 people diagnosed with psychosis-related disorders, using a model that integrated occupational therapy into sheltered or supported housing facilities. The narrative analysis showed positive results for participants, including an understanding of their personal transformations and the value of reaching goals as they re-entered society.

In another example, Perrins-Margalis, Rugletic, Schepis, Stepanski, and Walsh (2000) conducted a qualitative study to investigate the effects of purposeful activity on the performance of people with chronic mental illness. On the basis of their interpretation of a horticulture experience from the participants' perspective, these authors gained a more in-depth understanding of the effect of horticulture as a group-based activity on quality of life, which was a composition of life satisfaction, well-being, and self-concept. Carin-Levy, Kendall, Young, and Mead (2009) used a qualitative paradigm to see whether exercise and relaxation classes motivated participants to take part in other purposeful activities. They found that participants continued to use what they learned and perceived improvement in their own quality of life.

Reynolds, Vivat, and Prior (2008) studied 10 women with chronic fatigue syndrome or myalgic encephalopathy, using interviews and written narratives to learn about the meanings of art making. They determined that art making occurred as part of a broader acceptance and adjustment process. Isaksson, Josephsson, Lexell, and Skar (2007) used in-depth interviews of 13 women with spinal cord injuries to learn about their encounters in occupations. Results supported the finding that change for these women was complex because they struggled but were able to regain participation in occupations.

Future Research on Occupation-Based Intervention

Occupation-based interventions should be one of our future priorities for research. Occupations should be studied in the context of the body of knowledge that underlies this fundamental construct. Occupational science leadership identifies the importance of developing a discipline. Although developing a discipline is important, occupational therapy practitioners need to balance research to support the emerging discipline with research to support occupational therapy. Occupational therapy involves the use of a wide range of theoretical approaches and tools to bring about change. Occupational therapy scholars and researchers must provide a body of knowledge that supports the practice of the profession.

Occupational therapy practitioners consider activities to be essential in practice because they are the building blocks for occupation—the end goal of occupational therapy. Practitioners learn to select, adapt, modify, grade, and create activities that meet their clients' therapeutic needs. They understand that if the client understands the activities' purpose and focuses attention on their completion, occupational performance improves or behaviors change. The client is then able to synthesize or incorporate his or her occupational performance and behaviors into daily life occupations.

The health care delivery system and associated reimbursement structures have a direct influence on practitioners' attention to and use of activities and occupations. Occupational therapy practitioners must provide the most cost-effective intervention. In all cases, the intervention should be occupation based. At times, if addressing a specific occupational performance deficit, the practitioner may need to provide a preparatory activity that supports the performance of the occupation and its related activities.

We believe that the critical outcome of occupational therapy should be the client's ability to engage in occupational performance. Occupational therapy practitioners should provide an occupation-based intervention using a wide range of interventions, all of which are important and should be examined for their efficacy and effectiveness in creating environments in which clients' performance skills and behaviors improve. Such occupation-based intervention includes the three unique therapeutic modalities of (1) activity, (2) purposeful activity, and (3) occupation. Practitioners must keep in mind the central concern—occupation as an end.

Creating the Future of Occupational Therapy

As occupational therapy practitioners, we have to take responsibility for creating our own future. Many occupational therapy practitioners are interested in predicting and understanding what the future will hold. Shaping practice based on changes in health care and modern society as well as changes in human occupations makes good sense. In addition, many things that happen in the world and people's beliefs about them occur because of fears about current and future change. Here, we attempt to look at the future of human activity and how it may affect occupational therapy. We begin with some notions about change in Western society to provide some context and shape for these ideas.

Changes at the Societal Level

One of our first areas of focus for change must occur at the societal level. The future, as an unknown terrain, may seem inviting. One may anticipate the people, places, and events of the future with joy. The future may also seem fearsome, inhabited by unwanted changes, anticipated losses, and debility. In addition, people's views of future events will vary by age, circumstances, health, and system of belief. People often seek knowledge and understanding in a vain effort to control the future or at least make it less uncertain.

Vehicles for space travel and suits to protect a person from many environmental rigors do exist, but they usually do not resemble the stuff of car-

---

Exercise 19.1. Personal Reflection

Address each of the following in 3 sentences or fewer: (1) Who are you? (2) Who would you like to be? (3) Identify 3 similarities between the person you think you are and the person you would like to be, and be clear about the difference between who you think you are and who you want to be. (4) What have you learned from this reflection? (Insel & Roth, 1985)

---

toons or films depicting such travel or its dangers, including almost constant combat. Elements of a world of uncluttered spaces and rapid travel to near and distant places do exist, but along with traffic jams, tiny apartments, and problems associated with the accumulation of many objects. The world is more accurately a juxtaposition of startlingly new and strikingly innovative changes with the familiar, traditional elements of life.

People have no way to actually predict what will happen tomorrow, next week, next year, or in 2100. We do live with certain indicators of direction and possibility, such as knowledge of past and present human affairs, the acceleration of technological change, information about population trends, and data on global warming and climate change. Here, for some of these indicators, we discuss areas of the most important change. We explore how these changes affect human activity, but only as we can see them now, from our vantage point. Note that sudden and transforming change may be less likely than incremental change, but remember that it too can occur and possibly render all careful study of trends futile. Consider, for example, several recent natural events, including earthquakes and violent storms, and how massively they have affected human lives and habitation.

Changes in media and communication

Some of the most rapid changes during recent years have been in the modes and means of media and communication, as well as the content of people's communications. Some writing (Standage, 1998) has suggested that the introduction of telegraphy was seen to be as transforming in its day as Internet and telephone technology is perceived at present.

Since the introduction of the telegraph, however, the world has seen the development of all sorts of wireless communications, global print media losing its place to various online modes, and recording and film-making devices in rapidly proliferating forms. Computer technology spawns new applications, wonders, and intrusions into people's lives every day. This information age affects how people incorporate activity or inactivity into their lives.

Television, perhaps obsolescent, has many channels, and there are a wide range of other sources of information, including online news with chat options. These sources of information and entertainment have transformed people's lives in a very short span of time. Changes in media and modes of communication have also transformed people's occupation-driven lives. A few of these effects are that many people spend a good part of their workdays sitting at a monitor and keyboard and fill leisure hours taking part in other sedentary activities rather than physical activities. A current hot topic is widespread obesity related to these changing activity patterns and the importance of food in people's lives, as discussed in Chapter 3, "Dimensions of Occupations Across the Lifespan." The use of exercise equipment, yet another technology, is one way of balancing this lack of activity.

The ways in which people use their hands to accomplish tasks have radically changed. Technology has freed people from many manual tasks. For example, instead of writing letters and going to the post office to mail them, people send e-mails or text messages. Programs now allow people to talk into the computer rather than typing. In some cases, however, technological changes have created the need for more complex fine motor skills. The trends just described are likely to continue.

Other technological changes

Although communication technology has a primary effect on people's lives, general technological change also affects many aspects of people's existence. These changes primarily influence the lives of people in the developed world. Indeed, places still exist where it would be difficult to find a landline phone; many people cannot read; and hand tools take the foreground in the home, leisure, and work environments. How technological changes will move to new populations in the future is, in itself, a challenging issue to consider.

With rapidly developing and increasingly available technological devices and equipment, people have developed new ways of interacting with both the devices and each other. Today, many people have special skills to operate equipment, including digital satellite television and many household appliances; they learn the special skills and knowledge needed to operate modern cars; and even more expertise, training, and experience are needed to control the advanced equipment involved in flying or in information processing.

Now and in the future, changing technology will affect every aspect of people's lives, from smart phones and tablets to digital video recorders and programs on demand, to 3-dimensional copiers, to MRIs, to robotics, to mood- and activity-enhancing drugs, just to name a few. Technological change and new products will affect not only people's knowledge and interactions but also their bodies, how and why they move, and what they think and desire. In effect, this changing technology leads to transformations in people's daily activities.

Occupational therapy practitioners will have an increased need to understand and analyze these changes and new activity patterns. Exploring them with clients whose own lives will display altered activity patterns, newly emerging interests, and restructured circumstances is critical. Practitioners must also analyze how age and generation influence activity and activity choices, even before taking into account the influence of disability and possible new limitations on the lives of clients.

Technological change will add to the resources available in the rehabilitation process and may, like other societal changes, affect both the need for occupational therapy services and the way in which those services are offered. Technological change affects how practitioners carry out their daily activities, the way they feel about the things that they do, and the tools they use.

Changes in health and illness

In the developed world, increasing attention is paid to the maintenance and promotion of health. Attention to people's personal habits (e.g., smoking) and environmental factors (e.g., food additives) has led to changes in practices for some people and to legislation and social restriction in other cases. How people will define healthy practice and healthy living in the future remains to be seen, but occupational therapy practitioners and other health care practitioners are likely to continue giving attention to preventive measures and health-promoting activities.

Other recent health and illness trends that will probably extend into the future include the realization that newer, frequently more virulent communicable diseases often spread rapidly around the world because of increased international travel. The notion that a disease might be restricted to one community, one region, one nation, or even one continent is an illusion. Along with greater concern about the spread of such diseases, more attention will probably be paid to international public health measures.

In the United States, another notable health trend that is likely to extend into the future is the increasing use of pharmaceuticals in medicine. This development has already had a sizeable impact on the health care system. How the growth of pharmaceutical treatments will influence the future structure and practice of health care is still a matter of speculation but will no doubt have an effect on how health care is delivered.

Changes in resources

Recent history has indicated that the way in which money, goods, and other resources are generated, traded, and used in the world has also changed. This change will continue, and all segments of society will experience economic booms and busts and consequent adjustments. People seeking to improve their circumstances and find solutions for their own personal dilemmas will have difficulty doing so when the economy is faltering and will have more opportunities to meet their goals in prosperous times.

In the United States, fluctuating resources and a past that included no guaranteed health care coverage meant some types of health care were not readily available to a portion of society. This situation may be changing, through federal legislation and court action, but there is a strongly entrenched resistance to making health care widely available to all in society. If the changes proposed in the federal legislation do not take place, economic uncertainty and resulting shortages of services will lead to some people being unable to fulfill their personal goals for well-being. This situation, in turn, could lead to social unrest and anomie. In good times, more possibilities exist for addressing social ills and shortages, but the choices made will never address all social inequities.

Occupational therapy practitioners must consider issues of clients' resources, both current and future and how this affects people's lives when planning interventions. For example, for clients with few resources and pressing needs, practitioners will have to use creativity and ingenuity to develop useful and meaningful interventions and adaptive equipment.

Conversely, for clients with means, practitioners may, for example, need knowledge of how to invest online or how to use the latest sophisticated adapted equipment. Therefore, as much as practitioners need to be prepared to work in a world in which technology is ever-changing and continually more demanding, they also need to give more attention to their own adaptive skills and knowledge of the simplest and most rudimentary ways to solve problems of living and doing. In addition, practitioners will need to address their willingness to offer services pro bono when it is required to provide services in a more equitable fashion.

Tradition: The Pull of the Familiar

Most people would not be satisfied with a world filled only with objects and buildings constructed by people or objects that emphasize efficiency over other features. Within most people stirs a desire for the asymmetric, the familiar, even the traditional. Natural beauty sometimes reinforces the obverse of the electronic world at our fingertips. Yes, electricity, telephones, and a computer may be nearby, but our world is also shaped by family, expected behaviors, familiar foods, joys of work, and beautiful objects and vistas. Most people enjoy a world that combines the new and startling with the established and familiar (Friedman, 1999).

There is every reason to believe that the good and bad of people's past and present activity lives will follow them in some form into the future. Therefore, occupational therapy practitioners who emphasize the importance of the familiar by using, for example, arts and crafts in their reserve of purposeful activities, remind people that the drive to make things with their hands and to shape beauty

are human impulses. Practitioners should not only use technology in practice, but also incorporate natural and familiar activities into interventions.

Consequences of Change

Although change is a constant in human life, it always brings consequences. An examination of people's daily activities, both the mundane and the special, shows that adaptation to change is a requirement of the human condition. This requirement is true for the little child trying to overcome difficulties of movement, for the young adult coping with a devastating injury, and for the senior citizen dealing with the physical and mental changes caused by aging. People hold some aspects of their futures in their own hands, on the basis of their beliefs and actions. As stated earlier, some roads of the future are paved by past and current actions; most people make choices that shape their futures in clear ways. Nations, too, plan educational, transportation, and communication systems as well as relationships with other nations, thus influencing their futures.

Much, however, of what occurs in people's lives and in the larger world is unplanned and indeed unplannable. Most actions have unintended consequences. In the past, for example, the link between smoking tobacco and lung cancer was not known. Likewise, discernible but unintended connections exist among World Wars I and II and developments in the Balkans, and the history of European and U.S. relationships with the Middle East has led to upheavals in the world today. People's efforts to lead healthy lives do not invariably lead them to the outcomes they anticipate. Serendipity and tragedy can surprise and shock a person at any moment. These observations serve to remind us as occupational therapy practitioners that a good future is always uncharted and that even the best treatment plans need reconsideration.

The Life Course

Our knowledge of human development has expanded over time, and this helps the practitioner understand how interventions can be developed for people throughout the life course. Scientific knowledge of changes in human development have promoted the extension of the healthy human life span. For some people, the living environment has become cleaner over the past few centuries. It has also provided better nutrition, safer childbirth, fewer children per family, and the diminution of some diseases. Definitions and configurations of families also have changed radically, and they are expected to change more in the future (Collins, 2008). Some of these factors have permitted an extended life span for many people. The conscious plan and intent by some to move further in this direction hold tantalizing prospects of even longer and more successful lives.

Nonetheless, one major concern of occupational therapy practitioners (within their emphasis on normal and therapeutic occupation) must be enhancing and fulfilling an already extended life course. Practitioners must continue to attend to all the issues of human development, both healthy and deleterious, that they have made their focus. In the future, the promise of increased longevity, the issues of human development and aging, and the intersection of these factors with purposeful activities and occupation will continue to be a central theme. However, practitioners should not over- or underemphasize either end of the life cycle or neglect adolescence, young adulthood, or middle adulthood, no matter to what numerical ages these periods correspond. The transitions of life and aging, as normal and inexorable processes, will always color a person's activities and interests and will therefore influence the way in which practitioners apply activities therapeutically.

Belief Systems and Human Actions

People's personal beliefs affect their actions. Predictions of the future and generalizations about outcomes must take into account how ideology, convictions, and political actions affect human behavior. Neat plans not only become messy because of unintended consequences but also become complicated because the choices people make are dependent on their particular interpretations of the world. These interpretations are sometimes based on fervently held beliefs, religious traditions, political opinions, or ideological conditioning.

A portion of what makes the future unpredictable is those very belief systems that lead people to wage war, demand conformity with the tenets of their religion, promote new educational systems, fear change, or engage in new individual or shared activities (just to name a few possibilities). As a result, practitioners truly cannot know what the future will hold for occupational therapy. Still, it is our responsibility to stand for, promulgate, and adapt the tenets of the profession to the climate of the belief systems that develop.

Moreover, occupational therapy practitioners who have been engaged in this process must pave the way for future practitioners to draw from the knowledge and achievements of the past, avoid the pitfalls that experience has revealed, and trace indicators of how purposeful activities are changing. In doing so, practitioners will be as prepared as they can be to assist those who need assistance to lead fuller and more satisfying lives in the future.

Genetic Engineering

One area of knowledge that is bound to influence not only people's activities but the very nature of their beings is the burgeoning science of genetic engineering. Work to increase knowledge in this area has already been wildly successful and will no doubt continue in this direction. Alterations to the gene pool to treat illnesses and disabilities, promote fertility, or vary heritability are highly likely to affect the practice of occupational therapy and even who our clients will be. For example, future practice will no doubt include more twins and triplets. More complex multiple pregnancies and low birthweights will produce children in need of intervention. In the future, the profession will continue to see a changing human landscape resulting from increased knowledge and success in enhancing fertility. Changes in the field of fertility intervention are already garnering attention, but some commentators believe that they will affect a relatively small proportion of the population. Nonetheless, occupational therapy practitioners specializing in pediatrics will probably see many representatives of this portion of the population.

Cloning, efforts to modify genetic impairment, and even selective eugenics will be used by some to control reproduction, inform reproductive choices, and deal with heritable disease. As with other predictions for the future, some of these advances will have unintended consequences. Possibilities for new and as yet unimagined developments in the areas of genetics and reproductive technology probably form the most revolutionary changes in the society of the future. These developments will affect people's notions about family and definitions of human beings and relationships and will certainly affect occupational therapy practice.

Keeping Activities in Practice

As described in the chapters of this book, occupational therapy practitioners use activities with the ultimate goal that clients will engage successfully in occupations. Practitioners believe in the importance of activities and occupations. Practitioners are often unable or reluctant to use activities as part of their daily interventions. Why? When practitioners are asked what they do in practice, they often answer by describing specific intervention strategies or techniques. Many also describe specific hands-on manipulations or exercises that are performed during treatment sessions. The focus is on the result of the exercise rather than its meaningfulness. These kinds of answers reinforce the belief that the techniques for treatments are more important than the performance of the specific activity itself, even when the ability to perform a specific occupation is the end goal that the client is trying to achieve. What is missing from these answers is the heart of occupational therapy, which is the occupational basis of intervention.

Occupational therapy practitioners are ultimately concerned with the client's ability to engage in occupations. Engagement in occupations requires that the client be able to perform the many activities that are foundational to the specific occupations of his or her life. Therefore, practitioners should be comfortable explaining the outcomes of intervention in terms of the client's ability to engage in occupations. Practitioners' measures of success are the client's ability to perform the specific activities so that he or she can ultimately engage in occupations. Occupational therapy practitioners need to reaffirm the importance of the client's ability to perform occupations.

Demonstrating Occupational Therapy's Value in the Future

The future of occupational therapy is rich as society focuses on function, or the person's ability to engage in meaningful occupations, which is specifically the domain of occupational therapy. The challenge for occupational therapy practitioners is to move forward yet be true to the roots of the profession. Practitioners must value the client's

personal needs and desires and remember what is meaningful to him or her. They have to put aside their expectations of the client and focus on the client's expectations of himself or herself.

Practitioners need to collaborate with the client to learn to identify occupations consistent with the client's values. They must also be sensitive to and appreciate the client's culture and heritage. Focusing on the client's will, not on the practitioner's desires, is the art of occupational therapy practice. Once practitioners master artful practice that is true to the profession, they have to move forward in the world of science. Moving forward involves documenting what occupational therapy practitioners do and explaining the value of occupational therapy to each client and to society in general. Researchers can then conduct research to demonstrate the value and outcome of occupational therapy in a scientific manner.

Occupational therapy's concern with a person's ability to perform occupations is grounded in functional outcomes. In the therapeutic process, the practitioner first establishes *functional goals,* that is, goals that are meaningful to the client and will help him or her perform occupations and their related activities successfully. To determine whether the intervention has been effective, practitioners need to have clearly identified functional outcomes. Inherent in functional outcomes is the client's ability to perform activities so that he or she can engage in occupations.

Occupational performance is the ability to perform specific activities that allow the client to perform occupations and, thus, be a more functional person. What could be more functional than dressing oneself, feeding oneself, or being able to take care of one's children? In our view, occupational therapy is based on a concern for developing optimal function. The foci of future practice will be the measurement of an intervention's success through the demonstration of functional outcomes. Highlighting the person's ability to do something valued as the result of occupational therapy's interventions will demonstrate its value to society.

Occupational therapy practitioners' concern for the person's needs must be broadened to involve the context of the person's life. Practitioners need to focus not only on the person's needs and physical environment but also on how their chosen occupations occur in a much broader framework. A person's meaningful activities often involve other people. Thus, families, communities, and other social contexts must be included in interventions. The inclusion of client's families, significant others, and communities should be expanded. For example, children are treated with family-centered care, inpatient units often involve clients' families, and specific populations frequently live in community settings. As interventions move out of clinical settings, they become more meaningful to the client and the people in his or her life. It also brings the practice of occupational therapy into contact with a larger population and demonstrates its value to a broader public.

Another possible change in practice will be attending to populations. Currently, occupational therapy practitioners primarily use groups in intervention; however, the broader conceptualization of groups as target populations holds great potential for future practice.

For example, whereas now practitioners treat people with repetitive motion injuries, in the future more attention may be directed toward the prevention of such injuries by intervening with groups who may be prone to these problems. Practitioners might be involved in changing the environment, or they might try to change the way in which specific occupations are carried out. Prevention is just a small part of occupational therapy practice today, but it should become a bigger component in the future. In addition, the increasing aging population will demand practitioners' attention to help it adapt occupations for continued active community participation. This adaptation of activities on a larger and broader scale will become an essential component of practice.

To increase the scale of occupational therapy practice, the profession must focus on working with society at large to become more accommodating and inclusive of people with disabilities. This professional responsibility means that occupational therapy practitioners have to focus on the needs of a population and the community to identify the modifications and adaptations that will allow greater inclusion. If practitioners can help society address barriers that prevent inclusion, the goal of enhanced participation of people with disabilities can be reached.

Reflecting on future practice, we realize that the future is always unpredictable, sometimes exciting, and often threatening. Although we cannot predict what the future holds, we can reflect on whether occupational therapy has a sound foundation from which it can evolve. Shifts in practice sites and service delivery models are becoming evident in all areas of practice. Since the 1990s, occupational therapy services have shifted from clinic settings to more integrated community, classroom, and home settings. Occupational therapy's strength has always been its practitioners' willingness and ability to adapt and change in response to society. If occupational therapy is to continue to be viable, practitioners must continue to examine their interventions in light of a changing society. They must also examine society to set their intervention priorities and select the most appropriate tools for interventions, asking the questions, What occupations do people value? What occupations do people desire and need to engage in? Practitioners must know what activities are foundational to society's valued occupations to use occupation and related activities therapeutically. In addition, practitioners need to have an expanded appreciation of society that includes understanding the needs of minority, poor, chronically ill, and underserved elderly people. The future viability of occupational therapy may be determined by how these issues are addressed and how the evidence supports these practices.

Occupational therapy practitioners must become familiar with changes in the health care and education systems as they evolve. Moreover, practitioners cannot afford to continue to passively watch and attempt to respond to changes; rather, they must become their own advocates and actively shape newly emerging systems. Moving beyond direct services, practitioners must advocate for the concerns of individual clients and populations within managed services and participate in the creation of new service delivery models that ensure quality care in natural environments.

Summary

Many things in the world move in cycles; ideas come in and out of fashion just as skirt lengths, shoes, and hairstyles do. As professions grow and develop over time, they too experience a fluctuation of ideas. They respond to societal changes, or they become obsolete. When the profession of occupational therapy was founded, its basis was occupation, and it stressed the importance of engaging in occupation for a healthy and productive life. People may have used the term *occupation* differently then; however, they clearly recognized its importance to daily life. The term *occupation* has gone in and out of fashion in the profession and is currently widely used, with a renewed recognized focal importance.

Although little agreement exists among scholars on the definitions of *occupation* and *activity,* they do agree that these concepts are basic to occupational therapy. Discussions of the meanings of these terms to occupational therapy practitioners have consumed much attention around the world (Bauerschmidt & Nelson, 2011; Canadian Association of Occupational Therapists, 2002; Christiansen, Baum, & Bass-Haugen, 2005). The profession adopted a hierarchy in which *occupation* is the umbrella term, with *purposeful activities* being an important component under that umbrella (AOTA, 1997). It is critical that our profession continue to explore these terms, defining them and debating their relationship both to each other and to the practice of occupational therapy.

The challenge facing educators in the future is to encourage the exploration of these concepts, debate their meanings, and identify how they relate to practice. Students need to learn to think about the relationship among activity, purposeful activity, and occupation and how these concepts apply to intervention and to the profession as a whole. These concepts are the cornerstone of the profession and need our attention. Although the profession has grown extensively, it has also come full circle, moving closer to its roots. It is critical that we clarify the meaning and importance of *occupation* and *activities* and by doing so explain and describe both what we do and how it is important to society.

Mary Reilly claimed that "occupational therapy can be one of the greatest ideas of 20th-century medicine" (Reilly, 1962, p. 1). In the 21st century, occupational therapy continues to provide a very valuable service to people and society. The future will provide the practice of occupational therapy with many challenges, yet behind each challenge lies an opportunity to promote the importance of human activity and occupation.

References

Accreditation Council for Occupational Therapy Education. (2012). 2011 Accreditation Council for Occupational Therapy Education (ACOTE®) standards. *American Journal of Occupational Therapy, 66*(Suppl.), S6–S74. http://dx.doi.org/10.5014/ajot.2012.66S6

American Occupational Therapy Association. (1979). The philosophical base of occupational therapy. *American Journal of Occupational Therapy, 33,* 785.

American Occupation Therapy Association (1997). Statement—Fundamental concepts of occupational therapy: Occupation, purposeful activity, and function. *American Journal of Occupational Therapy, 51,* 864–866. http://dx.doi.org/10.5014/ajot.51.10.864

American Occupational Therapy Association. (2007). AOTA's *Centennial Vision* and executive summary. *American Journal of Occupational Therapy, 61,* 613–614. http://dx.doi.org/10.5014/ajot.61.6.613

American Occupational Therapy Association. (2012). Policy 1.11 The philosophical base of occupational therapy. *Policy manual.* Bethesda, MD: Author.

American Occupational Therapy Association. (2014). Occupational therapy framework: Domain and process (3rd ed.). *American Journal of Occupational Therapy, 68*(Suppl. 1), S1–S48. http://dx.doi.org/10.5014/ajot.2014.682006

American Occupational Therapy Association & American Occupational Therapy Foundation. (2011). Occupational therapy research agenda. *American Journal of Occupational Therapy, 65*(Suppl.), S4–S7. http://dx.doi.org/10.5014/ajot.2011.65S4

Bauerschmidt, B., & Nelson, D. L. (2011). The terms *occupation* and *activity* over the history of official occupational therapy publications. *American Journal of Occupational Therapy, 65,* 338–345. http://dx.doi.org/10.5014/ajot.2011.000869

Bravi, L., & Stoykov, M. E. (2007). New directions in occupational therapy: Implementation of the task-oriented approach in conjunction with cortical stimulation after stroke. *Topics in Stroke Rehabilitation, 14,* 68–73. http://dx.doi.org/10.1310/tsr1406-68

Canadian Association of Occupational Therapists. (2002). *Enabling occupation. An occupational therapy perspective* (rev. ed.). Ottawa: CAOT Publications ACE.

Carin-Levy, G., Kendall, M., Young, A., & Mead, G. (2009). The psychosocial effects of exercise and relaxation classes for persons surviving a stroke. *Canadian Journal of Occupational Therapy, 76,* 73–80. http://dx.doi.org/10.1177/000841740907600204

Christiansen, C. H., Baum, C. M., & Bass-Haugen, J. (Eds.). (2005). *Occupational therapy: Performance, participation, and well-being* (3rd ed.). Thorofare, NJ: Slack.

Clark, F., Azen, S. P., Zemke, R., Jackson, J., Carlson, M., Mandel, D.,... Lipson, L. (1997). Occupational therapy for independent-living older adults. A randomized controlled trial. *JAMA, 278,* 1321–1326. http://dx.doi.org/10.1001/jama.1997.03550160041036

Collins, G. (2008, July 17). Las Vegas envy. *The New York Times,* p. A21.

Creswell, J. W. (2012). *Qualitative inquiry and research design: Choosing among five approaches.* Thousand Oaks, CA: Sage.

Dickerson, A. E., & Brown, L. E. (2007). Pediatric constraint-induced movement therapy in a young child with minimal active arm movement. *American Journal of Occupational Therapy, 61,* 563–573. http://dx.doi.org/10.5014/ajot.61.5.563

Dirette, D. P. (2013). Letter From the Editor—The importance of frames of reference. *Open Journal of Occupational Therapy, 1*(2), 1–6. http://dx.doi.org/http://scholarworks.wmich.edu/ojot/vol1/iss2/1

Dunn, W. (1993). Useful research strategies for studying service provision in real life contexts. *Developmental Disabilities Special Interest Section Newsletter, 16,* 1–3.

Friedman, T. L. (1999). *The Lexus and the olive tree: Understanding globalization.* New York: Farrar, Straus & Giroux.

Gewurtz, R., Stergiou-Kita, M., Shaw, L., Kirsh, B., & Rappolt, S. (2008). Qualitative meta-synthesis: Reflections on the utility and challenges in occupational therapy. *Canadian Journal of Occupational Therapy, 75,* 301–308. http://dx.doi.org/10.1177/000841740807500513

Gillette, N. (1991). The challenge of research in occupational therapy. *American Journal of Occupational Therapy, 45,* 660–662. http://dx.doi.org/10.5014/ajot.45.7.660

Gutman, S. A. (2008). From Desk of the Editor—Research priorities of the profession. *American Journal of Occupational Therapy, 62,* 499–501. http://dx.doi.org/10.5014/ajot.62.5.499

Hammell, K. W. (2004). Dimensions of meaning in the occupations of daily life. *Canadian Journal of Occupational Therapy, 71,* 296–305. http://dx.doi.org/10.1177/000841740407100509

Hasselkus, B. R. (2002). *The meaning of everyday occupation.* Thorofare, NJ: Slack.

Hinojosa, J., Kramer, P., Royeen, C. B., & Luebben, A. (2003). The core concept of occupation. In P. Kramer, J. Hinojosa, & C. B. Royeen (Eds.), *Perspectives in human occupation: Participation in life* (pp. 1–17). Philadelphia: Lippincott Williams & Wilkins.

Howe, T.-H., & Wang, T.-N. (2013). Systematic review of interventions used in or relevant to occupational therapy for children with feeding difficulties ages birth–5 years. *American Journal of Occupational Therapy, 67,* 405–412. http://dx.doi.org/10.5014/ajot.2013.004564

Insel, G. M., & Roth, W. T. (1985). *Core concepts in health* (4th ed.). Palo Alto, CA: Mayfield.

Isaksson, G., Josephsson, S., Lexell, J., & Skar, L. (2007). To regain participation in occupations through human

encounters: Narratives from women with spinal cord injury. *Journal of Head Trauma Rehabilitation, 22,* 229–233. http://dx.doi.org/10.1097/01.HTR.0000281838.00344.03

Legg, L., Drummond, A., Leonardi-Bee, J., Gladman, J. R., Corr, S., Donkervoort, M., … Langhorne, P. (2007). Occupational therapy for patients with problems in personal activities of daily living after stroke: Systematic review of randomised trials. *British Medical Journal, 335,* 922–930. http://dx.doi.org/10.1136/bmj.39343.466863.55

Lindström, M., Sjöström, S., & Lindberg, M. (2013). Stories of rediscovering agency: Home-based occupational therapy for people with severe psychiatric disability. *Qualitative Health Research, 23,* 728–740. http://dx.doi.org/10.1177/1049732313482047

Lyons, M., Orozovic, N., Davis, J., & Newman, J. (2002). Doing–being–becoming: Occupational experiences of persons with life-threatening illnesses. *American Journal of Occupational Therapy, 56,* 285–295. http://dx.doi.org/10.5014/ajot.56.3.285

Mosey, A. C. (1996). *Applied scientific inquiry in the health professions: An epistemological orientation* (2nd ed.). Bethesda, MD: American Occupational Therapy Association.

Nielson, C., Youngstrom, M. J., Glantz, C., Henderson, M. L., Richman, N., … Peterson, M. (October 3, 2005). *Report of the Ad Hoc Workgroup on Implementing Occupation-Based Practice to the AOTA Board of Directors.* Bethesda, MD: American Occupational Therapy Association.

O'Toole, L., Connolly, D., & Smith, S. (2013). Impact of an occupation-based self-management programme on disease management. *Australian Occupational Therapy Journal, 60,* 30–38.

Paul, S., & Ramsey, D. (1998). The effects of electronic music-making as a therapeutic activity for improving upper extremity active range of motion. *Occupational Therapy International, 5,* 223–237. http://dx.doi.org/10.1002/oti.77

Perrins-Margalis, N. M., Rugletic, J., Schepis, N. M., Stepanski, H. R., & Walsh, M. A. (2000). The immediate effects of a group-based horticulture experience on the quality of life of persons with chronic mental illness. *Occupational Therapy in Mental Health, 16,* 15–32. http://dx.doi.org/10.1300/J004v16n01_02

Plante, E., Kiernan, B., & Betts, J. D. (1994). Method or methodolotry: The qualitative–quantitative debate. *Language, Speech, and Hearing Services in Schools, 25,* 52–54.

Polatajko, H. J., Cantin, N., Amoroso, B., McKee, P., Rivard, A., Kirsh, B., & Lin, N. (2007). Occupation-based enablement: A practice mosaic. In E. A. Townsend & H. J. Polatajko (Eds.), *Enabling occupation II: Advancing an occupational therapy vision for health, well-being, and justice through occupation* (pp. 177–202). Ottawa: CAOT Publications ACE.

Polatajko, H. J., & Davis, J. A. (2012). Advancing occupation-based practice: Interpreting the rhetoric. *Canadian Journal of Occupational Therapy, 79,* 259–262. http://dx.doi.org/10.2182/cjot.2012.79.5.1

Punch, K. F. (1998). *Introduction to social research: Quantitative and qualitative approaches.* Thousand Oaks, CA: Sage.

Reilly, M. (1962). Occupational therapy can be one of the great ideas of 20th-century medicine. *American Journal of Occupational Therapy, 16,* 1–9.

Reynolds, F., Vivat, B., & Prior, S. (2008). Women's experiences of increasing subjective well-being in CFS/ME through leisure-based arts and crafts activities: A qualitative study. *Disability and Rehabilitation, 30,* 1279–1288. http://dx.doi.org/10.1080/09638280701654518

Schepens, S., Sen, A., Painter, J. A., & Murphy, S. L. (2012). Relationship between fall-related efficacy and activity engagement in community-dwelling older adults: A meta-analytic review. *American Journal of Occupational Therapy, 66,* 137–148. http://dx.doi.org/10.5014/ajot.2012.001156

Skubik-Peplaski, C., Carrico, C., Nichols, L., Chelette, K., & Sawaki, L. (2012). Behavioral, neurophysiological, and descriptive changes after occupation-based intervention. *American Journal of Occupational Therapy, 66,* e107–e113. http://dx.doi.org/10.5014/ajot.2012.003590

Standage, T. (1998). *The Victorian Internet: The remarkable story of the telegraph and the nineteenth century's on-line pioneers.* New York: Walker.

Tamhane, A. C. (2009). *Statistical analysis of designed experiments: Theory and applications.* Hoboken, NJ: Wiley.

Teitelman, J., Raber, C., & Watts, J. (2010). The power of the social environment in motivating persons with dementia to engage in occupation: Qualitative findings. *Physical and Occupational Therapy in Geriatrics, 28,* 321–333. http://dx.doi.org/10.3109/02703181.2010.532582

Velleman, P. F., & Bock, D. E. (2008). *Stats: Data and models* (2nd ed.). Boston: Pearson/Addison-Wesley.

White, B. P., Mulligan, S., Merrill, K., & Wright, J. (2007). An examination of the relationships between motor and process skills and scores on the sensory profile. *American Journal of Occupational Therapy, 61,* 154–160. http://dx.doi.org/10.5014/ajot.61.2.154

World Health Organization. (2001). *International classification of functioning, disability and health.* Geneva: Author.

Yerxa, E. J. (1991). Seeking a relevant, ethical, and realistic way of knowing for occupational therapy. *American Journal of Occupational Therapy, 45,* 199–204. http://dx.doi.org/10.5014/ajot.45.3.199

Yoder, R. M., Nelson, D. L., & Smith, D. A. (1989). Added-purpose versus rote exercise in female nursing home residents. *American Journal of Occupational Therapy, 43,* 581–586. http://dx.doi.org/10.5014/ajot.43.9.581

SUBJECT INDEX

Note. Page numbers in *italics* indicate exhibits, figures, and tables.

CITATION INDEX

Note. Page numbers in *italics* indicate exhibits, figures, and tables.